Third Mobile Window Syndr

Gerard J. Gianoli • Philippa Thomson
Editors

Third Mobile Window Syndrome of the Inner Ear

Superior Semicircular Canal Dehiscence and Associated Disorders

Springer

Editors
Gerard J. Gianoli
Ear and Balance Institute
Covington, LA, USA

Philippa Thomson
North Berwick, East Lothian, UK

ISBN 978-3-031-16588-7 ISBN 978-3-031-16586-3 (eBook)
https://doi.org/10.1007/978-3-031-16586-3

This Springer imprint is published by the registered company Springer Nature Switzerland AG
The registered company address is: Gewerbestrasse 11, 6330 Cham, Switzerland

This book is dedicated to the memory of
James S. Soileau, M.D.
(7/24/1943–8/9/2022)

Mentor, role model, and friend.

He was a pioneer in the treatment of
vestibular disorders
and will be sorely missed.

Preface

> The more you know, the more you realize you don't know. (Attributed to Aristotle)

> There are known knowns. These are things we know that we know. There are known unknowns. That is to say, there are things that we know we don't know. But there are also unknown unknowns. There are things we don't know we don't know. (Donald Rumsfeld)

Welcome to the first textbook on Third Mobile Window Disorders (TMWD). We hope this is the first of many more to come. With the increased recognition of TMWD and the growing body of literature, the time is right to put together a single reference source for information related to TMWD. The title of this book (*Third Mobile Window Syndrome of the Inner Ear: Superior Semicircular Canal Dehiscence and Associated Disorders*) has been chosen after much consideration. Superior Semicircular Canal Dehiscence (SCD) is certainly the most recognized of the TMWD and the one that has been the subject of the most journal articles, but there is much more to TMWD than just SCD. To put a fine point on it, we define TMWD as a group of disorders. TMWD have a common clinical presentation including a combination of Tullio's phenomenon, pressure/strain-induced vertigo, and/or autophony—although there are certainly other associated symptoms. The "third window" effect results from the altered inner ear mechanics due to an additional defect in the inner ear or an aberration of its structural integrity.

In March 1998 Lloyd Minor published the first two patients to undergo surgery for SCD, improving their vestibular symptoms. Just two months prior to that publication, in January of 1998, I had performed my first SCD surgery with successful outcome and reported my first three surgical cases the following August 1999. (Not knowing that someone else had already discovered SCD, I thought I was the first!) At that time, the condition of SCD was unknown outside of a handful of people and the world of Neurotology believed SCD to be a rare disorder. In fact, when I submitted my first 24 surgical cases as part of my Thesis to the Triologic Society in the year 2000, it was rejected. The Thesis review committee believed the disorder was so rare, they distrusted my data. (They really would not believe my patient database now—I have probably seen more than 24 SCD patients in the last couple of weeks!) Despite the Triologic Thesis committee rejecting my paper, the surgical results spoke for themselves. The patients became advocates for the surgical correction of this disorder, regardless of the medical community lagging. Patients would show up at my office with typical TMWD, together with CT scans demonstrating SCD. Surgery would resolve their symptoms, and these patients would send more patients.

As patients with TMWD symptoms came through my office, it was apparent that many had symptoms of SCD but did not actually have SCD. Scrutinizing their CT scans, we identified several other areas of dehiscence—posterior semicircular canal dehiscence, cochlear facial dehiscence, large vestibular aqueduct, and others. However, there were also patients who had no identifiable bony defect or dehiscence on CT scan. These patients most likely either had (1) a dehiscence we just did not see/identify or (2) an oval or round window perilymph fistula. However, these patients had similar history and test profiles as the patients who had CT findings of a bony dehiscence.

Prior to 1998, SCD patients were routinely misdiagnosed with a variety of disorders including Ménière's disease, vestibular neuritis, patulous eustachian tube, otosclerosis, and other disorders. When an otologic disorder did not seem to fit, they were usually diagnosed with anxiety or panic disorder. This was obviously devastating to the patients. However, it was understandable since we simply had not yet identified SCD. That problem still exists. Many SCD patients are misdiagnosed with Migraine, Persistent Postural-Perceptual Dizziness, and Ménière's, among other things, but recognition of SCD has improved considerably over the 23 years I have been treating these patients. Unfortunately, the lesser known TMWD are suffering the fate of SCD patients in the 1990s. Many clinicians will appropriately recognize TMWD but will not look any further if the superior canal has a complete bony covering. Many of these patients have one of the lesser recognized TMWD.

As mentioned above, SCD was initially felt to be a rare disorder. I submit to you that SCD is not rare. The definition of a rare disease is well defined. The US Congress passed the Rare Disease Act of 2002 defining a rare disease as one that affects less than 200,000 Americans or roughly 0.06% of the population. The European Union defines a rare disease as one that afflicts less than 1 in 2000 people (0.05% of the population).

The Johns Hopkins temporal bone histology study [1] of >1000 temporal bones demonstrated 0.5% incidence of SCD and about 1.5% incidence of extreme bony thinning (<0.1 mm). That same temporal bone library demonstrated 0.6% incidence of cochlear-facial dehiscence [2] and 5% incidence of even more extreme thinning of bone in that area (<0.03 mm). So, CFD is actually more common than SCD, but it is not recognized or diagnosed nearly as frequently as SCD. When you add them together (SCD and CFD), we have a 1.1% incidence among the general population and approximately 6.5% incidence of extreme thinning (which could eventually lead to disease, i.e., "near dehiscence"). That 1.1% incidence does not include all the other types of dehiscences or new ones yet to be identified. Further, 1.1% is more than 20 times the upper limit of what defines a rare disease. When you consider all the different forms of TMWS (SCD, PCD, CFD, IAC-cochlear dehiscence, cochlear carotid dehiscence, large vestibular aqueduct, etc.), this is definitely not a rare problem. The NIH website still lists SCD as rare, but that post was submitted in May of 2015. It needs to be updated.

With this textbook we hope to spread awareness of TMWD as a diagnostic category which includes many entities. We also intend to provide tools for appropriate diagnosis and treatment. Along these lines, we have gathered a stellar cast of leaders in the neurotologic community to help write the book. While trying to be as comprehensive as we could, the topics included in this publication obviously aren't able to cover everything. As noted above by Aristotle, there is much more that we don't know. And as noted by Mr. Rumsfeld, there are unknown unknowns—those matters that we don't know we don't know, the ones that keep us up at night. Without doubt, the next textbook on this subject will include many things that we hadn't considered at this point in time. I shall look forward to seeing the future unfold.

References

1. Carey JP, Minor LB, Nager GT. Dehiscence or thinning of bone overlying the superior semicircular canal in a temporal bone survey. Arch Otolaryngol Head Neck Surg. 2000;126(2):137–47. https://doi.org/10.1001/archotol.126.2.137. PMID: 10680863.
2. Fang CH, Chung SY, Blake DM, Vazquez A, Li C, Carey JP, Francis HW, Jyung RW. Prevalence of cochlear-facial dehiscence in a study of 1,020 temporal bone specimens. Otol Neurotol. 2016;37(7):967–72. https://doi.org/10.1097/MAO.0000000000001057. PMID: 27203843.

Covington, LA, USA Gerard J. Gianoli

Contents

Contributors

Mitch F. Aquilina Jupiter Medical Center, ENT and Allergy Associates of Florida, Jupiter, FL, USA

Seilish C. Babu Michigan Ear Institute, Farmington Hills, MI, USA

Carey D. Balaban Department of Otolaryngology – Head and Neck Surgery, Rutgers Robert Wood Johnson Medical School, New Brunswick, NJ, USA

Rutgers Brain Health Institute, Piscataway, NJ, USA

Departments of Otolaryngology, Neurobiology, Communication Sciences and Disorders, and Bioengineering, University of Pittsburgh School of Medicine, Pittsburgh, PA, USA

Charlotte Barbier Department of Radiology, Centre Hospitalo-Universitaire de Caen, Caen, France

Lee M. Bauter Department of Otolaryngology-Head and Neck Surgery, Geisinger Medical Center, Danville, PA, USA

Dennis I. Bojrab Department of Neurotology, Michigan Ear Institute, Farmington Hills, MI, USA

Jonathan Choi Michigan Ear Institute, Farmington Hills, MI, USA

Ariana Chow Department of Neurosurgery, University of California, Los Angeles (UCLA), Los Angeles, CA, USA

Vince M. Desiato Department of Otolaryngology-Head and Neck Surgery, Geisinger Medical Center, Danville, PA, USA

Alan Desmond Wake Forest University Baptist Medical Center, Otolaryngology Head & Neck Surgery, Winston Salem, NC, USA

Karl W. Doerfer Department of Otolaryngology & Communication Sciences, Medical College of Wisconsin, Milwaukee, WI, USA

Courtney Duong Department of Neurosurgery, University of California, Los Angeles (UCLA), Los Angeles, CA, USA

Sarah Dwyer Michigan Ear Institute, Farmington Hills, MI, USA

Michael J. Eliason Department of Otolaryngology-Head and Neck Surgery, Naval Medical Center Portsmouth, Portsmouth, VA, USA

Debby Feinberg NeuroVisual Medicine Institute, Bloomfield Hills, MI, USA

Dennis Fitzgerald Otolaryngology Head and Neck Surgery, Jefferson Hospital, Philadelphia, PA, USA

Mark Frilling Department of Otolaryngology, University Hospitals Cleveland Medical Center, Cleveland, OH, USA

Arun K. Gadre Department of Otolaryngology-Head and Neck Surgery, Geisinger Medical Center, Danville, PA, USA

Gerard J. Gianoli Ear and Balance Institute, Covington, LA, USA

Quinton Gopen Department of Head and Neck Surgery, University of California, Los Angeles (UCLA), Los Angeles, CA, USA

David S. Haynes Department of Otolaryngology-Head and Neck Surgery, Vanderbilt University Medical Center, Nashville, TN, USA

Martin Hitier Department of Otolaryngology Head and Neck Surgery, Centre Hospitalo-Universitaire de Caen, Caen, France

Department of Anatomy, UNICAEN, Caen, France

Inserm, U 1075 COMETE, Caen, France

Normandie University, Caen, France

Robert S. Hong Michigan Ear Institute, Farmington Hills, MI, USA

Eugen Ionescu Paris Hearing Institute, Research Center of Pasteur Institute, Team Clinical and Translational Exploration of Sensorineural Hearing Loss, Inserm U1120, Paris, France

Department of Audiology and Neurotology, Lyon University Hospital, Lyon, France

Service d'Audiologie et d'Otoneurologie, CHU Lyon, Institute de l'Audition, Paris, France

Benjamin R. Johnson Department of Otolaryngology-Head & Neck Surgery, University Hospitals Cleveland Medical Center, Cleveland, Ohio, USA

Case Western Reserve University School of Medicine, Cleveland, Ohio, USA

Robert W. Jyung Department of Otolaryngology – Head and Neck Surgery, Rutgers New Jersey Medical School, Newark, NJ, USA

Karl Kado Department of Radiology, College of Human Medicine, Ascension Providence Hospital, Michigan State University, Southfield, MI, USA

Bradley W. Kesser UVA Health, Charlottesville, VA, USA

Nehzat Koohi Centre for Vestibular and Behavioural Neurosciences, Department of Clinical and Movement Neurosciences, UCL Institute of Neurology, University College London, London, UK

Stroke Services, National Hospital for Neurology and Neurosurgery, University College London Hospitals, London, UK

The UCL Ear Institute, University College London, London, UK

Shweta Kumar Department of Radiology, Geisinger Medical Center, Danville, PA, USA

J. Walter Kutz Jr. Otolaryngology and Neurological Surgery, The University of Texas Southwestern Medical Center, Dallas, TX, USA

Jenna J. Li Columbia University, New York, NY, USA

John C. Li Jupiter Medical Center, ENT and Allergy Associates of Florida, Jupiter, FL, USA

Cameron B. Lindemann Department of Otolaryngology-Head and Neck Surgery, Naval Medical Center Portsmouth, Portsmouth, VA, USA

Alexander L. Luryi Division of Otolaryngology-Head and Neck Surgery, Department of Surgery, Cooper University Hospital, Camden, NJ, USA

Natalie Mahgerefteh Department of Neurosurgery, University of California, Los Angeles (UCLA), Los Angeles, CA, USA

Gustavo A. Marino College of Medicine, University of Central Florida (UCF), Orlando, FL, USA

Surangi Mendis Department of Neuro-Otology, Royal National ENT and Eastman Dental Hospitals, UCLH, London, UK

Department of Audiovestibular Medicine, St Ann's Hospital, Whittington Health NHS Trust, London, UK

Gino Mongelluzzo Department of Radiology, Geisinger Medical Center, Danville, PA, USA

Daniel R. Morrison UVA Health, Charlottesville, VA, USA

Todd M. Mowery Departments of Otolaryngology, Neurobiology, Communication Sciences and Disorders, and Bioengineering, University of Pittsburgh School of Medicine, Pittsburgh, PA, USA

Department of Otolaryngology – Head and Neck Surgery, Rutgers Robert Wood Johnson Medical School, New Brunswick, NJ, USA

Rutgers Brain Health Institute, Piscataway, NJ, USA

Sarah Mowry Department of Otolaryngology-Head & Neck Surgery, University Hospitals Cleveland Medical Center, Cleveland, Ohio, USA

Case Western Reserve University School of Medicine, Cleveland, Ohio, USA

Department of Otolaryngology, Case Western Reserve University School of Medicine, Cleveland, OH, USA

Khashayar Mozaffari Department of Neurosurgery, University of California, Los Angeles (UCLA), Los Angeles, CA, USA

Arun Pajaniappane Department of Audiovestibular Medicine and Audiology, St George's University Hospitals NHS Foundation Trust, London, UK

Harley Street Audiovestibular Clinic, London, UK

Jay Patel Department of Neuro-Otology, Royal National ENT and Eastman Dental Hospitals, UCLH, London, UK

Ankita Patro Department of Otolaryngology-Head and Neck Surgery, Vanderbilt University Medical Center, Nashville, TN, USA

Paul Radomskij Department of Audiovestibular Medicine and Audiology, St George's University Hospitals NHS Foundation Trust, London, UK

UCL Ear Institute, London, UK

Pierre Reynard Department of Audiology and Neurotology, Centre Hospitalo-Universitaire Lyon, Lyon, France

Paris Hearing Institute, Research Center of Pasteur Institute, Team Clinical and Translational Exploration of Sensorineural Hearing Loss, Inserm U1120, Paris, France

Alejandro Rivas-Campo Department of Otolaryngology-Head & Neck Surgery, University Hospitals Cleveland Medical Center, Cleveland, Ohio, USA

Case Western Reserve University School of Medicine, Cleveland, Ohio, USA

Mark Rosner NeuroVisual Medicine Institute, Bloomfield Hills, MI, USA

Christopher A. Schutt Michigan Ear Institute, Farmington Hills, MI, USA

Michael D. Seidman Otolaryngology Head and Neck Surgery, University of Central Florida, Orlando, FL, USA

Otolaryngology Head and Neck Surgery, University of South Florida, Tampa, FL, USA

Department of Otolaryngology-Head and Neck Surgery, AdventHealth, Central Florida, Celebration, FL, USA

Maroun Semaan Department of Otolaryngology-Head & Neck Surgery, University Hospitals Cleveland Medical Center, Cleveland, Ohio, USA

Case Western Reserve University School of Medicine, Cleveland, Ohio, USA

Pedrom Sioshansi Wake Forest University Baptist Medical Center, Otolaryngology Head & Neck Surgery, Winston Salem, NC, USA

Miriam R. Smetak Department of Otolaryngology-Head and Neck Surgery, Vanderbilt University Medical Center, Nashville, TN, USA

James S. Soileau Ear and Balance Institute, Covington, LA, USA

Anette Sörlin ENT/Audiology, Sunderby Hospital, Luleå, Sweden

Donald Tan The University of Texas Southwestern, Dallas, TX, USA

Krister Tano ENT, Umeå University/Sunderby Hospital, Luleå, Sweden

Jordan M. Thompson Department of Otolaryngology – Head and Neck Surgery, Rutgers New Jersey Medical School, Newark, NJ, USA

Philippa Thomson North Berwick, East Lothian, UK

Francis Turjman Department of Neuroradiology, Centre Hospitalo-Universitaire Lyon, Groupement Hospitalier Est, Bron, France

Université Claude Bernard Lyon, Villeurbanne, France

UMR5515, INSERM U1206 Centre de Recherche en Acquisition et Traitement d'Images pour la Santé (CREATIS), Villeurbanne, France

P. J. Valigorsky III American University of Antigua College of Medicine, Osbourn, Antigua and Barbuda

P. Ashley Wackym New Jersey, USA

Rutgers Brain Health Institute, Piscataway, NJ, USA

Brady Workman Wake Forest University Baptist Medical Center, Otolaryngology Head & Neck Surgery, Winston Salem, NC, USA

Isaac Yang Department of Neurosurgery, University of California, Los Angeles (UCLA), Los Angeles, CA, USA

Part I
Understanding Third Mobile Window Syndrome

Gerard J. Gianoli

Introduction

In Part I of this book, we will elucidate the basics in the understanding of Third Mobile Window Disorders (TMWD). These are fundamental for anyone involved in the diagnosis, treatment, or research of TMWD. The history of TMWD is rich and winding. Pieces and parts to TMWD have arisen throughout the years and a clearer picture of what constitutes the disorder has emerged. The history of TMWD dates back to the experiments of Professor Pietro Tullio in 1929. It extends to the recognition of horizontal canal dehiscence by erosive cholesteatoma in early mastoid surgery experience, the identification of perilymph fistula after the advent of stapedectomy, Dr. Lloyd Minor's identification of superior canal dehiscence, and discovery of better tools for evaluation and management. Lastly, there is a growing identification of other areas of labyrinthine dehiscence that provoke Third Mobile Window Syndrome (TMWS).

Early on, many of the fundamental symptoms of TMWD were ignored such as Tullio's phenomenon and autophony. Some were often explained away as "something that just happens in some cases." Such is the case of "conductive inner ear hearing loss" that persisted after a minority of stapedectomy surgeries or the "pseudo-conductive hearing loss" of some Ménière's cases. We now know that those cases were in fact a different disorder than the otosclerosis cases and that the pseudo-conductive hearing loss of Ménière's was often TMWD. The theories on the pathophysiology and etiology of TMWD explain much of what was not understood back then. Further, many patients had been diagnosed with other otologic disorders before there was awareness of TMWD. The symptom overlap for Superior Semicircular Canal Dehiscence (SSCD) with other well-described otologic disorders is so pronounced that SSCD has been termed the Great Otologic Mimicker. A good understanding of the multiple manifestations of SSCD and TMWD is imperative to identifying these patients.

Until just recently, TMWD were a collection of random inner ear disorders without a good framework. A recently proposed classification system now inserts order among this chaos. Having this classification system may allow us to better compare diagnostic and treatment measures in future research. While we will certainly better refine our view of this entity, the advances in this field have certainly been immense in the past 24 years.

Chapter 1
History and Overview of Third Mobile Window Syndrome

P. Ashley Wackym, Carey D. Balaban, and Todd M. Mowery

Third mobile window syndrome (TMWS) (also known as third window syndrome [TWS] or otic capsule dehiscence syndrome [OCDS]) is a vestibular-cochlear disorder in humans in which a third mobile window of the inner ear creates changes to the flow of sound pressure level energy through the perilymph/endolymph. Sound transmission to the inner ear is normally through the oval and round window. Acoustic pressure enters through the oval window, is transmitted through the cochlea, and exits into the middle ear cavity via the round window [1]. The fluid in the cochlea through which sound is transmitted is functionally incompressible due to the surrounding osseous structures [2]. Movement of the cochlear fluid is thereby dependent on the mobility of the round and oval window membranes. Inward displacement of the oval window membrane via the stapes by ossicular vibration is matched by outward round window membrane displacement [2]. However, if a third mobile window is present, some of the acoustic pressure is shunted away from the cochlea and delivered to the vestibular receptors. Normally, sound pressure transduction by the stapes results in only cochlear hair cell transduction due to the round window, which dissipates cochlear vibration by impedance matching. Normally, because the vestibular labyrinth does not have a membrane or release valve to dissipate the introduced sound pressure, their pressure remains constant and the vestibular end-organs are not stimulated. However, if there is an additional fenestration,

P. A. Wackym (✉) · C. D. Balaban
Department of Otolaryngology – Head and Neck Surgery, Rutgers Robert Wood Johnson Medical School, New Brunswick, NJ, USA

Rutgers Brain Health Institute, Piscataway, NJ, USA
e-mail: wackym@neurotology.org; CBALABAN@pitt.edu

T. M. Mowery
Departments of Otolaryngology, Neurobiology, Communication Sciences and Disorders, and Bioengineering, University of Pittsburgh School of Medicine, Pittsburgh, PA, USA
e-mail: tm692@rwjms.rutgers.edu

G. J. Gianoli, P. Thomson (eds.), *Third Mobile Window Syndrome of the Inner Ear*, https://doi.org/10.1007/978-3-031-16586-3_1

the energy typically confined to the vestibule and cochlea escapes along a path of least resistance toward the defect or "third window" and during this the vestibular end-organs can be abnormally stimulated. The nature and location of this third mobile window can occur at many different sites (or multiple sites), which will be discussed later. The primary physiological symptoms include sound-induced and pressure-induced gravitational receptor dysfunction type of vertigo, migraine headaches (and variants), pseudoconductive hearing loss, autophony while speaking, and visual problems (nystagmus, oscillopsia). At the same time, individuals experience measurable deficits in basic decision-making, short-term memory, concentration, spatial cognition, and anxiety. In this chapter, the history of TMWS will be reviewed, but first a description of the clinical phenotype is essential to understand the spectrum of problems these patients experience.

Clinical Phenotype

The literature has been conflicted about the frequency of symptoms and diagnostic test findings in patients with TMWS. One illustrative summary that highlights the spectrum of the most common complaints from patients with perilymph fistula was published nearly a quarter century ago [3]. No doubt many of these patients had TMWS due to bony sites of dehiscence not yet discovered. Figure 1.1 shows the percentage of these patients reporting each of the 13 most common complaints. The three most frequent complaints were disequilibrium, headache, and dizziness. Other important clinical symptoms included cognitive dysfunction, nausea, visual

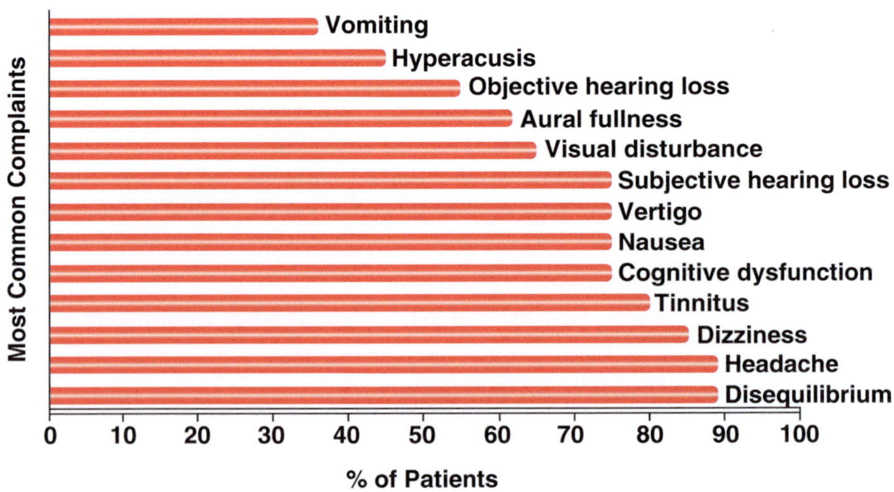

Fig. 1.1 Clinical phenotype of perilymph fistula (PLF). Percentage of 58 PLF patients reporting each of the most common complaints (created from the dataset of Black et al. [3]) Copyright © P.A. Wackym, used with permission

Table 1.1 Spectrum of symptoms, signs or exacerbating factors seen in third window syndrome

Category	Symptom, sign or exacerbating factors
Sound-induced	Dizziness or otolithic dysfunction (see vestibular dysfunction below); nausea; cognitive dysfunction; spatial disorientation; migraine/migrainous headache; pain (especially children); loss of postural control; falls
Autophony	Resonant voice; chewing; heel strike; pulsatile tinnitus; joints or tendons moving; eyes moving or blinking; comb or brush through hair; face being touched
Vestibular dysfunction	Gravitational receptor (otolithic) dysfunction type of vertigo (rocky or wavy motion, tilting, pushed, pulled, tilted, flipped, floor falling out from under); mal de débarquement illusions of movement
Headache	Migraine/migrainous headache; migraine variants (ocular, hemiplegic or vestibular [true rotational vertigo]); coital cephalagia; photophobia; phonophobia; aura; scotomata
Cognitive dysfunction	General cognitive impairment, such as mental fog, dysmetria of thought, mental fatigue; impaired attention and concentration, poor multitasking (women > men); executive dysfunction; language problems including dysnomia, agramatical speech, aprosodia, verbal fluency; memory difficulties; academic difficulty including reading problems and missing days at school or work; depression and anxiety
Spatial disorientation	Trouble judging distances; detachment/passive observer when interacting with groups of people; out of body experiences; perceiving the walls or floor moving
Anxiety	Sense of impending doom
Autonomic dysfunction	Nausea; vomiting; diarrhea; lightheadedness; blood pressure lability; change in temperature regulation; heart rate lability
Endolymphatic hydrops	Ear pressure/fullness not relieved by the Valsalva maneuver; barometric pressure sensitivity
Hearing	Pseudoconductive hearing loss (bone-conduction hyperacusis)

Adapted from Wackym et al. [4]. Used with permission, copyright © P.A. Wackym, MD

disturbance, and objective as well as subjective hearing loss. Review of Fig. 1.1 also demonstrates that these are extraordinarily similar to the spectrum of symptoms experienced by patients with SSCD, other TMWS sites of dehiscence and vestibular migraine. Table 1.1 outlines the contemporary spectrum of symptoms, signs or exacerbating factors seen in TMWS. It is important to understand that every patient with TMWS does not have all of the observed symptoms and that TMWS should be viewed as a spectrum of symptoms. Table 1.2 combines synonymous symptoms into common terms so that the reader can see a simplified framework illustrating these symptoms. As shown in Table 1.3 there are currently 15 known sites of dehiscence that can be seen using high-resolution temporal bone CT and in addition there are sites of dehiscence that cannot yet be seen with contemporary high-resolution temporal bone CT scans (CT– TMWS).

The more general term of TMWS is more appropriate than SSCD syndrome because the same spectrum of symptoms, signs on physical examination, and audiological diagnostic findings are encountered with superior semicircular canal dehiscence (SSCD), posterior semicircular canal dehiscence, posterior semicircular

Table 1.2 Combining synonymous symptoms into common terms

Common term	Symptoms
Anxiety	Anxiety; sense of impending doom
Aural pressure/ endolymphatic hydrops	Aural pressure; aural fullness; clogged sensation in ear; ear blocked, producing dizziness
Autonomic dysfunction	Nausea; vomiting; diarrhea; lightheadedness; blood pressure lability; change in temperature regulation; heart rate lability
Autophony	Autophony; echoing sensation in ear when talking; Kazoo character of voice
Cognitive dysfunction	General cognitive impairment, such as mental fog, dysmetria of thought, mental fatigue; impaired attention and concentration, poor multitasking (women > men); executive dysfunction; language problems including dysnomia, agrammatical speech, aprosodia, verbal fluency; memory difficulties; academic difficulty including reading problems and missing days at school or work; depression and anxiety
Drop attack	Drop attack; otolithic crisis of Tumarkin
Gaze-evoked tinnitus	Gaze-evoked tinnitus; head movement induced pulsatile tinnitus; disabling bilateral pulsatile tinnitus on changing head position; cricket-like tinnitus when head turned quickly
Headache, ear pain	Headache; ear pain; frequent headaches; migraine with or without migraine variants; otalgia
Hearing loss	Hearing loss; conductive hearing loss; mixed hearing loss; pseudoconductive hearing loss; sensorineural hearing loss
Hemifacial numbness	Hemifacial numbness
Hyperacusis to bodily sounds (such as hearing own eye balls move, own footsteps, eating/chewing)	Hyperacusis to bodily sounds; cochlear hypersensitivity to bone-conducted sounds; hear heel strike/footsteps; hearing own eye movements; hearing own eyelid blinking; hearing internal sounds; own chewing so loud that must stop to listen to others
Hyperacusis to environmental sounds	Hyperacusis; hypersensitivity to sound; intolerance to loud sound; phonophobia
Motion intolerance	Heightened sensitivity to motion; motion intolerance
Non-pulsatile tinnitus	Tinnitus; high-pitched tinnitus; continuous tinnitus
Positional vertigo/ instability/dizziness	Disequilibrium with rapid head motion; dizziness when inclining head upward or downward; imbalance when head moving quickly; positional vertigo/instability/dizziness; postural dyscontrol; vertigo following position change
Pulsatile oscillopsia	Pulsatile oscillopsia; pulse synchronous oscillopsia
Sound distortion	Sound distortion; distortion in ear
Spatial disorientation	Trouble judging distances; detachment/passive observer when interacting with groups of people; out of body experiences; perceiving the walls or floor moving; Mal de débarquement-type illusions of movement
Spontaneous oscillopsia/ tilting	Oscillopsia; oscillopsia during head movement; oscillopsia by specific activity or maneuver; oscillopsia during locomotion
Spontaneous pulsatile tinnitus	Pulsatile tinnitus; pulse synchronous tinnitus

Table 1.2 (continued)

Common term	Symptoms
Spontaneous dizziness (vertigo/disequilibrium/ nausea/dizziness/ instability)	Vertigo; vestibular migraine; sense that the world was spinning; sensation that the world was tilted; pulsion, pushed pulled, gravitational receptor dysfunction type of vertigo; dizziness; imbalance; disequilibrium; episodic disequilibrium; floating; floor falling out from under; intermittent disequilibrium; chronic disequilibrium; unsteadiness
Tinnitus aggravated by Valsalva maneuver	Tinnitus aggravated by Valsalva maneuver
Vertigo/disequilibrium/ nausea/ataxia/oscillopsia provoked by environmental sounds	Typically a gravitational receptor dysfunction type of vertigo; Vestibular hypersensitivity to air-conducted sounds; Vertigo triggered by low frequency train; Vertigo induced by loud noise; Vertigo by humming/singing; Vertigo/disequilibrium by sound; Oscillopsia induced by loud noise; Objects in visual surround moving + vertical diplopia when humming or loud noise; Eye flutter induced by loud noise; Tullio phenomenon; Discomfort to loud noise; Noise-induced dizziness; Dizziness worsened by loud sound; Imbalance induced by loud noise; Disequilibrium induced by loud sound; Disequilibrium and sound sensitivity when driving on freeway; Eyes jump when phone rang close to ear; Falling down when exposed to loud sound; Motion sickness sensation with nausea induced by loud sound (no real vertigo); Sound-induced nausea; Sound-induced sense of being overwhelmed
Vertigo/disequilibrium/ nausea/oscillopsia provoked by pressure/ Valsalva maneuver	Typically a gravitational receptor dysfunction type of vertigo; Vertigo induced by pressure; Vertigo/disequilibrium by pressure; Pneumatic speculum induced vertigo; Oscillopsia induced by pressure; Visual disturbances with sneezing; Blurred vision induced by pressure; Hennebert sign; Dizziness induced by pressure; Dizziness induced by exercise; Imbalance induced by pressure; Disequilibrium induced by pressure; Intolerance for vibration/slight oscillopsia when driving on freeway; Slight shift of the visual scene during Valsalva; Fistula sign

Adapted from Wackym et al. [4] and Naert et al. [5] Used with permission, copyright © P.A. Wackym, MD

canal-jugular bulb dehiscence, posterior semicircular canal-endolymphatic sac/vestibular aqueduct dehiscence, lateral semicircular canal dehiscence, lateral semicircular canal-facial nerve dehiscence, cochlea-facial nerve dehiscence (CFD), cochlea-internal carotid artery dehiscence, cochlea-internal auditory canal dehiscence, cochlear otosclerosis with internal auditory canal involvement, wide vestibular aqueduct, endolymphatic sac-jugular bulb dehiscence, posttraumatic hypermobile stapes footplate, vestibule-middle ear dehiscence, modiolus (X-linked stapes gusher), and CT– TWS (see review [4]). A common structural finding in all of these conditions is an otic capsule defect that creates a "third window." In the light of our recognition that there are multiple sites where third windows occur in the otic capsule, it is interesting to note that Kohut's definition of a PLF, from over a quarter century ago, still applies to all currently known sites producing a TWS [6]; "A perilymph fistula may be defined as an abnormal opening between the inner ear and the

Table 1.3 Location of third mobile window defects that can be seen with a CT scan and can result in third mobile window syndrome

Semicircular canals
Superior semicircular canal dehiscence
Posterior semicircular canal dehiscence
Posterior semicircular canal-jugular bulb dehiscence
Posterior semicircular canal-endolymphatic sac/vestibular aqueduct dehiscence
Lateral semicircular canal dehiscence
Lateral semicircular canal-facial nerve dehiscence
Cochlea
Cochlea-facial nerve dehiscence
Cochlea-internal auditory canal dehiscence
Cochlea-carotid artery dehiscence
Cochlear otosclerosis involving the internal auditory canal
Other labyrinthine sites
Wide vestibular aqueduct
Endolymphatic sac-jugular bulb
Posttraumatic hypermobile stapes footplate
Vestibule-middle ear dehiscence
Modiolus (X-linked stapes gusher)

external surface of the labyrinth capsule…." Hence, a fistula of the otic capsule (Kohut's definition) can occur in any location that is in communication with perilymph, whether a SSCD, CFD, or any of the well-established sites that can result in a TMWS.

Peripheral Vestibular Physiology and the Need for a Precise Lexicon

A central problem with understanding peripheral vestibular disorders or communicating associated symptoms is our use of poor, or at least imprecise, terminology. The terms vertigo, dizziness, and disequilibrium are frequently used; however, what do they mean? To best answer this question a brief review of peripheral vestibular function is necessary.

The role of the ten vestibular receptors is to transduce the forces associated with head acceleration and gravity into a biologic signal. Central nervous system integration of these data results in the subjective awareness of head position relative to the environment. Motor reflexes to maintain gaze and posture are generated in response to afferent vestibular input. Propulsion and orientation of the body in space depend on the vestibular system, on vision, and on the proprioceptive system. Most persons can manage with only two of these systems, but not with one. Accordingly, patients with vestibular dysfunction may have additional difficulty in maintaining equilibrium when vision or proprioception is impaired.

The vestibular system, through its signal transduction by the peripheral end-organs and their afferent neurotransmission, constantly signals the position of the head in space and effects a continuous adjustment of the musculature of the body. More specifically, it signals acceleration and deceleration of motion. The otolith organs are capable of signaling only linear acceleration or deceleration, whereas the cristae within the semicircular ducts are able to signal angular acceleration or deceleration. Constant motion/acceleration cannot be detected by the vestibular system.

The peripheral vestibular system represents a unique neurosensory system. At rest, the type I and type II vestibular hair cells and their primary afferent neurons have a relatively constant and symmetrical resting discharge rate of approximately 80 spikes/s. This discharge rate increases if the stereocilia are deflected toward the kinocilium of each type I or type II vestibular hair cell, and it decreases if they are deflected away from the kinocilium. Transduction of accelerated motion is brought about by movement of the endolymph, which is coupled to the stereocilia and kinocilia of the neuroepithelium. All the kinocilia are oriented in the same direction relative to the long axis of each crista, and flow of endolymph in one direction results in the same discharge characteristics for all the hair cells in each individual end-organ. A further level of redundancy exists in the push–pull organization between both sets of vestibular apparatus. For example, with rotation to the right in the horizontal plane, there is relative flow of endolymph to the left. The resting discharge rate from the right horizontal crista ampullaris is greatly increased as the cupula is deflected toward the vestibule (i.e., ampullipetal displacement), whereas the discharge rate from the left side decreases an equal amount as the cupula of the left horizontal crista ampullaris is deflected away from the vestibule (i.e., ampullifugal displacement). Normally, this bilateral system is constantly at work, receiving signals and passing them on to regulate posture and movement of the body, limbs, and eyes. Each of the five vestibular receptors on the left are paired with a specific receptor on the right. Under normal circumstances, the vestibular signals produced by each side are equal and opposite in magnitude bilaterally. The paired otolithic organs function by similar mechanisms, except that type I and type II vestibular hair cells are coupled to gravitational force through the otolithic membrane, and their overlying otoconia and the kinocilia are polarized relative to a region called the *striola*. Consequently, conscious perception of this normal vestibular activity does not occur. However, if there is an imbalance in the relative increase and decrease in afferent firing between paired vestibular receptors on both sides, patients experience vertigo.

Vertigo is an illusion of movement in any plane or direction. Patients are deceived so that they feel themselves move or see abnormal movement of their surroundings. For rotational receptor asymmetries, patients experience a true rotational or spinning movement. For gravitational receptor asymmetries, patients have a gravitational receptor dysfunction type of vertigo. They will often describe a “rocky, wavy, tilting” perception. Other descriptors include a sensation as “being on a moving boat, the floor falling out from under them or flipping." The terms dizziness, giddiness or disequilibrium do not accurately capture these experiences, yet they are often used, which leads to a poor understanding of TMWS otic capsule defect (e.g., SSCD) symptoms by most physicians. Patients with TMWS sites can experience true rotational vertigo; however, the dominant complaint is usually sound-induced gravitational receptor dysfunction type of vertigo. This clinical observation can be blurred by vestibular migraine with true rotational vertigo being superimposed on SSCD, CFD or other TMWS site of dehiscence. This will be discussed in greater detail in Chap. 25, "Migraine, Headache and Third Mobile Window Syndrome."

Central Nervous System Pathway Activation that Produce Secondary Symptoms

Most of the symptoms that disrupt the lives of patients with TMWS are related to the severe symptoms that are secondary to these gravitational receptor asymmetries [4, 7–20].

Autonomic Dysfunction

Autonomic dysfunction occurs to varying degrees with TMWS and/or vestibular migraine; however, it is extremely common. Autonomic dysfunction also occurs with rotational receptor asymmetries. These symptoms include nausea, "cold-clammy skin," decreased heart rate and vomiting. There have been many investigators who have studied the underlying mechanisms and pathways subserving this dysfunction [21–23].

Cognitive Dysfunction

Cognitive dysfunction is nearly universal in patients with TMWS due to the otolithic asymmetry. This is uncommon in rotational receptor dysfunction type of vertigo as seen with benign positional vertigo, vestibular neuronitis or other disorders producing true rotational vertigo. Patients with TMWS often use the following descriptors when describing their cognitive function: "fuzzy, foggy, spacey, out-of-it; memory and concentration are poor; difficulty reading—as if the words are floating on the page; trouble finding the right words; and forgetting what I wanted to say." This will be discussed in greater detail in Chap. 6, "The Cognitive/Psychological Effects of Third Mobile Window Syndrome."

Altered Spatial Orientation

Patients with TMWS and/or vestibular migraine often use the following descriptors when describing their altered spatial orientation: "trouble judging distances; feeling detached and separated or not connected, almost like watching a play when around other people; and even an out-of-body experience (in more severe gravitational receptor asymmetries)." Several groups have begun studying this phenomenon. Clinically, this spatial disorientation reverses after surgery; however, Baek and colleagues reported that spatial memory deficits following bilateral vestibular loss may be permanent [24]. There is also evidence that simulation of the vestibular system is necessary to maintain normal spatial memory [25]. Deroualle and Lopez have explored the visual-vestibular interaction and in their 2014 review of the topic conclude that vestibular signals may be involved in the sensory bases of self-other distinction and mirroring, emotion perception and perspective taking [26]. Clinically, patients with TMWS recognize changes in their personality. Smith and Darlington argue that these changes in cognitive and emotional occur because of the role the ascending vestibular pathways to the limbic system and neocortex play in the sense of spatial orientation [27]. They further suggest that this change in the sense of self is responsible for the depersonalization and derealization symptoms such as feeling "spaced out," "body feeling strange," and "not feeling in control of self."

Anxiety

Vestibular disorders can produce anxiety; however, the classic sense of impending doom only occurs with the most severe gravitational receptor asymmetries. It is none-the-less quite unnerving to patients because it is a unique type of anxiety and characteristically patients have no insight why they feel that way or what is making them feel that way. Much work has been completed to understand the underlying mechanisms and pathways subserving this dysfunction [18–23, 28, 29].

Sound-Induced Gravitational Receptor Dysfunction Type of Vertigo

In Minor's review of 65 patients with SSCD, 54 (83%) had vestibular symptoms elicited by loud sounds, and 44 (67%) had pressure-induced (sneezing, coughing, and straining) symptoms [30]. This is also characteristic of TMWS patients with other sites of dehiscence (Tables 1.1 and 1.2) [8–17].

Autophony

In TMWS one of the most disturbing auditory symptoms is autophony, an unpleasant subjective discomfort of one's own voice during phonation. Often patients describe their voice as "echo-like" or "resonant." This is also very common in TMWS. Just as in the case with SSCD [31], some patients with other sites of dehiscence can also hear their eyes move or blink [8–10]. There appears to be decreased hearing thresholds for bone-conducted sounds. Bhutta has postulated that patients who hear their eyes move do so via transdural transmission of extraocular muscle contraction [32]. If this is the case, further credence to the hypothesis that some cases of CT– TMWS represent an otic capsule defect in an area such as the modiolus creating a third window, just as is the case with SSCD and CFD [4, 18, 19].

Migraine and Gravitational Receptor Dysfunction Type of Vertigo

Migraine headache is nearly always present in patients with gravitational receptor dysfunction type of vertigo caused by a TMWS, but infrequently with rotational receptor dysfunction type of true rotational vertigo [4, 19–21]. This is an important concept as TMWS can induce or exacerbate migraine and the three variants of migraine—ocular migraine, hemiplegic migraine, and vestibular migraine in affected patients. This is why patients with TMWS, who normally only have gravitational receptor dysfunction type of vertigo (disequilibrium) can have episodes of vestibular migraine and infrequent true rotational vertigo attacks. Surgical management, based upon the procedure specific to the site of dehiscence typically resolves the migraine; however, sometimes there is a marked decrease of the frequency and intensity of the migraines, as migraine has a high incidence overall [4, 8–20]. This will be discussed in greater detail in Chap. 25, "Migraine, Headache and Third Mobile Window Syndrome."

The Experiments of Pietro Tullio

Pietro Tullio (1881–1941) was the director of the Laboratory of Experimental Physiology in Bologna during the early twentieth century. While other scientists of his time studying the nervous system preferred removing or lesioning a structure to deducing the singular function from the singular deficiency, Tullio preferred the direct stimulation of these parts to deduce function. He undertook most of his experiments on live pigeons. Pigeons had already been established as the classical test animal for labyrinth physiology because of their favorable semicircular canal anatomy. It was also well documented that head nystagmus was more prominent than ocular nystagmus in the pigeon, making observations of responses easier [33].

In 1929, Tullio presented "Some Experiments and Considerations on Experimental Otology and Phonetics" at the meeting of the Società dei Cultori delle Scienze Mediche e Naturali in 1929 [34]. These experiments described the eponymous Tullio phenomenon of sound-induced vertigo and/or eye movements. This work was nominated for the Nobel Prize in Physiology or Medicine in both 1930 and 1932; however, he was never awarded the prize. The body of this work was focused on surgically creating a third window in the semicircular canals of pigeons [35, 36]. Tullio hypothesized that the sound pressure reaching the ear affects all three canals at the same time, not just the opened canal. The difference in intensity in which the currents are distributed in the canals produces the head movement. By making an opening in a canal, its current of sound pressure would be dominant over the other canals, leading to visible movement in the plane of this canal. Tullio subsequently analyzed the movement made by pigeons on opening each canal. After the opening of the superior canal, the pigeon lifted its head and beak in the plane of the canal. With a single sound, the lifting and tilting of the head was about 45°; the extension of the movement attained 90° when the sound was prolonged. What he did not address was the otolithic function which is no doubt responsible for the head tilt visible in the figures that he published. When cocaine crystals were introduced into the osseous opening near the ampulla, so that the anesthetic reached the perilymph, the pigeon lifted its beak at every sound to successively decreasing heights, until it finally lowered. This phenomenon is due to the cocaine paralyzing the primary afferent dendrites of the ampulla in the superior semicircular canal, and likely the vestibule, so that the pigeon could no longer respond to this acoustic stimulation. The pigeon was still responsive to the currents in the lateral and posterior canals. This had a cumulative effect wherein the pigeon lowered its head in an intermediate plane to those canals. In a clever experimental design, Tullio attached a lever and marker to the pigeon's beak to provide a graphical plot of the reflexes made in response to the sound pressure stimulus. It was decades later that these basic experiments in pigeons were recognized to represent a clinical entity now known as TMWS. According to Cawthorne [37], the Tullio phenomenon only occurred in humans when more than one mobile window opened into the inner ear on the vestibular side of the inner ear.

Semicircular Canal Fenestration Operations for Otosclerosis

Antonio Maria Valsalva first described stapes ankylosis as a cause of hearing loss in 1704. Adam Politzer described the pathology as due to "new bone, overgrowing the oval window and stapes" in 1893. This corresponded with the first era of stapes surgery, which consisted of stapes mobilization, trephination, or removal. As these procedures became more common in Europe, complications of meningitis and death were recognized and led to the abandonment of the procedures around 1900 [37]. Following this, otologists continued to investigate alternative, safer methods of surgically correcting the conductive hearing loss from otosclerosis. Beginning in 1897, when Passow first postulated that perhaps it would be better to detour around the obstruction in the oval window rather than to mobilize or extract the stapes. Balance, Floderus, Bárány, Holmgren, Jenkins and Sourdille all contributed to refinement of multistage fenestration operations to create a new mobile window in the lateral semicircular canal. In 1938, Julius Lempert described a breakthrough single-stage technique creating a new mobile window that he termed "nov-ovalis" in the lateral semicircular canal fenestration via an endaural approach. About 50% of patients who had this procedure had improvement of their conductive hearing loss to a 20–25 dB air-bone gap with lasting results. This marked the rise of the fenestration era of otosclerosis surgery [38–40]. Shambaugh reviewed the postoperative problems that these fenestration patients experienced: wet fenestrated ear; meatal atresia; ballooning of the fenestra; closure of the fenestra; sensorineural hearing loss after fenestration; and progressive sensorineural hearing loss due to otospongiosis [39]. Interestingly, these patients, although susceptible to temperature-induced dizziness typically did not experience sound-induced dizziness. This is likely due to the fenestration operation recreating a second mobile window, as the oval window was not mobile. Cawthorne described the Tullio phenomenon in patients who had undergone fenestration procedures for otosclerosis in which the stapes was not fixed, creating a "third window" in the inner ear, which underscores this point [41].

Cholesteatoma

Labyrinthine fistulas creating a TMW constitute around 4–12% of complications due to cholesteatoma. In a large meta-analysis, the affected site of the labyrinthine fistula was lateral semicircular canal dehiscence in 87% of cases, promontory dehiscence in 8% of cases, SSCD in 6% of cases, and posterior semicircular canal dehiscence in 2% of cases [42]. Historically, management has been to leave the cholesteatoma matrix intact over the fistula; however, this results in frequent temperature and pressure related stimulation of inhibition of the affected side. More recently, removal of the entire cholesteatoma matrix from the fistula with immediate covering by autogenous material or after removal plugging the canal with autologous tissue [43]. Other authors have advocated the use of hydrodissection of the cholesteatoma matrix in the presence of labyrinthine fistula as a means of hearing preservation [44].

Early Stapedectomy Lessons Learned

Iatrogenic post-stapedectomy perilymph fistulas were first described a half-century ago. Steffen et al. [45] reported findings of gross perilymph flow at the oval window in post-stapedectomy patients with hearing loss, tinnitus, and vertigo. Fee [46] reported three patients who presented with vertigo, fluctuating hearing loss, and tinnitus, who also had known or suspected recent head trauma. Intraoperative findings showed perilymph leak at the oval window. Repair of the leak resulted in significant improvement in symptoms.

Perilymph Fistula

As shown in Fig. 1.1, the symptoms of perilymph fistula are observed in other TMWS known sites of dehiscence (Tables 1.1 and 1.2). This clinical entity will be discussed in greater detail in Chap. 8, "Perilymphatic Fistula."

Vestibular Evoked Myogenic Potentials

It was over a century ago that Robert Bárány began using caloric irrigation and his vertical axis rotational chair to assess horizontal canal function, yet it was not until 1994 that Colebatch and colleagues developed the sound-evoked cervical vestibular evoked myogenic potential (cVEMP) to study the gravitational receptors [47]. Sound-induced activation of the saccule leads to an inhibition of the sternocleidomastoid muscle and this inhibitory potential can be recorded as the cVEMP (for review see [48–50]). The evoked potentials recorded from a number of other muscles have been studied as well; however, it is the sternocleidomastoid muscle that is most consistently used in research and clinical applications. It has also been shown that both an ipsilateral and contralateral cVEMP can be recorded from the sternocleidomastoid muscle following ipsilateral stimulation [48, 51]. Bone-conducted stimuli have also been used to evoke cVEMP responses (for review see [49, 50]). All of these cVEMP methods depend on voluntary contraction of the sternocleidomastoid muscle so that the evoked inhibitory potential can be measured.

In patients with SSCD and other sites of dehiscence resulting in third window syndrome, cVEMPs are useful diagnostic indicators, with patients exhibiting abnormal responses to auditory clicks or tone bursts used in this test [4, 18–20, 52, 53]. The cVEMP amplitudes in the affected labyrinth are increased, and thresholds are reduced as the opening in the superior semicircular canal renders otolithic receptors more susceptible to stimulation by sound and vibration [4, 18–20, 30, 54–56]. The same cVEMP increased amplitude and decreased threshold has been reported in many other locations creating a TMWS including CT– TMWS and CFD [4, 18–20]. After surgical plugging of the SSCD, cVEMP thresholds and amplitudes normalize [56].

The ocular vestibular evoked myogenic potential (oVEMP) testing represents another diagnostic tool that can be important in the diagnosis of patients with TMWS. These potentials are excitatory and are recorded from surface electrodes over the inferior oblique muscles. Many have contributed to understanding the oVEMP response, particularly Ian Curthoys' group [49]. Both acoustic and bone-conduction stimuli activate the saccular and utricular otolithic receptors; however, the otolithic input to the sternocleidomastoid muscle is predominately from the saccular macula whereas the otolithic input to the inferior oblique muscle is predominately from the utricular macula [48–50]. Thus, quantitatively, cVEMP tests saccular function while oVEMP tests utricular function. Another practical extension of these relationships is that the cVEMP reflects inferior vestibular nerve function while the oVEMP reflects the superior vestibular nerve function. Clinically, the oVEMP amplitude is much smaller than the cVEMP amplitude and the response is often absent in older patients. Therefore, oVEMP thresholds are not typically measured but either a single 4 kHz or combination of 500 Hz and 4 kHz oVEMP response is measured [57]. With TMWS, the oVEMP amplitude is typically elevated [57].

Audiometry

Since TMWS patients suffer from auditory symptoms, all should undergo pure tone audiometry measuring both air-conduction and bone-conduction thresholds. If the difference between air- and unmasked bone-conduction thresholds is >10 dB, bone-conduction thresholds should be masked to accurately assess the left and right ear separately. The air-bone gap (ABG) is calculated by subtracting the bone-conduction threshold from the air-conduction threshold. Many, but not all, patients with TMWS, including SSCD, CFD CT– TMWS and many others suffer from low frequency air-bone gaps (ABG) of ≥10 dB, which can be due to low or negative bone-conduction thresholds and/or elevated air-conduction thresholds [4, 18–20, 54]. Obviously, ABGs are not unique to TMWS. They are a common finding in other otologic disorders causing conductive hearing loss, especially those with middle ear pathology [58]. Therefore, further evaluation of middle ear function using tympanometry and acoustic reflexes is warranted and aids in differentiating the various causes of the ABG [58, 59]. In contrast to ABG from middle ear pathology that causes abnormalities of tympanometry and/or loss of acoustic reflexes, TMWS cases with an ABG will exhibit normal tympanometry and preservation of acoustic reflexes. Therefore, the term pseudoconductive hearing loss is used in describing this ABG in TMWS patients.

High-Resolution Temporal Bone CT

The development and continued refinement of high-resolution temporal bone CT has been transformative in the identification of bony sites of TMWS. The ability to reformat the acquired data into axial, coronal, Stenvers and Pöschl planes, as well as utilization of gray-scale inversion has allowed the identification of small and unusual sites of a third mobile window resulting in TMWS [4, 60]. This will be discussed in greater detail in Chap. 12, “Imaging.”

Superior Semicircular Canal Dehiscence

While it was nearly a century ago that Tullio described the physiologic outcomes of creating a third mobile window in the semicircular canals of pigeons [33, 35, 36], it is approaching a quarter century ago that Minor et al. first described superior semicircular canal dehiscence (SSCD) in two patients [61]. However, this is not a new clinical entity as SSCD has been observed after CT imaging of Egyptian mummy heads [62].

Over the past 60 years, we have learned much regarding the clinical features, outcomes measured by validated survey instruments and neuropsychology testing as well as objective diagnostic studies in TMWS [54, 58, 59, 63–96]. Poe's group observed that 94% of patients with SSCD, or symptoms consistent with SSCD, experienced autophony and aural fullness, while 86% were found to have pseudo-conductive hearing loss [58, 75]. Interestingly, in their 2007 study, they included four cases of CT– TWS among their series of CT+ SSCD who had also had abnormally low cVEMP thresholds [58]. Because of their diagnostic dilemma, they did not manage these patients with surgical intervention. The University of Michigan group first described abnormal electrocochleography findings, usually associated with endolymphatic hydrops, in SSCD patients [96]. All four patients who were managed surgically had resolution of their abnormal ECoG findings. The Wackym group has used the Dizziness Handicap Inventory, the Headache Impact Test and comprehensive neuropsychology test batteries preoperatively and postoperatively to measure the cognitive dysfunction and migraine headache in TMWS patients to quantify their dysfunction and recovery outcomes [4, 18–20]. Crane et al. also reported the reduction of Dizziness Handicap Inventory scores after plugging the superior semicircular canal in patients with SSCD [92].

In addition, the Wackym group has reported a delayed development of CT– TWS after surgical plugging and resurfacing of CT+ SSCD TMWS [18–20]. In a series of near-SSCD patients undergoing plugging and resurfacing procedures at the Johns Hopkins Hospital, all patients noted initial improvement in at least one presenting TMWS symptom; however, five subjects (45%) reported the persistence or recurrence of at least one TMWS symptom at greater than one month after surgery [59]. In a larger series of SSCD patients, John Carey's group reported that among 222 patients who underwent plugging procedures for SSCD, there were 21 patients who underwent 23 revision surgeries for failure to resolve their TMWS symptoms [97]. After revision surgery, TMWS symptoms were completely resolved in eight (35%), partially resolved in seven (30%), and unresolved in seven (30%) [97]. One possible explanation of these findings is that in 14 (61%) of these patients, they also had CT– TMWS. It has been suggested that the modiolus may be one site for a CT– TMWS [4, 18–20], and Ilmari Pyykkö's and Dennis Poe's demonstration that intratympanic injection of gadolinium subsequently fills the perilymphatic space in mice [98], rats [99] and then exits the inner ear via the modiolus and into the internal auditory canal supports this possibility. Manzari and Scagnelli reported a patient with bilateral SSCD and bilateral dehiscent modioli experiencing bilateral TMWS; however, the patient was lost to follow up before surgical intervention [85]. Another possible etiology of "CT– TMWS" is an unrecognized CFD, as we reported recently [4].

Surgical management using plugging techniques via the middle cranial fossa or transmastoid approaches, as well as resurfacing techniques and round window reinforcement, have all been described (for review see [73]) and will be discussed in Chap. 15, "Surgical Intervention, Revision Surgery and Surgical Complications."

Spectrum of Known Sites Creating a Third Mobile Window

As shown in Table 1.3 there are currently 15 known sites of dehiscence that can be seen using high-resolution temporal bone CT and in addition there are sites of dehiscence that cannot yet be seen with contemporary high-resolution temporal bone CT scans (CT– TMWS). The 15 known visible by imaging sites of dehiscence are: superior semicircular canal dehiscence (SSCD), posterior semicircular canal dehiscence, posterior semicircular canal-jugular bulb dehiscence, posterior semicircular canal-endolymphatic sac/vestibular aqueduct dehiscence, lateral semicircular canal dehiscence, lateral semicircular canal-facial nerve dehiscence, cochlea-facial nerve dehiscence (CFD), cochlea-internal carotid artery dehiscence, cochlea-internal auditory canal dehiscence, cochlear otosclerosis with internal auditory canal involvement, wide vestibular aqueduct, endolymphatic sac-jugular bulb dehiscence, posttraumatic hypermobile stapes footplate, vestibule-middle ear dehiscence, modiolus (X-linked stapes gusher) plus CT– TWS (see review [4]).The prevalence of these TMWS sites in a cohort of 401 patients (802 temporal bones; 502 temporal bones associated with TMWS symptoms) with TMWS symptoms have been reported [4]. Of note, as shown in Table 1.4, there can be more than one site of dehiscence which has important implications for patients with persistent TMWS symptoms after surgical management of the most obvious site of dehiscence.

In general, surgical management involves plugging of the site of dehiscence when doing so introduces low to no morbidity; however, some sites of dehiscence such as a CFD could be plugged, but the resultant deafness and facial paralysis represent an unacceptable morbidity. For these sites, round window reinforcement has been an effective management strategy. Wackym et al. reported a series of CFD dehiscence patients managed with round window reinforcement using layered perichondrium, cartilage and minced perichondrium admixed with tissue glue [4]. Statistically there was no change in hearing postoperatively and a highly significant reduction in Dizziness Handicap Inventory scores (Fig. 1.2) [4].

This topic is covered in more detail in Chap. 7, "Other Sites of Dehiscence" and in Chap. 15, "Surgical Intervention, Revision Surgery and Surgical Complications."

Table 1.4 Prevalence of radiographic sites of dehiscence in 502 temporal bones associated with third mobile window syndrome in 401 patients (802 temporal bones)

Location(s)/site(s)	Prevalence (%)
Superior semicircular canal dehiscence	175/502 (34.9%)
Near-superior semicircular canal dehiscence	121/502 (24.1%)
CT– third window syndrome	97/502 (19.3%)
Cochlea-facial nerve dehiscence	52/502 (10.4%)
Superior semicircular canal dehiscence + cochlea-facial nerve dehiscence	30/502 (5.98%)
Cochlea-internal auditory canal dehiscence	5/502 (1.0%)
Cochlea-internal auditory canal dehiscence + cochlea-facial nerve dehiscence	4/502 (0.8%)
Lateral semicircular canal dehiscence	3/502 (0.6%)
Wide vestibular aqueduct	3/502 (0.6%)
Wide vestibular aqueduct + cochlea-facial nerve dehiscence	2/502 (0.4%)
Posterior semicircular canal dehiscence	2/502 (0.4%)
Superior semicircular canal-superior petrosal sinus dehiscence	2/502 (0.4%)
Superior semicircular canal dehiscence + posterior semicircular canal dehiscence + wide vestibular aqueduct	1/502 (0.2%)
Superior semicircular canal-subarcuate artery dehiscence	1/502 (0.2%)
Superior semicircular canal dehiscence + cochlea-internal auditory canal dehiscence	1/502 (0.2%)
Superior semicircular canal dehiscence + posterior semicircular canal dehiscence	1/502 (0.2%)
Posterior semicircular canal-jugular bulb dehiscence	1/502 (0.2%)
Modiolus	1/502 (0.2%)

CT- = High-resolution temporal bone computed tomography negative for visible site of dehiscence
Adapted from Wackym et al. [4]. Used with permission, copyright © P.A. Wackym, MD

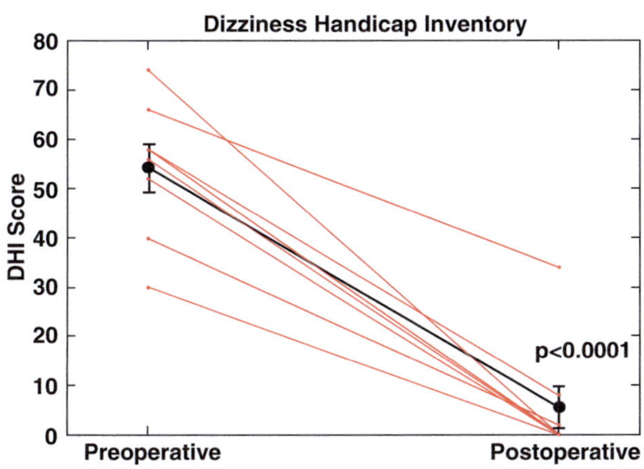

Fig. 1.2 For the cochlea-facial nerve dehiscence cohort who had round window reinforcement procedures performed, the preoperative mean Dizziness Handicap Inventory score was 54.25 (SE 4.9, range 30–74). The postoperative mean Dizziness Handicap Inventory score was 5.5 (SE 4.2, range 0–34). This improvement was highly statistically significant (paired t-test, $p < 0.0001$). These data are plotted as a single black line. Individual patients are plotted as separate lines (red). Copyright © P.A. Wackym, used with permission

Frontiers

The development of an experimental model for various TMWS sites, but especially SSCD, is essential for us to begin understanding the mechanisms responsible for the cognitive dysfunction, spatial disorientation, anxiety and migraine experienced by patients with TMWS. With this knowledge, better insight into the role peripheral vestibular dysfunction plays in disrupting central nervous system processing will emerge and thereby will open new avenues in clinical intervention in resolving these problems or accelerating recovery in these patients. It is also anticipated that advances will be made in refining surgical techniques (e.g., biological 3-D printed caps to cover SSCD defects) and improved diagnostic methods.

References

1. Merchant SN, Rosowski JJ. Conductive hearing loss caused by third-window lesions of the inner ear. Otol Neurotol. 2008;29:282–9. https://doi.org/10.1097/mao.0b013e318161ab24.
2. Stenfelt S, Goode RL. Bone-conducted sound: physiological and clinical aspects. Otol Neurotol. 2005;26:1245–6. https://doi.org/10.1097/01.mao.0000187236.10842.d5.
3. Black FO, Pesznecker S, Norton T, et al. Surgical management of perilymphatic fistulas: a Portland experience. Am J Otol. 1992;13:254–62.
4. Wackym PA, Balaban CD, Zhang P, Siker DA, Hundal JS. Third window syndrome: surgical management of cochlea-facial dehiscence. Front Neurol. 2019;10:1281. https://doi.org/10.3389/fneur.2019.01281.
5. Naert L, Van de Berg R, Van de Heyning P, et al. Aggregating the symptoms of superior semicircular canal dehiscence syndrome. Laryngoscope. 2018;128(8):1932–8. https://doi.org/10.1002/lary.27062.
6. Kohut RI, Perilymph fistulas. Clinical criteria. Arch Otolaryngol Head Neck Surg. 1992;118(7):687–92. https://doi.org/10.1001/archotol.1992.01880070017003.
7. Wackym PA. Vestibular migraine. Patient video describing symptoms before and after treatment with Topamax. https://www.youtube.com/watch?v=Zy7YjCDnLYM. https://doi.org/10.13140/RG.2.1.3096.2647. Published April 12, 2012. Accessed August 15, 2022. Copyright © P.A. Wackym, MD, used with permission.
8. Wackym PA. Right perilymph fistula not superior canal dehiscence. Patient video describing symptoms before and after surgical repair. https://www.youtube.com/watch?v=bDph0B0uLbg. https://doi.org/10.13140/RG.2.1.3097.8000. Accessed August 15, 2022. Copyright © P.A. Wackym, MD, used with permission.
9. Wackym PA. Right cochlea-facial nerve dehiscence: 16 year old thought to have conversion disorder. https://youtu.be/fTjsnnUALBw. https://doi.org/10.13140/RG.2.2.27418.90564. Published April 14, 2019. Accessed August 15, 2022. Copyright © P.A. Wackym, MD, used with permission.
10. Wackym PA. Perilymph fistula. https://www.youtube.com/watch?v=jSAM6h-7Mwc. https://doi.org/10.13140/RG.2.1.1000.6488. Published April 15, 2012. Accessed August 15, 2022. Copyright © P.A. Wackym, MD, used with permission.
11. Wackym PA. Right superior semicircular canal dehiscence repair: Symptoms and recovery. https://youtu.be/er4k8NZrG2I. https://doi.org/10.13140/RG.2.2.32032.79361. Published January 9, 2017. Accessed August 15, 2022. Copyright © P.A. Wackym, MD, used with permission.

12. Wackym PA. Recurrent third window syndrome co-morbidity: Functional neurological symptom disorder. https://youtu.be/AgUy07QxTxo. https://doi.org/10.13140/RG.2.2.15255.57763. Published January 9, 2017. Accessed August 15, 2022. Copyright © P.A. Wackym, MD, used with permission.
13. Wackym PA. Otic capsule dehiscence syndrome in one ear after a car accident. https://www.youtube.com/watch?v=1Nl9T6etxqM. https://doi.org/10.13140/RG.2.1.3359.9440. Published April 5, 2015. Accessed August 15, 2022. Copyright © P.A. Wackym, MD, used with permission.
14. Wackym PA. Cochlea-facial nerve dehiscence: traumatic third window syndrome after a snowboarding accident. https://youtu.be/NCDMD5FGf-w. https://doi.org/10.13140/RG.2.2.17283.76327. Published April 9, 2019. Accessed August 15, 2022. Copyright © P.A. Wackym, MD, used with permission.
15. Wackym PA. Surgery for cochlea-facial nerve dehiscence: Symptoms and tuning fork testing. https://youtu.be/lFR-zdYlIsY. https://doi.org/10.13140/RG.2.2.34129.79209. Published April 14, 2019. Accessed August 15, 2022. Copyright © P.A. Wackym, MD, used with permission.
16. Wackym PA. Tuning fork testing in otic capsule dehiscence syndrome. https://www.youtube.com/watch?v=Szp_kO8oVos. https://doi.org/10.13140/RG.2.1.4408.5204. Published April 21, 2015. Accessed August 15, 2022. Copyright © P.A. Wackym, MD, used with permission.
17. Wackym PA. Tuning fork testing before and after repair of two types of otic capsule dehiscence. https://www.youtube.com/watch?v=NIauJPbvSpA. https://doi.org/10.13140/RG.2.1.4365.7048. Published December 13, 2015. Accessed August 15, 2022. Copyright © P.A. Wackym, MD, used with permission.
18. Wackym PA, Wood SJ, Siker DA, Carter DM. Otic capsule dehiscence syndrome: Superior canal dehiscence syndrome with no radiographically visible dehiscence. Ear Nose Throat J. 2015;94(7):8–24. https://doi.org/10.1177/014556131509400802.
19. Wackym PA, Balaban CD, Mackay HT, et al. Longitudinal cognitive and neurobehavioral functional outcomes after repairing otic capsule dehiscence. Otol Neurotol. 2016;37(1):70–82. https://doi.org/10.1097/MAO.0000000000000928.
20. Wackym PA, Mackay-Promitas HT, Demirel S, et al. Comorbidities confounding the outcomes of surgery for third window syndrome: outlier analysis. Laryngosc Invest Otolaryngol. 2017;2(5):225–53. https://doi.org/10.1002/lio2.89.
21. Wackym PA, Balaban CD. Molecules, motion, and man. Otolaryngol Head Neck Surg. 1998;118:15–23.
22. Balaban CD, Thayer JF. Neurological bases for balance-anxiety links. J Anxiety Disord. 2001;15(1-2):53–79. https://doi.org/10.1016/s0887-6185(00)00042-6.
23. Balaban CD, McGee DM, Zhou J, Scudder CA. Responses of primate caudal parabrachial nucleus and Kölliker-fuse nucleus neurons to whole body rotation. J Neurophysiol. 2002;88:3175–93. https://doi.org/10.1152/jn.00499.2002.
24. Baek JH, Zheng Y, Darlington CL, Smith PF. Evidence that spatial memory deficits following bilateral vestibular deafferentation in rats are probably permanent. Neurobiol Learn Mem. 2010;94(3):402–13. https://doi.org/10.1016/j.nlm.2010.08.007.
25. Smith PF, Darlington CL, Zheng Y. Move it or lose it–is stimulation of the vestibular system necessary for normal spatial memory? Hippocampus. 2010;20(1):36–43. https://doi.org/10.1002/hipo.20588.
26. Deroualle D, Lopez C. Toward a vestibular contribution to social cognition. Front Integr Neurosci. 2014;8:16. https://doi.org/10.3389/fnint.2014.00016.
27. Smith PF, Darlington CL. Personality changes in patients with vestibular dysfunction. Front Hum Neurosci. 2013;7:678. https://doi.org/10.3389/fnhum.2013.00678.
28. Balaban CD. Projections from the parabrachial nucleus to the vestibular nuclei: potential substrates for autonomic and limbic influences on vestibular responses. Brain Res. 2004;996(1):126–37. https://doi.org/10.1016/j.brainres.2003.10.026.
29. Darlington CL, Goddard M, Zheng Y, Smith PF. Anxiety-related behavior and biogenic amine pathways in the rat following bilateral vestibular lesions. Ann N Y Acad Sci. 2009;1164:134–9. https://doi.org/10.1111/j.1749-6632.2008.03725.x.

30. Minor LB. Clinical manifestations of superior semicircular canal dehiscence. Laryngoscope. 2005;115:1717–27.
31. Crane BT, Lin FR, Minor LB, Carey JP. Improvement in autophony symptoms after superior canal dehiscence repair. Otol Neurotol. 2010;31(1):140–6.
32. Bhutta MF. Eye movement autophony in superior semicircular canal dehiscence syndrome may be caused by trans-dural transmission of extraocular muscle contraction. Int J Audiol. 2015;54(1):61–2.
33. Huizinga E. The physiological and clinical importance of experimental work on the pigeon's labyrinth. J Laryngol Otol. 1955;69:260–8. https://doi.org/10.1017/s0022215100050635.
34. Tullio P. Some experiments and considerations on experimental otology and phonetics: a lecture delivered at the meeting of the "Società dei cultori delle scienze e naturali" of Cagliari on 1st, July 1929: L. Cappelli 1929 ASIN: B0008B2T6Y
35. Tullio P. Das Ohr und die Entstehung der Sprache und Schrift. Berlin: Urban & Schwarzenberg; 1929. p. 1–455.
36. Addams-Williams J, Wu K, Ray J. The experiments behind the Tullio phenomenon. J Laryngol Otol. 2014;128(3):223–7. https://doi.org/10.1017/S0022215114000280.
37. Cawthorne T. Contributions of surgery to problems of neurootology. Br Med Bull. 1956;12:143–5.
38. Shea JJ Jr. A personal history of stapedectomy. Am J Otol. 1998;19(5):S2–12.
39. Shambaugh GE Jr. Julius Lempert and the fenestration operation. Am J Otol. 1995;16(2):247–52.
40. Lempert J. Lempert fenestra nov-ovalis for the restoration of practical unaided hearing in clinical otosclerosis; its present status. Proc R Soc Med. 1948;41(9):617–30.
41. Cawthorne T. Otosclerosis. J Laryngol Otol. 1955;69:437–56. https://doi.org/10.1017/S0022215100050933.
42. Copeland BJ, Buchman CA. Management of labyrinthine fistulae in chronic ear surgery. Am J Otolaryngol. 2003;24(1):51–60. https://doi.org/10.1053/ajot.2003.10.
43. Meyer A, Bouchetemblé P, Costentin B, Dehesdin D, Lerosey Y, Marie JP. Lateral semicircular canal fistula in cholesteatoma: diagnosis and management. Eur Arch Otorhinolaryngol. 2016;273(8):2055–63. https://doi.org/10.1007/s00405-015-3775-6.
44. Schmerber S, Baguant A, Fabre C, Quatre R. Surgical treatment of cholesteatomatous labyrinthine fistula by hydrodissection. Eur Ann Otorhinolaryngol Head Neck Dis. 2021;138(4):279–82. https://doi.org/10.1016/j.anorl.2020.11.004.
45. Steffen TN, Sheehy JL, House HP. The slipped strut problem. Ann Otol Rhinol Laryngol. 1963;72:191–205.
46. Fee GA. Traumatic perilymphatic fistulas. Arch Otolaryngol. 1968;88:477–80.
47. Colebatch JG, Halmagyi GM, Skuse NF. Myogenic potentials generated by click-evoked vestibulocollic reflex. J Neurol Neurosurg Psychiatry. 1994;57:190–7.
48. Welgampola MS, Colebatch JG. Characteristics and clinical applications of vestibular-evoked myogenic potentials. Neurology. 2005;64:1682–8.
49. Curthoys IS. A critical review of the neurophysiological evidence underlying clinical vestibular testing using sound, vibration and galvanic stimuli. Clin Neurophysiol. 2010;121(2):132–44.
50. Wackym PA, Ratigan JA, Birck JD, et al. Rapid cVEMP and oVEMP responses elicited by a novel head striker and recording device. Otol Neurotol. 2012;33(8):1392–400. https://doi.org/10.1097/MAO.0b013e318268d234.
51. McNerney KM, Burkard RF. The vestibular evoked myogenic potential (VEMP): air- versus bone-conducted stimuli. Ear Hear. 2011;32(6):e6–e15.
52. Hunter JB, Patel NS, O'Connell BP, et al. Cervical and ocular VEMP testing in diagnosing superior semicircular canal dehiscence. Otolaryngol Head Neck Surg. 2017;156:917–23. https://doi.org/10.1177/0194599817690720.
53. Brantberg K, Bergenius J, Tribukait A. Vestibular-evoked myogenic potentials in patients with dehiscence of the superior semicircular canal. Acta Otolaryngol. 1999;119:633–40. https://doi.org/10.1080/00016489950180559.

54. Pfammatter A, Darrouzet V, Gärtner M, et al. A superior semicircular canal dehiscence syndrome multicenter study: is there an association between size and symptoms? Otol Neurotol. 2010;31(3):447–54. https://doi.org/10.1097/MAO.0b013e3181d27740.
55. Streubel SO, Cremer PD, Carey JP, Weg N, Minor LB. Vestibular-evoked myogenic potentials in the diagnosis of superior canal dehiscence syndrome. Acta Otolaryngol Suppl. 2001;545:41–9. https://doi.org/10.1080/000164801750388090.
56. Welgampola MS, Myrie OA, Minor LB, Carey JP. Vestibular-evoked myogenic potential thresholds normalize on plugging superior canal dehiscence. Neurology. 2008;70:464–72. https://doi.org/10.1212/01.wnl.0000299084.76250.4a.
57. Tran ED, Swanson A, Sharon JD, et al. Ocular vestibular-evoked myogenic potential amplitudes elicited at 4 kHz optimize detection of superior semicircular canal dehiscence. Front Neurol. 2020;11:879. https://doi.org/10.3389/fneur.2020.00879.
58. Zhou G, Gopen Q, Poe DS. Clinical and diagnostic characterization of canal dehiscence syndrome: a great otologic mimicker. Otol Neurotol. 2007;28(7):920–6.
59. Ward BK, Wenzel A, Ritzl EK, et al. Near-dehiscence: clinical findings in patients with thin bone over the superior semicircular canal. Otol Neurotol. 2013;34:1421–8. https://doi.org/10.1097/MAO.0b013e318287efe6.
60. Schwartz T, Lindemann TL, Mongelluzzo G, Wackym PA, Gadre AK. Gray-scale inversion on HRCT: an adjunct to visualize fine structures of the temporal bone. Ann Otol Rhinol Laryngol. 2021;130(10):1125–31. https://doi.org/10.1177/0003489421996844.
61. Minor LB, Solomon D, Zinreich JS, Zee DS. Sound- and/or pressure-induced vertigo due to bone dehiscence of the superior semicircular canal. Arch Otolaryngol Head Neck Surg. 1998;124(3):249–58. https://doi.org/10.1001/archotol.124.3.249.
62. Dalchow CV, Schmidt C, Harbort J, Knecht R, Grzyska U, Muenscher A. Imaging of ancient Egyptian mummies' temporal bones with digital volume tomography. Eur Arch Otorhinolaryngol. 2012;269(10):2277–84. https://doi.org/10.1007/s00405-012-2011-x.
63. Wackym PA, Balaban CD, Ikezono T, Agrawal Y. Third window syndrome. Lausanne: Frontiers Media SA. 2021. https://doi.org/10.3389/978-2-88971-190-1. https://www.frontiersin.org/research-topics/12065/third-window-syndrome
64. Wackym PA, Agrawal Y, Ikezono T, Balaban CD. Editorial: Third window syndrome. Front Neurol. 2021;12:704095. https://doi.org/10.3389/fneur.2021.704095. PMID: 34220698; PMCID: 8250852.
65. Wackym PA. Round window reinforcement surgery for cochlea-facial nerve dehiscence: symptoms and testing. https://youtu.be/2z1RJEKZQ1A. Published April 15, 2019. https://doi.org/10.13140/RG.2.2.30617.06247. Accessed August 15, 2022.
66. Smullen JL, Andrist EC, Gianoli GJ. Superior semicircular canal dehiscence: a new cause of vertigo. J La State Med Soc. 1999;151(8):397–400.
67. Grieser BJ, Kleiser L, Obrist D. Identifying mechanisms behind the Tullio phenomenon: a computational study based on first principles. J Assoc Res Otolaryngol. 2016;17(2):103–18. https://doi.org/10.1007/s10162-016-0553-0.
68. Fox EJ, Balkany TJ, Arenberg IK. The Tullio phenomenon and perilymph fistula. Otolaryngol Head Neck Surg. 1988;98(1):88–9.
69. Pyykkö I, Ishizaki H, Aalto H, Starck J. Relevance of the Tullio phenomenon in assessing perilymphatic leak in vertiginous patients. Am J Otol. 1992;13(4):339–42.
70. Colebatch JG, Rothwell JC, Bronstein A, Ludman H. Click-evoked vestibular activation in the Tullio phenomenon. J Neurol Neurosurg Psychiatry. 1994;57:1538–40. https://doi.org/10.1136/jnnp.57.12.1538.
71. Ostrowski VB, Hain TC, Wiet RJ. Pressure-induced ocular torsion. Arch Otolaryngol Head Neck Surg. 1997;123(6):646–9.
72. Weinreich HM, Carey JP. Perilymphatic fistulas and superior semi-circular canal dehiscence syndrome. Adv Otorhinolaryngol. 2019;82:93–100. https://doi.org/10.1159/000490276.

73. Ward BK, Carey JP, Minor LB. Superior canal dehiscence syndrome: lessons from the first 20 years. Front Neurol. 2017;8:177. https://doi.org/10.3389/fneur.2017.00177.
74. Wackym PA. Cochlea-facial nerve dehiscence: third window syndrome after a car accident. https://youtu.be/eJX2RA3okKc. Published April 7, 2019. https://doi.org/10.13140/RG.2.2.12447.20646. Accessed August 15, 2022.
75. Mikulec AA, Poe DS, McKenna MJ. Operative management of superior semicircular canal dehiscence. Laryngoscope. 2005;115(3):501–7.
76. Young L, Isaacson B. Cochlear and petrous carotid canal erosion secondary to cholesteatoma. Otol Neurotol. 2010;31:697–8.
77. Meiklejohn DA, Corrales CE, Boldt BM, et al. Pediatric semicircular canal dehiscence: radiographic and histologic prevalence, with clinical correlations. Otol Neurotol. 2015;36(8):1383–9.
78. Park JJ, Shen A, Loberg C, Westhofen M. The relationship between jugular bulb position and jugular bulb related inner ear dehiscence: a retrospective analysis. Am J Otolaryngol. 2015;36(3):347–51.
79. Gopen Q, Zhou G, Poe D, Kenna M, Jones D. Posterior semicircular canal dehiscence: first reported case series. Otol Neurotol. 2010;31(2):339–44.
80. Bear ZW, McEvoy TP, Mikulec AA. Quantification of hearing loss in patients with posterior semicircular canal dehiscence. Acta Otolaryngol. 2015;135(10):974–7.
81. Elmali M, Poltat AV, Kucuk H, Atmaca S, Aksoy A. Semicircular canal dehiscence: frequency and distribution on temporal bone CT and its relationship with the clinical outcomes. Eur J Radiol. 2013;82(10):e606–9.
82. Blake DM, Tomovic S, Vazquez A, Lee HJ, Jyung RW. Cochlear-facial dehiscence–a newly described entity. Laryngoscope. 2014;124(1):283–9.
83. Fujita T, Kobayashi T, Saito K, Seo T, Ikezono T, Doi K. Vestibule-middle ear dehiscence tested with perilymph-specific protein cochlin-tomoprotein (CTP) detection test. Front Neurol. 2019;10:47.
84. Manzari L. Multiple dehiscences of bony labyrinthine capsule. A rare case report and review of the literature. Acta Otorhinolaryngol Ital. 2010;30(6):317–20.
85. Manzari L, Scagnelli P. Large bilateral internal auditory meatus associated with bilateral superior semicircular canal dehiscence. Ear Nose Throat J. 2013;92(1):25–33.
86. Fang CH, Chung SY, Blake DM, et al. Prevalence of cochlear-facial dehiscence in a study of 1,020 temporal bone specimens. Otol Neurotol. 2016;37(7):967–72.
87. Ho ML, Moonis G, Halpin CF, Curtin HD. Spectrum of third window abnormalities: semicircular canal dehiscence and beyond. AJNR Am J Neuroradiol. 2017;38(1):2–9. https://doi.org/10.3174/ajnr.A4922.
88. Koo JW, Hong SK, Kim DK, Kim JS. Superior semicircular canal dehiscence syndrome by the superior petrosal sinus. J Neurol Neurosurg Psychiatry. 2010;81:465–7. https://doi.org/10.1136/jnnp.2008.155564.
89. Ionescu EC, Al Tamami N, Neagu A, et al. Superior semicircular canal ampullae dehiscence as part of the spectrum of the third window abnormalities: a case study. Front Neurol. 2017;8:683. https://doi.org/10.3389/fneur.2017.00683.
90. Dasgupta S, Ratnayake SAB. Functional and objective audiovestibular evaluation of children with apparent semicircular canal dehiscence - a case series in a pediatric vestibular center. Front Neurol. 2019;10:306. https://doi.org/10.3389/fneur.2019.00306.
91. Hornibrook J. The balance abnormality of chronic perilymph fistula. https://www.youtube.com/watch?v=2DXgQMnlgbw. Published Nov 26, 2015. Accessed August 15, 2022.
92. Crane BT, Minor LB, Carey JP. Superior canal dehiscence plugging reduces dizziness handicap. Laryngoscope. 2008;118:1809–13. https://doi.org/10.1097/MLG.0b013e31817f18fa.
93. Gadre AK, Edwards IR, Baker VM, Roof CR. Membranous or hypermobile stapes footplate: a new anatomic site resulting in third window syndrome. Front Neurol. 2020;11:871. https://doi.org/10.3389/fneur.2020.00871.

94. Matsuda H, Tanzawa Y, Sekine T, et al. Congenital membranous stapes footplate producing episodic pressure-induced perilymphatic fistula symptoms. Front Neurol. 2020;11:585747. https://doi.org/10.3389/fneur.2020.585747.
95. Lin K, Lahey R, Beckley R, et al. Validating the utility of high frequency ocular vestibular evoked myogenic potential testing in the diagnosis of superior semicircular canal dehiscence. Otol Neurotol. 2019;40(10):1353–8. https://doi.org/10.1097/MAO.0000000000002388.
96. Arts HA, Adams ME, Telian SA, El-Kashlan H, Kileny PR. Reversible electrocochleographic abnormalities in superior canal dehiscence. Otol Neurotol. 2009;30(1):79–86.
97. Sharon JD, Pross SE, Ward BK, Carey JP. Revision surgery for superior canal dehiscence syndrome. Otol Neurotol. 2016;37(8):1096–103.
98. Zou J, Zhang W, Poe D, Zhang Y, Ramadan UA, Pyykkö I. Differential passage of gadolinium through the mouse inner ear barriers evaluated with 4.7T MRI. Hear Res. 2010;259(1-2):36–43.
99. Zou J, Poe D, Ramadan UA, Pyykkö I. Oval window transport of Gd-dOTA from rat middle ear to vestibulum and scala vestibuli visualized by in vivo magnetic resonance imaging. Ann Otol Rhinol Laryngol. 2012;121(2):119–28.

Chapter 2
Etiology

Karl W. Doerfer and Robert S. Hong

Background

Superior semicircular canal dehiscence (SSCD) syndrome, first described by Minor et al., results from bony dehiscence of the middle fossa overlying the superior semicircular canal, classically leading to symptoms of hearing loss, autophony, and sound-induced vertigo [1]. The mechanism behind this condition involves a pathophysiologic mobile window at the area of dehiscence. The two physiologic mobile windows, the oval and round windows, allow acoustic energy to travel through the cochlear scalae with only limited effect on the vestibular system. The addition of a third mobile window (TMW) provides another route for mechanical energy to traverse the inner ear, thus altering the normal function of both the cochlea and the vestibular organs. In terms of cochlear function, dissipation of acoustic energy through a TMW results in increased air conduction thresholds. Additionally, the impedance differential between the scala tympani and scala vestibuli increases, resulting in decreased bone thresholds. The resulting audiologic effect is a low-to-mid frequency air-bone gap, supranormal bone thresholds, and increased sensitivity to bodily sounds (e.g., autophony, pulsatile tinnitus). In terms of vestibular function, shunting of acoustic energy through the vestibule and superior semicircular canal leads to vestibular symptoms, most classically vertigo with loud sound (Tullio phenomenon). In addition to SSCD, less common areas of dehiscence between the otic capsule and surrounding structures have been reported, including the vestibular

K. W. Doerfer (✉)
Department of Otolaryngology and Communication, Medical College of Wisconsin, Milwaukee, WI, USA

R. S. Hong
Michigan Ear Institute, Farmington Hills, MI, USA
e-mail: rhong@med.wayne.edu

G. J. Gianoli, P. Thomson (eds.), *Third Mobile Window Syndrome of the Inner Ear*, https://doi.org/10.1007/978-3-031-16586-3_2

aqueduct, internal auditory canal, carotid canal, and facial nerve [2–6]. As with SSCD, these other foci of dehiscence have the potential to create a mobile third window, leading to hearing loss and vestibular dysfunction [2].

Symptoms of SSCD syndrome are variable and may be nonspecific. A study by Naert et al. aggregating symptoms reported spontaneous dizziness, sound- and pressure-induced vertigo, autophony, and hearing loss as occurring in >35% of affected patients. Other less specific symptoms included aural pressure, pulsatile tinnitus, hyperacusis to bodily or environmental sounds, and spontaneous or pulsatile oscillopsia [7]. Given the broad overlap of SSCD symptomatology with other conditions including Ménière's disease, vestibular migraine, patulous eustachian tube, conductive hearing loss, idiopathic intracranial hypertension, and other various causes of pulsatile tinnitus, alternative diagnoses should be considered when evaluating a patient with possible SSCD syndrome. Conversely, as growing evidence suggests a complex web of associations among vestibular disorders, including cohort studies showing an association between SSCD and migraine, the possibility of SSCD syndrome coinciding with other vestibular diagnoses should not be ignored [8–10].

Physical examination of patients with SSCD may show vertical torsional nystagmus with the fast-phase components directed downward and toward the affected ear with high-intensity acoustic stimuli, positive pressure applied to the tympanic membrane, or Valsalva maneuvers against pinched nostrils. These findings correspond to excitation of the superior canal afferents from ampullofugal deflection of the cupula. Nystagmus with opposite directionality may be seen with negative pressure in the external auditory canal, Valsalva against a closed glottis, and jugular venous compression, all of which cause ampullopetal deflection of the cupola and subsequent inhibition of tonic superior semicircular canal afferent activity. In addition to superior semicircular canal afferent modulation, otolith organ activation and inhibition may also occur, resulting in sound-induced ocular tilt mediated by the utricle and saccule as well as cardiovascular changes mediated by vestibulosympathetic reflexes.

Diagnostic evaluation of SSCD relies on both radiographic and audiologic testing. Assessing the bony integrity of the middle fossa requires high resolution computed tomography (HRCT) with ≤0.5 mm cuts performed perpendicular and parallel to the plane of the superior semicircular canal (Stenver and Poschl views). Audiologic evaluation involves audiogram as well as cervical and/or ocular vestibular evoked myogenic potentials (cVEMP and oVEMP), and electrocochleography (ECOG). Audiogram may show a hearing loss as described above, while cVEMP may show decreased thresholds, and oVEMP may show increased amplitude. ECOG may show an increased SP/AP ratio. Recently, oVEMP has been shown to be the most sensitive and specific test to confirm SSCD syndrome suspected from history, physical exam, audiogram, and HRCT [11–13].

Definitive diagnosis of SSCD syndrome can be challenging due to the inherent limitations of current imaging technology and variable patient factors. The incidence of SSCD syndrome in temporal bone histopathologic series is estimated to be between 0.5% and 0.6% [14, 15]. In contrast, radiographic studies suggest a dehiscence rate of 3.9–9% depending on the level of CT resolution and use of Stenver &

Poschl views [14]. This discrepancy arises from the inability of available CT technology to reliably detect extremely thin bone (i.e., <0.5 mm), thus raising the risk for false-positive results. Imaging limitations also may lead to false-negative results insofar as it cannot detect areas of increased bony compliance ("near dehiscence") or pinpoint areas of dehiscence, which have been shown to alter inner ear impedance [16, 17]. Other anatomic and patient factors may also complicate diagnosis. Several series describe patients with clear radiographic and audiovestibular evidence of SSCD who lack clear symptoms of SSCD syndrome [18–20]. One hypothesis suggests this is due to a tight dural seal over the area of dehiscence that prevents changes to inner ear impedance [15]. Alternatively, patients may have variable sensitivity to the auditory and vestibular effects of active dehiscence, raising the possibility that large areas of dehiscence may produce no noticeable symptoms for some, while others are exquisitely aware of symptoms produced by radiographically occult lesions. Finally, as noted earlier, SSCD-S may mimic or coincide with other similarly presenting conditions. These points underscore the importance of considering alternative diagnoses when evaluating a patient with possible SSCD-S, obtaining adequate objective testing to support a final diagnosis, and recommending appropriate management options based on the severity of symptoms.

Proposed Etiologies of Superior Canal Dehiscence

The etiology of SSCD syndrome is not fully understood. Early descriptions of the condition included anatomic and histopathologic studies that support an underlying developmental cause. However, other evidence suggests the condition may be acquired later in life due to various factors that cause thinning of the lateral skull base. Some researchers suggest a hybrid, multifactorial etiology for SSCD that incorporates a developmental basis for near dehiscence that later progresses to full-blown SSCD syndrome owing to acquired factors.

Abnormal Development and Congenital Factors

Several findings from histopathologic studies support a developmental etiology for SSCD. First, thinning of the middle fossa tends to be symmetric. Carey et al. showed that extremely thin bone (i.e., ≤0.10 mm) over one superior canal was strongly associated with middle fossa thinning on the contralateral side (0.07 ± 0.05 mm), which was significantly less than the average thickness found in adult controls (0.96 ± 0.61 mm). Similar rates of bilateral skull base attenuation have been described in studies evaluating the association between SSCD and spontaneous tegmen defects [14, 21–23]. Second, specimens with canal dehiscence show stable ossification patterns with lamellar bone on the margins of thin or dehiscent areas. Preservation of lamellae deposited during skull base ossification suggests that thinning occurs early in development rather than through a process that erodes through previously deposited bone. Third, samples from pediatric patients show that middle fossa thickness inversely correlates with age. In Anson and Donaldson's description of otic capsule development from a cartilage precursor, multiple, trilaminar ossification centers grow and fuse between the 15th and 21st weeks of development, eventually encasing the otic capsule in bone. The innermost, endosteal layer shows minimal growth following fusion. The middle layer develops into a dense, petrous layer approximately five months after birth, and the outer layer continues to grow and become pneumatized postnatally [24]. Carey et al. showed that average bone thickness in infants ≤1 year of age was only 0.15 ± 0.15 mm, while in the premature infant, the superior canal is covered only by the thin, inner periosteal layer until as late as ten months postnatally (Fig. 2.1) [15]. In adult specimens with thinning or dehiscence,

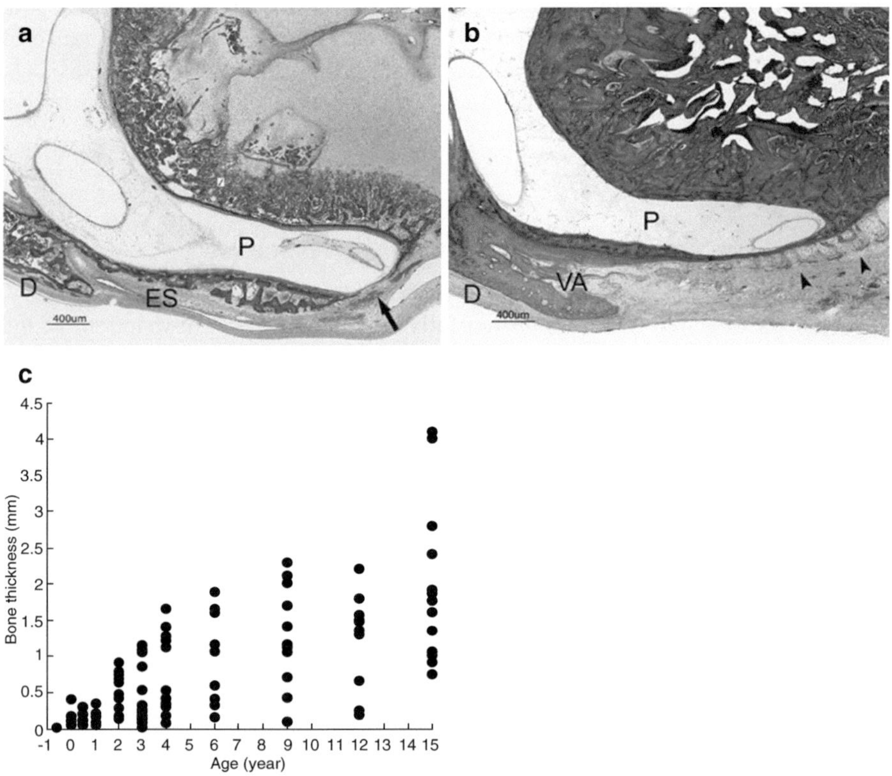

Fig. 2.1 (A) The posterior semicircular canal is not totally covered at gestational age of 24 weeks (arrow). (B) Mastoid development is not complete (arrowhead) in this thin bone from a neonate. (C) The correlation between age and bone thickness overlying the posterior semicircular canal in children ($\rho = 0.68$, $p < 0.01$; hematoxylin and eosin staining). *D* indicates dura, *ES* endolymphatic sac, *P* posterior semicircular canal, *VA* vestibular aqueduct. (**a**) Shows gestational age of 24 weeks, (**b**) a neonate, and (**c**) is a graph illustrating age and bvone thickness in children. (Republished with permission of Wolters Kluwer Health, Inc., from Nomiya S, Cureoglu S, Kariya S, et al. Posterior semicircular canal dehiscence: a histopathologic human temporal bone study. Otol Neurotol. 2010; 31(7):1122-1127. Permission conveyed through Copyright Clearance Center, Inc.) [25]

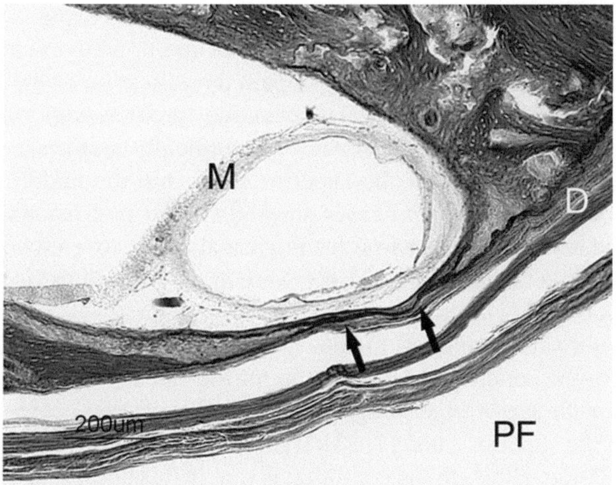

Fig. 2.2 The dehiscence of posterior semicircular canal in adult (male subject, right ear). The periosteum (arrow) remains between the canal and the dura (hematoxylin and eosin staining). D—indicates dura mater, M—membranous labyrinth, PF—posterior cranial fossa. (Republished with permission of Wolters Kluwer Health, Inc., from Nomiya S, Cureoglu S, Kariya S, et al. Posterior semicircular canal dehiscence: a histopathologic human temporal bone study. Otol Neurotol. 2010; 31(7):1122-1127. Permission conveyed through Copyright Clearance Center, Inc.) [25]

there is a similar appearance to infant specimens, suggesting a failure in postnatal development (Fig. 2.2) [15, 26].

In addition to developmental factors, other congenital comorbidities may play a role in canal dehiscence. Kuhn et al. showed an association between Chiari type I malformation and both posterior and superior canal dehiscence, although rates of posterior dehiscence were higher in these patients [27]. The authors proposed that overcrowding of the posterior fossa and elevated intracranial pressure, both fundamental elements of Chiari malformation, may contribute to bony remodeling or impaired development. Genetic factors have also been implicated, with mutations in the COCH and CDH23 genes being linked to SSCD in some reports [28, 29]. A small number of case reports have also shown a possible familial predisposition to SSCD syndrome [18, 23]. However, a clear inheritable cause has not been identified.

While temporal bone studies support a developmental etiology for SSCD, this theory is not well explained by the sequence of semicircular canal development. As the membranous labyrinth forms from the otocyst, the semicircular canals develop in a predictable sequence, beginning with the superior canal, followed by the posterior and horizontal canals. Ossification then follows this same sequence once the membranous labyrinth approaches adult dimensions [30, 31]. Thus, a purely developmental failure affecting the superior canal would also be expected to affect its posterior and lateral counterparts. However, such associations are rarely seen in patients with SSCD syndrome, with the vast majority showing otherwise normal otic capsule anatomy. One proposed explanation for this discrepancy is that protrusion of the developing superior canal into the cranium exposes this portion of the membranous labyrinth to contact with the dura and/or temporal lobe pulsations, which may lead to adhesion and focally impaired ossification of the superior canal during development [32]. A study by Hadi et al. may provide support for this theory. Authors of this study showed that that 92.3% of surgically confirmed cases of SSCD syndrome showed protrusion of the superior canal into the middle cranial fossa, while only 30% of non-dehiscent cases showed similar protrusion. These authors further reported that 28.6% of non-protruding canals were covered by supralabyrinthine air cells, while the remaining 71.4% were at the level of the tegmen and covered with thick bone [21].

Another major shortcoming of the developmental theory for SSCD syndrome is the tendency for the condition to manifest in mid-to-late adulthood, which suggests an association with age or other longstanding conditions that decrease bony thickness overlying the superior canal [1, 33]. Canal dehiscence has been reported in the pediatric population, although the condition is rare in this age-group [34]. In a series of HRCT scans performed on children with hearing loss, Chen et al. reported a radiographic dehiscence rate of 4% and 11%, respectively [35]. However, these patients lacked other symptoms of SSCD syndrome and the established high rate of false positives using imaging alone makes it difficult to interpret the results of this study. For infants with radiographic dehiscence, the lack of objective findings may be due to limitations associated with newborn hearing screening and audiometric testing coupled with postnatal middle fossa thickening and vestibular maturation that occur before more detailed testing is possible.

Acquired Factors

Age and Gender

The role of age and gender in the development of SSCD syndrome has been evaluated by several studies. Davey et al. evaluated 140 temporal bones from 121 patients ranging from six to 86 years of age. These authors found a statistically significant difference in bone thickness when comparing females 45 years old and younger vs. 45 years old and above. This difference was mostly due to a significant decline in average thickness in females over 70. Similar findings were seen in male patients, although average bone thickness was higher. In addition, a linear regression model using age and gender as independent variables showed a loss of 0.005 mm of bone over the superior canal for every year increase in age [36]. Similarly, in a radiographic study, Nadgir et al. categorized patients in increasing, 20-year age groups. These researchers found a 93% increase in radiographic SSCD with each successively older age category (Fig. 2.3) [37]. Other investigations have shown evidence for progressive thinning with increasing age and even direct observation of radiographic progression [38, 39], although in some studies, significant bone loss was only apparent in female patients [14, 40]. Authors suggested age-related bone

Table 1: Age group of patients with SSCD		
Age Group (yr)	Total Patients Reviewed	Total Patients with SSCD
0–20	46	1
21–40	92	5
41–60	120	9 (3[a])
61–80	40	7 (3[a])
81–100	6	2

[a] Number of patients with bilateral dehiscence.

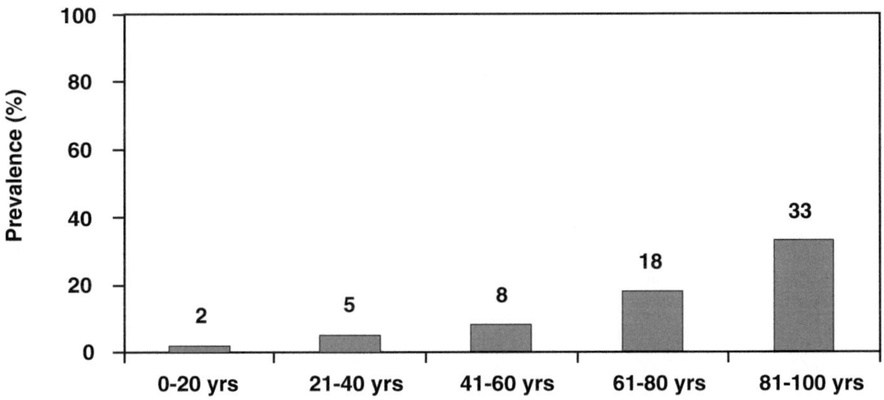

Fig. 2.3 Prevalence of patients with SSCD and age (Republished with permission of American Society of Neuroradiology, from Nadgir RN, Ozonoff A, Devaiah AK, Halderman AA, Sakai O. Superior Semicircular Canal Dehiscence: Congenital or Acquired Condition? Am J Neuroradiol. 2011; 32(5):947-949. Permission conveyed through Copyright Clearance Center, Inc) [37]

demineralization, which is more pronounced in menopausal women, as a possible cause for these findings. The progressive thinning with each successive decade in life is in sharp contrast to the progressive thickening seen during the first four years of life [15]. This suggests that the natural course of bone thickness over the superior semicircular canal is relatively rapid thickening during early childhood with slow progressive thinning over the rest of an individual's life with perhaps an acceleration of this process in the 7th to 9th decades.

Chronic Conditions

Several chronic conditions have also been proposed to lead to acquired dehiscence, including idiopathic intracranial hypertension (IIH), and chronic otitis media. These factors have all been implicated more broadly with middle fossa erosion leading to cerebrospinal fluid leak (CSF) and encephalocele formation [41–43]. By extension, it is thought they may also contribute to thinning of the otic capsule over the superior canal. This is borne out by the literature, which does seem to support an association between tegmen defects and SSCD syndrome, with rates of coinciding defects ranging from 14 to 76% [14, 21, 38, 44, 45]. A retrospective study by Oh et al. found that patients with lateral skull base encephalocele and CSF leak had a 5.7 times greater likelihood of having SSCD syndrome compared to controls [22].

IIH has been linked to skull base attenuation, encephalocele formation, and CSF leak in multiple studies [14, 15, 46]. Mechanistically, this is thought to be due to increased force of dural pulsations resulting in bony erosion of the middle fossa. However, the association between IIH and SSCD proper is less clear. In their large temporal bone series, Carey et al. found no association between SSCD and a clinical history of elevated intracranial pressure [15]. More recent studies investigating the role of intracranial pressure have been equivocal. Several series have found an association with tegmen thinning and/or dehiscence and a history of IIH or high opening pressure on lumbar puncture [47, 48]. However, while some studies showed associated thinning over the superior canal, others found otic capsule bone to be unaffected [49–51]. Obesity, considered a risk factor for IIH and lateral skull base defects, has also been evaluated by several studies, but its association with SSCD specifically is unclear [22, 50, 52, 53]. Obstructive sleep apnea (OSA), which is closely linked to obesity, has been linked to radiographic SSCD [54]. One proposed theory for this association involves dramatic increases in intracranial pressure, with CSF pressures transiently rising between 50 and 750 mm H_2O during apneic events [55]. However, as with other studies reporting only rates of radiographic dehiscence, it is difficult to make firm conclusions about an association with SSCD syndrome proper.

The role of chronic inflammation in SCCD has also been evaluated. In a large retrospective study, Cho et al. compared rates of radiologic SSCD in ears with a history of unilateral chronic otitis media (COM), using the healthy ears as controls. The authors found that ears affected by COM had significantly higher rates of both definite and suspicious SSCD compared to ears without COM (3.4% vs. 0.3% and 3.2% vs. 0.9%, respectively). Furthermore, authors found reduced mastoid volumes with intact tympanic membranes in patients with SSCD, suggesting that a past history of otitis media without active inflammation may have a role in the development of dehiscence [56]. Other studies have also shown smaller temporal volumes, as well as reduced pneumatization and density, in patients with SSCD compared to controls [14, 57, 58].

Other Causes for Acquired Dehiscence Associations

Other less common causes of acquired dehiscence have been reported. Temporal bone fracture has been implicated in several reports of SSCD syndrome, as have acute infection, fibrous dysplasia, neoplasm, vascular anomalies, and erosion from the superior petrosal sinus [39, 59–64]. Other acquired foci of labyrinthine dehiscence have also been described. Lateral canal dehiscence is a well-known entity, with the most common causes being cholesteatoma, infection, and iatrogenic injury. Additionally, posterior semicircular canal dehiscence has been described in several reports, with symptoms mimicking SSCD syndrome but vestibular findings consistent with a posterior canal lesion [65, 66].

Multifactorial Etiology

Competing evidence for a developmental and an acquired etiology for SSCD may be reconciled by a multifactorial model that incorporates both sets of factors. In this model, developmentally thin middle fossa bone is subjected to long-term, progressive thinning that ultimately results in development of SSCD syndrome. This hypothesis could account for the observation that radiographic thinning and dehiscence appears to be present in a subset of patients who lack symptoms or other acquired risk factors for SSCD syndrome. Exposure to such risk factors need only cause sub-millimeter reductions in bone thickness to cause frank dehiscence and development of SSCD symptoms. One line of evidence that may support this theory is the relatively high rate of patients with SSCD syndrome who report a specific, often innocuous, precipitating event prior to developing symptoms. In their original article, which included both surgical and non-surgical patients, Minor et al. reported that 23% experienced a precipitating event leading to onset of symptoms, including minor head trauma, falls without head trauma, lifting, and straining [1]. In a later meta-analysis of surgically managed patients, Watters et al. observed a second event, including acute pressure changes, in 48% of patients [67]. That such common, often low-intensity events could lead to dehiscence suggests that these patients were already predisposed to developing dehiscence, due to developmental thinning, acquired attenuation, or a combination of both. This phenomenon also underscores research showing that even pinpoint areas of dehiscence can alter inner ear impedance, leading to development of a third mobile window [16, 68].

Conclusion

SSCD is a TMW phenomenon with unclear etiology, although there is evidence supporting both developmental and acquired causes. Evidence for a developmental etiology largely comes from histopathologic studies showing a high rate of symmetric middle fossa attenuation, stable bone deposition, and progressive middle fossa thickening in infants. Evidence of SSCD as an acquired phenomenon stems from its manifestation in later life, as well as studies showing associations between middle fossa thinning with factors including advancing age, female gender, and IIH. These competing theories may be reconciled by a multifactorial model wherein developmentally thin bone over the superior canal is subjected to further thinning from acquired causes, ultimately leading to frank dehiscence and development of SSCD syndrome. Regardless of its cause, clear diagnosis may be challenging due to nonspecific symptomatology, limitations of current radiologic technology, and variable patient factors. Thorough patient evaluation and appropriate testing are required to both establish a diagnosis of SSCD and to properly assess symptom burden before recommending treatment.

References

1. Minor LB. Superior canal dehiscence syndrome. Am J Otol. 2000;21(1):9–19.
2. Merchant SN, Nakajima HH, Halpin C, et al. Clinical investigation and mechanism of air-bone gaps in large vestibular aqueduct syndrome. Ann Otol Rhinol Laryngol. 2007;116(7):532–41. https://doi.org/10.1177/000348940711600709.
3. Blake DM, Tomovic S, Vazquez A, Lee HJ, Jyung RW. Cochlear-facial dehiscence–a newly described entity. Laryngoscope. 2014;124(1):283–9. https://doi.org/10.1002/lary.24223.
4. Karlberg M, Annertz M, Magnusson M. Mondini-like malformation mimicking otosclerosis and superior semicircular canal dehiscence. J Laryngol Otol. 2006;120(5):419–22. https://doi.org/10.1017/S0022215106000934.
5. Kim HHS, Wilson DF. A third mobile window at the cochlear apex. Otolaryngol Head Neck Surg Off J Am Acad Otolaryngol-Head Neck Surg. 2006;135(6):965–6. https://doi.org/10.1016/j.otohns.2005.04.006.
6. Lund AD, Palacios SD. Carotid artery-cochlear dehiscence: a review. Laryngoscope. 2011;121(12):2658–60. https://doi.org/10.1002/lary.22391.
7. Naert L, Berg R, Heyning P, et al. Aggregating the symptoms of superior semicircular canal dehiscence syndrome. Laryngoscope. 2018;128(8):1932–8. https://doi.org/10.1002/lary.27062.
8. Zhu RT, Van Rompaey V, Ward BK, Van de Berg R, Van de Heyning P, Sharon JD. The interrelations between different causes of dizziness: a conceptual framework for understanding vestibular disorders. Ann Otol Rhinol Laryngol. 2019;128(9):869–78. https://doi.org/10.1177/0003489419845014.
9. Chung LK, Ung N, Spasic M, et al. Clinical outcomes of middle fossa craniotomy for superior semicircular canal dehiscence repair. J Neurosurg. 2016;125(5):1187–93. https://doi.org/10.3171/2015.8.JNS15391.
10. Jung DH, Lookabaugh SA, Owoc MS, McKenna MJ, Lee DJ. Dizziness is more prevalent than autophony among patients who have undergone repair of superior canal dehiscence. Otol Neurotol Off Publ Am Otol Soc Am Neurotol Soc Eur Acad Otol Neurotol. 2015;36(1):126–32. https://doi.org/10.1097/MAO.0000000000000531.
11. Zhang L, Creighton FX, Carey JP. A cohort study comparing importance of clinical factors in determining diagnosis and treatment for superior semicircular canal dehiscence syndrome. Otol Neurotol Off Publ Am Otol Soc Am Neurotol Soc Eur Acad Otol Neurotol. 2021;42(9):1429–33. https://doi.org/10.1097/MAO.0000000000003274.
12. Zuniga MG, Janky KL, Nguyen KD, Welgampola MS, Carey JP. Ocular versus cervical VEMPs in the diagnosis of superior semicircular canal dehiscence syndrome. Otol Neurotol Off Publ Am Otol Soc Am Neurotol Soc Eur Acad Otol Neurotol. 2013;34(1):121–6. https://doi.org/10.1097/MAO.0b013e31827136b0.
13. Janky KL, Nguyen KD, Welgampola M, Zuniga MG, Carey JP. Air-conducted oVEMPs provide the best separation between intact and superior canal dehiscent labyrinths. Otol Neurotol Off Publ Am Otol Soc Am Neurotol Soc Eur Acad Otol Neurotol. 2013;34(1):127–34. https://doi.org/10.1097/MAO.0b013e318271c32a.

14. Crovetto M, Whyte J, Rodriguez OM, Lecumberri I, Martinez C, Eléxpuru J. Anatomo-radiological study of the superior semicircular canal dehiscence. Eur J Radiol. 2010;76(2):167–72. https://doi.org/10.1016/j.ejrad.2009.05.038.
15. Carey JP, Minor LB, Nager GT. Dehiscence or thinning of bone overlying the superior semicircular canal in a temporal bone survey. Arch Otolaryngol Neck Surg. 2000;126(2):137. https://doi.org/10.1001/archotol.126.2.137.
16. Pisano DV, Niesten MEF, Merchant SN, Nakajima HH. The effect of superior semicircular canal dehiscence on intracochlear sound pressures. Audiol Neurotol. 2012;17(5):338–48. https://doi.org/10.1159/000339653.
17. Ward BK, Wenzel A, Ritzl EK, et al. Near-dehiscence: clinical findings in patients with thin bone over the superior semicircular canal. Otol Neurotol. 2013;34(8):1421–8. https://doi.org/10.1097/MAO.0b013e318287efe6.
18. Mikulec AA, McKenna MJ, Ramsey MJ, et al. Superior semicircular canal dehiscence presenting as conductive hearing loss without vertigo. Otol Neurotol Off Publ Am Otol Soc Am Neurotol Soc Eur Acad Otol Neurotol. 2004;25(2):121–9. https://doi.org/10.1097/00129492-200403000-00007.
19. Erdogan N, Songu M, Akay E, et al. Posterior semicircular canal dehiscence in asymptomatic ears. Acta Otolaryngol. 2011;131(1):4–8. https://doi.org/10.3109/00016489.2010.502184.
20. Berning AW, Arani K, Branstetter BF. Prevalence of superior semicircular canal dehiscence on high-resolution CT imaging in patients without vestibular or auditory abnormalities. AJNR Am J Neuroradiol. 2019;40(4):709–12. https://doi.org/10.3174/ajnr.A5999.
21. El Hadi T, Sorrentino T, Calmels MN, Fraysse B, Deguine O, Marx M. Spontaneous tegmen defect and semicircular canal dehiscence: same etiopathogenic entity? Otol Neurotol Off Publ Am Otol Soc Am Neurotol Soc Eur Acad Otol Neurotol. 2012;33(4):591–5. https://doi.org/10.1097/MAO.0b013e31824bae10.
22. Oh MS, Vivas EX, Hudgins PA, Mattox DE. The prevalence of superior semicircular canal dehiscence in patients with mastoid encephalocele or cerebrospinal fluid otorrhea. Otol Neurotol. 2019;40(4):485–90. https://doi.org/10.1097/MAO.0000000000002155.
23. Brantberg K, Bergenius J, Mendel L, Witt H, Tribukait A, Ygge J. Symptoms, findings and treatment in patients with dehiscence of the superior semicircular canal. Acta Otolaryngol. 2001;121(1):68–75. https://doi.org/10.1080/000164801300006308.
24. Anson BJ, Donaldson JA. Surgical anatomy of the temporal bone. 3rd ed. Philadelphia: Saunders; 1981.
25. Nomiya S, Cureoglu S, Kariya S, et al. Posterior semicircular canal dehiscence: a histopathologic human temporal bone study. Otol Neurotol. 2010;31(7):1122–7. https://doi.org/10.1097/MAO.0b013e3181eb3309.
26. Whyte Orozco J, Martínez C, Cisneros A, Obón J, Gracia-Tello B, Angel CM. Defect of the bony roof in the superior semicircular canal and its clinical implications. Acta Otorrinolaringol Esp. 2011;62(3):199–204. https://doi.org/10.1016/j.otorri.2010.11.009.
27. Kuhn JJ, Clenney T. The association between semicircular canal dehiscence and Chiari type I malformation. Arch Otolaryngol Neck Surg. 2010;136(10):1009. https://doi.org/10.1001/archoto.2010.169.
28. Hildebrand MS, Tack D, Deluca A, et al. Mutation in the COCH gene is associated with superior semicircular canal dehiscence. Am J Med Genet A. 2009;149(2):280–5. https://doi.org/10.1002/ajmg.a.32618.
29. Niesten MEF, Lookabaugh S, Curtin H, et al. Familial superior canal dehiscence syndrome. JAMA Otolaryngol Neck Surg. 2014;140(4):363. https://doi.org/10.1001/jamaoto.2013.6718.
30. Nemzek WR, Brodie HA, Chong BW, et al. Imaging findings of the developing temporal bone in fetal specimens. AJNR Am J Neuroradiol. 1996;17(8):1467–77.
31. Satar B, Mukherji SK, Telian SA. Congenital aplasia of the semicircular canals. Otol Neurotol Off Publ Am Otol Soc Am Neurotol Soc Eur Acad Otol Neurotol. 2003;24(3):437–46. https://doi.org/10.1097/00129492-200305000-00014.
32. Takahashi N, Tsunoda A, Shirakura S, Kitamura K. Anatomical feature of the middle cranial fossa in fetal periods: possible etiology of superior canal dehiscence syndrome. Acta Otolaryngol. 2012;132(4):385–90. https://doi.org/10.3109/00016489.2011.637234.

33. Karimnejad K, Czerny MS, Lookabaugh S, Lee DJ, Mikulec AA. Gender and laterality in semicircular canal dehiscence syndrome. J Laryngol Otol. 2016;130(8):712–6. https://doi.org/10.1017/S0022215116008185.
34. Lagman C, Ong V, Chung LK, et al. Pediatric superior semicircular canal dehiscence: illustrative case and systematic review. J Neurosurg Pediatr. 2017;20(2):196–203. https://doi.org/10.3171/2017.3.PEDS1734.
35. Chen EY, Paladin A, Phillips G, et al. Semicircular canal dehiscence in the pediatric population. Int J Pediatr Otorhinolaryngol. 2009;73(2):321–7. https://doi.org/10.1016/j.ijporl.2008.10.027.
36. Davey S, Kelly-Morland C, Phillips JS, Nunney I, Pawaroo D. Assessment of superior semicircular canal thickness with advancing age: SSC thickness and age. Laryngoscope. 2015;125(8):1940–5. https://doi.org/10.1002/lary.25243.
37. Nadgir RN, Ozonoff A, Devaiah AK, Halderman AA, Sakai O. Superior semicircular canal dehiscence: congenital or acquired condition? Am J Neuroradiol. 2011;32(5):947–9. https://doi.org/10.3174/ajnr.A2437.
38. Lookabaugh S, Niesten MEF, Owoc M, Kozin ED, Grolman W, Lee DJ. Audiologic, cVEMP, and radiologic progression in superior canal dehiscence syndrome. Otol Neurotol Off Publ Am Otol Soc Am Neurotol Soc Eur Acad Otol Neurotol. 2016;37(9):1393–8. https://doi.org/10.1097/MAO.0000000000001182.
39. Bae JS, Lim HW, An YS, Park HJ. Acquired superior semicircular canal dehiscence confirmed by sequential CT scans. Otol Neurotol Off Publ Am Otol Soc Am Neurotol Soc Eur Acad Otol Neurotol. 2013;34(6):45–6. https://doi.org/10.1097/MAO.0b013e31828d6753.
40. Sood D, Rana L, Chauhan R, Shukla R, Nandolia K. Superior semicircular canal dehiscence: a new perspective. Eur J Radiol Open. 2017;4:144–6. https://doi.org/10.1016/j.ejro.2017.10.003.
41. Kemink JL, Graham MD, Kartush JM. Spontaneous encephalocele of the temporal bone. Arch Otolaryngol Head Neck Surg. 1986;112(5):558–61. https://doi.org/10.1001/archotol.1986.03780050082015.
42. Stucken EZ, Brown K, Selesnick SH. Clinical and diagnostic evaluation of acoustic neuromas. Otolaryngol Clin N Am. 2012;45(2):269–84, vii. https://doi.org/10.1016/j.otc.2011.12.001.
43. Sdano MT, Pensak ML. Temporal bone encephaloceles. Curr Opin Otolaryngol Head Neck Surg. 2005;13(5):287–9. https://doi.org/10.1097/01.moo.0000179247.51476.f5.
44. Nadaraja GS, Gurgel RK, Fischbein NJ, et al. Radiographic evaluation of the tegmen in patients with superior semicircular canal dehiscence. Otol Neurotol Off Publ Am Otol Soc Am Neurotol Soc Eur Acad Otol Neurotol. 2012;33(7):1245–50. https://doi.org/10.1097/MAO.0b013e3182634e27.
45. Teixido M, Kung B, Rosowski JJ, Merchant SN. Histopathology of the temporal bone in a case of superior canal dehiscence syndrome. Ann Otol Rhinol Laryngol. 2012;121(1):7–12. https://doi.org/10.1177/000348941212100102.
46. Yu A, Teich DL, Moonis G, Wong ET. Superior semicircular canal dehiscence in East Asian women with osteoporosis. BMC Ear Nose Throat Disord. 2012;12:8. https://doi.org/10.1186/1472-6815-12-8.
47. Kutz JW, Husain IA, Isaacson B, Roland PS. Management of spontaneous cerebrospinal fluid otorrhea. Laryngoscope. 2008;118(12):2195–9. https://doi.org/10.1097/MLG.0b013e318182f833.
48. Brainard L, Chen DA, Aziz KM, Hillman TA. Association of benign intracranial hypertension and spontaneous encephalocele with cerebrospinal fluid leak. Otol Neurotol Off Publ Am Otol Soc Am Neurotol Soc Eur Acad Otol Neurotol. 2012;33(9):1621–4. https://doi.org/10.1097/MAO.0b013e318271c312.
49. Berkiten G, Gürbüz D, Akan O, et al. Dehiscence or thinning of bone overlying the superior semicircular canal in idiopathic intracranial hypertension. Eur Arch Otorhinolaryngol. 2021;279(6):2899–904. https://doi.org/10.1007/s00405-021-07020-z.
50. Kuo P, Bagwell KA, Mongelluzzo G, et al. Semicircular canal dehiscence among idiopathic intracranial hypertension patients: SSCD among IIH patients. Laryngoscope. 2018;128(5):1196–9. https://doi.org/10.1002/lary.26795.

51. Handzel O, Brenner-Ullman A, Niry D, et al. Tegmen attenuation in patients with idiopathic intracranial hypertension is progressive. Laryngoscope. 2020;130(12):28490. https://doi.org/10.1002/lary.28490.
52. Rizk HG, Hatch JL, Stevens SM, Lambert PR, Meyer TA. Lateral skull base attenuation in superior semicircular canal dehiscence and spontaneous cerebrospinal fluid otorrhea. Otolaryngol Head Neck Surg Off J Am Acad Otolaryngol. 2016;155(4):641–8. https://doi.org/10.1177/0194599816651261.
53. Jan TA, Cheng YS, Landegger LD, et al. Relationship between surgically treated superior canal dehiscence syndrome and body mass index. Otolaryngol Head Neck Surg Off J Am Acad Otolaryngol-Head Neck Surg. 2017;156(4):722–7. https://doi.org/10.1177/0194599816686563.
54. Schutt CA, Neubauer P, Samy RN, et al. The correlation between obesity, obstructive sleep apnea, and superior semicircular canal dehiscence: a new explanation for an increasingly common problem. Otol Neurotol Off Publ Am Otol Soc Am Neurotol Soc Eur Acad Otol Neurotol. 2015;36(3):551–4. https://doi.org/10.1097/MAO.0000000000000555.
55. Sugita Y, Iijima S, Teshima Y, et al. Marked episodic elevation of cerebrospinal fluid pressure during nocturnal sleep in patients with sleep apnea hypersomnia syndrome. Electroencephalogr Clin Neurophysiol. 1985;60(3):214–9. https://doi.org/10.1016/0013-4694(85)90033-1.
56. Cho YW, Shim BS, Kim JW, et al. Prevalence of radiologic superior canal dehiscence in normal ears and ears with chronic otitis media: radiologic SCD in normal versus COM ears. Laryngoscope. 2014;124(3):746–50. https://doi.org/10.1002/lary.24281.
57. Shim BS, Kang BC, Kim CH, Kim TS, Park HJ. Superior canal dehiscence patients have smaller mastoid volume than age- and sex-matched otosclerosis and temporal bone fracture patients. Korean J Audiol. 2012;16(3):120. https://doi.org/10.7874/kja.2012.16.3.120.
58. de Jong MA, Carpenter DJ, Kaylie DM, Piker EG, Frank-Ito DO. Temporal bone anatomy characteristics in superior semicircular canal dehiscence. J Otolaryngol. 2017;12(4):185–91. https://doi.org/10.1016/j.joto.2017.08.003.
59. Crane BT, Carey JP, McMenomey S, Minor LB. Meningioma causing superior canal dehiscence syndrome. Otol Neurotol Off Publ Am Otol Soc Am Neurotol Soc Eur Acad Otol Neurotol. 2010;31(6):1009–10. https://doi.org/10.1097/MAO.0b013e3181a32d85.
60. Goddard JC, Go JL, Friedman RA. Imaging case of the month: fibrous dysplasia causing superior canal dehiscence. Otol Neurotol Off Publ Am Otol Soc Am Neurotol Soc Eur Acad Otol Neurotol. 2013;34(1):1–2. https://doi.org/10.1097/MAO.0b013e3182355642.
61. Koo JW, Hong SK, Kim DK, Kim JS. Superior semicircular canal dehiscence syndrome by the superior petrosal sinus. J Neurol Neurosurg Psychiatry. 2010;81(4):465–7. https://doi.org/10.1136/jnnp.2008.155564.
62. Parlea E, Georgescu M, Calarasu R. Superior canal dehiscence syndrome – case report. Romanian J Neurol. 2012;11:142–6.
63. Peng KA, Ahmed S, Yang I, Gopen Q. Temporal bone fracture causing superior semicircular canal dehiscence. Case Rep Otolaryngol. 2014;2014:1–4. https://doi.org/10.1155/2014/817291.
64. Aladham Y, Ahmed O, Hassan SAS, Francis-Khoury E. Traumatic superior semicircular canal dehiscence syndrome: case report and literature review. J Surg Case Rep. 2021;2021(1):592. https://doi.org/10.1093/jscr/rjaa592.
65. Cremer PD, Migliaccio AA, Pohl DV, et al. Posterior semicircular canal nystagmus is conjugate and its axis is parallel to that of the canal. Neurology. 2000;54(10):2016–20. https://doi.org/10.1212/wnl.54.10.2016.
66. Krombach GA, DiMartino E, Schmitz-Rode T, et al. Posterior semicircular canal dehiscence: a morphologic cause of vertigo similar to superior semicircular canal dehiscence. Eur Radiol. 2003;13(6):1444–50. https://doi.org/10.1007/s00330-003-1828-5.
67. Watters KF, Rosowski JJ, Sauter T, Lee DJ. Superior semicircular canal dehiscence presenting as postpartum vertigo. Otol Neurotol. 2006;27(6):756–68. https://doi.org/10.1097/01.mao.0000227894.27291.9f.
68. Merchant SN, Rosowski JJ. Conductive hearing loss caused by third-window lesions of the inner ear. Otol Neurotol Off Publ Am Otol Soc Am Neurotol Soc Eur Acad Otol Neurotol. 2008;29(3):282–9. https://doi.org/10.1097/mao.0b013e318161ab24.

Chapter 3
Pathophysiology of Third Mobile Window Syndrome

John C. Li, Mitch F. Aquilina, and Jenna J. Li

Pathophysiology is a discipline that studies how and why patients present with certain signs and symptoms of a disease process. To understand the pathophysiology of third mobile window syndrome (TMWS), the normal vestibular and normal cochlear physiology must first be explored. Then, one will be able to see what can go wrong with these systems.

Some of the manifestations of TMWS vestibular symptoms may include dizziness in response to loud sounds (Tullio phenomenon) or in response to pressure changes (Hennebert sign); common TMWS cochlear symptoms include autophonia (hearing echoes in one's own voice), pulsatile tinnitus, hyperacusis, or hearing loss (that can mimic conductive hearing loss with elevated Bone Conduction responses). Pathophysiology dictates that the characteristics of the dizziness and other symptoms are directly related to the location of the dehiscence.

For instance, semicircular canal dehiscence syndrome can involve any of the three semicircular canals. Although the superior canal seems to have garnered a lot of attention recently, it is important to recognize that the posterior and lateral canals can also be affected. Activation of the horizontal canal will cause horizontal nystagmus, whereas superior or posterior canal perturbations cause rotational nystagmus [1, 2].

In addition to this, there are other areas of the labyrinth other than the semicircular canals that can be defective. There could be defects in the cochlea, as well as the valvular aqueducts and natural windows that service the cochlea and vestibule. The correlation between these defects and following clinical syndromes hopefully can be explained by the pathophysiology outlined in this chapter. Entities such as

J. C. Li (✉) · M. F. Aquilina
Jupiter Medical Center, ENT and Allergy Associates of Florida, Jupiter, FL, USA

J. J. Li
Columbia University, New York, NY, USA
e-mail: jjL2217@columbia.edu

G. J. Gianoli, P. Thomson (eds.), *Third Mobile Window Syndrome of the Inner Ear*, https://doi.org/10.1007/978-3-031-16586-3_3

enlarged vestibular aqueduct, cochlear deformities, X-linked stapes gusher, bone dyscrasias, and perilymphatic fistulae are all part of the family of TMWS pathologies [3, 4].

To make sense of how things work, one must start by first looking at structure (which is the anatomy). Next, we need to understand how that structure functions (physiology). And finally, we need to explore what happens when the structure doesn't function properly. What can go wrong with any particular structure and its components. (That is pathophysiology.) When studying labyrinthine pathophysiology, it will be helpful to review the neuroanatomy of the inner ear and understand how it functions in nonpathological cases.

Inner Ear Anatomy: Structure and Function

Semicircular Canals

In basic terms, the inner ear is a single structure that houses two compartments: one for hearing and one for spatial orientation. Both functions reside in a single structure, and there is overlap between them. The structure of the inner ear can be compared to a snail with a spiral-shaped shell and an unusual head (instead of two optic tentacles proceeding from the snail's head, there are three loops that are the semicircular canals).

The hearing function occurs within the spiral, snail-shell cochlea (Fig. 3.1), while the spatial orientation function occurs in the unusual snail head, the three-looped labyrinth. Each loop is a semicircular canal and detects rotational movement. The arrangement of the loops perpendicular to one another along *xyz* axes allows the system to capture and resolve three-dimensional angular motion in any plane of motion, even if the motion is not directly along the axis of one of the canals [6].

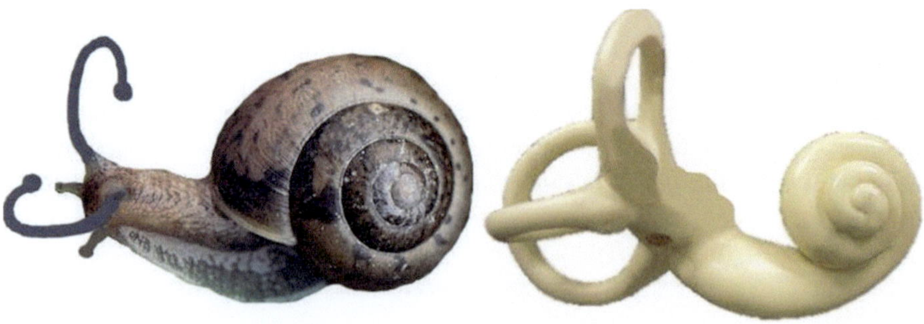

Fig. 3.1 Cochleae and snail shells are visually similar due to their spiral shape. Although this comparison is useful for visualization, unlike many natural mollusk shells, the cochlear spiral does not actually conform to the logarithmic Fibonacci spiral, and it is suspected that the spiral seen in cochlear geometry is due to the spatial constraints of the inner ear [5]

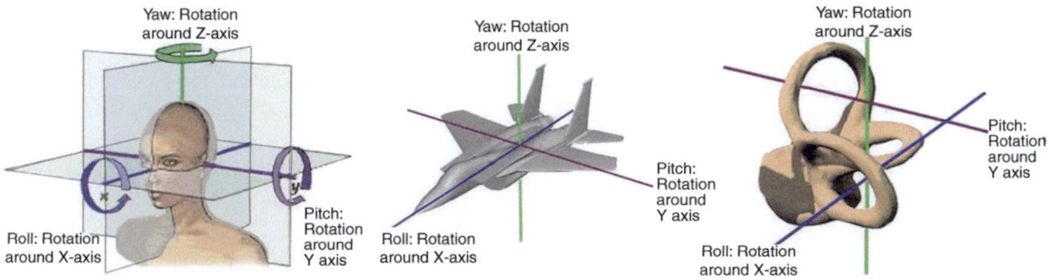

Fig. 3.2 Planes of rotation of the human head are like that of an airplane and are mediated by the three semicircular canals which are oriented at perpendicular axes to each other

The semicircular canals track rotational motion and can be understood with a comparison to the flight control system of an aircraft. The rotational movement of the aircraft can be analyzed in the components of "roll," "pitch," and "yaw", based on the *xyz* axes (Fig. 3.2). The three canals, horizontal (lateral), superior (anterior), and posterior (inferior) correspond to each of these dimensions. (Note: The lead author of this chapter is an Air Force Flight Surgeon, general aviation pilot, CEO of an aerospace company, as well as a neurotologist. That might explain why in this chapter one might see a multitude of comparisons and references to aviation flight control systems and the vestibular system.)

Motion on the *z*-axis is perhaps easiest to understand. Conventionally, rotational movement on the *z*-axis refers to a horizontal spinning motion around a vertical *z*-axis (although some texts flip *y* and *z* motion, this is the standard *z* direction). In an airplane, this rotational motion is called "yaw." Yaw is activated by the plane's rudder; the rudder is used to point the aircraft to turn right or left.

In the human ear, the horizontal semicircular canal detects horizontal rotational movement. Specifically, the horizontal canal detects the motion of shaking one's head from right to left, as if saying "no." Note that eye movements are tied to the semicircular canal movements. This constitutes the vestibular-ocular reflex. As one rotates the head from right to left, the eye reflexively moves in the opposite direction from left to right. This reflex gives image stability. The horizontal canal is slave to horizontal eye movements.

It should be noted that the "horizontal" canal is not exactly horizontal in the skull, it is actually tilted about 30° up (Fig. 3.3). One theory for this is that the human head was designed to consistently look down at a 30-degree angle to forage for food or to avoid stepping on snakes. This downward gaze would put the horizontal canal back at a true horizontal [8–11].

The *x*- and *y*- axes represent "roll" and "pitch" in an airplane. A "snap roll" is activated by the airplane's ailerons and rotates the plane like a corkscrew in the *x*-axis in line with the nose (Fig. 3.4).

"Pitch," controlled by the airplane's elevator, points the nose of the airplane up or down, in motion along the *y*-axis. Nodding the head is a change in pitch.

Hybrid motions require a combination of *x*- and *y*-inputs, such as in a "barrel roll."

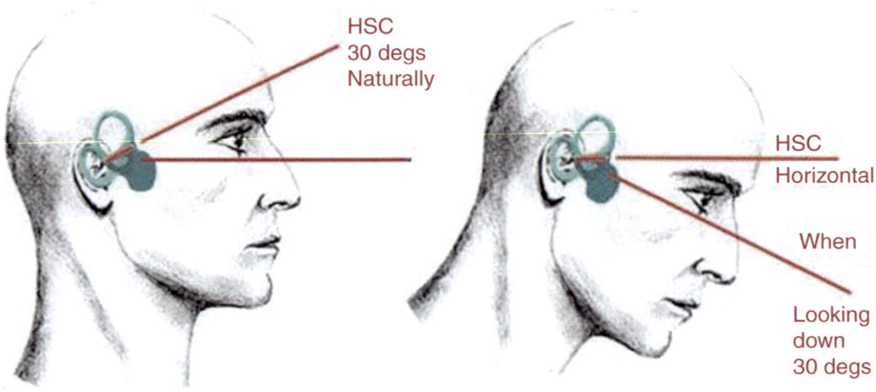

Fig. 3.3 The horizontal semicircular canal is actually tilted upward by about 30° when the head is looking off into the distance. However, it is postulated that the human head was designed to be tilted down 30° scanning the ground for danger, which then puts the horizontal canal in the true horizontal position [7]

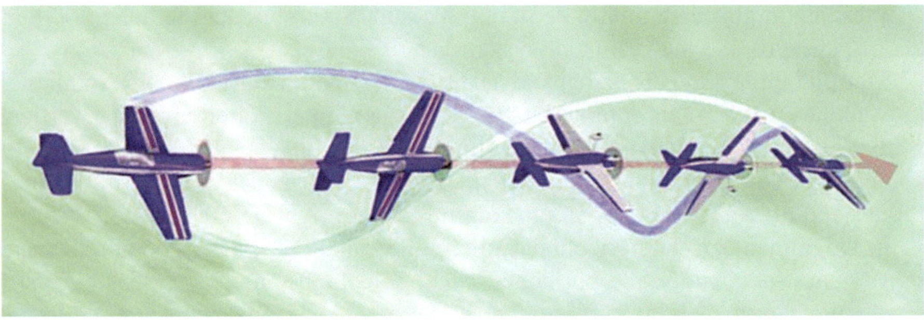

Fig. 3.4 "Snap Roll" aka "Aileron Roll" is a rotation around the x-axis in a straight linear path

As a jet barrel rolls about the x-axis (see Fig. 3.5), there are times when the nose points up and times when the nose points down. This type of motion requires manipulation of the y-axis to achieve. When two axes are involved in the motion, the resultant vector is a hybrid combination of the motion along two planes.

Most of the movement of the human head stimulates more than one semicircular canal at any given time. If the human head were oriented exactly like a fighter jet, then nodding up and down, is like "pitching" up and down in the y-axis and should only stimulate one semicircular canal (the canal show in purple). However, superior and posterior semicircular canals are actually oriented about 45 degrees off the conventional x- and y-axes. Thus, nodding up and down actually affects two canals (both the purple and the blue canals) (Fig. 3.6).

If one nods one's head up and down as if saying "yes," the motion in the y-axis stimulates *both* the superior canal and the posterior canal simultaneously. The brain

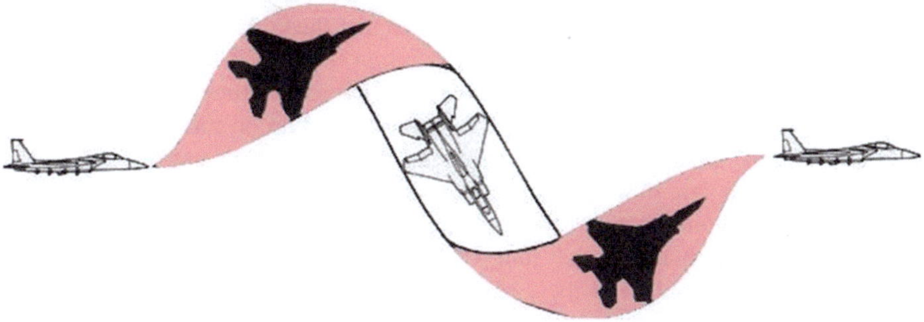

Fig. 3.5 A "Barrel Roll" is a rotation around the x-axis combined with some up pitch and down pitch around the y-axis in a corkscrew path

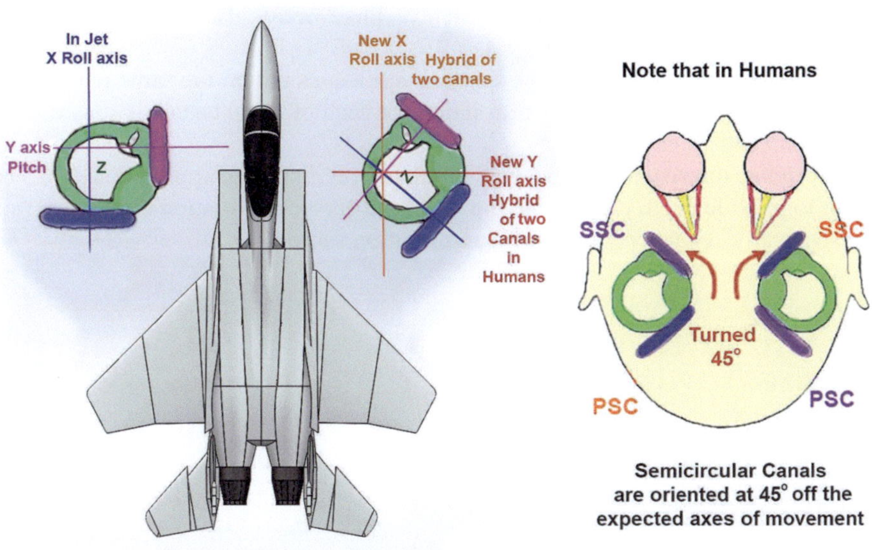

Fig. 3.6 If the semicircular canals were oriented like an airplane, then pure roll would be detected by one canal and pitch by a different canal. However, in humans, the axis is twisted by 45° so that pitch (as well as roll) changes stimulate both superior and posterior canals

interprets the relative contributions from each canal and resolves the vector so that one feels the nod.

Similarly, if one did cartwheels in the *x*-axis, the motion would also stimulate *both* the superior canal and the posterior canal simultaneously. This movement would create a different vector giving the sensation of an aileron roll. If one did balletic pirouettes in *z*-axis motion, the motion would primarily stimulate the horizontal canal, though it would also affect both superior and posterior canals a little bit.

Again, the eye movements are tied to the movements of the vertical canals. Head rolling actions will give rise to counter-torsional eye movements. The system is a little more complex due to the 45° offset of the vertical canals, however, the oblique muscles of the eye have adapted to the offset so that the entire system works flawlessly [12].

Moreover, the alignment of the canals allows for redundancy in the neuroanatomy. Each semicircular canal has a corresponding backup on the opposite side of the body. That is, the two horizontal semicircular canals provide backup orientation input, because they are in the same plane of rotation. The *Right* superior semicircular canal is in the same plane as the posterior canal on the *left* side. The acronym RALP refers to this plane. RALP stands for right anterior (same as superior canal) and left posterior canal. And the *Left* superior semicircular canal is in the same plane as the posterior canal on the *right* side. This plane is called the LARP plane. LARP stands for left anterior (same as superior canal) and right posterior canal. Thus, if a patient loses function on one side, they have a backup sensory system in the same plane (Fig. 3.7).

In addition to back up functionality, there may also be some additive functionality.

Note that although each of the semicircular canals are on the same plane as the corresponding mate, the center of rotation for each of those canals is separated by approximately 10 cm.

Much like the visual system which uses two eyes displaced approximately 6.3 cm apart to provide depth perception, the displaced centers of rotation might give "stereoscopically" enhanced movement and position sense [13].

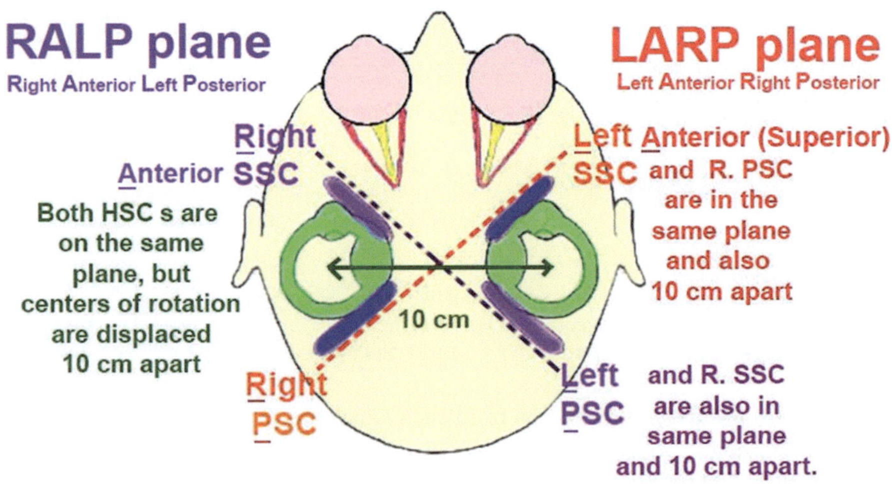

Fig. 3.7 Note that the *R*ight *A*nterior (superior) canal is in the same plane as the *L*eft *P*osterior canal. This is the RALP plane. Similarly the *L*eft *A*nterior (superior) canal is in the same plane as the *R*ight *P*osterior canal and thus redundant. This is the LARP plane. Note the 10 cm (approx.) displacement

Otolith Organs

The otolith organs of the inner ear are the saccule and the utricle (Fig. 3.8). These organs are located at the vestibule and function as encoders for linear acceleration. Working as non-rotational motion detectors in the inner ear, they can detect acceleration forward, backward, side-to-side, and up-and-down. The saccule is sensitive to motion in the sagittal plane and therefore detects vertical or up-and-down acceleration, as one would experience when riding in an elevator. The saccule is generally the gravity detector when one is upright.

Acceleration in the horizontal plane, such as a sudden start and stop in an automobile, is detected by the utricle. It is also sensitive to head tilt.

The acceleration detecting systems in the utricle and the saccule are composed of calcium carbonate deposits embedded on top of a gelatinous layer, which rests on top of motion-detecting hair cells. When the body experiences a sudden lurch forward, the relatively heavier calcium particles resting on the "jello" are the last to

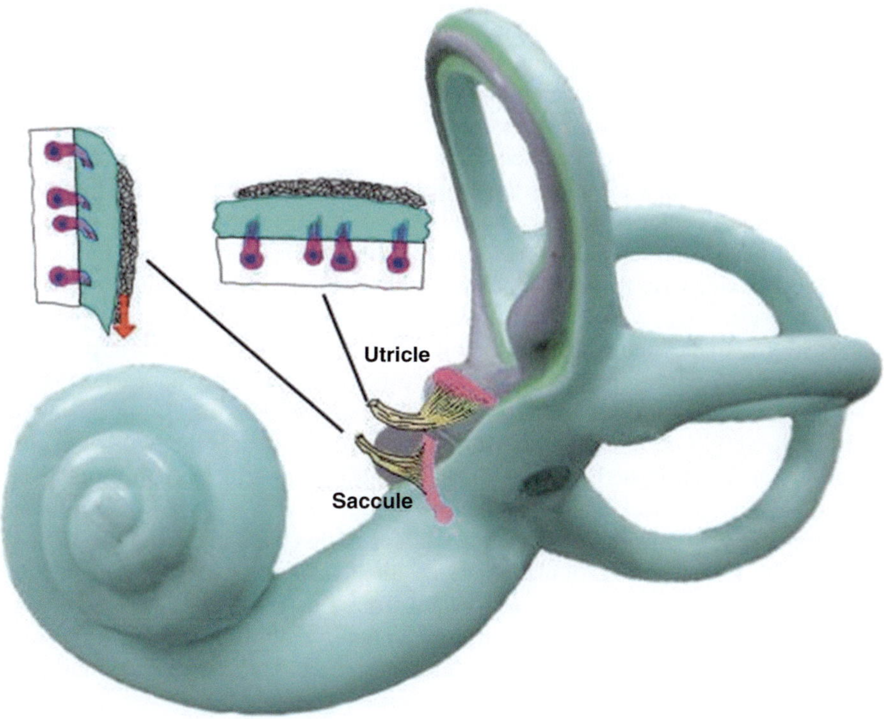

Fig. 3.8 The otolithic organs detect linear motion. The Saccule senses vertical movement, and the Utricle senses horizontal translational movement

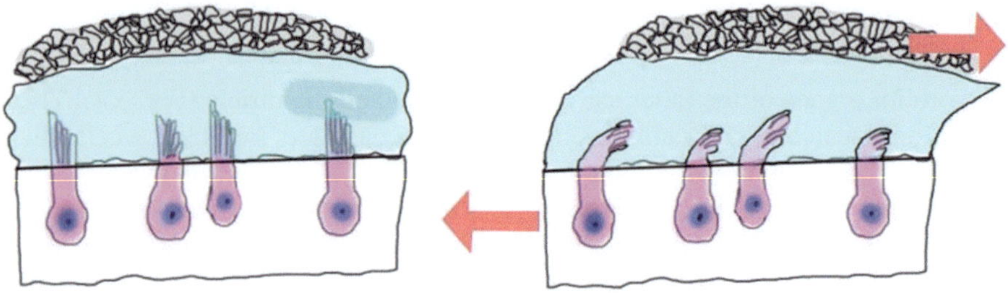

Fig. 3.9 The otolithic organs are comprised of sensory cells embedded in a gelatinous material with otoliths on top. The gelatin padding moves opposite the direction of the motion, while the mass effect of the otoliths accentuates the shearing effect. The lower arrow shows the direction of the motion. The upper arrow shows the relative direction of the gelatinous displacement of the hair cells

move due to inertia (Fig. 3.9). This lag pulls the jello and the hair cells backward with respect to the rest of the body, thus triggering the sense of acceleration. Once the motion settles into constant velocity, the lagging particles will catch up to the jello on the hair cells, turning off the sensation of acceleration. If there were a sudden stop, the particles would slingshot forward and trigger a hair cell signal that would indicate the sudden deceleration [14].

Since gravity is also a form of acceleration, it should be noted that the otolithic organs can be stimulated by head position as well as motion. Remember that accelerating the utricle forward slings the otoliths posteriorly. When the macular nerve "switch" detects posterior displacement, the subject feels as though he is accelerating forward. So what happens when a patient lies supine? The heavy otoliths will displace posteriorly (in the supine position, this is downwardly) because of gravity. Why does he not feel as though he were being propelled upwardly at a rapid rate? The answer is that concurrent visual input reframes vestibular input. Our brains are wired to trust visual reference points over vestibular input. The inner ear information augments what we see. We have learned that when we are lying down, our otoliths are SUPPOSED to be posteriorly displaced, and that is the NORMAL sensation of being still in bed. Our vision and proprioception of the comfortable bed pressing against the back augments this sensation.

Interestingly, flight simulators take advantage of this phenomenon by manipulating both the visual and vestibular input simultaneously. For example, to give the illusion of a fighter jet accelerating forward from a catapult launch off an aircraft carrier, the simulator simply rotates upward so that the otoliths displace posteriorly while simultaneously displaying the rushing of scenery. This visual vestibular combination culminates in a very realistic experience [15–17].

Also of note is the fact that otolithic movement (or non-movement) that is out of sync from the expected visual input can cause nausea and disorientation. This happens in simulators that do not do a good job coupling the vestibular input to the visual, or on boats where the sensation of movement does match an apparently (visually) stable environment, or other situations where vestibular and visual inputs become convoluted [18].

In the past, the otolithic organs were difficult to assess. Now, utricular function can be evaluated with the video ocular counter roll test and also subjective visual vertical testing. The utricular response to head tilt to one side and then the other can be asymmetric when one side is damaged [19, 20].

Semicircular Canals Mechanics

The fluid-filled semicircular canals have a different mechanism for detecting motion. Although one might think that a swirling flow of fluid in the canals would move the hair cells of the "nerve switch" (cupula) to give a sensation of rotational movement, the opposite is true. Due to inertia, the fluid within the canal stays relatively still, while the bony semicircular canal revolves around the fluid.

Picture a pattern in the foam on top of a frothy latte. If the latte cup is quickly spun clockwise, the pattern on the liquid would appear to stay relatively still from the perspective of the viewer. However, from the cup's point of view, there would be a relative counterclockwise flow of fluid (Fig. 3.10).

The same is true for the tubular semicircular canal: the relative flow of fluid is detected by a cupula and is reported to the brain as a sensation of rotation. The greater the movement, the greater the flow of fluid and the greater the deflection of the cupula will be. If the relative flow of fluid is appropriate, the brain interprets the cupular stimulus as normal movement. If the cupular deflection is disproportionate

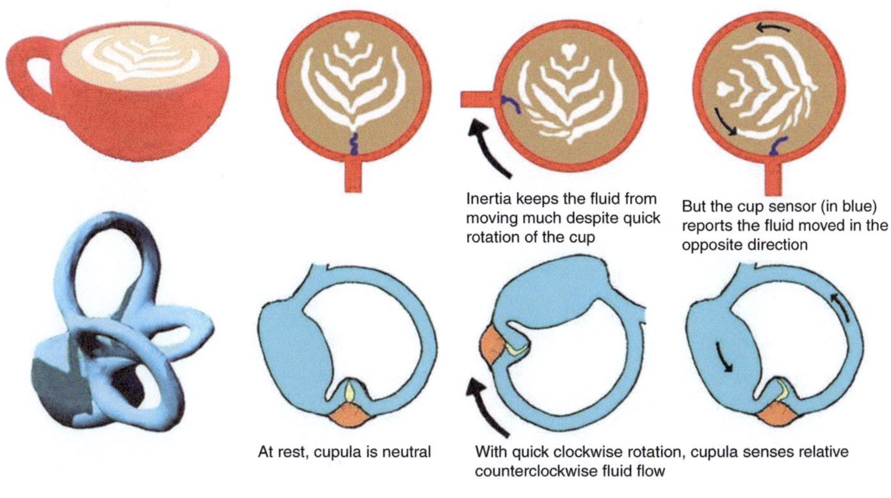

Fig. 3.10 If the cup is quickly rotated clockwise, the blue motion detector (cupula) deflects opposite to the cup motion. Inertia keeps the coffee still. However, from the cup's frame of reference, it seems as though the fluid moved counterclockwise. Similarly, the fluid inside the semicircular canal stays relatively still as the head rotates around the fluid. The relative motion between the fluid and the semicircular canal deflects the cupula, triggering a sense of motion

to the movement experienced, then the subject will feel "dizzy" or vertiginous. There are certain conditions where the cupular deflections do not match the actual head movements. For example in Benign Positional Vertigo, loose particles can slow the movement of the endolymph giving a lag time between commencement of actual movement to perceived movement. Cupulolithiasis (heavy cupula) creates inappropriate gravitational cupular movement with respect to position changes giving the sense of motion when there is no motion.

TMWS can also cause inappropriate cupular deflection and thus cause vertigo.

Third Mobile Window Syndrome: Fluid Dynamics and the Balloon/Box Model

It can be useful to understand fluid dynamics in a nonpathological system in order to contrast it with the dynamics of a pathological system.

Imagine taking a water balloon and putting it inside of a box. The balloon is protected by the box, which acts as a shell or outer skeleton. Similarly, the inner ear structures are protected by the labyrinthine bone.

Now imagine exposing the balloon at the top of the box and cutting a hole at the bottom of the box, exposing the membrane of the water balloon. If one pressed a finger into the membrane at the top, the membrane at the bottom would bulge out. If a similar pressure were exerted on the membrane at the bottom, the membrane at the top would bulge out (Fig. 3.11). This is a two-window system, the natural configuration of the inner ear; the two apertures are the oval and round windows.

Due to the incompressibility of liquid, a pressure exerted inward on the balloon's membrane through the top aperture which displaces, for example, one cubic millimeter of fluid results in a bulge in the bottom window of a corresponding one cubic

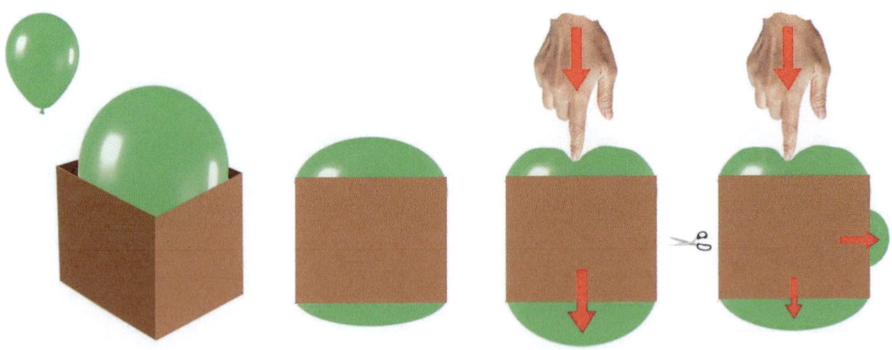

Fig. 3.11 The inner ear oval and round windows can be analogous to a balloon in a box with two openings at the top and the bottom. The balloon is filled with perilymph. Pressure applied to the top bulges the bottom. If you cut a third window in the side of the box, then the balloon will share the bulging between the new window and the bottom bulge

millimeter. If the top membrane is subjected to vibrations, the oscillations of the bottom membrane will match the oscillations of the top membrane. The fluid inside oscillates with respect to the casing. The amount of energy exerted on the top is functionally equal to the energy output on the other side, as nearly all the energy is transferred via the fluid to the second window.

Now, imagine what might happen if an additional hole is cut into the box somewhere else. If the same pressure were exerted on the balloon's membrane at the top, the bottom hole would still bulge, but it would bulge less. The new hole would also bulge. Some of the energy or fluid displacement would be lost at the other window, as the fluid displacement of the top membrane would be distributed among the other holes in the system. This balloon in box analogy describes the theory of Third Window Syndrome.

The ear's anatomy is slightly more complex but can be understood with similar mechanics. First, imagine taking the box, turning it on its side and stretching it like a tube, so that the left opening is now much farther away from the right opening. Fold the long tube in half into a "U" shape so that the ends of the tube are right next to each other (Fig. 3.12).

This system looks like a double-barreled shotgun on one end, and a U-shaped loop of pipe on the other end. In this configuration, the oval window and the round window sit next to each other on the double-barreled shotgun end. The U-shaped (helicotrema) end of the tube is rolled up like a snail, 2½ turns. This system describes the shape of the cochlea.

When the stapes bone exerts pressure inward on the oval window, a fluid pulse travels through the tube, through the 2 1/2 turns of the cochlea and the scala vestibuli, makes a U-turn at the helicotrema, comes back down to another 2 1/2 turns through the scala tympani, and creates a bulge at the round window. There is a "push me, pull you" effect. The windows move opposite of each other. When the oval

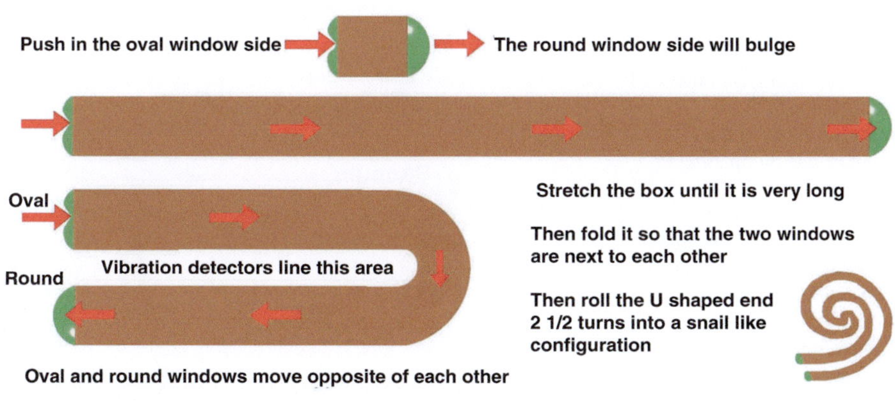

Fig. 3.12 Water balloon in a box analogy of Cochlear anatomy. The box is elongated and then doubled up into a U-shaped configuration. Then the U shape is rolled up like a snail 2.5 turns. The ends represent the oval window and the round window. The windows move in opposite directions as pulses of fluid flow through the long tube

window is pushed in, the round window bulges out and then vice versa. These fluid pulses carry the sound energy that drives hearing.

Anything that restricts the motion of this fluid will diminish hearing.

The Vestibule

The cochlear system and the semicircular canal system overlap at a structure known as the vestibule, which is essential to the function of both systems. The vestibule is a chamber from which all of the semicircular canals arise. Picture a coffee mug with three handles coming off at 90° angles. Each of these handles has a cupula at one end (Fig. 3.13).

The otolithic organs also reside in the vestibule. The saccule and utricle output to the inferior vestibular nerve.

The vestibule is connected to the outside world through the oval window via the stapes on one end, and the other end connects to the cochlea, terminating at the round window [14].

The importance of the vestibule is that it houses components of both hearing and balance systems and yet, in normal conditions, it allows the two systems to function independently without significant crossover. However, in pathological situations, the close proximity of these two systems allows for misdirection and thus inappropriate actuation or degradation of both systems.

Also note that the vestibule only has two openings. One is the oval window and the other one leads to the cochlea which ultimately terminates at the round window.

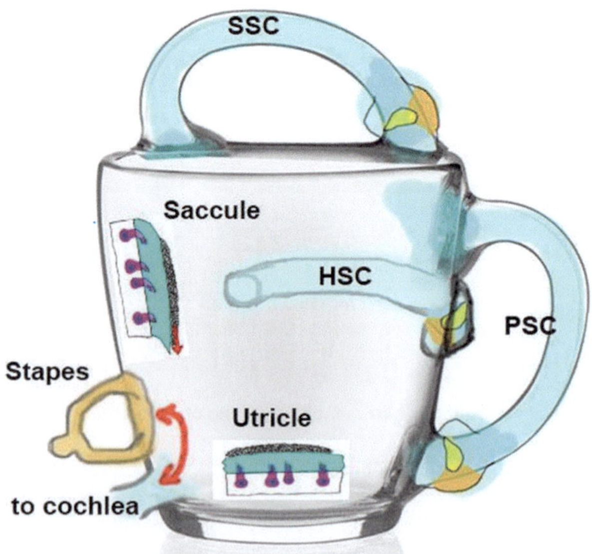

Fig. 3.13 The vestibule is like a busy coffee mug with three handles (semicircular canals), otolithic organs, and two ports that lead to the outside world: an oval window and an opening to the cochlea (which ultimately leads to the round window). Movement of the stapes creates a fluid flow (in red) between the oval and round windows, leaving the other structures undisturbed

This means that any vibrations that come into the vestibule through the oval window get directed out through the cochlea to the round window. The rest of the structures in the vestibule remain undisturbed.

What is a Dehiscence? Mechanics of a Mobile Third Window

In a nonpathological system, the inner ear and semicircular canals are entirely encased in bone with the exception of the round and oval windows. In a normal system, there is a layer of bone overlying the superior canal (and all the other canals for that matter) separating it from the middle fossa dura. However, in some cases, this bone is eroded and becomes very thin or even perforates, exposing the perilymphatic membrane (the water balloon's skin in the balloon/box analogy). This creates the third window.

Pressure Misdirection in TMWS Causing Abnormal Stimulation

TMWS will allow pressure misdirection between the round window and the third window. This is most easily explained by taking the superior canal dehiscence as an example. The abnormal window between the inner ear and the dura can cause pressure shunting to areas not used to pressure fluctuations.

If intracranial pressure fluctuates for any reason, the pressure pulse can cause the membrane of the dehiscent area to be pressed inward, squeezing the endolymphatic space, which would send a fluid pulse traveling down *both* arms of the superior semicircular canal. The fluid flow would stimulate the cupula, deflecting a "Nerve Switch," ampullopetally, or towards the ampulla, in a way that makes the patient feel like they are tumbling head over heels. This will reflexively be accompanied by an associated torsional nystagmus, where the top of the eye rotates towards the affected ear. Increased intracranial pressure can be triggered by a Valsalva maneuver (lifting heavy weights, straining during bowel movements) or simply by head movements (Fig. 3.14).

An increase in middle ear pressure would have an effect opposite to that of increased intracranial pressure. Increased pressure in the middle ear would apply a force that presses in on the round and oval window simultaneously. Normally, simultaneous pressure on a two window system creates zero pressure gradient and there is no net movement. However, if there is a dehiscence, the middle ear pressure pulse will generate a pressure wave upward, towards the dehiscence (Fig. 3.15). As the wave passes the ampulla, the cupula is deflected ampullofugally, (away from the ampula) and the patient would experience a backflip-like sensation. The eyes would demonstrate an opposite beating rotational nystagmus with the top of the eye moving away from the affected ear. This is why auto insufflation, pneumo-otoscopy, and altitude changes can result in barotraumas related vertigo [21].

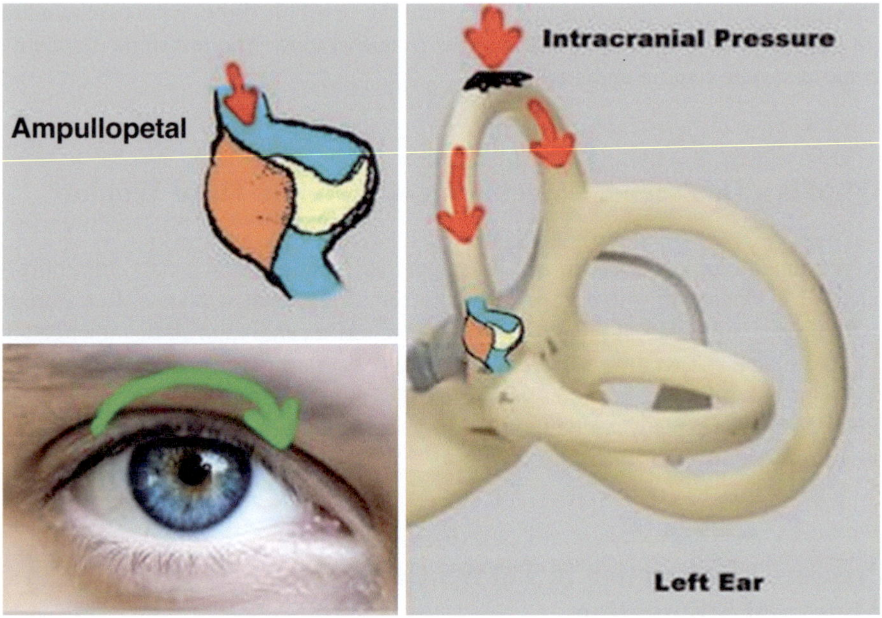

Fig. 3.14 Intracranial pressure pulses through the dehiscence, traveling down both arms of the SSC on its way to the round window. Pressure down the ampullar side can cause ampulloPETAL deflection of the cupula and trigger a torsional nystagmus where the top of the eye rotates towards the affected ear

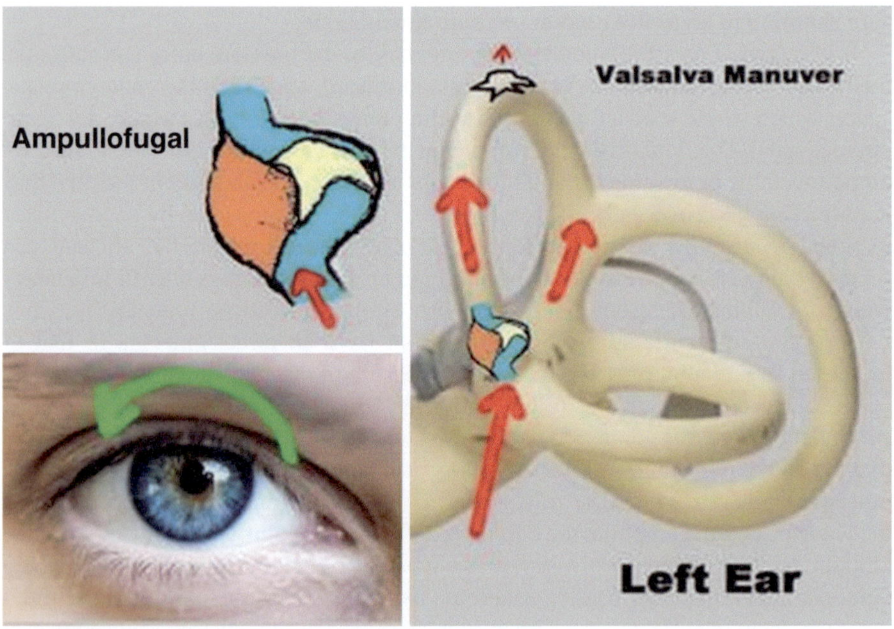

Fig. 3.15 Middle ear pressure pulses via the round and oval windows travel up through the vestibule on its way to the dehiscence. Pressure UP the ampullar side can cause ampulloFUGAL deflection of the cupula and trigger a torsional nystagmus where the top of the eye rotates away from the affected ear

Loss of Sound Energy

Consider the labyrinthine system and the balloon/box model again. A labyrinth with a normal physiology has the usual two windows, and all the pressure directed at the oval window (first window) travels through the tube and is transferred to the round window (second window). In the case of pathological physiology, if there is a third opening anywhere along the way, some of that pressure would be divided between the second window and third window. In this case, the sound energy would be stolen by the third window and wasted on vibrating the dura above, or some other opening below. This pathological model would result in less transference of the vibrational energy traveling through the cochlea, and thus cause hearing loss [21, 22] (Fig. 3.16).

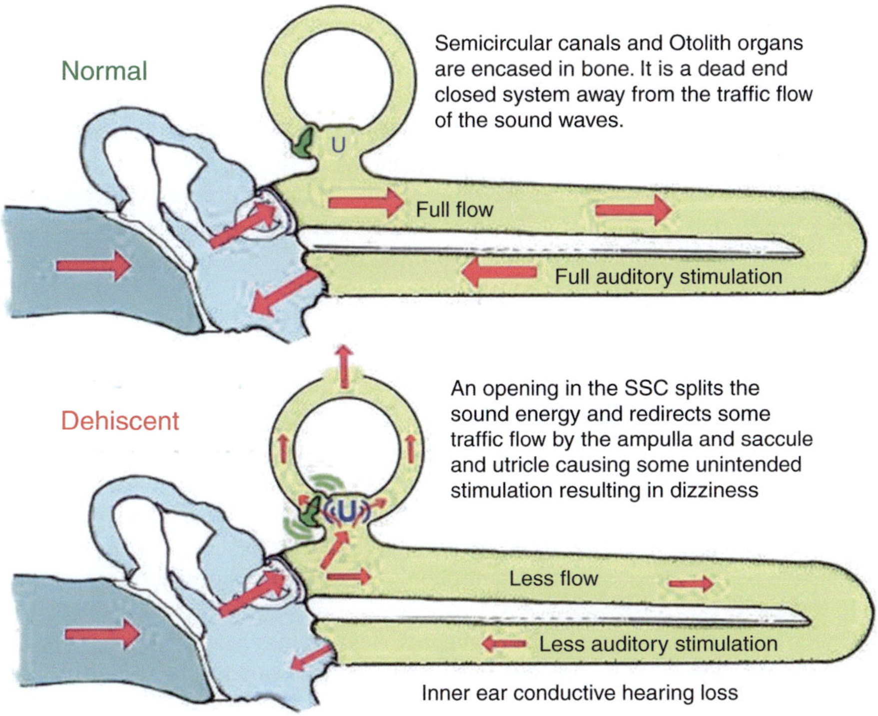

Fig. 3.16 The upper diagram shows the normal configuration of the inner ear in a simplified fashion, with an unrolled cochlea. Full stimulation of the tympanic membrane is transmitted to the oval window, and the full flow of energy is detected by the cochlear hair cells giving full auditory stimulation. The lower diagram shows a dehiscent superior canal creating a 3rd window. The full energy of the oval window stimulation is now divided between the dehiscence and the round window. The redirected flow to the dehiscence stimulates the ampulla and otolithic organs causing dizziness. This leaves less energy flow in the cochlea so there is less auditory stimulation, which is manifested as an inner conductive hearing loss

Inner Ear Conductive Hearing Loss

In the normal configuration, the tympanic membrane, malleus and incus are tied via the stapes to the oval window. Sound vibrations are funneled down the ear canal directly to the inner ear through this chain. The pressure wave is captured by the drum then via the malleus and incus, received by the stapes and transmitted between the oval window and round window.

As the stapes footplate vibrates in and out, it makes the incompressible fluid also flow back and forth, moving the round window (second window) in and out in synchrony with the first window.

It is the movement of the inner ear fluid that stimulates the hearing hair cells in between the two windows to fire and generate sound perception. The stronger the vibrations, the louder the perception.

The presence of a third window will steal vibrational energy from the second window and thereby cause a loss of sound energy. This loss is perceived as a loss of volume and is considered a conductive loss. Most conductive losses are due to middle ear problems, specifically restriction of ossicular mobility or drum issues. A conductive loss despite the presence of an intact eardrum and normal vibrating hearing bones is puzzling. Years ago, before the concept of TMWS was elucidated, these types of hearing loss were called "inner ear conductive hearing loss."

Many ill-fated stapedectomies have been done in efforts to correct mysterious hearing losses that turned out to be "inner ear conductive losses." Unfortunately, most of these surgeries did not work and often made the patient more dizzy and symptomatic [23].

Autophonia and Amplification of Internal Body Sounds

It is well known that conductive hearing loss can cause bone conduction sound to be perceived greater than air conduction sound. When patients with conductive hearing loss hum to themselves, they hear the humming louder in the ear with the loss. Conductive hearing loss can cause autophonia as well as amplification of internal body sounds.

On the Weber test, subjects with conductive hearing loss hear the tuning fork the loudest on the side with the greatest loss. There are two general theories as to why this happens.

One theory states that because the ear with the conductive hearing loss is mostly receiving input from the bone conduction with little air conduction contribution, the bone conduction is heard louder [24].

This phenomenon occurs because the conduction problem of the external and middle ear masks the ambient noise of the room, while the well-functioning inner ear (cochlea) picks the sound up via the bones of the skull, causing it to be perceived as a louder sound in the affected ear.

Another theory is based on the occlusion effect described by Tonndorf et al. Lower frequency sounds (as made by the tuning forks) that are transferred through the skull and through the hearing bones escape from the canal. If an "occlusion" is present, the sound cannot escape and appears louder on the ear with the conductive hearing loss [25].

The author postulates a deeper underlying mechanism regarding the amplification of internal noises as it pertains to TWMS.

The tympanic membrane is coupled to the oval window in a way that amplifies the sound through a series of boney lever mechanisms. Smaller forces using longer levers can move larger components, similar to the way a lighter person could move a heavier person on a seesaw more easily if the fulcrum of the seesaw is nearer to the heavier person. In a healthy system, the ossicular chain acts like an amplifier feeding the cochlea, and each step of the chain contributes to maximizing the ear's sensitivity to sound coming from the outside world into the inner ear. The same principle is seen in a snowshoe where the force of a person's foot is spread out over a larger area to stop the individual from sinking into the snow. In the middle ear, the area differential of the larger tympanic membrane to the smaller round window creates a larger mechanical force on the smaller window.

The system typically does not work as well going backwards. It is easier to move the light person a longer distance than it is to move the heavy person a short distance due to leverage; a small force requires a long lever arm over a fulcrum to move a heavy object. If one tries to apply the small force directly to the heavy object, it will not be sufficient to move the heavy object, the seesaw will not move. So in a sense, the lever mechanism acts almost as a one-way valve (although not entirely one way since it is still possible for energy to flow the other way). Sounds can easily travel through the drum and get amplified through the ossicular chain to get into the inner ear. However, sounds originating internally will have a harder time backdriving the system. Do note that backdriving is possible, but just harder.

While it is possible that one can actually hear normal unamplified internal body sounds, these sounds will not be as loud as the external sounds being funneled into the ear canal and amplified through the malleus, incus and stapes. External sounds move the inner ear fluid by plunging the stapes in and out like a piston. Internal sounds vibrate the boney shell of the inner ear around the stationary fluid, resulting in a similar relative motion.

However, this motion is dampened because as stated before, it is more difficult to vibrate the stapes footplate than it is to vibrate the tympanic membrane. The ossicular chain acts like an encumbrance to the oval window when sound is moving the "wrong way." The internal sounds waste energy to "backdrive" the oval window that is encumbered by the hearing bones and drum.

If the oval window and the stapes were disconnected, the encumbrance would be released. This would allow the fluid to move more freely between the two windows (oval and round windows). Thus, internal sounds would seem much louder in ossicular chain discontinuity.

When a third window superior semicircular canal dehiscence is present and the normal ossicular chain encumbering the oval window remains intact, the fluid can move freely between the round window and the dehiscence, better stimulating the hearing hair cells. This accounts for why TMWS patients might complain of hearing internal noises at annoyingly loud volumes, hear themselves talk and breathe, or why they might find their heel strike on hard floors as exceptionally loud [26].

VEMP Physiology

A full discussion of VEMPs is outside the scope of this chapter. However, in brief, the concept of VEMP (vestibular-evoked myogenic potential) is based on the fact that the inner ear has some cross reactivity when it comes to sound sensation and movement sensation. It is possible to trigger the inner ear motion detectors using a sound burst. This reflex is measured by EMG response either in an obicularis oculi muscle (o-VEMP) or the sternocleidomastoid muscle (c-VEMP) after a tone is presented to the ear in question [27].

To understand the overlap between auditory and vestibular sensations, we need to understand the frequency spectrum. It all boils down to speed of movement and cycles per second. Consider a large fan. As it starts up, at one revolution per min, it moves silently. At 60 RPM, (1 cycle per second) or 1 Hz, the fan still remains in silent motion. Somewhere at about 20 Hz, the fan might give off a low tone rumble… and at higher RPMs it may start to give off a higher pitched whine. One can see that at some point the movement becomes fast enough to generate sound.

The electromagnetic vibration chart is very fascinating. The spectrum is very large, ranging from sound to radio waves, to light, to X-rays and gamma radiation. It is interesting that our sensory organs can only detect energy in three tiny parts of the spectrum. We can detect movement starting at the slowest frequencies with our vestibular system. Next we can detect sound energy in the next bracket of frequencies with our cochlear apparatus. Then there is a gap of frequencies that humans cannot detect that contain ultrasound, radio waves, microwaves and infrared energy. Then, finally light energy is detected by our eyes (Fig. 3.17).

Human auditory frequency detection is said to fall between 20 cycles per second and 20,000 cycles per second. That means that we have specialized hair cells that detect vibrations between this range of frequencies. These cells live in the cochlea. These vibrations are detected as sound [28].

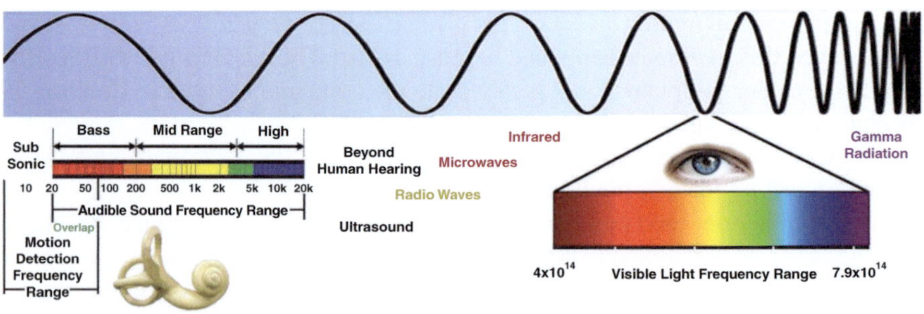

Fig. 3.17 Whether a signal is detected as a movement or sound, or light, it is all about how fast something vibrates. The electromagnetic spectrum from low frequency to high frequency vibrations spans from simple motion to sound, to ultrasound, to radio waves, to microwaves, to light, all the way to X-rays and gamma radiation. We have somatosensory and vestibular receptors that detect motion of vibrations from 0 to 70 Hz. We have auditory receptor cells that detect vibrations from 20 to 20,000 Hz. And we have light receptors that detect the 4×10^{14} to 7.9×10^{14} Hz range

What about vibrations lower than 20 cycles per second? Humans detect the lower frequencies as movement. These movement detectors are special sensory cells located in the saccule and utricle in the vestibule, and the cupula of the semicircular canals. If one shakes the head side to side at one cycle in one second, then the sensory organ (the cupula) of the horizontal canals detect a frequency of one Hertz.

While there is no overlap between hearing and vision frequencies so that one cannot see musical tones and hear green lights, there is actually significant overlap of the auditory and vestibular senses. This results in cross-sensory stimulation. That means that it is possible to stimulate both the hearing and the otolithic organs with tones presented in the overlap frequencies.

Prior studies of the vestibular system's contribution to postural control have been limited to frequency bandwidths below 20 Hz. More recent work, however, suggests that vestibular contributions to postural muscles can be measured up to 25 Hz in appendicular muscles and 70 Hz in neck muscles [29, 30].

Then there are other papers that show that the vestibular system and the auditory system have overlapping sensitivities in the 200–750 Hz range or more. This means sounds presented in these frequencies may trigger a sensation of movement, which then trigger a reflexive muscle twitch to counter that movement [31].

Why Are VEMP Thresholds Affected in SCD?

So as one can see, there is natural overlap between vestibular sensory organs and sound sensation. This means that low frequency sounds have the potential to trigger vestibular sensations in a "normal" fashion and we can measure that threshold with VEMPS.

Typically the VEMP test is done with a 500 Hz tone. That 500 Hz tone has to be presented at a certain threshold loudness for a normal human otolithic organ to detect it.

In patients with SCD, the threshold for the electrical event is decreased, meaning that it takes less powerful sound stimulation for the electrical activity to trigger. Additionally, if the same 500 Hz sound stimulation is used, patients with SCD will have a larger response than those who don't have SCD.

The logical explanation for this is, again, the fact that the sound pressure waves that used to be entirely directed between the oval and round windows is now redirected through the vestibular system and thus affects the saccule and utricle more than it would have when the vibrations were mostly isolated in the cochlea. That redirection stimulates the otolithic organs more, and the auditory system less [27].

However, there is relatively new evidence that there may be more reasons for positive o-VEMPs in SCD than just the misdirected vibrations to the otolithic organs. It is generally known that the VEMP response is tied to the saccule and utricle which are enervated by the inferior vestibular nerve. Thus the thought came about that VEMPs test the inferior vestibular system exclusively. However, there is evidence that there is another neural input contributing to the enhanced responses after SCD. Superior canal afferent neurons project indirectly to both contralateral inferior oblique via the contralateral III nerve nucleus (the source of o-VEMPs) and also to the ipsilateral sternocleidomastoid. It was not previously known that these neurons were sensitive to sounds up to 4000 Hz, until experimentation done by Leonardo Manzari. His work showed that in dehiscences, the superior vestibular nerve can be involved. In addition to that, the frequency response can go as high as 4000 Hz. In fact, the 4000 Hz stimulation might be a better, more specific o-VEMP test for SCD than 500 Hz stimulation. [32, 33].

Fistula Test and Hennebert's Sign

The Fistula Test and Hennebert's sign are tests for perilymphatic fistula or third window syndrome. They can be done quite informally with subjective observation of nystagmus or more formally with VNG tracings. Fistula testing basically involves putting positive and negative pressure on the eardrum to drive the stapes back and forth to see if the pressure changes cause dizziness. Hennebert's sign is one way of doing an informal fistula test. It is done by closing off the external ear canal by compressing the tragus with a finger and watching for nystagmus.

The Hennebert's sign is characterized by a few beats of horizontal nystagmus. Characteristically it is a low frequency and low amplitude nystagmus. Most patients indicate a sensation of dizziness as the test is being done.

Other ways of doing a fistula test involve pneumotoscopy or a tympanogram machine using VNG. Clearly these tests move the fluid within the inner ear. Based on the pathophysiology described in this chapter, patients with TWMS will get misdirected flow over the vestibular end organs and trigger dizziness [34, 35].

Tullio's Phenomenon

Tullio's phenomenon is the elicitation of dizziness and nystagmus from acoustic stimulation. This was generally seen in patients diagnosed with fistulas and enlarged vestibular aqueduct syndromes. Now it is quite recognized to be associated with SCD and TMWS.

As we have seen, sound pulses that are redirected through the vestibular system by the third window dehiscence trigger an otolithic response. The louder the sound is, the stronger the response. This is the natural response to sensory nerve cell stimulation. However, it is also possible to stimulate a nerve in a way that the sensory organ was not designed to sense. For example, even though eyes were designed to detect light, a mechanical jolt like a punch in the eye can cause a flash of shooting stars. Thus a mechanical wave may likewise trigger the vestibular hair cells in an abnormal fashion, resulting in dizziness. So although the exact cellular mechanism of Tullio's phenomenon is not perfectly understood, it does make sense that the redirection of fluid flow over the vestibular organs is to blame [36–38].

Advanced Pathophysiology

The Third Window Theory and Balloon/Box Model explain why some signs and symptoms are present in the case of TMWS. However, some situations remain unexplained.

For instance, the theory does not explain why some patients are asymptomatic. For example, there are many patients who are incidentally noted to have SSCD while undergoing CT scans for reasons not related to dizziness. Many of these patients have no neurotologic complaints. According to the Third Window Theory, the third window allows intracranial pressure to create abnormal flow of fluid in the superior canal, triggering hair cells that detect motion, and resulting in symptoms such as conductive hearing loss, autophonia, and pressure-induced vertigo. Why wouldn't all patients with a labyrinthine dehiscence on CT scans present with neurotologic complaints?

There are several potential explanations:

- Remaining thin bone layer that cannot be seen on CT scan
- Near dehiscence or incomplete dehiscence and the second event theory
- Alteration of intracranial pressure may increase compliance of the round window and all the windows
- Brain/cognitive compensation
- Dense brain sitting on top of a fistula, phase shifts, and the inertial orientation of the fluid column

Remaining Thin Bone Layer

The simplest explanation for an asymptomatic patient would be that even though a CT scan may seem to show a defect, a defect is not actually present. It is possible that the resolution of the CT scan may not be sufficient to detect the presence of a thin layer of bone that remains over the alleged dehiscence. As long as the otic capsule is intact, even by the thinnest bone, the subject should have no symptoms. The presence or absence of thinned intact bone is difficult to prove in a living patient since asymptomatic patients are unlikely to consent to exploratory craniotomies. Of course, the postmortem finding of a frank SCD in a patient who never complained about SCD symptoms cannot be posthumously questioned about their condition. However, there are some cases that are radiographically convincing for a frank dehiscence where the patient has few, if any, symptoms.

Near Dehiscence, Incomplete Dehiscence, and the Second Event Theory

Some asymptomatic patients may only experience intermittent symptoms. In these cases, it is hypothesized that there is extreme thinning of the bone layer to the point where the bone is semi flexible. The bone layer may hold up under normal circumstances, but succumb to major pressure loads.

The Second Event Theory refers to the thought that a secondary traumatic event is often the instigator of the symptoms. One might have a near dehiscence for a long time, and then a Valsalva-type maneuver or barotrauma breaks the thin bone and initiates the syndrome and accompanying pathological symptoms. This is the so-called straw that breaks the camel's back.

Intracranial Pressure and Increased Compliance

Gianoli and Soileau [39] proposed the theory that the alteration of intracranial pressure may result in increased compliance at the round and oval windows and, if pressure changes were extreme, potential disruption of the windows might occur, resulting in a frank middle ear perilymphatic fistula.

They also further proposed a grading system for SSCD:

Stage 1: Asymptomatic
Stage 2: Minor's Syndrome—Tullio's phenomenon and Valsalva induced vertigo correlating with increased compliance of the cochlear windows
Stage 3: Ménière's syndrome—vertigo and hearing loss mimicking Ménière's disease correlating with frank oval or round window perilymph fistula
Stage 4: End stage—profound hearing loss and or vestibular areflexia as a result of repeat damage from Stage 3

In medical terms, high compliance means low resistance, low elastic recoil, floppy thin tissue. Conversely, low compliance implies high resistance, thick, firm tissue. Returning to the balloon analogy, one might assume that the compliance of all three windows is the same. However, it is possible that in some cases the round and oval windows are highly compliant and the pathological third window is non-compliant, making the path of least resistance between the natural two windows. Thus, in some cases, if the third window is highly resistant to distension, it won't bulge much, resulting in less flow over the ampulla and fewer or no symptoms.

This theory could explain why some patients have no symptoms even though they appear to have a third window syndrome. It may also explain why round window reinforcement has been noted to resolve SSCD symptoms (at least temporarily) in many patients [40].

Neurological Insensitivity

On the other hand, it is also possible that the patient, despite a frank dehiscence, is simply neurologically insensitive. Perhaps they have had a pre-existing vestibular disorder like Ménière's disease or vestibular neuritis. Perhaps there has been prior surgery or a congenital abnormality. In any of these cases, the pressure waves of the SCD still travel past the vestibular system, however, because the nerve has been "numbed," a nerve signal is not generated. Thus the dehiscence appears to be asymptomatic.

Cognitive Adaptation

Brain/cognitive adaptation and compensation might occur in some patients, especially if the problem began at an early age. There are many examples of individuals who have what seem to be obvious disabilities, who function as if they had no problems at all. For example, some patients present with a congenital nystagmus but are not dizzy, despite their eyes exhibiting a strong resting nystagmus.

Fluid Dynamics, Phase Shifts, and Dense Brain Resting on Fistula

Other explanations for the asymptomatic patient with radiographic SSCD might lie in non-Newtonian fluid dynamics, fluid wave phase shifts that cause amplitude cancelation, or the simple possibility that the temporal lobe of the brain rests over and covers the SCD.

Dense Brain Resting on Fistula

Gerard Gianoli notes several cases where frank obvious SCDs were found in asymptomatic patients who were undergoing craniotomies to repair encephaloceles [39]. John Carey and Lloyd Minor have proposed the idea of "auto plugging" of the SCD by the temporal lobe in some cases with a very large SCD. (These cases, however, were symptomatic and the vHIT results for the superior canal demonstrated reduced gain which led to their conclusions.) It is still hypothesized that the pressure of the temporal lobe of the brain into the SCD can plug the SCD and ameliorate symptoms [26, 41].

Phase Shifts

Any wave can be canceled by another wave of equal amplitude and frequency by phase shifting it 180°. The phase shift phenomenon can be seen applied in noise cancelation headphones. The phase shift phenomenon can also be seen in the case of a TM perforation over the round window, which causes sound waves to hit the drum and the round window at the same time. In a natural configuration, as the drum pushes in the oval window, the round window bulges out. Thus, in the natural condition, the round window and the drum are out of phase by 180° by design, and the drum shields the round window from incoming sound waves.

A TM perforation over the round window allows sound waves to push on the drum and round window simultaneously. The round window then receives incoming sound as well as the input from the oval window 180° out of phase with the incoming sound, resulting in a canceling effect. This phenomenon results in a significant conductive hearing loss. Extrapolating the phase shift phenomenon to an SCD situation, it is possible that phase shifts could theoretically mitigate the autophony and amplification of internal sounds via the phase cancelation effect.

Symptomatic Patients Without Evidence of SCD

On the other end of the spectrum, some patients present with symptoms but do not have clinical or X-ray evidence of SCD. This can possibly be explained by the notion that there are areas in the otic capsule that could be thin or dehiscent other than the superior canal. For instance, the posterior semicircular canal could be dehiscent at the posterior fossa dura or at the jugular bulb. Horizontal canal dehiscence, usually eroded by cholesteatoma, can happen in the middle ear. The horizontal canal can also be thinned near the second genu of the facial nerve. Cochlear dehiscence can happen at the labyrinthine segment of the facial nerve, or at the level of the carotid artery. A defect in any of these areas can result in symptoms similar to SCD.

Other Sites Outside of the Semicircular Canals

Enlarged Vestibular Aqueduct/Jugular Bulb Dehiscence

An enlarged vestibular aqueduct is defined as Enlargement of the vestibular operculum by >1.5–2 mm. A dilated Vestibular Aqueduct opening would act as a third window, allowing sound energy to escape from the inner ear and intracranial pressure shifts to be detected by the vestibular system causing dizziness [42, 43].

A Jugular bulb dehiscence into the vestibular aqueduct can cause a similar third window situation.

X-Linked Stapes Gusher Syndrome It is due to an X-linked mutation affecting males. They are born with a mixed hearing loss which progresses to severe deafness in the first decade. They have a mixed hearing loss from cochleovestibular malformation. The "inner ear" conductive hearing loss is due to a dehiscence between the basal turn of the cochlea and the internal auditory canal. There is direct communication between perilymph and the subarachnoid fluid due to the absence of the lamina cribrosa. When surgeons unwittingly attempt stapedectomy, these patients "gush" perilymph which accounts for the name [44, 45].

Bone Dyscrasias Metabolic bone disease such as Paget's, Osteogenesis Imperfecta, and Otospongiosus can cause conductive hearing loss in multiple ways. In some cases, abnormal deposition of bone can cause restriction of vibrations. In other cases, there have been post mortem studies showing microscopic fistulae too small for CT to detect, causing TMWS [46].

Perilabyrinthine Fistula This refers to a constellation of neoplastic or inflammatory processes that can erode into the bony labyrinth. One of the most common is cholesteatoma. Cholesteatoma is often seen eroding the lateral semicircular canal, but it can also affect the labyrinth at the oval window, as well as the other semicircular canals.

Temporal bone fractures from trauma can also create a TMWS. Labyrinthine bone does not tend to heal with boney union. It tends to fill in the fracture line with fibrous tissue to seal off leakage of perilymph. However, that only serves to turn the entire fracture line into a soft dehiscent mobile third window to the outside world [47].

Sometimes it takes a good detective to find the dehiscence. Much like if one has water intrusion into the house, one might ask "where is the leak?" In working up a patient who has "inner ear conductive hearing loss" or pressure evoked dizziness, the physician must be mindful in asking open mindedly "where is the weak spot?" Understanding the anatomy and physiology will help the clinician find the source.

Summary

The pathophysiology of third mobile window syndrome (TMWS) seems to be well explained by the water balloon in a box analogy. Normal anatomy and physiology is based on the fact that there are only two natural windows between which the inner ear fluids flow. This fluid movement stimulates the hearing hair cells in between the windows resulting in auditory perception. If at any time a third window develops, then some of the fluid flow is misdirected to the new window. If some of the energy flow is misdirected to the labyrinthine section, then the flow will stimulate the vestibular organs and give a false sense of motion. This causes dizziness. The sharing of sound energy between three windows instead of two means that each window will get less energy. If the vibrational energy between the original two windows in the cochlea is reduced, then the hearing perception will be less. This is the reason for the so-called inner ear conductive hearing loss.

The third window can couple audiovestibular disturbances to things that cause intracranial pressure to fluctuate, changes in middle ear pressure as well as abnormal reactions to a wide variety of sound stimulation.

It is important to remember that there are some patients who have symptoms that do not have superior canal dehiscence. This can be due to several reasons. TMWS can occur albeit rarely in areas outside the semicircular canals such as the cochlea and the vestibule. This accounts for the symptoms due to pathologies ranging from temporal bone fractures to enlarged vestibular aqueduct. It is the misdirection of flow that also accounts for the various other variants of TMWS.

It is also important to realize that even strong CT evidence of what looks to be a dehiscence may be completely asymptomatic in some patients.

Conclusions

TMWS is a collection of inter-related symptoms due to abnormal windows (bone openings) in the bone encased labyrinth. Pathophysiology helps explain why patients who have a third window might have symptoms like "inner ear conductive hearing loss," autophonia, Hennebert's sign, Tullio's phenomenon, dizziness upon straining, and barotrauma related vertigo.

References

1. Minor LB, Solomon D, Zinreich JS, Zee DS. Sound- and/or pressure-induced vertigo due to bone dehiscence of the superior semicircular canal. Arch Otolaryngol Head Neck Surg. 1998;124:249–58.
2. Ward BK, Carey JP, Minor LB. Superior canal dehiscence syndrome: lessons from the first 20 years. Front Neurol. 2017;8:177.
3. Ho ML, Moonis G, Halpin CF, Curtin HD. Spectrum of third window abnormalities: semicircular canal dehiscence and beyond. Am J Neuroradiol. 2017;38(1):2–9.
4. Krombach GA, DiMartino E, Schmitz-Rode T, et al. Posterior semicircular canal dehiscence: a morphologic cause of vertigo similar to superior semicircular canal dehiscence. Eur Radiol. 2003;13:1444–50.
5. Pietsch M, Aguirre Dávila L, Erfurt P, Avci E, Lenarz T, Kral A. Spiral form of the human cochlea results from spatial constraints. Sci Rep. 2017;7(1):7500.
6. Ades HW, Engström H. Anatomy of the inner ear. In: Keidel WD, Neff WD, editors. Auditory system. Handbook of sensory physiology, vol. 5. Berlin: Springer; 1974.

7. Spoor F, Wood B, Zonneveld F. Implications of early hominid labyrinthine morphology for evolution of human bipedal locomotion. Nature. 1994;369:645–8.
8. Carey JP, Della SC. Principles of applied vestibular physiology. In: Flint PW, et al., editors. Cummings otolaryngology - Head and neck surgery. 5th ed. Philadelphia: Elsevier; 2010. p. 2276–304.
9. Migliaccio AA, Della Santina CC, Carey JP, Minor LB, Zee DS. The effect of binocular eye position and head rotation plane on the human torsional vestibuloocular reflex. Vis Res. 2006;46(16):2475–86.
10. Solomon D, Zee DS, Straumann D. Torsional and horizontal vestibular ocular reflex adaptation: 3-dimensional eye movement analysis. Exp Brain Res. 2003;152(2):150–5.
11. Della Santina CC, Potyagaylo V, Migliaccio AA, Minor LB, Carey JP. Orientation of human semicircular canals measured by 3-dimensional multiplanar CT reconstruction. J Assoc Res Otolaryngol. 2005;6(3):191–206.
12. Leigh RJ, Zee DS. The neurology of eye movements. Oxford: Oxford University Press; 2015.
13. Cremer PD, et al. Posterior semicircular canal nystagmus is conjugate and its axis is parallel to that of the canal. Neurology. 2000;54(10):2016–20.
14. Kingma H, Van De Berg R. Anatomy, physiology and physics of the peripheral vestibular system. In: Furman JM, Lempert T, editors. Handbook of clinical neurology, vol. 137. New York: Elsevier; 2016. p. 1–16.
15. Newman MC, Lawson BD, Rupert AH, McGrath BJ. The role of perceptual modeling in the understanding of spatial disorientation during flight and ground-based simulator training. In: Proceedings of the AIAA modeling and simulation of technologies conference. Minneapolis: AIAA; 2012. p. 14.
16. Mittelstaedt H. Somatic graviception. Biol Psychol. 1996;42:53–74.
17. Ito Y, Gresty MA. Subjective postural orientation and visual vertical during slow pitch tilt for the seated human subject. Aviat Space Environ Med. 1997;68:3–12.
18. Kennedy RS, Fowlkes JE, Berbaum KS, Lilienthal MG. Use of a motion sickness history questionnaire for prediction of simulator sickness. Aviat Space Environ Med. 1992;63(7):588–93.
19. Otero-Millan J, Treviño C, Winnick A, Zee DS, Carey JP, Kheradmand A. The video ocular counter-roll (vOCR): a clinical test to detect loss of otolith-ocular function. Acta Otolaryngol. 2017;137(6):593–7.
20. Manzari L, Burgess AM, MacDougall HG, Curthoys IS. Superior canal dehiscence reveals concomitant unilateral utricular loss (UUL). Acta Otolaryngol. 2015;135:557–64.
21. Cremer PD, Minor LB, Carey JP, Della Santina CC. Eye movements in patients with superior canal dehiscence syndrome align with the abnormal canal. Neurology. 2000;55:1833–41.
22. Minor LB, et al. Dehiscence of bone overlying the superior canal as a cause of apparent conductive hearing loss. Otol Neurotol. 2003;24:270–8.
23. Merchant SN, Rosowski JJ, McKenna MJ. Superior semicircular canal dehiscence mimicking otosclerotic hearing loss. Adv Otorhinolaryngol. 2007;65:137–45.
24. Kelly EA, Li B, Adams ME. Diagnostic accuracy of tuning fork tests for hearing loss: a systematic review. Otolaryngol Head Neck Surg. 2018;159(2):220–30.
25. Tonndorf J. Bone conduction. In: Tobias JV, editor. Foundations of modern auditory theory, vol. 2. New York: Academic Press; 1972. p. 195–237.
26. Eberhard KE, Chari DA, Nakajima HH, Klokker M, Cayé-Thomasen P, Lee DJ. Current trends, controversies, and future directions in the evaluation and management of superior canal dehiscence syndrome. Front Neurol. 2021;12:638574.
27. Streubel SO, Cremer PD, Carey JP, Weg N, Minor LB. Vestibular-evoked myogenic potentials in the diagnosis of superior canal dehiscence syndrome. Acta Otolaryngol. 2001;545:41–9.
28. Fettiplace RHCT. Tuning, and synaptic transmission in the mammalian cochlea. Compr Physiol. 2017;7:1197–227.
29. Viviani P, Berthoz A. Dynamic of the head-neck system in response to small perturbations: analysis and modelling in the frequency domain. Biol Cybern. 1975;19:19–37.

30. Pozzo T, Berthoz A, Lefort L. Head stabilization during various locomotor tasks in humans. Exp Brain Res. 1990;82:97–106.
31. Manzari L, Burgess AM, MacDougall HG, Curthoys IS. Enhanced otolithic function in semicircular canal dehiscence. Acta Otolaryngol. 2011;131:107–12.
32. Manzari L, Burgess AM, McGarvie LA, Curthoys IS. An indicator of probable semicircular canal dehiscence: ocular vestibular evoked myogenic potentials to high frequencies. Otolaryngol Head Neck Surg. 2013;149:142–5.
33. Curthoys IS. The new vestibular stimuli: sound and vibration-anatomical, physiological and clinical evidence. Exp Brain Res. 2017;235:957–72.
34. Hennebert C. A new syndrome in hereditary syphilis of the labyrinth. Presse Med Belg Brux. 1911;63:467–70.
35. Nadol JB Jr. Positive "fistula sign" with intact tympanic membrane. Arch Otolaryngol. 1974;100:273–8.
36. Ostrowski VB, Byskosh A, Hain TC. Tullio phenomenon with dehiscence of the superior semicircular canal. Otol Neurotol. 2001;22:61–5.
37. Kaski D, Davies R, Luxon L, et al. The Tullio phenomenon: a neurologically neglected presentation. J Neurol. 2012;259:4–21.
38. Iversen MM, Zhu H, Zhou W, et al. Sound abnormally stimulates the vestibular system in canal dehiscence syndrome by generating pathological fluid-mechanical waves. Sci Rep. 2018;8:10257.
39. Gianoli GJ, Soileau JS. Superior canal dehiscence. In: Dizziness and vertigo across the lifespan. Amsterdam: Elsevier; 2011.
40. Gianoli G. Superior semicircular canal dehiscence repair. In: Babu S, editor. Practical otology for the otolaryngologist. San Diego: Plural Publishing; 2013. p. 287–96.
41. Carey JP, Migliaccio AA, Minor LB. Semicircular canal function before and after surgery for superior canal dehiscence. Otol Neurotol. 2007;28:356–64.
42. Valvassori G, Clemis J. The large vestibular aqueduct syndrome. Laryngoscope. 1978;88:273–8.
43. Hourani R, Carey J, Yousem DM. Dehiscence of the jugular bulb and vestibular aqueduct: findings on 200 consecutive temporal bone computed tomography scans. J Comput Assist Tomogr. 2005;29:657–62.
44. Talbot JM, Wilson DF. Computed tomographic diagnosis of X-linked congenital mixed deafness, fixation of the stapedial footplate, and perilymphatic gusher. Am J Otol. 1994;15:177–82.
45. Sennaroglu L, Saatci I. A new classification for cochleovestibular malformations. Laryngoscope. 2002;112:2230–41.
46. Santos F, McCall AA, Chien W, et al. Otopathology in osteogenesis imperfecta. Otol Neurotol. 2012;33:1562–6.
47. Kang HM, Kim MG, Boo SH, et al. Comparison of the clinical relevance of traditional and new classification systems of temporal bone fractures. Eur Arch Otorhinolaryngol. 2012;269:1893–9.

Chapter 4
Classification of Third Mobile Window Anomalies

Eugen Ionescu, Gerard J. Gianoli, and P. Ashley Wackym

Introduction

While superior semicircular canal dehiscence (SSCD) is relatively well-known in the medical community, there are many other sites of otic capsule dehiscence (OCD) which create a third mobile window resulting in third window syndrome (TWS). Over the past quarter century, there has been tremendous expansion of the depth of our knowledge and understanding of TWS; however, the identification of lesser-known sites of OCD remains an important diagnostic and therapeutic challenge. This is all the more so as in our experience TWS, including SSCD, remains under-diagnosed. Therefore, the development of a unitary anatomical-clinical and radiological classification would be an important step for a better understanding of these pathologies by neurotologists, otologists, neurologists, auditory-vestibular specialists, otolaryngologists, and neuroradiologists. Thus, the probability of being left without an etiological diagnosis in case of "mysterious" pseudo-conductive hearing loss, with or without obvious associated vestibular phenomena, should become lower. Furthermore, due to the progressive increase in new reported variants of OCD, the characterization of the anatomical structures involved, as well as the size and location of the TW, has become essential for a better understanding of the various mechanisms associated with this pathology. This allows us not only to

E. Ionescu (✉)
Service d'Audiologie et d'Otoneurologie, CHU Lyon, Institute de l'Audition, Paris, France
e-mail: eugen.ionescu@chu-lyon.fr

G. J. Gianoli
Ear and Balance Institute, Covington, LA, USA

P. A. Wackym
New Jersey, USA

G. J. Gianoli, P. Thomson (eds.), *Third Mobile Window Syndrome of the Inner Ear*, https://doi.org/10.1007/978-3-031-16586-3_4

systematize the different known variants but also to propose new, eventually less invasive or more pathophysiological therapeutic strategies. Based on the experience of the authors of this chapter, who have considered not only personal case studies but also other relevant publications on the subject, this chapter is the result of collaborative collegial work.

We are aware that there are several valuable articles in which an anatomical or radiological systematization of the lesions of the third window has already been proposed [1–6], however, in our opinion these authors did not propose a comprehensive unitary anatomical-clinical and radiological classification as presented here.

Please note that the authors have voluntarily excluded to review the tumoral, infectious, metabolic, or traumatic pathologies of the petrosal bone which can generate secondarily a TWS (e.g. glomus tumors, middle ear cholesteatoma, Paget's disease, perylimphatic fistula after fracture of the petrosal bone, etc.). It seems to us that it is easier to look for an area where the labyrinth is opened by a pathological process (thus generating a secondary TW), in the case of tumor or traumatic pathology of the petrosal bone, than to look for a "primary" OCD that is much less known or suspected by ENT specialists or radiologists.

Material and Methods

In the original paper proposing a unitary classification of third mobile window abnormalities [7], clinical and radiological data of 259 patients presenting a conductive hearing loss were retrospectively reviewed. Patients with degenerative processes or chronic infection of the petrosal bone, whether they underwent surgery or not, were excluded.

Due to the didactic purpose of this chapter, some other documented radiological data were used as well as audio-vestibular details from different relevant sources published previously.

Vestibular and Audiological Evaluation

Standard neurotological examination, including cranial nerve evaluation and otomicroscopy, was routinely performed in all patients. Pure tone audiometry (PTA; Madsen Astera-Otometrics), middle ear reflexes (Madsen Zodiac 901 tympanometer), videonystagmography including bone vibratory test (BVT) and valsalva maneuver (VNG, Ulmer SystemR; Synapsis SA), video head impulse test (VHIT, ICS Impulse R; GN Otometrics), cervical vestibular evoked potentials (cVEMPs), and ocular vestibular evoked potentials (oVEMPS) (Bio-Logic RNav-Pro system) in air conduction with 750 Hz stimuli were systematically performed in all patients.

Radiological Assessment

(a) Petrous bone high-resolution CT (GE GSI Revolution, GE Healthcare, USA) was performed in all patients. Slices were acquired helically in the axial plane at a nominal thickness of 0.625 mm with a 50% overlap of 0.312 mm, as recommended [8–10]. Images were obtained in ultra-high resolution at 140 kV and 200 mAs/section. The primary images were reworked in the axial and coronal planes of the lateral CSC at a 60 mm field of view with a 512 matrix for an isometric voxel. Pöschl plane (i.e., superior SCC plane) using Advantage Workstation (AW) Server visualization software (GE Healthcare, USA) was also employed.
(b) Additionally, 3 Tesla MRI (3T MRI; GE Healthcare, Philips Ingenia, Philips healthcare) of the petrous bone and inner ear structures was also performed if associated pathologies were suspected, or when vestibular and/or vascular structures appeared to be involved at the TW's interface. 3D T1-weighted contrast enhanced sequences allowed for confirmation of the vascular nature of the involved structure, and the HR 3D T2 labyrinth sequence DRIVE (DRIVEN Equilibrium pulse, TE 157, TR 1000, slice thickness 0.4, Turbo factor 40, Matrix 500 × 500, voxel size: 0.4 × 0.4 isotropic) highlighted, when necessary, the morphology and permeability of the membranous labyrinth. Fused images between CT slices in Pöschl plane and 3D T1 weighted contrast enhanced sequence obtained with post-processing software (AW Server, GE Healthcare) were performed to assess the TW interface.

Results

Following this analysis, a classification of OCD was proposed based on the anatomic structures and radiological features involved at the TW partition (Table 4.1). A list of the most frequent symptoms from the initial series was included.

Table 4.1 Third mobile window abnormalities (TMWA): classification and clinical elements

	Interface	Type	Number of patients	Clinical features	cVEMP thresholds
Extralabyrinthine TMWA (OCD)	OC-Meningeal	I	48	Vertigo (42%) Auditory symptoms (35%)	Decreased (20%)
	OC-Vascular	II	28	Vertigo (64%) Auditory symptoms (64%)	Decreased (14%)
	OC-Petrosal	III	17	Vertigo (47%) Auditory symptoms (52%)	Decreased (21%)
Intralabyrinthine TMWA -like	Vestibular aqueduct - Posterior SC		4	Vertigo (50%) Auditory symptoms (25%)	Decreased (0%)
Multiple OCD	Multiple locations (on the same ear)	/	11	Vertigo (80%) Auditory symptoms (100%)	Decreased (40%)

SC, Semicircular Canal; OCD, Otic Capsule Dehiscence

Type I: OCD-Meningeal

This type (Fig. 4.1) includes two main subsets that were historically the first cases of dehiscence described in the literature:

Subtype Ia

This type refers to the SSCD described by Minor, in which the SSC is typically in contact with the dura of the middle cerebral fossa (Fig. 4.1a, b).

Subtype Ib

This type of dehiscence involves the posterior SC (PSC), which can be in contact with, or very close to, the dura of the posterior fossa (Fig. 4.1c, d). As in the Type Ia, Type Ib may be present bilaterally. The pathophysiological mechanism for this type, including its two sub-variants, was largely described previously.

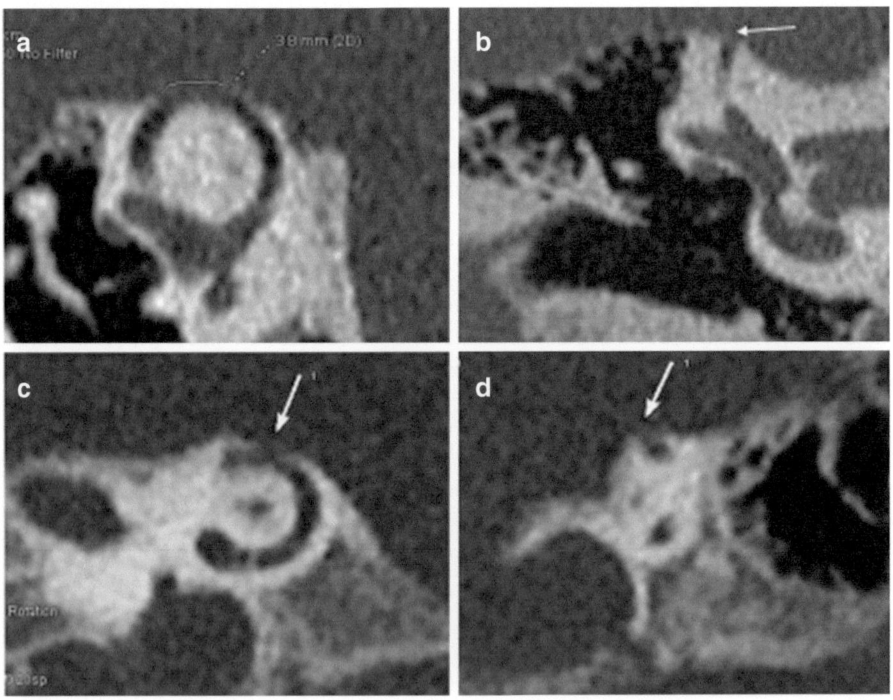

Fig. 4.1 Type I otic capsule dehiscence (OCD) (OC-meningeal interface). (**a**, **b**) Superior semicircular canal dehiscence (SSCD); (**c**, **d**) Posterior semicircular canal dehiscence (PSCD)

In air conduction (sounds frequencies ranging from 500 to 2000 Hz) the perilymph-driven hydraulic acoustic pressure, which normally reaches the round window, dissipates toward the dehiscence where a drop in impedance occurs, resulting in increased audiometric thresholds [11–13]. According to Iversen and Rabbit [11], the resultant biomechanical phenomena in the membranous SC can lead to an opposite neural vestibular response at the level of the cupula depending on the frequency of the stimulus, with a decrease and increase of the afferent firing rate for low and high frequencies, respectively. In bone conduction, the decrease in impedance favors the gradient between the vestibular and tympanic ramps and leads to a lowering of the thresholds. Application of a loud sound or pressure in the external auditory canal (EAC) potentially gives rise to an excitatory ampullofugal flow in the SSC. In addition, performing a Valsalva maneuver, by pinching the nostrils, classically results in ampullofugal movement [14]. Ampullopetal (inhibitory) flow is then attained by applying negative pressure in the EAC, or from a closed glottis Valsalva maneuver (increased intracranial pressure) (Fig. 4.2a, b).

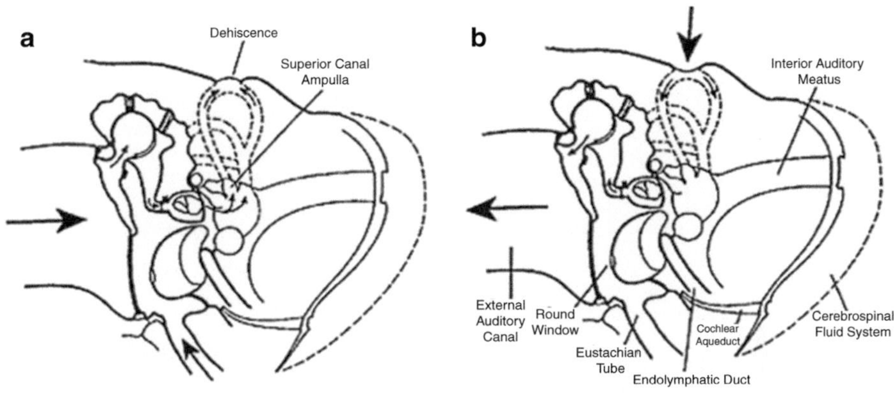

Fig. 4.2 Type I OCD's mechanism: (**a**) Sound, positive pressure in the external canal, and Valsalva maneuver against pinched nostrils evoke pressure changes that result in expansion of the membranous canal with corresponding outward movement in the area of dehiscence. Such pressure within the membranous canal causes ampullofugal deflection of the superior canal cupula that results in excitation of vestibular-nerve afferents innervating the ampulla. (**b**) Valsalva maneuver against a closed glottis, bilateral jugular venous compression, and negative pressure in the external canal result in inward movement in the area of dehiscence of the superior canal. Such pressure leads to ampullopetal deflection of the cupula and inhibition of the superior canal. *Reproduction with permission from Lloyd Minor [14]

Type II: OCD-Vascular

This type (Fig. 4.3) of dehiscence correlates with a contact between the membranous vestibular or cochlear labyrinth and a vascular venous or, less frequently, arterial structure. It includes subtypes IIa, IIb, and IIc.

Subtype IIa

This type involves vasculo-vestibular contact between the membranous SSC and the superior petrous sinus (SPS) (Fig. 4.3a–c). Interestingly, in our reported series [7] there was no evidence of a "true" Tullio phenomenon, including nystagmus elicited by loud sound stimulation, in this group of patients. Moreover, the Valsalva maneuver against the closed glottis did not cause true vertigo except for slight "dizziness" in a few cases. Instead, during this maneuver, an increase in the intensity of their pulsatile tinnitus was constantly reported. This subtype can also integrate SSCD-subarcuate artery dehiscence and SSCD-superior petrosal vein dehiscence variants [15].

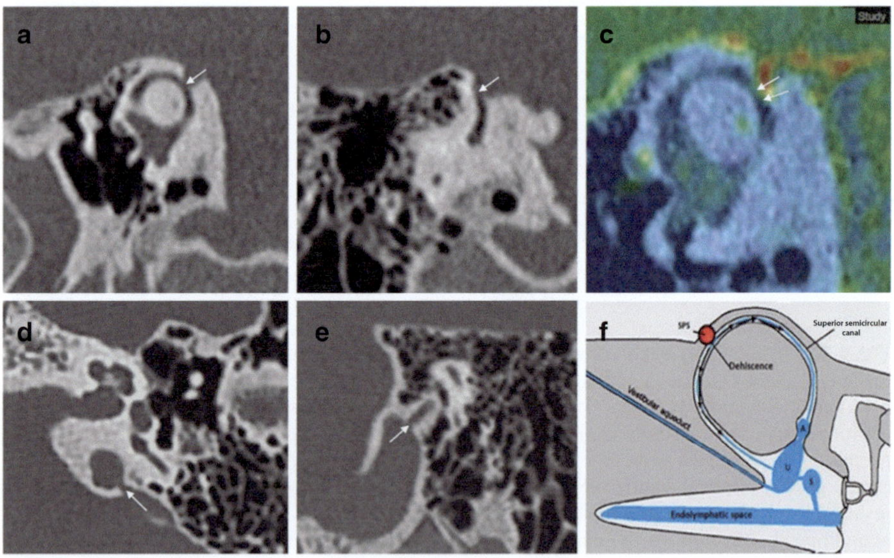

Fig. 4.3 Type II extralabyrinthine OCD (OC-vascular interface). HRCT in the plane of the superior (Poschl) denuded SSC (white arrows) (**a**, **b**), 3T MRI labyrinthine, fused image between 3DT1-weighted contrast enhanced sequence and 3DT2 DRIVE sequence: Mass effect exerted by the Superior Petrosal Sinus (SPS) against the membranous SSC (yellow arrows) (**c**). High-resolution CT (HRCT) in axial plane (**d**), coronal plane (**e**): contact between the denuded VA and the IJV (white arrows). Proposed schematization of the mechanism of vestibulo-vascular TW. Pulsations of the interested vascular wall in intimate contact with the otic capsule membrane would cause non-physiological stimulation of the cochlea and/or the nearest vestibular sensory organs (**f**): Membranous SSC in contact with the SPS

Subtype IIb

This concerns OCD involving the internal jugular vein (IJV) and various vestibular structures. A dehiscence involving the vestibular aqueduct (VA) in contact with the IJV (Fig. 4.3d, e) was the second most prevalent variant series as it was diagnosed in 19 out of 97 patients [7]. This presentation may be bilateral as well. Variant between IJV and PSC was identified in fewer patients. A dehiscence involving the IJV and the cochlear aqueduct (CA) was found to be rarer since in the above-mentioned study only three ears (left-sided) in two patients, age varying from 12 to 53 (1M, 1F) was diagnosed. In subtype IIb OCD, vertigo and/or pulsatile tinnitus induced by exertion were constantly reported. Positional vertigo was also a commonly reported symptom with no evidence for true benign positional paroxysmal vertigo (BPPV) episodes.

Subtype IIc

In this subtype the OCD is localized between the membranous cochlea and the intrapetrous carotid artery [16]. Pulsatile tinnitus exerted by physical exercise synchronous with the peripheral pulse is specific for this variant. The pathomechanism of the inner ear ends structures' stimulation does not seem obvious. However, it can be hypothesized that, compared to type I dehiscences, in type II dehiscences non-physiological audio-vestibular stimulation can be produced by the vascular structure pulsations [17] (Fig. 4.3f). Thus, the vibrations generated by the vascular wall, in contact with the perilymphatic space, will generate symptoms of intensity (pulsating tinnitus and/or dizziness) depending on the location, surface, and importance of any mass effect exerted by the vessel on the labyrinthine structure at the TW level [5].

Type III: OCD-Petrosal Bone

This type encompasses all OCD variants (with to date only three reported subtypes) in which the membranous labyrinth is in direct contact with pneumatic elements of the temporal bone. The difference between this OCD type and a perilymphatic fistula (PLF), which may generate similar symptoms, consists in the integrity of the labyrinthine membrane which is disrupted allowing endolymphatic fluid leak in the case of PLF.

Subtype IIIa

It involves a communication between the cochlea and the facial nerve canal - or cochlear-facial dehiscence (CFD) (Fig. 4.4a, b). In these patients, autophony and slight conductive hearing loss were predominant. Dizziness related to loud sounds

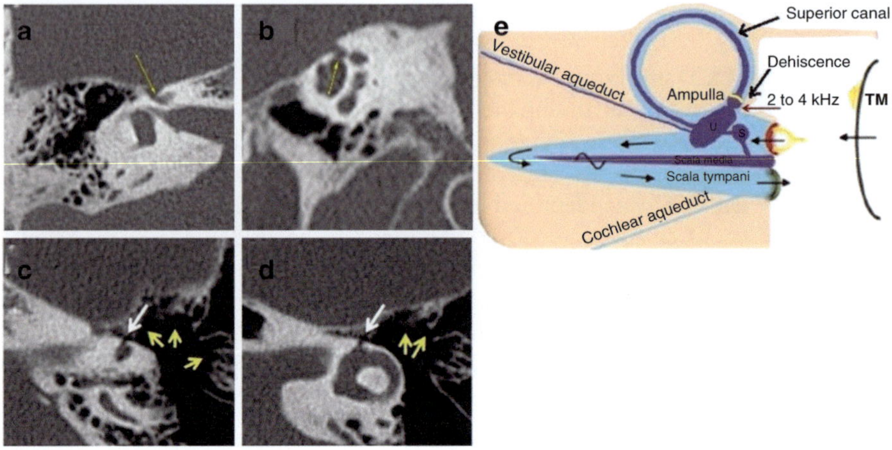

Fig. 4.4 Type III extralabyrinthine OCD (OC-petrosal interface). Right ear cochleo-facial dehiscence (CFD): the second turn of the cochlea dehiscent on the facial nerve canal in its geniculate zone (or the first segment of the facial nerve canal) on axial section or coronal oblique section (**a**, **b**). Ampullary dehiscence (white arrow) localized on the LSC (**c**, **d**). Note the hyper pneumatization of the mastoid and attical regions (yellow arrows). Proposed mechanism's schema in this variant of ampullary dehiscence, which relies on a principle similar to a Helmholtz resonator. T M, tympanic membrane (**e**). *Modified with permission from Rosowski [1] and from Ho [3]

or physical exercise was frequently described. Affected attention, difficulty judging distances, and migraines or chronic equivalents have also been reported frequently [16, 18].

Subtype IIIb

It includes a dehiscent surface between the membranous labyrinth and some hyperpneumatized mastoid air cells freely communicating with the tympanic cavity. This variant was for the first time reported in one 60-year-old male patient [19] in which a strong Tullio phenomenon, associated with a typical down-beating nystagmus indicating a stimulation of the left SSC, was highlighted by a left auditory stimulation at 120 dB between 2 and 4 kHz, although there was no conductive hearing loss. Hyperpneumatization of the petrous bone appears to play an important role in the pathomechanism of this rare OCD. HRCT showed a significant number of large mastoid air cells communicating with the tympanic cavity (Fig. 4.4c, d) and they appear to be in intimate contact with the membranous SSC and the lateral SC (LSC), respectively, via an ampullary located dehiscence of maximum 1.5 mm width. The disposition of these mastoid air cells would act as an acoustic amplifier like the physical principle of a Helmholtz resonator (Fig. 4.4e). Thus, the sound vibrations transmitted via the tympanic cavity and amplified at the mastoid cell/ampullary vestibular membrane interface will directly stimulate the cupula of the concerned SSC. As this hypothesis does not imply a significant acoustic energetic shunt toward the posterior labyrinth, it could therefore explain the absence of conductive hearing loss. Although the lateral SC ampulla also appeared dehiscent (Fig. 4.4c, d), most likely the air cells adjacent to this structure did not communicate with the tympanic cavity, and the above SSC therefore remained asymptomatic.

Subtype IIIc

It includes cochlear (or labyrinthine) dehiscence over the internal auditory canal (IAC), a "near" dehiscence of this subtype is indicated in Fig. 4.6a.

Intralabyrinthine Third Mobile Window-Like Variants

This subgroup corresponds to an abnormal contact between two membranous parts of the same labyrinth being constantly associated with limited inner ear anomalies. For example, dehiscence involving a dilated endolymphatic sac (Fig. 4.5a, b) or a similar presentation involving an EVA in contact with the ampulla of the PSC. Some anatomical variants or other forms of intralabyrinthine TMWA sharing similar

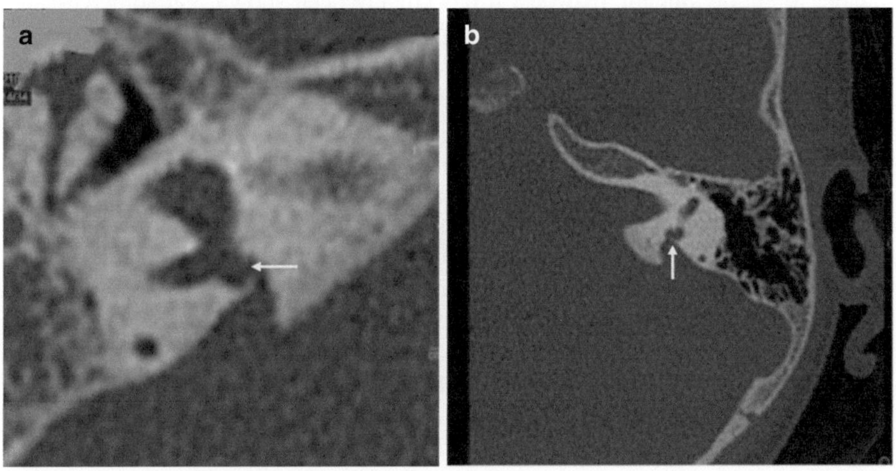

Fig. 4.5 Intralabyrinthine TMWA-like. (**a**), Vestibulo-vestibular dehiscence: between the vestibular aqueduct (VA) widened to 3 mm (white arrow) and the right posterior SC (white arrow) - right ear; a similar variant on the left ear between an enlarged VA and the SSC at the level of the common crus (**b**)

symptoms could be included in this subtype. Pathophysiological mechanisms, including changes in endolymphatic flow caused by the presence of dilatation of the vestibular organs or the presence of intralabyrinthine obstacles (fibrosis, tumors), primary or secondary endolymphatic hydrops, may be included. Matsuda et al. [20] recently reported the case of a congenital dehiscence of the stapes footplate in a patient presenting a sudden right-sided hearing loss and severe vertigo that occurred immediately after nose-blowing. These last-mentioned variants, associated with challenging clinical pictures, allow us to insist and emphasize the importance of careful and collaborative study of audio-vestibular exams and imagery for the sake of finding the diagnosis in certain "unexplained" symptoms. Some authors considered an isolated EVA or enlarged cochlear aqueduct as a distinct TW, since the perilymphatic normal flow transporting the acoustic energy to the cochlear end receptors is disrupted [1]. We agree with this vision although these pathological conditions are not generated by a "true" OCD, but the intimate mechanism seems quite similar to that of a third mobile window. Therefore, we could include these cases in the class "intralabyrinthine TMW" or having a TMW-like mechanism, in addition to intracochlear schwannomas (ICS) that could induce modifications of the endolymphatic flow. Indeed, in a cohort of 19 patients with ICS, Fröhlich et al. measured the cVEMPS thresholds [21]. On the affected side, the threshold was unexpectedly lowered in 21% of patients mimicking the presence of a TMW. The authors suggested that individualizing the management of these patients with a detailed functional evaluation of the labyrinth is paramount for proposing treatment options and predicting outcomes. As a physiological explanation, the authors mentioned changes in endolymphatic flow secondary to tumor obstruction in a similar manner to endolymphatic hydrops. It has already been shown that some cases of endolymphatic hydrops can mimic the TW syndrome with a similar clinical presentation [22–25]. Besides, primary overpressure in the endolymphatic or perilymphatic spaces could explain a limited conductive hearing loss as previously reported [26–28]. It is worth adding here that the notion of "inner ear conductive hearing loss," considered lately as specific to TW lesions, was already used by Muchnik et al. to describe the air bone gap (ABG) observed in some patients with Ménière's disease [26]. Other TMWA-like pathologies may include perilymphatic fistula (PLF). Although it may appear anatomically like type III extralabyrinthine OCD, clinical evidence indicates the involvement of other endolymphatic flows generating nystagmus with different characteristics [8]. Some authors have reconciled PLF with OCD because of similar pathophysiological elements [9, 16]. The explanation for some clinical differences may lie in the fact that in PLF, the vestibular membrane is compromised at this level while in type III, it remains intact. Hence, PLFs have not been considered in our classification as "true TW" because they involve an opening of the membranous labyrinth that allows the leakage of perilymph and/or endolymph with the obvious direct negative impact on the vestibulocochlear micromechanics.

Multiple OCD Localizations

There is more and more evidence that multiple OCD localizations (Fig. 4.6a–c) are not rare. See Table 4.2 for the most common symptoms found in multiple localization series as well as the most common associations on the same ear; the most important audiological and vestibular data are also displayed. Besides an accurate and complete diagnosis, the main challenge in multiple OCDs in the same ear is to select an appropriate therapeutic strategy for patients with disabling symptoms. It also involves establishing the order in which these multiples dehiscences should be treated. At the time of publication, according to our knowledge there are no available data or consensus in the literature to council practitioners about the approach of multiple OCDs.

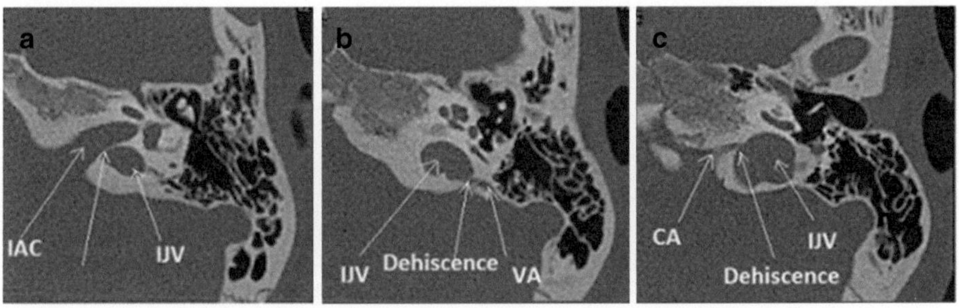

Fig. 4.6 Multiple localization OCD: high riding left IJV at the origin of two type II of OCD. Near dehiscent jugular bulb in the IAC (White arrow), a thin bone lamina is remaining (**a**); Dehiscence between IJV interface and VA (**b**); Dehiscence between IJV interface and CA (**c**). *IJV* internal jugular vein, *IAC* internal auditory canal, *VA* vestibular aqueduct, *CA* cochlear aqueduct

Table 4.2 Clinical characteristics of patients with multiple localization OCD (all OCD were ipsilateral)

Age	Ear	1st OCD dehiscence	2nd OCD dehiscence	Symptoms	Audiometry findings	oVEMPs	oVEMPs
16	RE	PSC-IJV	CFD	Tinnitus with head movement Noise-induced vertigo	Mild Hearing loss ABG = 5 (RE)	Bilateral threshold (x2)	Higher amplitude (RE)
37	RE	SSC-SPS	CFD	Pulsatile tinnitus (RE)	Normal	Higher amplitude (LE)	Absent
48	LE	SSC-Meningeal	CFD	Noise-induced autophonia pulsatile tinnitus (LE)	Bilateral low-frequency hearing loss ABG = 5 bilateral	Higher amplitude (LE) Threshold 60 dB (LE)	Higher amplitude (LE) Threshold 60 dB (LE)
73	RE	SSC-Meningeal	CFD	Decreased hearing Tinnitus Autophonia Cough-induced vertigo	ABG = 30 dB (RE)	Higher amplitude (RE) Threshold 60 dB (RE)	Higher amplitude (RE) Absent (LE)
68	LE	SSC-Meningeal	Cochlea-Carotid	Decreased hearing	Mixed HL ABG = 50 dB (RE) SNHL (LE)	NA	NA
59	LE	IJN-Vestibular aqueduct	CFD	Tinnitus (tapping) (LE) Instability and vertigo	ABG = 10 dB (RE) 20 dB (LE)	Normal	NA
67	LE	IJV-Vestibular aqueduct	IJV-IAC	Pulsatile tinnitus (RE)	Normal	Normal (RE) Absent (LE)	NA
46	LE	SSC-Meningeal	CFD	Bilateral HL Tinnitus (RE) Effort-induced vertigo	ABG = 20 dB (RE) Bilateral SNHL	Absent (RE) Decreased threshold 60 dB (LE)	Absent (RE) Decreased threshold 70 dB (LE)
72	RE	SSC-Meningeal	IJV-Vestibular aqueduct	Autophonia Pulsatile tinnitus Effort-induced vertigo	Bilateral SNHL	Threshold 50 dB (RE) Normal (LE)	NA
13	LE	IJV-Vestibular aqueduct	IJV-Cochlear aqueduct	Effort-induced vertigo	Normal	Normal	NA

CT-OCD or Not Identified OCD (NIOCD)

As introduced by Shuknecht [10] at the early age of deafness surgery, Wackym et al. [29, 30] reported patients with a group of symptoms suggestive of OCD, even if the imaging was negative. In these patients, the presence of a possible OCD may also be indicated by the presence of cervical or ocular VEMPs below the normal threshold. According to these newly described (or future) variants of OCD, performing temporal bone HRCT with infra-millimetric slice thickness as recommended can be of great benefit in the diagnostic process in such symptomatic patients, and in search of all possible types of OCD [14, 31].

A particular subtype that can be included here is the "Near Dehiscence Syndrome" (NDS). As described by several authors [32, 33] the third mobile window syndrome may be present, even partially, in the case of significant bone thinning of confirmed SSC either by HRCT or when no frank dehiscence was found intraoperatively. Although NDS has not yet been reported at other sites, physiologically there is no reason to think that this could not be present elsewhere.

Perspectives

Superior semicircular dehiscence has been the subject of numerous articles codifying its surgical management [34]. Concomitantly, with a better understanding of the OCD pathophysiology, new therapeutic procedures have emerged to diminish operative risks. Creighton et al. described the case of a patient with a SSCD who benefited from an endoscopic "underwater" procedure in a balanced salt solution [35]. This attempt was aimed at limiting the risk of PLF by injecting fluid into the mastoid, as a counter pressure method during the plugging procedure. From our perspective, the major principle to be considered in the future for the treatment of TW lesions would be to find the most appropriate methods that aim at reducing the abnormal transmission of sound vibrations through the abnormal window to the vestibular and/or to cochlear end organs, without excluding any highly functional labyrinthine segment. A step forward would possibly be the manufacturing of a physical or a numerical semicircular model, which would allow for a better pathophysiological approach and management of these challenging pathologies. With the actual constraints and ethical considerations in clinical medical research, this method could be promising. Such a model could allow researchers to obtain a "near real" simulation of volumetric and pressure changes in the endolymphatic system generated by the various surgical procedures proposed in this pathology. This could avoid certain negative postoperative outcomes seen in a number of patients and, most likely, new surgical techniques or improvement of existing ones. Furthermore, it may be the ideal way to manage and possibly resolve certain complex pathophysiological and treatment dilemmas, such as therapeutic choice in multiple OCD locations.

Conclusions

Based on anatomo-radiologic data of the inner ear structures involved, a classification of TMWA is proposed in this chapter (Fig. 4.7a, b). Although some systematizations of this pathology have been proposed previously, we believe that this new classification that considers not only the anatomical structures involved in the TW interface, but also their precise topographic localization, would lead to a better further understanding of the underlying pathophysiological mechanisms of this pathology. Moreover, the present classification could allow ENT specialists, researchers,

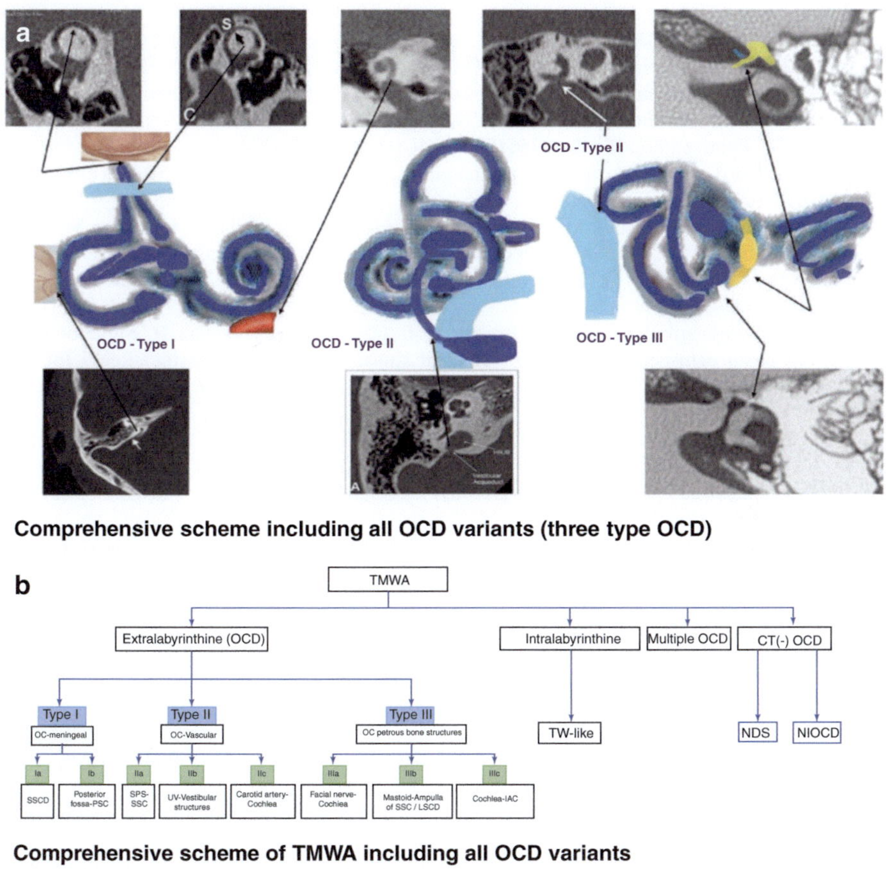

Fig. 4.7 (**a**) 3 type extra labyrinthine OCD classification in images—correspondence between imagery and anatomic variants. (**b**) Comprehensive algorithm of third mobile window (TMWA) anomalies classification. *IAC* internal auditory canal, *IJV* internal jugular vein, *LSCD* lateral semicircular canal, *OC* otic capsule, *OCD* otic capsule dehiscence, *SSCD* superior semicircular canal dehiscence, *NDS* near dehiscence syndrome, *NIOCD* non-identified otic capsule dehiscence, *SPS* superior petrosal sinus, *PSC* posterior semicircular canal, *SSC* superior semicircular canal, *TW* third window

radiologists, and/or clinical audiologists to better understand some OCD variants and related TMWA, as well as to imagine possible innovative therapeutic approaches in the future. In some OCD variants, especially in those involving vascular structures (Type II OCD), MRI has greatly contributed to a better visualization of the anatomical elements in contact at the level of the TW, which has been an essential element for the current classification and for the development of new endovascular treatment techniques.

References

1. Merchant SN, Rosowski JJ. Conductive hearing loss caused by third-window lesions of the inner ear. Otol Neurotol. 2008;29(3):282–9. https://doi.org/10.1097/MAO.0b013e318161ab24.
2. Ho ML, Moonis G, Halpin CF, Curtin HD. Spectrum of third window abnormalities: semicircular canal dehiscence and beyond. AJNR Am J Neuroradiol. 2017;38(1):2–9. https://doi.org/10.3174/ajnr.A4922. PMID: 27561833; PMCID: PMC7963676.
3. Ho ML. Third window lesions. Neuroimaging Clin N Am. 2019;29(1):57–92. https://doi.org/10.1016/j.nic.2018.09.005.
4. Scarpa A, Ralli M, Cassandro C, Gioacchini FM, Greco A, Di Stadio A, Cavaliere M, Troisi D, de Vincentiis M, Cassandro E. Inner-ear disorders presenting with air-bone gaps: a review. J Int Adv Otol. 2020;16(1):111–6. https://doi.org/10.5152/iao.2020.7764. PMID: 32401207; PMCID: PMC7224429.
5. Ionescu E, Reynard P, Coudert A, Roiban L, Boudrigua AL, Thai-Van H. Superior semicircular canal dehiscence by superior petrosal sinus: proposal for classification. J Int Adv Otol. 2021;17(1):35–41. https://doi.org/10.5152/iao.2020.9384. PMID: 33605219; PMCID: PMC7901425.
6. Waldeck S, Lanfermann H, von Falck C, Froelich MF, Chapot R, Brockmann M, Overhoff D. New classification of superior semicircular canal dehiscence in HRCT. PLoS One. 2022;17(1):e0262758. https://doi.org/10.1371/journal.pone.0262758. PMID: 35051221; PMCID: PMC8775191.
7. Reynard P, Idriss S, Ltaief-Boudrigua A, Bertholon P, Pirvan A, Truy E, Thai-Van H, Ionescu EC. Proposal for a unitary anatomo-clinical and radiological classification of third mobile window abnormalities. Front Neurol. 2022;12:792545. https://doi.org/10.3389/fneur.2021.792545. PMID: 35087471; PMCID: PMC8786803.
8. Helmchen C, Gehrking E, Gottschalk S, et al. Persistence of perilymph fistula mechanism in a completely paretic posterior semicircular canal. J Neurol Neurosurg Psychiatry. 2005;76:280–2. https://doi.org/10.1136/jnnp.2004.038083.
9. Weinreich WM, Carey JP. Perilymphatic fistulas and superior semi-circular canal dehiscence syndrome. Adv Otorhinolaryngol. 2019;82:93–100. https://doi.org/10.1159/000490276.
10. Schuknecht HF. Otologic mystery. Am J Otol. 1987;8:182–3.
11. Iversen MM, Rabbitt RD. Wave mechanics of the vestibular semicircular canals. Biophys J. 2017;113:1133–49. https://doi.org/10.1016/j.bpj.2017.08.001.
12. Iversen MM, Rabbitt RD. Biomechanisms of third window syndrome. Front Neurol. 2020;11:891. https://doi.org/10.3389/fneur.2020.00891.
13. Grieser BJ, Kleiser L, Obrist D. Identifying mechanisms behind the tullio phenomenon: a computational study based on first principles. J Assoc Res Otolaryngol. 2016;17:103–18. https://doi.org/10.1007/s10162-016-0553-0.
14. Ward BK, Carey JP, Minor LB. Superior canal dehiscence syndrome: lessons from the first 20 years. Front Neurol. 2017;8:177. https://doi.org/10.3389/fneur.2017.00177.

15. Lund AD, Palacios SD. Carotid artery-cochlear dehiscence: a review. Laryngoscope. 2011;121(12):2658–60. https://doi.org/10.1002/lary.22391.
16. Wackym PA, Balaban CD, Zhang P, Siker DA, Hundal JS. Third window syndrome: surgical management of cochlea-facial nerve dehiscence. Front Neurol. 2019;10:1281. https://doi.org/10.3389/fneur.2019.01281.
17. Liu Z, Bi W, Li J, Li Q, Dong C, Zhao P, et al. Superior semicircular canal dehiscence in relation to the superior petrosal sinus: a potential cause of pulsatile tinnitus. Clin Radiol. 2015;70:943–7. https://doi.org/10.1016/j.crad.2015.04.017.
18. Wackym PA, Mackay-Promitas HT, Demirel S, Gianoli GJ, Gizzi MS, Carter DM, Siker DA. Comorbidities confounding the outcomes of surgery for third window syndrome: outlier analysis. Laryngosc Investig Otolaryngol. 2017;2(5):225–53. https://doi.org/10.1002/lio2.89. PMID: 29094067; PMCID: PMC5654938.
19. Ionescu EC, Al Tamami N, Neagu A, Ltaief-Boudrigua A, Gallego S, Hermann R, Truy E, Thai-Van H. Superior semicircular canal ampullae dehiscence as part of the spectrum of the third window abnormalities: a case study. Front Neurol. 2017;8:683. https://doi.org/10.3389/fneur.2017.00683. PMID: 29312118; PMCID: PMC5742101.
20. Matsuda H, Tanzawa Y, Sekine T, Matsumura T, Saito S, Shindo S, et al. Congenital Membranous stapes footplate producing episodic pressure-induced perilymphatic fistula symptoms. Front Neurol. 2020;11:585747. https://doi.org/10.3389/fneur.2020.585747.
21. Fröhlich L, Curthoys IS, Kösling S, Obrist D, Rahne T, Plontke SK. Cervical and ocular vestibular-evoked myogenic potentials in patients with intracochlear schwannomas. Front Neurol. 2020;11:549817. https://doi.org/10.3389/fneur.2020.549817.
22. Young YH, Wu CC, Wu CH. Augmentation of vestibular evoked myogenic potentials: an indication for distended saccular hydrops. Laryngoscope. 2002;112:509–12. https://doi.org/10.1097/00005537-200203000-00019.
23. Taylor RL, Zagami AS, Gibson WP, Black DA, Watson SR, Halmagyi MG, et al. Vestibular evoked myogenic potentials to sound and vibration: characteristics in vestibular migraine that enable separation from Menière's disease. Cephalalgia. 2012;32(3):213–25.
24. Wen MH, Cheng PW, Young YH. Augmentation of ocular vestibular-evoked myogenic potentials via bone-conducted vibration stimuli in ménière disease. Otolaryngol Neck Surg. 2012;146:797–803. https://doi.org/10.1177/0194599811433982.
25. Manzari L, Tedesco AR, Burgess AM, Curthoys IS. Ocular and cervical vestibular-evoked myogenic potentials to bone conducted vibration in Ménière's disease during quiescence vs during acute attacks. Clin Neurophysiol. 2010;121:1092–101. https://doi.org/10.1016/j.clinph.2010.02.003.
26. Muchnik C, Hildesheimer M, Rubinstein M, Arenberg IK. Low frequency air-bone gap in Menière's disease without middle ear pathology. A preliminary report. Am J Otol. 1989;10:1–4.
27. Yetişer S, Kertmen M. Cochlear conductive hearing loss in patients with Meniere's disease. Kulak Burun Bogaz Ihtis Derg. 2007;17:18–21.
28. Sugimoto S, Yoshida T, Teranishi M, Okazaki Y, Naganawa S, Sone M. The relationship between endolymphatic hydrops in the vestibule and low-frequency air-bone gaps. Laryngoscope. 2018;128:1658–62. https://doi.org/10.1002/lary.26898.
29. Wackym PA, Wood SJ, Siker DA, Carter DM. Otic capsule dehiscence syndrome: superior semicircular canal dehiscence syndrome with no radiographically visible dehiscence. Ear Nose Throat J. 2015;94:8–24. https://doi.org/10.1177/014556131509400802.
30. Wackym PA, Agrawal Y, Ikezono T, Balaban CD. Editorial: third window syndrome. Front Neurol. 2021;12:704095. https://doi.org/10.3389/fneur.2021.704095.
31. Curtin HD. Imaging of conductive hearing loss with a normal tympanic membrane. AJR Am J Roentgenol. 2016;206:49–56. https://doi.org/10.2214/AJR.15.15060.
32. Ward BK, Wenzel A, Ritzl EK, Gutierrez-Hernandez S, Della Santina CC, Minor LB, et al. Near-dehiscence: clinical findings in patients with thin bone over the superior semicircular canal. Otol Neurotol. 2013;34(8):1421–8. https://doi.org/10.1097/MAO.0b013e318287efe6.

33. Baxter M, McCorkle C, Trevino Guajardo C, Zuniga MG, Carter AM, Della Santina CC, Minor LB, Carey JP, Ward BK. Clinical and physiologic predictors and postoperative outcomes of near dehiscence syndrome. Otol Neurotol. 2019;40(2):204–12. https://doi.org/10.1097/MAO.0000000000002077. PMID: 30570606; PMCID: PMC6326856.
34. Mau C, Kamal N, Badeti S, Reddy R, Ying YM, Jyung RW, et al. Superior semicircular canal dehiscence: diagnosis and management. J Clin Neurosci. 2018;48:58–65. https://doi.org/10.1016/j.jocn.2017.11.019.
35. Creighton F Jr, Barber SR, Ward BK, Sharon JD, Carey JP. Underwater endoscopic repair of superior canal dehiscence. Otol Neurotol. 2020;41:560. https://doi.org/10.1097/MAO.0000000000002277.

Chapter 5
The Otologic Mimicker: Vestibular and Auditory Symptoms

Mark Frilling and Sarah Mowry

Introduction

It is said that third mobile window disorders (TMWD) are the great otologic mimicker, presenting with vestibular and auditory symptoms mimicking some of the more common otologic disorders making the accurate diagnosis of a TMWD all the more difficult. This chapter will help differentiate the classic symptoms of common and less common otologic disorders to help the clinician make accurate diagnoses. We will discuss the classic findings and symptoms found in a patient with a TMWD and the testing that will assist in ruling out other disorders to make the correct diagnosis.

Vestibular Symptoms

Without exception, history taking is the single most important diagnostic tool for a patient that presents with vertigo or dizziness. An accurate diagnosis can be obtained 80% of the time based on history alone [1, 2]. Some of the important aspects of the

M. Frilling
Department of Otolaryngology, University Hospitals Cleveland Medical Center, Cleveland, OH, USA
e-mail: Mark.frilling@uhhospitals.org

S. Mowry (✉)
Department of Otolaryngology, University Hospitals Cleveland Medical Center, Cleveland, OH, USA

Department of Otolaryngology, Case Western Reserve University School of Medicine, Cleveland, OH, USA
e-mail: Sarah.Mowry@uhhospitals.org

G. J. Gianoli, P. Thomson (eds.), *Third Mobile Window Syndrome of the Inner Ear*, https://doi.org/10.1007/978-3-031-16586-3_5

history to ascertain are description of events, duration, frequency, triggers, changes in hearing, exacerbating factors, and what resolves the events. True vertigo is generally broken down into central vs. peripheral. Other common etiologies can cause vertigo-like symptoms including cardiac, neurologic, metabolic disorders, or medication side effects that patients may perceive as vertigo. Physical exam and further vestibular testing can help elucidate the true underlying etiology of a patient's vertigo.

Subjective Findings

Possibly the most integral part of a patient's history is the description of their "dizzy" episodes. Dizziness can have varying meanings to different people. Is it a true room spinning vertigo with a sensation of movement indicating a likely peripheral etiology? Or is it a disequilibrium, "feels like my balance is off," that may suggest a central etiology? Central disorders classically include retrocochlear or cerebellar dysfunction/lesions. Peripheral vertigo can be seen in numerous conditions including unilateral vestibular weakness, benign paroxysmal positional vertigo (BPPV), Mal de Débarquement syndrome, Ménière's Disease, or TMWD. Patients describing lightheadedness/presyncope or vague "mental fog" suggests a non-vestibular disorder and more of a systemic etiology including arrhythmias, cardiogenic, anemia or poor circulation, neurogenic, thyroid issues, orthostatic hypotension, etc. A thorough non-vestibular workup should be performed in these patients by their primary care provider. In the patient that describes rotary vertigo, their description of the events should include queries regarding duration, frequency, and associated symptoms such as changes in hearing, aural fullness, and headaches. Triggering or exacerbating factors are particularly important to explicate such as movement induced symptoms, noise induced symptoms, Valsalva triggers, recent upper respiratory infections, stress, high-salt diet, allergies, barotrauma, or weather changes. Equally important is what helps to abort the episodes: eye fixation, going to a dark quiet room, or medications.

TMWD represent areas of dehiscence of the bony labyrinth or inner ear (including the round and oval windows) that creates a characteristic vertigo triggered when the area of dehiscence is subjected to pressure change. External pressure can be presented in different forms. Sound-induced vertigo is the classically described Tullio phenomenon while pressure-induced vertigo from pneumatic otoscopy describes the Hennebert sign or "fistula sign." Both of these signs result in a vertical nystagmus first described by Minor and colleagues in 1998 with respect to superior semicircular canal dehiscence (SSCD) [3]. Tullio phenomenon was described by an Italian biologist, Pietro Tullio, in 1929 when he discovered that a fistula created in the horizontal semicircular canal of pigeons resulted in the birds quickly turning their heads in the contralateral direction when exposed to loud sounds [4]. This first became clinically relevant when Hennebert made the connection between pressure-induced vestibular changes and inner ear dysfunction in patients with congenital syphilis. Later temporal bones of syphilitic patients were found to have gummatous osteomyelitis and fistulas of the labyrinth [5]. Vertigo in TMWDs with meningeal exposure, as occurs in SSCD, can also be triggered by a Valsalva maneuver or any acute change in intracranial pressure. Provocative or exacerbating factors of a patient's vertigo are particular symptoms that may clue a provider into a possible TMWD diagnosis.

Vestibular symptoms from SSCD were divided into four categories by Minor with associated prevalence [6]:

- Tullio phenomenon, eye movement evoked by sound: 82%.
- Valsalva-induced, eye movement evoked by internal pressure: 75%.
- Hennebert sign, eye movement evoked by external pressure on the tympanic membrane: 45%.
- Sound-induced head tilt in the plane of the affected canal: 20%.

In addition to episodic vertigo, chronic disequilibrium is a common complaint of patients suffering from a TMWD—affecting up to 76% in one case series [7]. The disequilibrium may or may not worsen with sound or external pressure. Patients often have a difficult time describing their vestibular symptoms, which can be quite debilitating. The wide variety of patient descriptions of vestibular symptoms in TMWD is one of the reasons it is called the otologic mimicker.

Physical Exam Findings

Vestibular examination can help to differentiate TMWD from other common vestibular disorders. Most patients with small to moderately sized TMWD will demonstrate normal and symmetric vestibulo-ocular reflexes on head thrust testing and the absence of nystagmus after horizontal or vertical head shaking. Defects greater than or equal to 5 mm in SSCD will start to show nystagmus on head thrust testing [3]. Spontaneous nystagmus is not typically seen in TMWD although it has been described in rare cases due to large defects in the superior semicircular canal (SSC) that allow intracranial pressure variations to create a pulsatile stimulus [8].

Findings characteristic of a peripheral vestibular origin include spontaneous nystagmus with the head still, decreased nystagmus with visual fixation, and/or increased nystagmus when fixation is absent [9]. Infrared video goggles or Frenzel glasses can help facilitate testing, allowing the practitioner to better assess nystagmus characteristics by preventing visual fixation. Misalignment of the eyes, i.e., strabismus, while not a vestibular disorder can certainly produce symptoms of vertigo/dizziness and may be apparent with use of Frenzel lenses. Ophthalmology referral is indicated for such patients.

A Dix-Hallpike test should be performed on all patients presenting with vestibular symptoms to assess for possible BPPV, the most common cause of peripheral vertigo. Testing should be performed even if symptoms appear non-positional. The Dix-Hallpike maneuver is performed by rotating the patient's head 30–45° towards the ear being tested, starting in the sitting position and quickly placing the patient in

Table 5.1 Vestibular mimickers

Signs/symptoms of TWS	Differential diagnosis
Vertigo/dizziness	BPPV; migraine; Ménière's disease; labyrinthitis; AIED; mass lesions (vestibular schwannoma); TWS; Mal de Débarquement; central etiology (stroke/TIA)
Tullio's phenomenon (vertigo with loud sounds)	Ménière's disease; otosyphilis; TWS; idiopathic; vestibulocochlear fibrosis; postsurgical; lyme disease; otosclerosis
Hennebert's sign (pressure induced vertigo through the EAC)	Ménière's disease; otosyphilis; TWS
Visual-spacial disorientation	Migraine; multiple sclerosis; multisensory balance dysfunction; cognitive dysfunction (Alzheimer's disease)
Valsalva induced vertigo	Vertebrobasilar insufficiency; TWS

the supine position. A positive test will evoke a geotropic rotary nystagmus indicating otolith presence in the testing ear's posterior semicircular canal. The test can conveniently be transitioned into a canalith repositioning maneuver (i.e., Epley maneuver) to reposition the otoliths out of the posterior SCC.

Table 5.1 outlines common vestibular symptoms associated with TMWD and a possible differential diagnosis for each symptom. Exploration of diagnostic vestibular testing related to TMWD can be explored in Chap. 11.

Auditory Symptoms

As in the patient presenting with vestibular complaints, a thorough history is the centerpiece to working up a patient presenting with auditory symptoms. The presence of otalgia, otorrhea, tinnitus, aural fullness, hearing loss, and fluctuation of hearing must all be explored in the patient interview. The duration and frequency of symptoms, a history of ear infections or prior ear surgeries, exposure to ototoxic medications or loud noise, and a history of head trauma are additional and essential aspects of the history to obtain. A tuning fork exam can be performed in the office, but ultimately a full audiogram should be performed.

Subjective Findings

Auditory findings in TMWD, like vestibular findings, can vary widely. Common symptoms often described by TMWD patients include autophony, hearing internal bodily movements, aural fullness, hearing loss, hyperacusis, and pulsatile tinnitus. In addition to hearing one's voice, some patients may describe being able to hear their eyeballs move or their feet hit the floor; this description differs from the autophony observed in patulous eustachian tube dysfunction (ETD) that is exacerbated by respiration and correlates with coordinated tympanic membrane movement on exam. Patients with negative pressure ETD sometimes also describe autophony but this is differentiated from TMWD by retracted tympanic membrane or middle ear effusion on physical exam and abnormal tympanogram findings. Aural fullness is a common complaint in a number of disorders including low frequency sensorineural hearing loss (LFSNHL), Ménière's disease, ETD, and temporomandibular myofascial disorders. TMWDs with either meningeal or vascular bony dehiscence can both present with pulsatile tinnitus, which can also present in vascular lesions (arteriovenous malformation (AVM)/arteriovenous fistula (AVF)), idiopathic intracranial hypertension (IIH), glomus tumors, venous hum, sigmoid sinus diverticulum, and carotid pseudoaneurysm. Appropriate imaging modalities will help to differentiate these underlying etiologies. Conductive hyperacusis including a feeling or hearing the pulse in the affected ear, has been described in up to 39% of patients with SSCD [10]. Ultimately, it is less common for TMWD to present with auditory symptoms alone without any coexisting vestibular complaints.

Physical Exam Findings

Patients with TMWD will classically demonstrate a conductive hearing loss on tuning fork examination with a 512 Hz Weber test lateralizing to the ipsilateral ear [3, 11]. 54% of patients will demonstrate a vertical–torsional nystagmus on pneumatic otoscopy [10]. On otoscopy, in an absence of a history of ear disease, the external auditory canal, tympanic membrane, and mesotympanic space will appear normal. An abnormal otoscopic examination should lead the practitioner down the diagnostic pathway for the visualized lesion.

Table 5.2 outlines common audiologic symptoms associated with TMWD and a possible differential diagnosis for each symptom. Diagnostic audiometric findings associated with TMWD are further explored in Chap. 11.

Table 5.2 Audiologic mimickers

Signs/symptoms	Differential diagnosis
Autophony	CSOM, ETD; TMWD
Aural fullness	LFSNHL, endolymphatic hydrops/Ménière's disease, ETD, temporomandibular myofascial disorders
Pulsatile tinnitus	Vascular lesions (AVM/AVF), IIH, glomus tumors, venous hum, sigmoid sinus diverticulum, carotid pseudoaneurysm; TMWD
Conductive hearing loss	Any disorder affecting the EAC, TM or ossicular chain including otosclerosis, ETD, etc.

Imaging

The next step in the workup of a patient presenting with audiovestibular symptoms concerning for a TMWD is to obtain a high-resolution temporal bone CT scan, specifically with direct axial images, accompanied by Poschl and Stenvers reconstructions. This remains the gold standard in identifying the location of dehiscence. MRI is typically normal in SSCD but may be useful when evaluating for concurrent CSF leak or meningoencephalocele and in ruling out retrocochlear pathology [12]. Further discussion of the imaging of TMWD can be found in Chap. 12.

Differential Diagnosis for the Otologic Mimicker

Otologic Mimickers

Benign Paroxysmal Positional Vertigo (BPPV)

BPPV is the most common vestibular disorder with an incidence of 10–64 per 100,000, with an increasing 38% incidence with each decade of life [13, 14]. The disorder may be even more common than once suspected, with one study showing positive results in 9% of randomly selected geriatric patients undergoing positional testing with no former diagnosis of BPPV [15]. Vertigo provoked by position changes with quick resolution with eye fixation is the hallmark description of BPPV. 94% of cases involve the posterior semicircular canal [16]. Vertigo is typically triggered with movement towards the affected ear. A diagnostic Dix-Hallpike maneuver will incite an ipsi-directional torsional nystagmus after a short latency, resolves in 10–30 s, and diminishes with repeated positional testing (i.e., fatigues) [17]. Canalith repositioning maneuvers (i.e., Epley maneuver in posterior SSC involvement) are highly effective in treating the current episode, however does not prevent recurrent episodes, which occurs at a rate of approximately 15% per year [18]. The other semicircular canals can certainly be affected by dislodged otoconia as well. Horizontal canal BPPV is seen in up to 10% patients with positional vertigo and can be provoked with a head roll maneuver. Superior canal BPPV is considered quite rare, affecting less than 2% of positional vertigo patients. It is important to note that patients can have multiple affected canals simultaneously and if the posterior canal CRM does not resolve the symptoms, the patient should be tested for horizontal or superior canal BPPV in addition to expanding the differential diagnosis of the vertigo symptom.

BPPV and TMWD share the symptom of vertigo. The vertigo for both disorders may be provoked by head movement and in both disorders there can be a sense of disequilibrium between the vertigo attacks. However, BPPV is by definition positional and has characteristic head movements that provoke the vertigo—rolling over in bed, looking up (top shelf vertigo), and bringing the head up from a dependent position. TMWD patients do not often have a specific positioning maneuver that will induce vertigo but may describe dizziness with rapid head turning. In posterior canal BPPV, the vertigo and characteristic nystagmus will be induced by the

Dix-Hallpike maneuver. In TMWD the positioning maneuvers do not produce nystagmus but the patient may report a sense of "dizziness" when they move from supine to the seated upright position but will not have an "unwinding nystagmus" as seen with pcBPPV. Additionally, TMWD are often accompanied by auditory symptoms which are not seen in BPPV. A diagnosis of BPPV is a purely clinical diagnosis based on exam findings whereas additional diagnostic testing is required to identify the TMWD diagnosis. Failure to provoke nystagmus with positioning testing should prompt the practitioner to expand their differential diagnosis. However, one should keep in mind that the presence of BPPV or TMWD does not preclude the concomitant existence of the other.

Eustachian Tube Dysfunction

Eustachian tube dysfunction (ETD) is very common and accounts for more than 2 million patient visits per year in the adult population in the United States alone [19]; in pediatric patients, ETD is strongly associated with chronic otitis media with effusion [20]. Disorders of the Eustachian tube (ETD) can be classified as either obstructive or patulous, and both have significant symptomatic overlap with each other and TMWDs. ETD often manifests as reports of aural fullness and pressure, autophony, and muffled hearing.

Patients with obstructive ETD experience symptoms due to failure of equalization of the middle ear pressure to barometric pressure. The dynamic opening of the ET orifice in the nasopharynx allows air to travel from the nose to the middle ear; mucosal edema within the ET or anatomic variants of the ET, or both, result in failure to replenish the middle ear aeration. Failure to ventilate the middle ear cleft results in retraction of the tympanic membrane due to absorption of the nitrogen by the mucosa of the ear. Acute negative pressure on the TM is painful, as reported by those who experience barochallenged ETD (pain with air travel or scuba diving). Patients may report the need for frequent Valsalva maneuvers to forcefully open the ET in the nasopharynx and push air into the middle ear cleft.

Treatment of obstructive ETD revolves around mitigation of mucosal edema with topical steroids, ventilation tube placement, or mechanically crushing the tissue with balloon dilation. Anatomic variability can contribute to obstructive ETD but is not amenable to treatment medically or surgically. Obstructive ETD can mimic TMWDs with regard to aural fullness and muffled hearing. However, obstructive ETD patients do not experience episodic vertigo and have stigmata of chronic tympanic membrane retraction on otoscopy. Audiometrically, both groups may have a conductive hearing loss with preserved cochlear function; however, obstructive ETD patients will have abnormal tympanograms with pressures in negative excess of –150 dPa (Type C) [21].

Patulous ETD refers to an ET which is "too open." Although the atmospheric pressure is equal between the middle ear and nasopharynx, patients with patulous ETD report muffled hearing, fullness and autophony. The autophony in patulous ETD is often particularly prominent with breathing, and patients report hearing and feeling their breath in their ear. This symptom is particularly bothersome to many patients and can sometimes be mitigated by lying flat and using gravity to pull the ET orifice closed; consequently it is important to observe the TM for respiratory movement in both the seated and the supine positions. The aural symptoms of patulous ETD can be improved by forceful sniffing to apply negative pressure to the ET orifice for temporary closure. However, the symptoms recur quickly in many patients and they may develop a habit of sniffing. Patulous ETD can occur in patients who experience a significant and rapid weight loss, such as after bariatric surgery [22]. Treatment for patulous ETD is focused on increasing tissue mass at the ET orifice in the nasopharynx and may involve irritative solutions applied via the nose (premarin nose drops) or injection of material into the torus tubarius to increase tissue bulk.

As with obstructive ETD, the symptom overlap with TMWD is considerable as both patient groups will experience aural fullness, autophony, and muffled hearing. However unlike TMWD patients, patulous patients do not report episodic vertigo, nor sound or pressure-induced symptoms. On exam, patulous patients have a normal appearing tympanic membrane on cursory evaluation; however, on closer inspection the tympanic membrane can be seen to move with the respiratory cycle. A small paper patch can be placed on the TM in the office in the patient suspected of having patulous ETD which often improves or resolves the symptoms; the added weight on the TM will not resolve the symptoms for patients with TMWD.

Ménière's Disease

Ménière's Disease (MD) is a commonly recognized cause of peripheral vertigo. Incidence ranges from 7 to 515 per 100,000 based on several studies depending on the country [23]. The classic episodic symptoms include aural fullness, fluctuating low to mid-frequency sensorineural hearing loss (SNHL), roaring tinnitus, and rotatory vertigo. Only one third of cases present with this full quadrad of symptoms, however [24]. Ménière's disease may be due to overproduction or inadequate absorption of the endolymph within the membranous labyrinth, although a full understanding of the pathophysiology is not known. In an acute attack, vertigo lasts several minutes to several hours followed by a post-vertiginous disequilibrium. Patients generally report normal balance function between episodes.

Diagnostic criteria has been set forth by the American Academy of Otolaryngology-Head and Neck Surgery (AAO-HNS) Foundation which distinguishes between definite and probable MD [25, 26]. MD is characterized by two or more spontaneous attacks of vertigo, each lasting 20 min to 12–24 h and fluctuating aural symptoms (hearing loss, tinnitus, or fullness) in the affected ear, and exclusion of other causes with testing. Definite MD has the additional criteria of audiometrically documented fluctuating low to mid-frequency SNHL in the affected ear before, during, or after an attack. ECOG findings can show an SP/AP ratio of >45%. ENG testing can show a decreased vestibular response to caloric stimulation in the affected ear. Abnormal VEMP testing can be seen with a reduction in amplitude of >40% [27]. While all of these vestibular tests may help confirm a diagnosis of MD, sensitivity is limited in all. Therefore, vestibular testing is not required for a diagnosis of MD. The AAO-HNS recently published updated Clinical Practice Guidelines in 2020 which thoroughly dissects the prophylactic, medical and surgical treatment options available to patients with MD [28]. The overriding philosophy of MD treatment centers around noninvasive and nondestructive management for as long as possible due to the possibility of bilateral involvement.

Ménière's Disease and TMWD have significant overlap in symptomatology and exam findings. Both disorders are characterized by episodic vertigo, aural fullness, tinnitus, and hearing loss. In MD, the vertiginous episodes last for minutes to hours and the patient is often prostrate during these episodes—having severe nausea and vomiting and often unable to walk. These spells are often unprovoked and happen with little to no warning. TMWD patients usually describe a provoking trigger for their vertigo such as loud noise or straining. MD patients may notice sensitivity to salt in the diet whereas TMWD patients do not have a dietary trigger. Tinnitus associated with MD also differs in quality compared to TMWD; MD patients often describe low pitched noise in the ear (ocean, jet engine, roaring) whereas TWMD patients often have pulsatile tinnitus. The hearing loss experience by MD patients is classically a low frequency sensorineural loss with loss of clarity. By comparison, the TMWD hearing loss is low frequency but conductive in nature with preserved word understanding. TMWD can be identified on diagnostic testing (imaging and VEMP testing are most well reported) but there is no confirmatory diagnostic test for MD. There may be significant overlap between endolympatic hydrops and TMWD based on recent MRI imaging, however, the implications of these findings is not entirely clear. The reader is encouraged to further explore the association of endolymphatic hydrops, Ménière's Disease and TMWD in Chap. 18.

Otosclerosis

Otosclerosis is a disorder affecting the enchondrial bone of the otic capsule. The histopathology of this disorder is specific to the otic capsule and is termed "otospongiosis." In otosclerosis, the enchondrial bone throughout the otic capsule can undergo increased rates of bone turnover, abnormal bone deposition, and vascular proliferation [29]. Radiographically, this abnormal bone turnover results in areas of radiolucency at the fissula ante fenestram or, in patients with cochlear involvement, demineralization around the cochlear duct—referred to as a "halo sign." Otosclerosis often presents with progressive hearing loss, autophony and tinnitus. The tinnitus in otosclerosis is subjective and non-pulsatile in nature whereas TMWD patients often report pulsatile tinnitus. Patients may also have a family history of the disease or have family members who have "had surgery for their hearing." To differentiate between TMWD and otosclerosis, the practitioner may be able to utilize both physical exam findings and diagnostic testing differences. On examination, both disorders may cause tuning fork abnormalities. Also, both disorders often have a normal otoscopic examination of the tympanic membrane and middle ear cleft. In very active otosclerosis, the cochlear promontory may have increased vascularity which appears with a red hue without mass lesion (Schwartze sign). The promontory in TMWD should appear normal. On audiometric testing both groups have a conductive hearing loss. In SSCD, patients may demonstrate a supra-threshold bone line in the low frequencies, often with closure of the air bone gap in the mid to high frequencies. Otosclerosis often demonstrate closure of their air-bone gap at 2000 Hz (Carhart's notch) due to a dip in the bone scores, whereas TMWD does not. Acoustic reflexes are particularly helpful in distinguishing the two groups. Otosclerosis demonstrates absent acoustic reflexes due to fixation of the stapes footplate whereas TMWD does not lose this reflex. Of note, there are case reports of patients having both otosclerosis and SSCD, where the SSCD was unmasked by correction of the otosclerosis [30, 31]. The reader should consider concurrent disorders if corrective surgery for otosclerosis fails to close the air bone gap or results in episodic vertigo.

Autoimmune Inner Ear Dysfunction

Autoimmune inner ear disease (AIED) occurs secondary to an immunologically mediated attack onto the audiovestibular system. Originally described by McCabe as purely audiologic in nature, patients can experiences vestibular symptoms as well [32]. AIED is uncommon, accounting for <1% of all cases of hearing loss and dizziness [32]. Symptoms include fluctuating, rapidly progressive bilateral SNHL often accompanied by tinnitus, and aural fullness. Patients are more likely to present with mild ataxia and episodic lightheadedness than true vertigo. AIED occurs more commonly in females between 20 and 50 years of age. 30% of patients with AIED will have another systemic autoimmune disorder present [33]. The inner ear is not exposed to many antigens, leading theories on the pathogenesis of AIED include cross reaction, bystander damage, intolerance, and genetic factors related to the immunologic response. Presentation can be similar to MD and TMWD but with bilateral involvement being a key distinguishing feature of AIED, though AIED can be asymmetric early in the disease process. 16% of bilateral and 6% of unilateral MD may be caused by immune dysfunction [33]. Serological testing can give mixed results [34]. Initial treatment includes systemic vs. intratympanic steroids while immunomodulatory agents are often prescribed for long-term treatment [35]. The rapidly progressive symptoms and response to steroid medications help to distinguish AIED from TWMDs.

Labyrinthitis

Labyrinthitis describes inflammation of the inner ear, commonly divided into serous vs. suppurative labyrinthitis. Suppurative labyrinthitis describes a pyogenic infection of the inner ear, which can produce severe symptoms resulting in permanent hearing loss and vestibular dysfunction and can be rapidly progressive and life-threatening if intracranial complications occur. Serous labyrinthitis describes inflammation of the inner ear without frank bacterial infection, which also can present with severe symptoms although often long-term sequela are not always observed. Both serous and suppurative labyrinthitis can be isolated to the ear (tympanogenic) or extend intracranially.

Labyrinthitis is a clinical diagnosis and can occur in the setting of acute or chronic otitis media. Inflammation can spread via an acquired pathway between the middle and inner ear spaces, notably temporal bone fracture, iatrogenic from otologic surgery, or cholesteatoma erosion (most commonly fistula formation of the horizontal SSC). However, there is often no apparent inner-middle ear communication in many cases of tympanogenic labyrinthitis. Meningitis can be a source of inflammatory and infectious spread from the meninges into the inner ear in cases of meningogenic labyrinthitis. 5–35% of patients who survive bacterial meningitis will have bilateral SNHL [36]. MRI is the preferred modality to assess patients with labyrinthitis commonly showing hyperintense labyrinthine signal on T1 post-contrast imaging sequences.

The differentiation between TWMD and labyrinthitis is based on history and audiometry. In most cases of labyrinthitis the vertigo is sudden in onset, intense in nature and continuous initially but gradually improves as central compensation occurs. The hearing loss is predominantly sensorineural in nature after resolution of a middle ear effusion; these symptoms are in contradiction to TMWD patients who experience provokable episodic vertigo and generally have a conductive hearing loss. Additionally, TMWD patients do not often experience resolution of the vestibular symptoms with time.

Mass Lesions Involving the Labyrinth

Vestibular schwannomas (VS) are tumors arising from Schwann cells within the internal auditory canal (IAC) and can present with a constellation of vertigo, SNHL, and/or facial nerve palsy depending on its location and size within the IAC. Schwann cells are also found more distally within the inner ear labyrinth itself, which can produce tumors termed intralabyrinthine schwannomas (ILS). ILS are much more rare compared to VS and are often mistaken for inflammation of the labyrinth on MRI [37]. Symptoms vary based on specific location of the ILS anatomically described by the revised Kennedy classification system [38]. Nearly all patients present with some form of hearing loss and may describe disequilibrium vs. vertigo. ILS interruption of intralabyrinthine fluid mechanics make these lesions difficult to clinically differentiate from MD and TMWD. The characteristic MRI findings of intralabyrinthine hyperintensity on post-contrast T1 weighted imaging is diagnostic [39]. Treatment is dictated by patient symptoms, tumor size, and location.

Secondary third windows are a well known complication of other masses in the temporal bone, namely cholesteatoma and petrous apex lesions. Cholesteatomas can be particularly erosive and result in fistulization of any of the labyrinthine structures although the HSCC is the most commonly involved, as the cholesteatoma sac expands into the antrum and mastoid air cells. Like TMWD patients, cholesteatoma patients will often report aural fullness, autophony, hearing loss and occasionally episodic dizziness/vertigo. Rates of occult or symptomatic fistulas in cholesteatoma vary widely with rates as high as 15% in some early series prior to routine use of pre operative imaging; current series report rates of labyrinthine fistulas between 2 and 8% [40–42]. Dizziness/vertigo in a patient with cholesteatoma is highly suggestive of a fistula [43]. The key differentiator in this group of patients is the history or discovery of chronic inflammatory otitis media and identification of cholesteatoma. The cholesteatomatous fistula patient will most likely have an abnormal otoscopic exam belying either active disease or the stigma of prior surgery for cholesteatoma. Additionally, unlike TMWD patients, cholesteatoma patients will likely report long standing ear problems, otorrhea, non-pulsitile tinnitus, and occasionally pain.

Of note, it is possible that a patient with cholesteatoma also has an unrelated TMWD. Imaging of the temporal bone is critical in this situation as cholesteatoma surgery will not address those symptoms caused by the TWMD. To identify two distinct diagnoses, the CT imaging would need to identify the dehiscence in an anatomically separate location from the cholesteatoma and this separation would need to be confirmed at surgery as the CT images in cholesteatoma may not detect thin layers of matrix over a secondary fistula.

Petrous apex lesions may also result in otologic symptoms mimicking TMWD [44]. Cholesterol granulomas of the petrous apex will often present with aural fullness, hearing loss and dizziness. Key features that distinguish petrous apex lesions include headache, lack of episodic symptoms, and stereotypical findings on CT and MRI imaging. Other lesions of the petrous bone, such as meningioma and endolymphatic sac tumors may also present with symptoms mimicked by TMWD including aural fullness, hearing loss and vertigo. Often these symptoms are not provokable and progressive in patients with mass lesions; the hearing loss is sensorineural in nature; and they do no report autophony. Imaging will clearly differentiate a mass lesion from a TMWD.

Neurologic Mimickers

Multisensory Balance Dysfunction

Neurologic findings can vary based on the etiology of a patient's dizziness. Cranial nerves, motor and sensory findings, cerebellar testing, coordination, and mental status are all important aspects of the physical exam that may help lead towards an underlying etiology. Particular attention should be made when evaluating extraocular movements during the cranial nerve exam as previously discussed. Both motor and sensory neuropathies can contribute to vestibular symptoms. Certain neurologic findings, including dysarthria, visual disturbances, extremity weakness, or ataxia, indicate a central etiology to vertigo symptoms. Romberg and gait testing helps to assess the visual, vestibular and somatosensory coordination necessary to maintain balance.

With age and cognitive decline, the prevalence of "dizziness" increases. Dizziness is the most common complaint among patients older than 75 years presenting to a doctor's office [45]. Many studies have revealed age-related changes in the vestibular organs, together coupled with peripheral neuropathy, decreased visual acuity, impaired cognitive function, and a decline in neuroplasticity. All of these changes contribute to the increased prevalence of this multisensory balance dysfunction—"dizziness." Increased fall risk and the associated morbidity and mortality that comes with falls are a serious health concern in the elderly population. However, the misconception that all dizziness in the elderly population is age-related can result in a delay in diagnosis of treatable etiologies [46, 47]. A thorough evaluation for treatable causes of dizziness in the aging population is imperative, along with appropriate referrals for non-peripheral causes. Many patients will benefit from practical interventions such as vestibular physical therapy, exercise programs, and falls risk reduction.

Migraine

Vertigo and migraine are two common neurologic complaints often coexistent in the general population. In one large population-based study, the lifetime prevalence of migraine was 14% and vestibular vertigo 7%, giving an expected absolute chance coincidence of 1%, though actual coincidence was found to be 3.2% [48]. Significantly less patients with tension headache reported vertigo compared to patients with migraine, 8% vs. 27% respectively [49, 50]. Many different subtypes of migraine exist including generalized with or without aura, ocular, menstrual, abdominal, vestibular, and migraine without headache. Many patients with TMWD also have coincident migraines, but this may be simply related to the high prevalence of migraines in the general population. For some patients, TMWD symptoms can be migraine triggers. Dietary and environmental triggers can be present in all types of migraine.

Vestibular migraine is the second most common cause of vertigo and the most common cause of spontaneous episodic vertigo. The description of a patient's vertigo can be spontaneous and positional along with ataxia of variable duration lasting seconds to days. Most episodes of vertigo have no sequential relationship with the headache [50]. A diagnostic criteria for vestibular migraine was created by the Migraine Classification Committee of the International Headache Society and is included below:

1. At least 5 episodes fulfilling criteria 3 and 4 (listed below).
2. A current or past history of migraine without aura or migraine with aura.
3. Vestibular symptoms of moderate or severe intensity, lasting between 5 min and 72 h.
4. At least 50% of episodes are associated with at least one of the following three migrainous features:
   (a) Headache with at least two of the following four characteristics:
      - Unilateral location
      - Pulsating quality
      - Moderate or severe intensity
      - Aggravation by routine physical activity

   (b) Photophobia and phonophobia
   (c) Visual aura
5. Not better accounted for by another ICHD-3 diagnosis or by another vestibular disorder.

Migraine is a clinical diagnosis and treatment focuses around dietary modifications, trigger avoidance and pharmacologic therapy, both prophylactic and abortive. Suspicion or diagnosis of migraine should prompt a neurology referral.

Migraine and TMWD disorders have significant symptomatic overlap but the patient history will give clues to help differentiate the two disorders. Additionally, because migraine has a high prevalence in the population, there is a strong possibility that both patient groups can present with aural fullness, tinnitus, and episodic balance dysfunction. Tinnitus in migraine disorders is non-pulsatile and may be unilateral or bilateral, whereas TMWD patients more often experience pulsatile tinnitus in just the affected ear. Often the balance dysfunction in migraine is variable in its manifestation such that patients may have both episodic true vertigo as well as a sense of disequilibrium at different times. Balance dysfunction in migraine does not have to occur temporally associated with head pain, however, other migraine associated symptoms are associated as noted above in the IHS criteria. The balance dysfunction of TMWD is not associated with headache but the associated symptoms of hyperacusis/phonophobia and nausea/vomiting are similar between the two disorders. Often patients will have symptoms consistent with both migraine and TMWD. In these cases, optimal control of migraine is imperative prior to consideration of surgical treatment of TMWD when they are coexistent. Failure to treat common migraine or vestibular migraine prior to surgery may result in prolonged recovery times or overt surgical failure to treat the TMWD associated balance dysfunction [51]. We strongly recommend maximal medical treatment of migraine in those with concomitant TWMD prior to any attempts at repair of the dehiscence. Further exploration of migraine disorders and SSCD can be found in Chap. 25.

Mal de Débarquement Syndrome

Mal de Débarquement (MDD) is characterized by the persistent feeling of dizziness and disequilibrium lasting longer than one month after prolonged sea voyage though can occur after air travel, train rides, space flight, and even skiing. MDD should be distinguished from land sickness, which is much more short-lived resolving spontaneously within two days. In the majority of patients with MDD, symptoms are not experienced until after disembarking [52]. MDD affects mostly females between 30 and 50 years of age with a mean duration of 3.5 years [53]. The pathophysiology of MDD remains controversial and in general is considered a variant of motion sickness, though this does not explain the female and age predominance. Others believe it to be related to migraine or a form of anxiety. Treatment is often medical and largely ineffective, aimed primarily at keeping the patient comfortable until spontaneous remission [52]. MDD has a clear inciting/index event and the majority of TMWD do not (traumatic TMWD being the exception). MDD symptoms are constant and can be perceived at rest and in motion. TMWD patients may have some disequilibrium, however the majority have episodic vertigo which does not improve over time and many have audiologic symptoms as well, which MDD does not.

Psychiatric Mimickers

Prior to Minor and colleagues' landmark description of SSCD in 1998, patients suffering from SSCD and other TMWDs were inappropriately labeled "crazy" and "difficult" as they did not fall within the categories of known vestibular disorders at that time [3]. Patients with TMWDs can still face these preconceived designations due to its relatively new and unknown familiarity amongst primary care providers. The DSM-V criteria for "panic attack" include four or more of the following symptoms which occur suddenly and are accompanied by fear or a "sense of discomfort" [54]:

1. Palpitations, pounding heart, or accelerated heart rate
2. Sweating
3. Trembling or shaking
4. Sensations of shortness of breath or smothering
5. Feeling of choking
6. Chest pain or discomfort
7. Nausea or abdominal distress
8. Feeling dizzy, unsteady, lightheaded, or faint
9. Derealization (feelings of unreality) or depersonalization (being detached from oneself)
10. Fear of losing control or "going crazy"
11. Fear of dying
12. Paresthesias (numbness or tingling sensation)
13. Chills or hot flushes.

Many of the symptoms above accompany TMWD as well, so when patients present to the emergency room and report dizziness, nausea, disorientation and a feeling of "going crazy," the TMWD patient will often receive the wrong diagnosis. Additionally, it is easy to imagine how descriptions like "hearing my eyeballs move" and other internal bodily sounds may trigger a psychiatry referral amongst physicians unaware of the TMWD entity. Anecdotally, many patients experience a sense of relief to the anxiety surrounding their symptoms when the correct diagnosis of a TMWD is made. A careful otologic history in these patients can often differentiate panic attacks from TWMD. TMWD patients may certainly experience nausea, palpitations and sweating immediately following a vertigo episode. The timing of the vertigo in relation to the other symptoms is an important feature. Other clues to the TMWD diagnosis include a history of pulsatile tinnitus and nonfluctuating hearing loss. TMWD symptoms are often triggered by a physical activity such as straining, applying pressure to the ear canal or exposure to loud impulse noise. Panic attacks may have no inciting event or can be triggered by intrusive thoughts. There is certainly overlap between TMWD and anxiety as many patients will avoid, or have significant anxiety about, activities which have triggered symptoms in the past. Thus TMWD can cause or exacerbate preexisting anxiety and panic disorders [51]. The reader can explore patient stories about the TMWD journey in Chap. 27. Unfortunately for these patients, incorrect psychiatric diagnoses are still commonplace.

Table 5.3 lists the comparisons of similar and different symptoms and findings for the disorder mimicked by TMWD.

Table 5.3 Symptom differentiation for mimicking disorders

Mimicker disorder	Similar symptoms	Different symptoms/signs
Ménière's Disease	Aural fullness, episodic vertigo, muffled hearing	Non-pulsatile tinnitus, sensorineural hearing loss, no autophony
Otosclerosis	Conductive hearing loss, normal tympanogram findings	Absence of vertigo, absent acoustic reflexes
Obstructive Eustachian tube dysfunction	Aural fullness, autophony, conductive hearing loss	Absence of vertigo, abnormal otoscopic exam findings, abnormal tympanogram findings
Patulous Eustachian tube dysfunction	Aural fullness, autophony	History of rapid weight loss, absence of vertigo, respiratory mobility of the TM on otoscopy
BPPV	Positional vertigo, disequilibrium	Absence of hearing loss, no aural fullness, no autophony
Labyrinthitis	Vertigo, hearing loss	Rapid onset of symptoms, unilateral SNHL
Autoimmune inner ear disease	Vertigo, hearing loss	Rapid onset of symptoms, responsive to steroids
Secondary labyrinthine fistulas	Vertigo, aural fullness, hearing loss	History of ear disease, characteristic imaging findings, abnormal otoscopic exam
Schwannomas	Vertigo/disequilibrium, hearing loss	SNHL, characteristic imaging findings, non-pulsatile tinnitus
Migraine	Episodic vertigo/disequilibrium, tinnitus	Headaches, non-pulsatile tinnitus, dietary triggers
Mal de Débarquement	Disequilibrium	History of sea voyage/inciting event, no aural fullness, no hearing loss, no autophony, no hearing loss
Multisensory balance dysfunction	Disequilibrium	Absence of hearing loss, vision changes, peripheral neuropathy
Panic disorder	Somatic symptoms with events, anxiety	Triggered by intrusive thoughts

Asymptomatic Labyrinthine Dehiscence

The true incidence of labyrinthine dehiscence is hard to quantify. It is possible that a patient may have several of the symptoms of TMWD and a dehiscence seen on radiography but whose symptoms are not caused by the radiographic dehiscence. Additionally, there are certainly patients who have a radiographically identified dehiscence who do not have symptoms of TMWD. Several studies including an examination of 1000 adult temporal bones by Carey et al. revealed a 0.5% incidence of dehiscence and an additional 1.4% incidence of markedly thinned bone overlying the SSC [55]. Similar radiographic studies have demonstrated a 3–9% rate of radiographic SSCD though this is likely overestimated due to resolution limitations and absence of Poschl or Stenvers reconstructions [56–59]. Others have reported a 3% rate of radiographic dehiscence but just 0.6% had clinical manifestations consistent with SSCD [59]. The incidence/prevalence of symptomatic SSCDs is unclear, and the incidence of other less common TMWDs is even less clear as most descriptions of other windows are limited to case reports or small case series. It is possible that TMWD symptoms may occur on a spectrum, though further studies are necessary to determine what factors make a labyrinthine dehiscence symptomatic vs. asymptomatic.

Ockham's Razor

In training, we are often told to not make two diagnoses when one will suffice. However, it bears mentioning that TMWD can exist concurrently with any of the above mentioned disorders. For example, there is emerging evidence that many patients with SSCD also have hydrops identified on MRI. The prevalence of migraine is quite high in the general population and many symptoms of migraine overlap with TMWD. The literature is rife with reports of patients undergoing stapes surgery only to develop TMWD syndrome after the oval window fixation is corrected because they had an undiagnosed dehiscence somewhere else in the otic capsule. It is important to try to identify which disorder is causing the primary symptom for the patient and attempt treatment for that disorder. For instance, vestibular migraine should be controlled before surgery for a radiographic SSCD, as untreated vestibular migraine will likely lead to symptomatic failure of SSCD surgery.

Bilateral Third Mobile Windows

The congenital theory of SSCD argues thin bone overlying the SSC either causes a persistent dehiscence vs. predisposition to dehiscence later in life. This may explain why up to 50% of patients with SSCD will have bilateral defects [59]. Those with bilateral SSCD may develop oscillopsia [8]. Many patients are only symptomatic on one side, therefore treatment should center around addressing the more symptomatic ear and monitoring for resolution of symptoms before possibly proceeding with treatment of the contralateral.

Diagnostic Algorithm

When a patient presents for evaluation of various otologic complaints, it is helpful to organize the workup oftentimes on the most prominent symptoms experienced by the patient. Figure 5.1 outlines possible workup algorithms based on the most bothersome/prominent symptom reported by the patient on presentation.

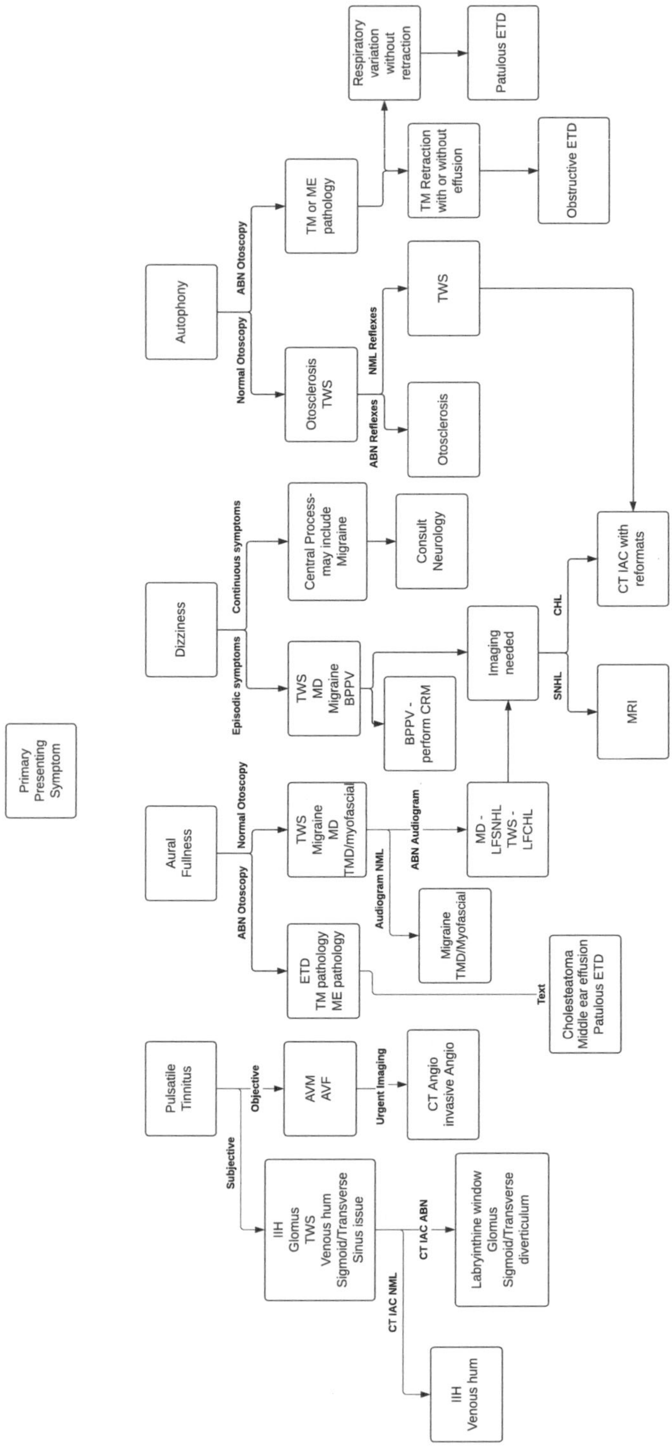

Fig. 5.1 Workup algorithms

Conclusion

Third window syndrome has a variety of presenting symptoms and signs. There is no "one thing" that points the practitioner to the correct diagnosis but a constellation of symptoms and findings that, when taken together, suggest the correct course of action. Practitioners must maintain a high index of suspicion for TMWD in patients who present with audiovestibular complaints; the differential diagnosis is broad but with a careful evaluation the correct diagnosis can be made.

References

1. Roland LT, Kallogjeri D, Sinks BC, et al. Utility of an abbreviated dizziness questionnaire to differentiate between causes of vertigo and guide appropriate referral: a multicenter prospective blinded study. Otol Neurotol. 2015;36(10):1687–94.
2. Friedland DR, Tarima S, Erbe C, Miles A. Development of a statistical model for the prediction of common vestibular diagnoses. JAMA Otolaryngol Head Neck Surg. 2016;142(4):351–6.
3. Minor LB, Solomon D, Zinreich JS, Zee DS. Sound- and/or pressure-induced vertigo due to bone dehiscence of the superior semicircular canal. Arch Otolaryngol Head Neck Surg. 1998;124(3):249–58.
4. Tullio P. Das Ohr und die Enstehung der Sprache und Schrift. Berlin: Urban & Schwartzenberg; 1929.
5. Hennebert C. A new syndrome in hereditary syphilis of the labyrinth. Presse Med Belg Brux. 1911.
6. Minor LB. Clinical manifestations of superior semicircular canal dehiscence. Laryngoscope. 2005;115(10):1717–27.
7. Minor LB. Superior canal dehiscence syndrome. Am J Otol. 2000;21(1):9–19.
8. Tilikete C, Krolak-Salmon P, Truy E, Vighetto A. Pulsesynchronous eye oscillations revealing bone superior canal dehiscence. Ann Neurol. 2004;56(4):556–60.
9. Hullar T, Zee D, Minor L. Evaluation of the patient with dizziness. In: Cummings otolaryngology head and neck surgery. 6th ed. Philadelphia: Saunders Elsevier Inc.; 2015. p. 2525–47.
10. Minor LB, Cremer PD, Carey JP, della Santina CC, Streubel SO, Weg N. Symptoms and signs in superior canal dehiscence syndrome. Ann N Y Acad Sci. 2001;942:259–73.
11. Baloh RW. Superior semicircular canal dehiscence syndrome: leaks and squeaks can make you dizzy. Neurology. 2004;62(5):684–5.
12. Suryanarayanan R, Lesser TH. 'Honeycomb' tegmen: multiple tegmen defects associated with superior semicircular canal dehiscence. J Laryngol Otol. 2010;124(5):560–3.
13. Mizukoshi K, Watanabe Y, Shojaku H, et al. Epidemiological study on benign paroxysmal positional vertigo. Acta Otolaryngol. 1988;447:67–72.
14. Froehling D, Silverstein MD, Mohr DN, Beatty CW, Offord KP, Ballard DJ. Benign positional vertigo: incidence and prognosis in a population-based study in Olmsted County Minnesota. Mayo Clin Proc. 1991;66:596–601.
15. Oghalai JS, Manolidis S, Barth JL, Stewart MG, Jenkins HA. Unrecognized benign paroxysmal positional vertigo in elderly patients. Otolaryngol Head Neck Surg. 2000;122(5):630–4.
16. Honrubia V, Baloh RW, Harris MR, Jacobson KM. Paroxysmal positional vertigo syndrome. Am J Otol. 1999;20(4):465–70.
17. Dix MR, Hallpike CS. The pathology, symptomatology and diagnosis of certain common disorders of the vestibular system. Proc R Soc Med. 1952;45(6):341–54.

18. Epley JM. The canalith repositioning procedure: for treatment of benign paroxysmal positional vertigo. Otolaryngol Head Neck Surg. 1992;107(3):399–404.
19. Vila PM, Thomas T, Liu C, Poe D, Shin JJ. The burden and epidemiology of eustachian tube dysfunction in adults. Otolaryngol Head Neck Surg. 2017;156(2):278–84. https://doi.org/10.1177/0194599816683342.
20. Stenström C, Bylander-Groth A, Ingvarsson L. Eustachian tube function in otitis-prone and healthy children. Int J Pediatr Otorhinolaryngol. 1991;21(2):127–38. https://doi.org/10.1016/0165-5876(91)90143-y.
21. Jerger JF. Suggested nomenclature for impedance audiometry. Arch Otolaryngol. 1972;96(1):1–3. https://doi.org/10.1001/archotol.1972.00770090039002.
22. Eravci FC, Yildiz BD, Özcan KM, et al. Analysis of the effect of weight loss on eustachian tube function by transnasal video endoscopy. J Craniofac Surg. 2022;33(3):219–21. https://doi.org/10.1097/SCS.0000000000007965.
23. Havia M, Kentala E, Pyykkö I. Prevalence of Menière's disease in general population of Southern Finland. Otolaryngol Head Neck Surg. 2005;133(5):762–8.
24. Kentala E. Characteristics of six otologic diseases involving vertigo. Am J Otol. 1996;17(6):883–92.
25. Committee on Hearing and Equilibrium. Committee on Hearing and Equilibrium guidelines for the diagnosis and evaluation of therapy in Ménière's disease. Otolaryngol Head Neck Surg. 1995;113(3):181–5.
26. Alford B. Committee on Hearing and Equilibrium. Report of Subcommittee on equilibrium and its measurement. Ménière's disease: criteria for diagnosis and evaluation of therapy for reporting. Trans Am Acad Ophthalmol Otolaryngol. 1972;76(6):1462–4.
27. Magliulo G, Cianfrone G, Gagliardi M, Cuiuli G, D'Amico R. Vestibular evoked myogenic potentials and distortion-product otoacoustic emissions combined with glycerol testing in endolymphatic hydrops: their value in early diagnosis. Ann Otol Rhinol Laryngol. 2004;113(12):1000–5.
28. Basura GJ, Adams ME, Monfared A, et al. Clinical practice guideline: ménière's disease. Otolaryngol Head Neck Surg. 2020;162(2):1–55. https://doi.org/10.1177/0194599820909438.
29. Quesnel AM, Ishai R, McKenna MJ. Otosclerosis: temporal bone pathology. Otolaryngol Clin N Am. 2018;51(2):291–303. https://doi.org/10.1016/j.otc.2017.11.001.
30. Maxwell AK, Slattery WH, Gopen QS, Miller ME. Failure to close the gap: concomitant superior canal dehiscence in otosclerosis patients. Laryngoscope. 2020;130(4):1023–7. https://doi.org/10.1002/lary.28167.
31. McClellan J, Nguyen A, Hamilton B, Jethanamest D, Hullar TE, Gupta S. Stapes surgery outcomes in patients with concurrent otosclerosis and superior semicircular canal dehiscence. Otol Neurotol. 2020;41(7):912–5. https://doi.org/10.1097/MAO.0000000000002673.
32. McCabe BF. Autoimmune sensorineural hearing loss. Ann Otol Rhinol Laryngol. 1979;88(5 Pt 1):585–9. https://doi.org/10.1177/000348947908800501.
33. Frejo L, Soto-Varela A, Santos-Perez S, et al. Clinical subgroups in bilateral Meniere disease. Front Neurol. 2016;7:182. https://doi.org/10.3389/fneur.2016.00182.
34. Bovo R, Ciorba A, Martini A. Vertigo and autoimmunity. Eur Arch Otorhinolaryngol. 2010;267(1):13–9.
35. Harris JP, Weisman MH, Derebery JM, et al. Treatment of corticosteroid-responsive autoimmune inner ear disease with methotrexate: a randomized controlled trial. JAMA. 2003;290(14):1875–83.
36. Baldwin RL, Sweitzer RS, Freind DB. Meningitis and sensorineural hearing loss. Laryngoscope. 1985;95(7 Pt 1):802–5.
37. van Abel KM, Carlson ML, Link MJ, et al. Primary inner ear schwannomas: a case series and systematic review of the literature. Laryngoscope. 2013;123(8):1957–66.
38. Green J. Intralabyrinthine schwannoma. In: Jackler RK, Driscoll CLW, editors. Tumors of the ear and temporal bone. Philadelphia: Lippincott Williams & Wilkins; 2000. p. 146–55.

39. Donnelly MJ, Daly CA, Briggs RJ. MR imaging features of an intracochlear acoustic schwannoma. J Laryngol Otol. 1994;108(12):1111–4.
40. Sheehy JL. Management of the labyrinthine fistula. Clin Otolaryngol Allied Sci. 1978;3(4):405–14. https://doi.org/10.1111/j.1365-2273.1978.tb00721.x.
41. Gormley PK. Surgical management of labyrinthine fistula with cholesteatoma. J Laryngol Otol. 1986;100(10):1115–23. https://doi.org/10.1017/s0022215100100684.
42. Meyer A, Bouchetemblé P, Costentin B, Dehesdin D, Lerosey Y, Marie JP. Lateral semicircular canal fistula in cholesteatoma: diagnosis and management. Eur Arch Otorhinolaryngol. 2016;273(8):2055–63. https://doi.org/10.1007/s00405-015-3775-6.
43. Rosito LPS, Canali I, Teixeira A, Silva MN, Selaimen F, Costa SS. Cholesteatoma labyrinthine fistula: prevalence and impact. Braz J Otorhinolaryngol. 2018;85(2):222–7. https://doi.org/10.1016/j.bjorl.2018.01.005.
44. Hoa M, House JW, Linthicum FH, Go JL. Petrous apex cholesterol granuloma: pictorial review of radiological considerations in diagnosis and surgical histopathology. J Laryngol Otol. 2013;127(4):339–48. https://doi.org/10.1017/S0022215113000091.
45. Sloane PD. Dizziness in primary care. J Fam Pract. 1989;29(1):33–8.
46. Lawson J, Johnson I, Bamiou DE, Newton JL. Benign paroxysmal positional vertigo: clinical characteristics of dizzy patients referred to a falls and syncope unit. QJM. 2005;98(5):357–64.
47. Neuhauser HK, von Brevern M, Radtke A, et al. Benign paroxysmal positional vertigo: clinical characteristics of dizzy patients referred to a falls and syncope unit. Neurology. 2005;65(6):989–04.
48. Akdal G, Baykan B, Ertaş M, et al. Population-based study of vestibular symptoms in migraineurs. Acta Otolaryngol. 2015;135(5):435–9.
49. Kayan A, Hood JD. Neuro-otological manifestations of migraine. Brain. 1984;107(4):1123–42.
50. Bisdorff A. Migraine and dizziness. Curr Opin Neurol. 2014;27(1):105–10.
51. Wackym PA, Mackay-Promitas HT, Demirel S, et al. Comorbidities confounding the outcomes of surgery for third window syndrome: outlier analysis. Laryngosc Investig Otolaryngol. 2017;2(5):225–53. https://doi.org/10.1002/lio2.89.
52. Hain TC. Mal de Debarquement syndrome (MDD or MdDS). Internet.
53. Gordon CR, Shupak A, Nachum Z. Mal de debarquement. Arch Otolaryngol Head Neck Surg. 2000;126(6):805–6.
54. Substance Abuse and Mental Health Services Administration (US). Substance abuse and mental health services administration. Impact of the DSM-IV to DSM-5 changes on the national survey on drug use and health. Mental illness.
55. Carey JP, Minor LB, Nager GT. Dehiscence or thinning of bone overlying the superior semicircular canal in a temporal bone survey. Arch Otolaryngol Head Neck Surg. 2000;126(2):137–47.
56. Williamson RA, Vrabec JT, Coker NJ, Sandlin M. Coronal computed tomography prevalence of superior semicircular canal dehiscence. Otolaryngol Head Neck Surg. 2003;129(5):481–9.
57. Bremke M, Luers JC, Anagiotos A, et al. Comparison of digital volume tomography and high-resolution computed tomography in detecting superior semicircular canal dehiscence—a temporal bone study. Acta Otolaryngol. 2015;135(9):901–6.
58. Branstetter BF IV, Harrigal C, Escott EJ, Hirsch BE. Superior semicircular canal dehiscence: oblique reformatted CT images for diagnosis. Radiology. 2006;238(3):938–42.
59. Masaki Y. The prevalence of superior canal dehiscence syndrome as assessed by temporal bone computed tomography imaging. Acta Otolaryngol. 2011;131(3):258–62.

Chapter 6
The Cognitive/Psychological Effects of Third Mobile Window Syndrome

Todd M. Mowery, Carey D. Balaban, and P. Ashley Wackym

As reviewed in Chap. 1, "*History and Overview of Third Mobile Window Syndrome*" there are currently 15 known sites of dehiscence that can be seen using high-resolution temporal bone CT and in addition there are sites of dehiscence that cannot yet be seen with contemporary high-resolution temporal bone CT scans (CT– TMWS). Table 6.1 outlines the contemporary spectrum of symptoms, signs or exacerbating factors seen in third mobile window syndrome (TMWS) (also known as third window syndrome [TWS] or otic capsule dehiscence syndrome [OCDS]) and diagnostic tools and metrics available to measure these clinically observed phenomenon. This chapter will focus on the cognitive and psychological dysfunction induced by TMWS as well as recovery after surgical management of the specific site(s) of bony dehiscence.

T. M. Mowery · P. A. Wackym (✉)
Department of Otolaryngology – Head and Neck Surgery, Rutgers Robert Wood Johnson Medical School, New Brunswick, NJ, USA

Rutgers Brain Health Institute, Piscataway, NJ, USA
e-mail: tm692@rwjms.rutgers.edu; wackym@neurotology.org

C. D. Balaban
Departments of Otolaryngology, Neurobiology, Communication Sciences and Disorders, and Bioengineering, University of Pittsburgh School of Medicine, Pittsburgh, PA, USA
e-mail: CBALABAN@pitt.edu

G. J. Gianoli, P. Thomson (eds.), *Third Mobile Window Syndrome of the Inner Ear*, https://doi.org/10.1007/978-3-031-16586-3_6

Table 6.1 Spectrum of symptoms, signs or exacerbating factors seen in third window syndrome and diagnostic tools and metrics available to measure these clinically observed phenomenon

Category	Symptom, sign or exacerbating factors	Diagnostic tools and metrics
Sound-induced	Dizziness or otolithic dysfunction (see vestibular dysfunction below); nausea; cognitive dysfunction; spatial disorientation; migraine/migrainous headache; pain (especially children); loss of postural control; falls	History; 128 Hz and 256 Hz tuning forks applied to ankles, knees, and/or elbows heard or felt in the ear or head; pneumatic otoscopy; cVEMP/oVEMP with reduced threshold with or without increased amplitude, auditory stimuli inducing symptoms; Romberg test while pure tones delivered to individual ear or low frequency tuning fork applied to elbow
Autophony	Resonant voice; chewing; heel strike; pulsatile tinnitus; joints or tendons moving; eyes moving or blinking; comb or brush through hair; face being touched	History
Vestibular dysfunction	Gravitational receptor (otolithic) dysfunction type of vertigo (rocky or wavy motion, tilting, pushed, pulled, tilted, flipped, floor falling out from under); mal de débarquement illusions of movement	History; Dizziness handicap inventory (DHI); cVEMP/oVEMP; computerized dynamic posturography; Romberg/ sharpened Romberg; head tilt; nuchal muscle tightness
Headache	Migraine/migrainous headache; migraine variants (ocular, hemiplegic or vestibular [true rotational vertigo]); coital cephalalgia; photophobia; phonophobia; aura; scotomata	History; Headache impact test (HIT-6); migraine disability assessment test (MIDAS)
Cognitive dysfunction	General cognitive impairment, such as mental fog, dysmetria of thought, mental fatigue; Impaired attention and concentration, poor multitasking (women > men); Executive dysfunction; Language problems including dysnomia, agramatical speech, aprosidia, verbal fluency; Memory difficulties; Academic difficulty including reading problems and missing days at school or work; Depression and anxiety	History *Cognitive screen*: MoCA and Schmahmann syndrome scale *IQ*: WRIT or WAIS2 *Attention*: NAB, Attention Module and/or CPT3 *Memory*: CVLT2, WMS4, or WRAML2 *Executive functioning*: WCST, TMT, D-KEFS *Language*: NAB, Naming *Visuospatial*: Benton JLO *Mood/personality*: Clinical interview, PHQ-9, GAD-7, ACES, BDI2, BAI, personality assessment inventory (PAI), or Millon behavioral diagnostic
Spatial disorientation	Trouble judging distances; detachment/passive observer when interacting with groups of people; out of body experiences; perceiving the walls or floor moving	History; subjective visual vertical

Table 6.1 (continued)

Category	Symptom, sign or exacerbating factors	Diagnostic tools and metrics
Anxiety	Sense of impending doom	History; GAD-7; BAI
Autonomic dysfunction	Nausea; vomiting; diarrhea; lightheadedness; blood pressure lability; change in temperature regulation; heart rate lability	History; autonomic testing
Endolymphatic hydrops	Ear pressure/fullness not relieved by the Valsalva maneuver; barometric pressure sensitivity	History; electrocochleography, tympanometry
Hearing	Pseudo-conductive hearing loss (bone-conduction hyperacusis)	Comprehensive audiometric evaluation including tympanometry, stapedial reflex testing, speech perception testing, air-conduction and bone-conduction thresholds; magnitude varies by site of dehiscence

ACES adverse childhood experiences scale, *BAI* beck anxiety inventory, *BDI2* Beck depression inventory, 2nd edition, *Benton JLO* Benton judgment of line orientation, *CPT3* continuous performance test, 3rd edition, *CVLT2* California Verbal Learning Test, 2nd edition, *D-KEFS* Delis-Kaplan executive function system, *DHI* dizziness handicap inventory, *GAD-7* generalized anxiety disorder screener, *HIT-6* headache impact test, *MoCA* Montreal cognitive assessment, *NAB* neuropsychological assessment battery, *PAI* personality assessment inventory, *PHQ-9* patient health questionnaire, *TMT* trail making test, *WAIS2* Wechsler adult intelligence scale, 2nd edition, *WCST* Wisconsin card sorting test, *WMS4* Wechsler memory scale, 4th edition, *WRAML2* wide range assessment of memory and learning, 2nd edition, *WRIT* wide range intelligence test
Adapted from Wackym et al. [1] used with permission, copyright © P.A. Wackym, MD

Central Nervous System Pathway Activation that Produce Secondary Symptoms

Most of the symptoms that disrupt the lives of patients with TMWS are related to the severe symptoms that are secondary to these gravitational receptor asymmetries [1–16].

Autonomic Dysfunction

Autonomic dysfunction occurs to varying degrees with the specific location producing the TMWS and/or vestibular migraine; however, it is extremely common. Autonomic dysfunction also occurs with rotational receptor asymmetries. These symptoms include nausea, "cold-clammy skin," decreased heart rate and vomiting. There have been many investigators who have studied the underlying mechanisms and pathways subserving this dysfunction [17–20].

Cognitive Dysfunction

In the past there has been some debate concerning the causal relationship between vestibular disease and cognitive dysfunction (e.g., see [21]). More recently, a growing body of research indicates a very complex relationship between vestibular function and cognition [22, 23], with a nearly universal presence in patients with TMWS [1–13].

These studies report that this is uncommon in rotational receptor dysfunction type of vertigo as seen with benign positional vertigo, vestibular neuronitis or other disorders producing true rotational vertigo. Patients with TMWS often use the following descriptors when describing their cognitive function: "fuzzy, foggy, spacey, out-of-it; memory and concentration are poor; difficulty reading—as if the words are floating on the page; trouble finding the right words; and forgetting what I wanted to say." To understand the complexity of the connection between vestibular dysfunction and cognitive impairment we must turn to behavioral (e.g., lesion) and anatomical (neural tracing) studies in animals. An excellent review by Hitier et al. carefully outlines the neuroanatomical pathways from the vestibule to the central nervous system in rodents, cats, and non-human primates [24]. They describe five major pathways by which vestibular information is integrated throughout the brain. These include (1) a vestibulo-thalamic-cortical pathway for environmental spatial integration, (2) a tegmental-thalamic-entorhinal pathway for calculating head direction, (3) a reticularis pontis oralis-supramammillary-septal pathway to the hippocampus involved with spatial memory and object recognition, (4) a cerebellar-thalamic-cortical pathway that supports spatial learning, and (5) a vestibular-thalamic-striatal pathway that supports spatial learning and memory. The detailed anatomical pathways are beyond the scope of this review; however, there is no doubt that vestibular dysfunctions, such as those associated with TMWS, will influence normal activity along these major pathways and would subsequently impact cognitive functions governed by them. The debate surrounding vestibular function and cognition arises from the complexity of the vestibular system's non-classical sensory function. Classic sensory systems (e.g., vision) have modal specific inputs with straightforward pathways from the brainstem and/or midbrain to the thalamus, and then the cortex. Within each brain region, sensory stimuli are represented by external maps held in stable receptive fields. That is, the peripheral receptors of the retina, cochlea, and skin are represented as retinotopic, tonotopic, and somatotopic maps throughout each modality specific neuraxis. Vestibular pathways integrate heavily with these modalities through direct vestibular nucleus projections and higher-order brain regions in the midbrain and thalamus. The core regions integrate environmental spatial auditory and visual information, as well as proprioceptive somatotopic information about limb position and posture with vestibular information about head direction, angular velocity, and momentum. Vestibular information is constantly updating, and lacks a classical map to probe with neurophysiological techniques, so these types of data have been difficult to interpret and studied far less than the classic sensory systems. Despite this limited body of rigorous investigation in animal research, a growing amount of human data do offer interesting clues as to how vestibular dysfunction induces cognitive impairment in these individuals.

Third Mobile Window Syndrome and Cognitive Impairment (Human Studies) Gurvich and colleagues published an excellent review of the role of the vestibular system on cognition and psychiatry [25]. As reported in the animal literature, two key anatomical regions that provide links between the vestibular system and neural networks involved in cognitive and emotional processing are the parabrachial nucleus and the hippocampus [17–20]; however, many of the neuroanatomical regions that are linked to the vestibular system are also implicated in several psychiatric illnesses. The past decade has seen an increased interest in the relationship between the vestibular system and mood, cognition and psychiatric symptoms with studies demonstrating vestibular stimulation can produce changes in mood, cognition and psychiatric symptoms [26–28]. We have also seen many individuals with TMWS assigned a psychiatric diagnosis before their vestibular disorder was diagnosed and have observed resolution of their "psychiatric disorder" following surgical intervention. This, unfortunately, is common with children [4, 5, 10, 11]. The hippocampus is consistently implicated in cognition and models of psychiatric disorders and there is a large body of evidence supporting vestibular–hippocampal interactions [29–33].

Another possible hypothesis of why TMWS patients experience their cognitive dysfunction and spatial disorientation and recovery of function after surgical intervention is that intermittent aberrant otolithic input to the cerebellum creates an episodic but reversible cerebellar cognitive affective syndrome [34–38]. Schmahmann conceptualizes cerebellar cognitive affective syndrome as dysmetria of thought and emotion. He describes impairment of executive function (planning, set-shifting, verbal fluency, abstract reasoning, and working memory); spatial cognition (visual spatial organization and memory); personality change (blunting of affect or disinhibited and inappropriate behavior); and language deficits (agrammatism and aprosodia) [34–38]. These clinical features closely fit what TMWS patients describe and their neuropsychology testing measures [1, 4–11, 14–16]. Table 6.2 summarizes the clinical features of the cerebellar cognitive affective syndrome in adults.

Table 6.2 Clinical features of the cerebellar cognitive affective syndrome in adults

Cognitive function	Clinical features
Executive function	Planning, set-shifting, verbal fluency, abstract reasoning, working memory
Spatial cognition	Visual spatial organization and memory
Personality change	Blunting of affect or disinhibited and inappropriate behavior
Language deficits	Agrammatism and aprosodia

Adapted from Schmahmann [34]. Used with permission, copyright © P.A. Wackym, MD

Smith et al. and Zheng et al. have reported that modulation of memory, but not spatial memory, occurs with vestibular lesions and can be influenced by galvanic vestibular stimulation [39, 40]. These findings may lead to additional treatment strategies that may accelerate or maximize recovery after repairing an otic capsule defect resulting in TMWS.

We published a study incorporating pre- and postoperative quantitative measurement of cognitive function in a cohort of patients with CT– TMWS and/or SSCD [15]. There were 17 patients (13 adults, four children) with clinical SSCD spectrum who underwent surgical management. We completed neuropsychology test batteries preoperatively and every three months postoperatively for up to one year. These included: Beck's Depression Inventory-II (BDI-II); Delis-Kaplan Executive Function System (D-KEFS); Wide Range Intelligence Test (WRIT FSIQ); and Wide Range Assessment of Memory and Learning (WRAML-2), including the four domains of verbal memory, visual memory, attention/concentration and working memory. We statistically compared pre- versus three months postoperative (post-1) and post-1 versus most recent cognitive and neurobehavioral function (post-2). As shown in Fig. 6.1, there was a highly significant improvement in BDI-II at pre- versus post-2 ($p = 0.0006$) but no further improvement at most recent ($p = 0.68$). As shown in Fig. 6.2, there was a statistically significant improvement of D-KEFS at post-2 ($p = 0.023$) as well as at most recent ($p = 0.023$). For the WRAML-2 (pre- vs post-1; post-1 vs most recent): verbal ($p = 0.02$; $p = 0.008$); visual ($p = 0.24$; $p = 0.10$); attention/concentration ($p = 0.05$; $p = 0.048$); and working memory ($p = 0.27$; $p = 0.007$). Overall there was a marked improvement in cognitive and neurobehavioral function postoperatively. The delay in performance improvement measured in some domains may represent brain reorganization. Delayed improvement in specific domains may represent an opportunity for additional intervention to accelerate recovery. These interventions may include galvanic stimulation, the use of a ketogenic diet or neurocognitive therapy approaches.

We also published a comorbidity study and noted a high rate of psychological comorbidity ($n = 6$) [16]. The Millon Behavioral Medicine Diagnostic (MBMD) and the clinical psychology examinations were the most useful in identifying these comorbidities [16]. Factitious disorder, functional neurologic symptom disorder (formerly conversion disorder) dissociative motor disorder variant, somatic symptom disorder, attention deficit hyperactivity disorder (ADHD), dissociative identity disorder (DID), major depressive disorder (MDD), and post-traumatic stress disorder (PTSD) were represented in 6 of the 12 participants in the comorbidity cohort. Suicidal ideation was also common ($n = 6$) [16]. These findings underscore the challenges in sorting out the TMWS symptoms caused by the dehiscence, those resulting from other comorbid conditions, or those resulting from interactions between the two factors.

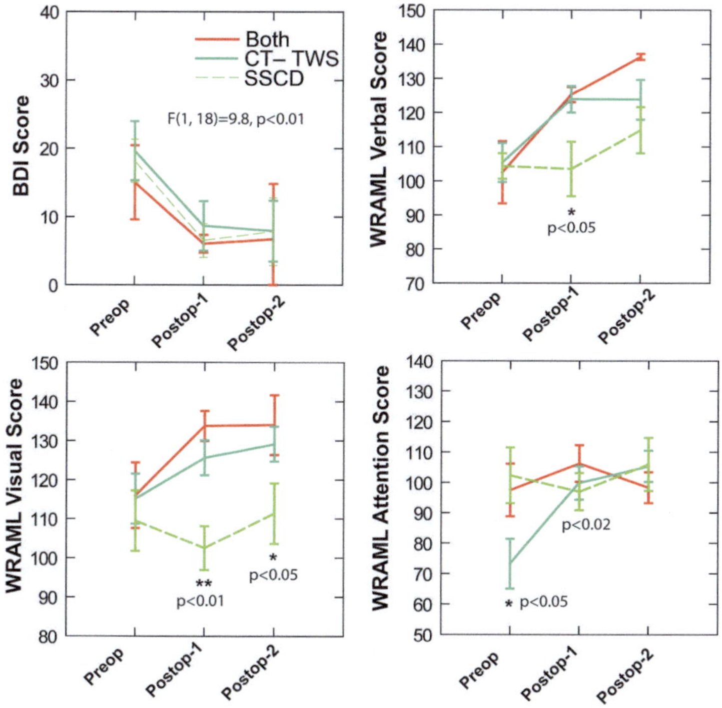

Fig. 6.1 Top left, the preoperative scores from the Beck Depression Index-II (BDI) indicated mild depression in all three groups. There was significant and parallel improvement to the minimal depression range after surgery in all three groups ($F(1,18) = 9.8$, $p < 0.01$), which appeared on the first postoperative test session. Note that this recovery is rapid and significantly better, even a few months after surgical intervention. Adapted from Wackym et al. [15] Copyright © P.A. Wackym, MD, used with permission. Top right, for the Wide Range Assessment of Memory and Learning-2 (WRAML) verbal subtest, the SSCD only group treated with SSCD plugging showed a delayed improvement on the WRAML verbal subtest; it was significantly lower than the CT– TWS only group treated with RWR and the both SSCD and subsequent CT– TWS group treated with RWR and SSCD plugging for the first postoperative test (ANOVA followed by least significant differences tests). All three groups showed statistically significant improvement in the verbal subtest by the most recent neuropsychology test battery assessment. (* means $p < 0.05$ by least significant differences tests. Only the between groups differences are indicated). Bottom left, for the WRAML visual subtest, unlike patients with CT– TWS only treated with RWR or both SSCD and CT– TWS treated with SSCD plugging and RWR surgeries, the SSCD only group treated with SSCD plugging did not show statistically significant improvement at either the initial or most recent postoperative testing session, and remained significantly lower than either of the other groups (analysis of variance with repeated measures on test times and a between groups factor of operative history, followed by least significant difference tests). There was a statistically significant improvement in the visual subtest for the CT– TWS only group treated with RWR and the both CT– TWS and SCD group treated with RWR and SSCD plugging, respectively, at both the initial postoperative assessment as well as at the most recent assessment. (* means $p < 0.05$ and ** $p < 0.01$ by least significant differences tests. Only the between groups differences are indicated). Bottom right, for the WRAML attention concentration subtest, preoperatively, the CT– TWS group treated with RWR only showed abnormally low scores on the WRAML attention/concentration subtest (in this figure, 95% confidence interval of 55.271–91.229 re: normal of 100); however, the performance normalized after surgery. There were significant test time effects overall (improvement in all groups), initially (preoperative) worse in the CT– TWS only than the SSCD only and the both SSCD and CT– TWS patients ($p < 0.02$, Fisher's Least Significant Difference [LSD] test), but the same afterwards. (* means $p < 0.05$ by least significant differences tests. Only the between groups differences are indicated)

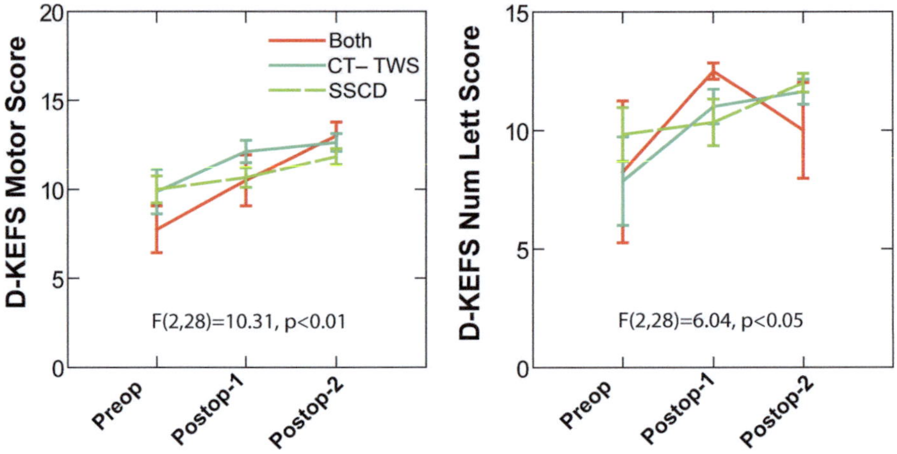

Fig. 6.2 Analysis of variance showed that there was significant postoperative improvement in both the Delis-Kaplan Executive Function System (D-KEFS) motor score ($F(2,28) = 10.31$, $p <$ 0.0.01) and the number and letter score ($F(2,28) = 6.04$, $p < 0.05$). There were no significant differences between the treatment responses for all three groups (CT– TWS only treated with RWR, both SSCD and CT– TWS treated with SSCD plugging and RWR surgeries, and SSCD only treated with SSCD plugging only). Adapted from Wackym et al. [15] Copyright © P.A. Wackym, MD, used with permission

Altered Spatial Orientation

Patients with TMWS and/or vestibular migraine often use the following descriptors when describing their altered spatial orientation: "trouble judging distances; feeling detached and separated or not connected, almost like watching a play when around other people; and even an out-of-body experience (in more severe gravitational receptor asymmetries)." Several groups have begun studying this phenomenon. Clinically, this spatial disorientation reverses after surgery; however, Baek and colleagues reported that spatial memory deficits following bilateral vestibular loss may be permanent [41]. There is also evidence that simulation of the vestibular system is necessary to maintain normal spatial memory [42]. Deroualle and Lopez have explored the visual-vestibular interaction and in their 2014 review of the topic conclude that vestibular signals may be involved in the sensory bases of self-other distinction and mirroring, emotion perception and perspective taking [43]. Clinically, patients with TMWS recognize changes in their personality. Smith and Darlington argue that these changes in cognitive and emotional states occur because of the role the ascending vestibular pathways to the limbic system and neocortex play in the sense of spatial orientation [44]. They further suggest that this change in the sense of self is responsible for the depersonalization and derealization symptoms such as feeling "spaced out," "body feeling strange," and "not feeling in control of self."

Anxiety

Vestibular disorders can produce anxiety; however, the classic sense of impending doom only occurs with the most severe gravitational receptor asymmetries. It is none-the-less quite unnerving to patients because it is a unique type of anxiety and characteristically patients have no insight why they feel that way or what is making them feel that way. Much work has been completed to understand the underlying mechanisms and pathways subserving this dysfunction [1, 14–20, 45].

Unfortunately, many patients with TMWS and other peripheral vestibular disorders are assigned a diagnosis of panic disorder (PD). The DSM V characterizes PD as episodic, unexpected panic attacks that occur without a clear trigger. Panic attacks are defined by the rapid onset of intense fear (typically peaking within about 10 minutes) with at least four (or more) of the following symptoms occurring: (1) palpitations, pounding heart, or accelerated heart rate; (2) sweating; (3) trembling or shaking; (4) sensations of shortness of breath or smothering; (5) feelings of choking; (6) chest pain or discomfort; (7) nausea or abdominal distress; (8) feeling dizzy, unsteady, light-headed, or faint; (9) chills or heat sensations; (10) paresthesias (numbness or tingling sensations); (11) derealization (feelings of unreality) or depersonalization (being detached from oneself); (12) fear of losing control or "going crazy;" and/or (13) fear of dying. At least five of the symptoms above can be caused by the autonomic dysfunction associated with vestibular asymmetries and several more of the symptoms can result from the altered spatial orientation observed in patients with these vestibular disorders.

Frontiers

To move our understanding of vestibular influence on behavior, cognition, and symptomology associated with central brain processes forward we will need to pursue the systematic investigation of vestibular disorder in analogous animal models. This will allow us to design experiments that replicate the peripheral cause of vestibular dysfunction and investigate the central changes along the five pathways discussed above. Our group has recently designed an animal model of TMWS that will provide the foundation for the thorough investigation of the symptomology described in this chapter [46]. In this model, a fenestration in the superior semicircular canal produces a pseudoconductive hearing loss (elevated ABR thresholds), and sound evoked changes to myogenic potentials (cervical positive vestibular evoked myogenic potentials [c+VEMPs]) that parallel the cVEMP elevated amplitude and decreased threshold phenomenon observed in humans with TMWS. This model also exhibits significant decision making impairments that we can exploit to investigate the vestibular injury induced maladaptive central plasticity that drives cognitive dysfunction. Modern innovative tools such as adeno-associated viruses (e.g., optogenetics; channelrhodopsin-2 [ChR2], designer receptors exclusively activated by designer drugs [DREADDs]; G-protein inhibitory DREADDs based on human muscarinic receptor [HM4Di]) coupled with advances in awake behaving neurophysiology, and in vitro whole-cell recording can be used to isolate and manipulate selective brain circuits. This will allow us to ask highly interpretative questions concerning the influence of vestibular function on physiology (e.g., balance), emotional states (e.g., anxiety, fear), and cognitive-behavioral processes. By unraveling the complexity of vestibular influence on central brain function, we should gain novel insights into the etiology of symptomology in humans that hopefully lead to new treatment approaches for chronic TMWS symptoms and other vestibular related disorders in the coming decades.

Summary

Patients with peripheral vestibular disorders, particularly TMWS patients, often experience central nervous system processing problems that can be overwhelming and difficult to understand for many clinicians. Most of the symptoms that disrupt the lives of patients with TMWS are related to the severe symptoms that are secondary to these vestibular asymmetries, including: autonomic dysfunction; spatial disorientation; and anxiety. Cognitive impairment and recovery after surgical management of TMWS has also been measured using neuropsychology test instruments. Statistically significant improvement in scores associated with depression, executive function and several domains related to verbal memory, visual memory, attention/concentration, and working memory have been observed. However, to further complicate the diagnosis and management of these TMWS patients with cognitive dysfunction, comorbidities can occur and we have identified TMWS patients with: factitious disorder; functional neurologic symptom disorder (formerly conversion disorder) dissociative motor disorder variant; somatic symptom disorder; attention deficit hyperactivity disorder; dissociative identity disorder; major depressive disorder; and post-traumatic stress disorder. Suicidal ideation was also common. These findings underscore the challenges in sorting out the TMWS symptoms caused by the dehiscence, those resulting from other comorbid conditions, or those resulting from interactions between the two factors.

References

1. Wackym PA, Balaban CD, Zhang P, Siker DA, Hundal JS. Third window syndrome: surgical management of cochlea-facial dehiscence. Front Neurol. 2019;10:1281. https://doi.org/10.3389/fneur.2019.01281.
2. Ward BK, Carey JP, Minor LB. Superior canal dehiscence syndrome: lessons from the first 20 years. Front Neurol. 2017;8:177. https://doi.org/10.3389/fneur.2017.00177.
3. Wackym PA. Vestibular migraine. Patient video describing symptoms before and after treatment with Topamax. https://doi.org/10.13140/RG.2.1.3096.2647. https://www.youtube.com/

watch?v=Zy7YjCDnLYM. Published April 12, 2012. (Accessed August 15, 2022). Copyright © P.A. Wackym, MD, used with permission.
4. Wackym PA. Right perilymph fistula not superior canal dehiscence. Patient video describing symptoms before and after surgical repair. https://doi.org/10.13140/RG.2.1.3097.8000. https://www.youtube.com/watch?v=bDph0B0uLbg. Accessed August 15, 2022. Copyright © P.A. Wackym, MD, used with permission.
5. Wackym PA. Right cochlea-facial nerve dehiscence: 16 year old thought to have conversion disorder. https://doi.org/10.13140/RG.2.2.27418.90564. https://youtu.be/fTjsnnUALBw. Published April 14, 2019. Accessed August 15, 2022. Copyright © P.A. Wackym, MD, used with permission.
6. Wackym PA. Perilymph fistula. https://doi.org/10.13140/RG.2.1.1000.6488. https://www.youtube.com/watch?v=jSAM6h-7Mwc. Published April 15, 2012. Accessed August 15, 2022. Copyright © P.A. Wackym, MD, used with permission.
7. Wackym PA. Right superior semicircular canal dehiscence repair: symptoms and recovery. https://doi.org/10.13140/RG.2.2.32032.79361. https://youtu.be/er4k8NZrG2I. Published January 9, 2017. Accessed August 15, 2022. Copyright © P.A. Wackym, MD, used with permission.
8. Wackym PA. Recurrent third window syndrome co-morbidity: functional neurological symptom disorder. https://doi.org/10.13140/RG.2.2.15255.57763. https://youtu.be/AgUy07QxTxo. Published January 9, 2017. Accessed August 15, 2022. Copyright © P.A. Wackym, MD, used with permission.
9. Wackym PA. Otic capsule dehiscence syndrome in one ear after a car accident. https://doi.org/10.13140/RG.2.1.3359.9440. https://www.youtube.com/watch?v=1Nl9T6etxqM. Published April 5, 2015. Accessed August 15, 2022. Copyright © P.A. Wackym, MD, used with permission.
10. Wackym PA. Cochlea-facial nerve dehiscence: traumatic third window syndrome after a snowboarding accident. https://doi.org/10.13140/RG.2.2.17283.76327. https://youtu.be/NCDMD5FGf-w. Published April 9, 2019. Accessed August 15, 2022. Copyright © P.A. Wackym, MD, used with permission.
11. Wackym PA. Surgery for cochlea-facial nerve dehiscence: symptoms and tuning fork testing. https://doi.org/10.13140/RG.2.2.34129.79209. https://youtu.be/lFR-zdYlIsY. Published April 14, 2019. Accessed August 15, 2022. Copyright © P.A. Wackym, MD, used with permission.
12. Wackym PA. Tuning fork testing in otic capsule dehiscence syndrome. https://doi.org/10.13140/RG.2.1.4408.5204. https://www.youtube.com/watch?v=Szp_kO8oVos. Published April 21, 2015. Accessed August 15, 2022. Copyright © P.A. Wackym, MD, used with permission.
13. Wackym PA. Tuning fork testing before and after repair of two types of otic capsule dehiscence. https://doi.org/10.13140/RG.2.1.4365.7048. https://www.youtube.com/watch?v=NIauJPbvSpA. Published December 13, 2015. Accessed August 15, 2022. Copyright © P.A. Wackym, MD, used with permission.
14. Wackym PA, Wood SJ, Siker DA, Carter DM. Otic capsule dehiscence syndrome: superior canal dehiscence syndrome with no radiographically visible dehiscence. Ear Nose Throat J. 2015;94(7):E8–24. https://doi.org/10.1177/014556131509400802.
15. Wackym PA, Balaban CD, Mackay HT, et al. Longitudinal cognitive and neurobehavioral functional outcomes after repairing otic capsule dehiscence. Otol Neurotol. 2016;37(1):70–82. https://doi.org/10.1097/MAO.0000000000000928.
16. Wackym PA, Mackay-Promitas HT, Demirel S, et al. Comorbidities confounding the outcomes of surgery for third window syndrome: outlier analysis. Laryngosc Invest Otolaryngol. 2017;2(5):225–53. https://doi.org/10.1002/lio2.89.
17. Wackym PA, Balaban CD. Molecules, motion, and man. Otolaryngol Head Neck Surg. 1998;118:S15–23.
18. Balaban CD, Thayer JF. Neurological bases for balance-anxiety links. J Anxiety Disord. 2001;15(1-2):53–79. https://doi.org/10.1016/s0887-6185(00)00042-6.
19. Balaban CD, McGee DM, Zhou J, Scudder CA. Responses of primate caudal parabrachial nucleus and Kölliker-fuse nucleus neurons to whole body rotation. J Neurophysiol. 2002;88:3175–93. https://doi.org/10.1152/jn.00499.2002.

20. Balaban CD. Projections from the parabrachial nucleus to the vestibular nuclei: potential substrates for autonomic and limbic influences on vestibular responses. Brain Res. 2004;996(1):126–37. https://doi.org/10.1016/j.brainres.2003.10.026.
21. Gizzi M, Zlotnick M, Cicerone K, Riley E. Vestibular disease and cognitive dysfunction: no evidence for a causal connection. J Head Trauma Rehabil. 2003;18(5):398–407. https://doi.org/10.1097/00001199-200309000-00002.
22. Ferrè ER, Haggard P. Vestibular cognition: state-of-the-art and future directions. Cogn Neuropsychol. 2020;37:413–20. https://doi.org/10.1080/02643294.2020.1736018.
23. Smith PF. The vestibular system and cognition. Curr Opin Neurol. 2017;1:84–9. https://doi.org/10.1097/WCO.0000000000000403.
24. Hitier M, Besnard S, Smith PF. Vestibular pathways involved in cognition. Front Integr Neurosci. 2014;8:59. https://doi.org/10.3389/fnint.2014.00059.
25. Gurvich C, Maller JJ, Lithgow B, Haghgooie S, Kulkarni. Vestibular insights into cognition and psychiatry. Brain Res. 2013;1537:244–59. https://doi.org/10.1016/j.brainres.2013.08.058.
26. Dodson MJ. Vestibular stimulation in mania: a case report. J Neurol Neurosurg Psychiatry. 2004;75:168–9.
27. Levine J, Toder D, Geller V, et al. Beneficial effects of caloric vestibular stimulation on denial of illness and manic delusions in schizoaffective disorder: a case report. Brain Stimul. 2012;5:267–73. https://doi.org/10.1016/j.brs.2011.03.004.
28. Winter L, Kruger TH, Laurens J, et al. Vestibular stimulation on a motion-simulator impacts on mood states. Front Psychol. 2012;3:499. https://doi.org/10.3389/fpsyg.2012.00499.
29. Besnard S, Machado ML, Vignaux G, et al. Influence of vestibular input on spatial and nonspatial memory and on hippocampal NMDA receptors. Hippocampus. 2012;22:814–26. https://doi.org/10.1002/hipo.20942.
30. Brandt T, Schautzer F, Hamilton DA, et al. Vestibular loss causes hippocampal atrophy and impaired spatial memory in humans. Brain. 2005;128:2732–41. https://doi.org/10.1093/brain/awh617.
31. Hüfner K, Hamilton DA, Kalla R, et al. Spatial memory and hippocampal volume in humans with unilateral vestibular deafferentation. Hippocampus. 2007;17(6):471–85. https://doi.org/10.1002/hipo.20283.
32. Sharp PE, Blair HT, Etkin D, Tzanetos DB. Influences of vestibular and visual motion information on the spatial firing patterns of hippocampal place cells. J Neurosci. 1995;15:173–89. https://doi.org/10.1523/JNEUROSCI.15-01-00173.1995.
33. Smith PF, Horii A, Russel N, et al. The effects of vestibular lesions on hippocampal function in rats. Prog Neurobiol. 2005;75(6):391–405. https://doi.org/10.1016/j.pneurobio.2005.04.004.
34. Schmahmann JD. Disorders of the cerebellum: ataxia, dysmetria of thought, and the cerebellar cognitive affective syndrome. J Neuropsychiatry Clin Neurosci. 2004;16(3):367–78. https://doi.org/10.1176/jnp.16.3.367.
35. Hoche F, Guell X, Vangel MG, Sherman JC, Schmahmann JD. The cerebellar cognitive affective/Schmahmann syndrome scale. Brain. 2018;141(1):248–70. https://doi.org/10.1093/brain/awx317.
36. Schmahmann JD. The cerebellum and cognition. Neurosci Lett. 2019;688:62–75. https://doi.org/10.1016/j.neulet.2018.07.005.
37. Argyropoulos GPD, van Dun K, Adamaszek M, et al. The cerebellar cognitive affective/Schmahmann syndrome: a Task Force Paper. Cerebellum. 2020;19(1):102–25. https://doi.org/10.1007/s12311-019-01068-8.
38. Van Overwalle F, Manto M, Cattaneo Z, et al. Consensus paper: cerebellum and social cognition. Cerebellum. 2020;19(6):833–68. https://doi.org/10.1007/s12311-020-01155-1.
39. Smith PF, Geddes LH, Baek JH, Darlington CL, Zheng Y. Modulation of memory by vestibular lesions and galvanic vestibular stimulation. Front Neurol. 2010;1:141. https://doi.org/10.3389/fneur.2010.00141.
40. Zheng Y, Geddes L, Sato G, Stiles L, Darlington CL, Smith PF. Galvanic vestibular stimulation impairs cell proliferation and neurogenesis in the rat hippocampus but not spatial memory. Hippocampus. 2014;24(5):541–52. https://doi.org/10.1002/hipo.22247.

41. Baek JH, Zheng Y, Darlington CL, Smith PF. Evidence that spatial memory deficits following bilateral vestibular deafferentation in rats are probably permanent. Neurobiol Learn Mem. 2010;94(3):402–13. https://doi.org/10.1016/j.nlm.2010.08.007.
42. Smith PF, Darlington CL, Zheng Y. Move it or lose it–is stimulation of the vestibular system necessary for normal spatial memory? Hippocampus. 2010;20(1):36–43. https://doi.org/10.1002/hipo.20588.
43. Deroualle D, Lopez C. Toward a vestibular contribution to social cognition. Front Integr Neurosci. 2014;8:16. https://doi.org/10.3389/fnint.2014.00016.
44. Smith PF, Darlington CL. Personality changes in patients with vestibular dysfunction. Front Hum Neurosci. 2013;7:678. https://doi.org/10.3389/fnhum.2013.00678.
45. Darlington CL, Goddard M, Zheng Y, Smith PF. Anxiety-related behavior and biogenic amine pathways in the rat following bilateral vestibular lesions. Ann N Y Acad Sci. 2009;1164:134–9. https://doi.org/10.1111/j.1749-6632.2008.03725.x.
46. Wackym PA, Balaban CD, Van Osch OJ, et al. New model of superior semicircular canal dehiscence with reversible diagnostic findings characteristic of patients with the disorder. Front Neurol. 2022.

Chapter 7
Other Kinds of Dehiscences

Jordan M. Thompson and Robert W. Jyung

Introduction

In 1986, Wadin et al. illustrated the connection between an otic capsule dehiscence and auditory/vestibular symptoms: they described a 54-year-old man with sudden right-sided sensorineural hearing loss (SNHL) after a severe fit of coughing, which progressed to deafness within a few days, associated with severe tinnitus and unsteadiness. Vertigo and nystagmus could be provoked with tragal pressure (Hennebert's sign), and computed tomography showed a high-riding jugular bulb adjacent to the medial aspect of the posterior semicircular canal, with suspected dehiscence [1, 2]. However, the synthesis of the Tullio phenomenon and Hennebert's sign as manifestations of superior semicircular canal dehiscence (SSCD), under the concept of the third mobile window, is credited to Minor et al. in 1998 [3]. In 2008, Merchant and Rosowski established an explanation common to all third window abnormalities: when a bony defect results in an additional mobile window of the inner ear, the normal low impedance pressure gradient between the oval and round windows is disrupted. In contrast, various "normal third window" structures such as vestibular aqueduct, cochlear aqueduct, and nearby blood vessels have exceptionally high impedances to flow and thus, do not generally transmit sound energy to cause symptoms. They found that the classic conductive hearing loss (CHL) of third window defects resulted from both worsened air-conduction threshold and improved bone conduction thresholds [4]. Various studies have expanded on this concept including a 2010 study done with rats, in which a small third window was drilled into the cochlea. Interestingly, a third window drilled over the scala vestibuli, but not over the scala tympani, resulted in a significant increase in air-conduction

J. M. Thompson · R. W. Jyung (✉)
Department of Otolaryngology – Head and Neck Surgery, Rutgers New Jersey Medical School, Newark, NJ, USA
e-mail: jt979@njms.rutgers.edu; jyungrw@njms.rutgers.edu

G. J. Gianoli, P. Thomson (eds.), *Third Mobile Window Syndrome of the Inner Ear*, https://doi.org/10.1007/978-3-031-16586-3_7

auditory thresholds [5]. Since Minor's landmark study in 1998, a variety of third window abnormalities have been described, including specific anatomic lesions such as cochlear dehiscences (facial canal, internal carotid artery, internal auditory canal, and jugular bulb), semicircular canal dehiscences (posterior and lateral), and large vestibular aqueducts. Furthermore, there is now a growing list of lesions causing otic capsule dehiscences which result in similar third window symptoms, including neoplasms, venous malformations, congenital malformations, and otosclerosis [6]. Additionally, third window syndrome (TWS) has been described that results from diffuse lesions (ex. Paget's disease) which cause a distributive effect. This chapter will review these other types of third window abnormalities, while other topics such as X-linked stapes gushers and perilymphatic fistulas will be discussed in detail elsewhere.

Cochlear-Facial Canal Dehiscence

History

The first case of cochlear-facial dehiscence (CFD) reported was actually embedded within a study of eight cases of facial nerve stimulation after cochlear implant activation [7]: a 69-year-old man with idiopathic but possibly noise-induced SNHL experienced immediate facial nerve stimulation after left cochlear implantation with a 22-channel nucleus device. Review of his preoperative CT showed "minimal bone to actual dehiscence of bone between the cochlea and labyrinthine segment of the facial nerve bilaterally" as the underlying cause. However, in 2014 Blake et al. provided the first formal description of CFD as a symptomatic entity, reporting two cases, each with bilateral CFD: a 69-year-old man with bilateral hearing loss, pulsatile tinnitus, and autophony for his voice, and a 42-year-old woman with left-sided hearing loss and left pulsatile tinnitus [8]. The first pediatric case of CFD was described in 2020 by Koroulakis et al. [9]. Since 2014, there have been several additional case reports, yet CFD has been only rarely reported.

Demographics and Prevalence

In 2016, Fang et al. conducted a histological examination of more than 1000 temporal bone specimens from the Johns Hopkins Crowe-Guild temporal bone collection, which was ideal for CFD analysis by virtue of being sectioned in the coronal plane. They measured the cochlear facial partition width (CFPW), defined as the bony width between the cochlear basilar turn to the facial nerve labyrinthine segment, as well as variables such as facial canal width (FC), facial nerve width (FN), and otic capsule area (OCA). They discovered six CFD cases, for a prevalence of 0.59%

[10]. Of the six CFD specimens, four contained data on the contralateral ear; while none of these four cases showed bilateral dehiscences, the mean contralateral CFPW was very thin at a mean of 0.045 mm, compared to the 0.23 mm average CFPW of all specimens. *Importantly, OCA was the most powerful positive predictor of CFPW*, and surprisingly, greater FC also predicted thicker CFPW. The mean OCA for the six CFD cases was significantly smaller than non-dehiscent specimens and even cases with very thin CFPW cases (<0.1 mm) showed smaller OCA compared with the rest. In contrast, increasing age significantly and negatively correlated with CFPW. In 2017, Schart-Moren conducted another prevalence study in Sweden using 113 archival temporal bones micro-CT scans and 334 corrosion casts of human temporal bones. They found a higher rate of CFD, roughly 1.4%. Interestingly, the CFPW in silicone molds was found to be 0.20 mm and 0.22 mm in the resin molds [11], which is very similar to the CFPW values reported previously by Fang et al. Bigelow et al. dissected eight temporal bone specimens and found a similar average width of 0.29 mm between the labyrinthine segment of the facial nerve and the scala tympani of the basal turn [7].

Pathogenesis

As an isolated entity, the pathogenesis of CFD may depend on two variables: the ossification process of the fallopian canal and the overall development of the otic capsule. In 1981, Marquet established that fallopian canal dehiscences were common adjacent to the vestibule but rare adjacent to the cochlea [12]. Expanding on this, Declau et al. reported that facial canal development was more complex than simple ossification of the otic capsule. Using light and scanning electron microscopy, they examined the ossification pattern of the facial canal across 22 fetal temporal bones, ranging from 14 to 25 weeks (estimated gestational age). They concluded that the final architecture of the facial canal was dependent on an intramembranous ossification of inner and outer connective tissue sheaths around the nerve and *not* dependent on the endochondral ossification of the otic capsule. Final closure of the canal required intramembranous ossification of the outer connective tissue sheath; therefore, facial canal dehiscences occurred at sites where this process was impaired, consistently at sites with proximity to epithelium such as the middle ear mucosa or arachnoid membrane [13]. However, since the bony partition between the cochlea and the facial nerve is not in immediate contact with such epithelium, and since fallopian canal dehiscences are rare adjacent to the cochlea, failure of intramembranous ossification may not fully explain how CFD occurs. Fang et al. demonstrated that otic capsule development was a critical predictor of CFPW in temporal bone histology and therefore its development (or lack thereof) must be considered in the pathogenesis of CFD [10].

Bone loss due to chronic inflammation or other osteopenic conditions such as menopause or chronic HIV infection could be considered in the pathophysiology of

CFD, as with other dehiscences. Individuals with these conditions superimposed on thin native CFPW might be at increased risk for CFD; while this has not been specifically demonstrated yet, such a mechanism would be consistent with the negative impact of age on histologic CFPW and the significant reduction of bone thickness over the superior semicircular canal in women aged >45 years versus <45 years [10, 14]. However, in a much earlier study that measured the CFPW in 24 temporal bone histopathology specimens of patients ranging from 6 to 76 years old (all with documented normal hearing), no clear decrement of CFPW with age was seen [15]. One group has even suggested that chronic intracranial hypertension and pressure-induced bone loss could result in CFD [16].

Bone erosion by facial nerve tumors at the geniculate ganglion can directly cause CFD. In 1998, Chung et al. reported three cases of facial nerve schwannomas that eroded into the cochlea, illustrating with a case of a 58-year-old man with a left-sided tumor that eroded not only the cochlea but also the ossicles and the middle fossa floor [17]. Symptoms and audiometric findings were not provided in that report. In 2019, Loos et al. reported a 60-year-old woman who presented with vertigo and falling, without other symptoms, and her initial audiogram showed mild symmetric high-frequency SNHL. A VNG demonstrated right caloric areflexia. A 3T MRI scan revealed a right facial nerve schwannoma centered at the geniculate ganglion, with extension into the labyrinthine segment. She then sustained a sudden right profound SNHL, and cone beam CT detected a 2.8 mm dehiscence of the middle turn of the cochlea. Her hearing loss did not respond to steroids and CO_2 inhalation [18]. It is important to acknowledge that tumor-related CFD may present differently from isolated CFD, given additional factors such as multifocal labyrinthine erosion by some tumors, conductive components caused by middle ear extension, as well as the unique ways that tumor biology can affect cochlear function [19].

Symptoms

It appears that the presenting symptoms of CFD can vary considerably, based on whether CFD results from a developmental deficiency versus an erosive process such as tumor growth. Therefore, it may be reasonable to differentiate "primary" CFD, where no direct cause is apparent, from "secondary" CFD, where a facial nerve tumor has eroded into the cochlea or systemic illness has resulted in bone loss at the cochlear-facial partition. This is complicated by the fact that CFD can coexist with sensorineural hearing loss (SNHL) or other disease entities such as chronic otitis media (COM), where the symptoms resulting from the coexisting pathology may override or mask symptoms related to the CFD itself. As with other forms of otic capsule dehiscence, some CFD cases could be asymptomatic.

Blake et al. detailed the symptoms which can be associated with CFD, presenting two cases. Presumably, Case 1 was a primary case: a 69-year-old man presented with pulsatile tinnitus, autophony, no vertigo and with an intact facial nerve exam. He reported an abnormal ability to hear sounds from his car engine when placing his hands on the steering wheel. Case 2 was a 42-year-old woman with HIV-related meningitis who presented with left-sided pulsatile tinnitus and conductive hearing loss (CHL), along with an ipsilateral tympanic membrane perforation [8]. In theory, Case 2 could represent a secondary case, given the known issue of accelerated bone loss in chronic HIV infection [20].

Radiology

In the senior author's experience (RWJ), careful inspection of axial images of the junction of the basal turn of the cochlea and the labyrinthine segment of the fallopian canal can reveal a "double-shadow" sign, where a greater lucency appears at the point of overlap, relative to the lucency of the basal turn or fallopian canal individually. In both cases presented by Blake et al., the CT confirmed no bony margin in the axial, coronal, and Stenvers planes between the superior portion of the basal turn of the cochlea and the intersecting point with the labyrinthine segment of the facial nerve, resulting in an apparent fusion of the fallopian canal and cochlear basal turn. In both cases, this dehiscence was bilateral but larger on the left side [8]. Perhaps importantly, both cases showed very thin/dehiscent tegmen plates, reminiscent of those seen with SSCD. In 2018, Song et al. reported a radiographic prevalence study from two academic centers: they examined CT scans of 206 patients, with a total of 406 ears (excluding six ears with prior surgery or other confounding issues). They found an overall CFD prevalence rate of 5.4% (22/406 ears), with 9.2% of patients demonstrating unilateral or bilateral CFD (19/206) and 1.4% demonstrating bilateral CFD (3/206) [21, 22]. Their average radiographic CFPW was 0.6 ± 0.2 mm, notably thicker than the histologic/anatomic studies. Additionally, they found that older age, traditional CT scans with more volume averaging, and thinner CT slice thickness were significant predictors for radiographic CFD, but the presence of SSCD or dehiscences along other segments of the facial nerve did not. While the authors noted that only 1 out of 19 patients with radiographic CFD had mixed hearing loss without any discernable cause of hearing loss (other than CFD) and only a single episode of vertigo, the retrospective nature of their study did not include a standardized documentation of third window symptoms and therefore the exact prevalence of TWS in radiographic CFD is unknown. They point out that radiographic CFD, having a relatively higher prevalence compared with histologic CFD, may include incidental cases without clinical implications. It is a given that histologic assessment would always be more accurate than radiographic methods for detecting CFD, and Fang et al. had already predicted that the high rate (35%) of histologic cases with sufficiently thin (<0.1 mm) CFPW might falsely appear dehiscent on CT imaging [10]. One possible interpretation of the radiographic data is that the clinical syndrome associated with CFD entity might require (1) full dehiscence and (2) dehiscence beyond a certain dimension in order to generate TWS. Furthermore, imaging may be overdiagnosing near dehiscences as true CFD. Importantly, Song et al. did not report the *dimension* of the dehiscences they detected. However, it is unclear currently how often CFD is present without clinical manifestations or at which thresholds these symptoms begin.

Audiometry and VEMP Findings

Both CFD cases described by Blake et al. showed striking audiometric features: the audiogram for Case 1 showed unique bilateral, symmetric "air-conduction notches" at 1 kHz, while in Case 2, bilateral bone conduction notches were seen, at 3 kHz on the right side and at 2 kHz on the left. VEMP testing in both cases showed absent waveforms at lower thresholds, bringing into question VEMP utility for CFD [8]. In a study assessing efficacy of round window reinforcement (RWR) to control TWS symptoms of CFD, Wackym et al. discovered that within the operated CFD patients, there was a statistically significant lower cVEMP threshold in the operated ears (average 75 dB) compared to non-operated ears (85.7 dB). However, there was no statistical difference in cVEMP threshold between the CFD and non-CFD ears of the cohort not treated with RWR [23]. Overall, there is a paucity of audiometric and VEMP data on primary CFD cases outside of these two studies, since many papers have focused on histology, radiology, or secondary CFD cases, as well as the relevance of CFD to cochlear implantation, where the degree of hearing loss masks any audiometric characteristics specific to the dehiscence.

Special Considerations

In the setting of cochlear implantation, CFD may lead to problematic facial nerve stimulation (FNS). In the cochlear implant case described by Bigelow et al., FNS due to CFD was traced to two electrodes but eventually required elimination of seven electrodes, and a postoperative CT scan confirmed the implant array was abutting the labyrinthine segment of the facial nerve [7]. For this reason, they emphasized the need to assess for CFD on preoperative CT imaging. Following their cautioning, a number of authors have reported CFD as the underlying cause of non-auditory percepts in CI patients, including dysgeusia [24]. In 2017, Fang et al. reported three cochlear implant cases with CFD identified on preoperative CT scans. Cases 1 and 2 experienced FNS after implant activation but Case 3 did not experience any FNS despite the presence of a right CFD measuring 1.8 mm [25]. In Case 1, four of the five offending electrodes were later re-introduced without eliciting FNS by globally reducing dynamic range and changing the pulse width, and in Case 2, all five offending electrodes were successfully re-introduced with smaller dynamic ranges. All three cases achieved excellent speech discrimination ability with no facial palsies. In contrast, Kaufman et al. reported a single case of CFD with problematic FNS after CI activation, within a large series of 497 CI cases. They highlighted the significantly increased risk of non-auditory percepts (NAP) and FNS with lateral wall electrodes versus peri-modiolar arrays, and their lone CFD case ultimately required explantation of a lateral wall electrode and reimplantation with a perimodiolar electrode array [26]. Zellhuber et al. reported a case of severe FNS from a left CI in a 32-year-old man with bilateral CFD. He had suffered from chronic headaches and visual disturbance related to hydrocephalus caused by a pineocytoma, prompting craniotomies at ages 9 and 12. He developed repeated bilateral sudden SNHL and later required CI placement with a lateral wall electrode array. However, multiple interventions to limit FNS as well as eventual device failure resulted in such poor performance that he required reimplantation with a different manufacturer: this device was selected specifically for its multi-mode grounding scheme and monophasic passive discharge stimulation, which eliminated the FNS and his performance dramatically improved [16].

In 2020, Camerin et al. reported a transient facial palsy which developed one week after uneventful cochlear implantation in a 23-year-old woman with auditory neuropathy (House-Brackmann IV). Her facial nerve recovered within one week after a course of oral steroids; following implant activation, she had no facial activation or recurrent paresis. In comparing preoperative and postoperative CT imaging, a CFD was confirmed on the preoperative scan and the CI electrode was found in close proximity to the labyrinthine segment of facial nerve [27]. In contrast, Koroulakis et al. reported a 15-month-old male toddler born small for gestational age, with bilateral severe to profound sensorineural hearing loss (SNHL). CT revealed bilateral 0.8 mm bone defects between the labyrinthine segment of fallopian canal and the adjacent cochlea. At age three, he underwent bilateral cochlear implantation with subsequent improvements to speech and hearing, and no issues with facial nerve stimulation [9]. Schart-Morén have identified a large late myogenic potential at 6 and 7.5 ms latency, seen on intraoperative electrically evoked ABRs in two patients with CFD undergoing cochlear implant placement. They suggested that its presence might predict facial nerve stimulation at implant activation [11].

In summary, while CFD increases the risk of FNS after CI activation, the mere presence of a CFD does not always result in FNS and should not deter CI placement. However, preoperative detection of CFD will allow better patient counseling regarding risks and may influence the choice of both manufacturer and type of electrode array [28]. Garaycochea et al. described a patient with bilateral Ménière's disease found to have both a right cochlear-internal auditory canal dehiscence (CIACD) and right CFD during clinical work-up following a CSF gusher encountered during right cochlear implantation. As in the original cases, VEMPs did not confirm a TWS [29].

Treatment

Literature on surgical management of CFD is limited. Having demonstrated efficacy of round window reinforcement (RWR) for otic capsule dehiscence syndrome (in which no radiographically visible dehiscence can be identified), Wackym et al. compared surgical outcomes of eight patients with clinical TWS and radiological confirmed CFD with a similar group of eight patients who did not undergo surgical intervention [23, 30]. Eight patients (five children, three adults) underwent round window reinforcement (RWR) using a thinned perichondrial graft followed by a

2 mm punched out conchal cartilage graft split in half. The Dizziness Handicap Inventory (DHI) and Headache Impact Test (HIT-6) were assessed pre- and postoperatively. In each respective cohort, 75% had sound-induced dizziness, however, in the group which did not undergo RWR, the symptoms were subjectively not as bothersome. There was no statistical difference in hearing outcomes after RWR in the CFD cohort. For CFD patients who underwent RWR, there was a highly significant improvement in both the mean DHI score and the HIT-6 score. Based on this work, patients with TWS symptoms related to CFD may benefit from surgical management.

Cochlear-Carotid Dehiscence

History

In 2004, Modugno et al. first reported a dehiscence of the bony plate between the basal turn of the cochlea and the adjacent carotid canal. They described a 63-year-old man with bilateral, nonpulsatile tinnitus, and bilateral mid- and high-frequency SNHL, as well as decreased VEMP thresholds bilaterally. High-resolution CT imaging revealed bilateral cochlear-carotid dehiscences (CCD), and they hypothesized that the associated SNHL could result from inner hair cell damage due to chronic pressure from the internal carotid artery (ICA) [31].

Prevalence

In 2006, Young et al. examined 30 temporal bone CT scans and measured the cochlear-carotid interval (CCI), defined as the minimal distance between the basal turn of cochlea and petrous internal carotid artery. They found that the CCI had a wide range; the mean value of the right ear was 1.2 ± 0.8 and 1.2 ± 0.9 mm on the left. They reported a single case of CCD, with a CCI of 0.0 m on the left and 0.2 mm on the right [32]. A much larger multi-detector CT study of the CCI was completed on 1105 patients by Gunbey et al. in 2011. This study found a mean CCI of 1.0 ± 0.8, consistent with Young's earlier measurements. Notably, they found eight patients (0.7%) with unilateral CCD and two patients (0.1%) with bilateral CCD. A limitation of this study was that they were unable to correlate imaging with symptoms. There was no significant difference in CCI with sex or laterality, but there was a positive correlation between the right and left CCI [33]. Another study of 155 temporal bone CT scans (310 ears) showed a mean CCI 1.9 mm ± 1.1, including one case of complete CCD (0.3%). They showed a negative correlation between CCI and age [34]. As in the prior study, they found a positive correlation between the patients' right and left CCI.

Pathogenesis and Relationship with Other Otologic Pathology

While the initial case report by Modugno et al. represents a primary CCD, dehiscences in this location can also occur secondary to other diseases which degrade the otic capsule [31]. In 2006, Kim and Wilson reported a 62-year-old man with progressive right hearing loss and classic tuning fork and audiometric findings of otosclerosis, including a Carhart notch. Following a small fenestra stapedotomy, the patient noted sound- and pressure-provoked vertigo as well as occasional pulse-synchronous tinnitus, and his audiogram showed an 18 dB average air-bone gap from 500 to 2 kHz. CT evaluation showed a cochlear-carotid dehiscence; close inspection of the images shows a rounded lucency bridging between the apex of the cochlea and the carotid canal, rather than a primary dehiscence. The lucency could represent otosclerosis or some other lesion, but regardless, a TWS mechanism could explain his symptoms [35]. In 2011, a similar case report described a patient with stapes fixation, however, this patient was found to have bilateral CCD at the apical turn at the cochlea [36]. Importantly, Young and Isaacson described a case of CCD caused by cholesteatoma eroding into the vestibule, basal turn, and middle turns of the cochlea [37].

Symptoms

The presence of symptoms from CCD, as with other dehiscences, may depend on the size. Oliver et al. reported a case of an apical CCD with persistent unilateral pulsatile tinnitus. In contrast to prior case reports, this patient had severe low frequency SNHL and normal c- and oVEMPs. Of note, despite this patient having unilateral symptoms and unilateral pathology on audiogram, the patient had evidence of bilateral dehiscences on CT imaging. Her symptoms correlated with the ear which had a larger width of deficient bone of 1.5 mm (compared to the contralateral ear at 0.8 mm) [38].

CCD can manifest as fluctuating symptoms. Young et al. presented a single case of CCD: a 56-year-old man with recurrent episodes of reduced hearing in both ears provoked with strenuous exercise, such as weightlifting or running, as well as riding on a train through an underground tunnel or traveling to high altitude. During each episode, he noted an increase in his baseline tinnitus and aural fullness, and his hearing loss would resolve over 5–10 days without intervention, alternating between his ears every 2–3 weeks [32].

In 2013, Cetin et al. assessed the influence of the CCI on hearing loss in 90 subjects (180 ears) who had presented with varying complaints of hearing loss, tinnitus, vertigo, and Bell's palsy. They measured the CCI using reformatted axial FIESTA images from a 1.5 T MRI system. The CCI did not show any significant differences between gender (mean 2.31 in woman, 2.28 in men) or laterality, nor was there any relationship with age. Surprisingly, when subjects were grouped according to *mid-frequency* hearing loss versus normal hearing, a statistically greater CCI was found in the hearing loss group, rather than the normal hearing group [39]. Limitations of the study include its retrospective design and inclusion of patients with varied pathology as well as the utilization of MRI images to assess a bony dehiscence.

An interesting study by Gunbey et al. in 2016 looked at 25 patients with tinnitus (and CCD) and correlated tinnitus perception scores with CCI (determined by temporal MRI). There was no statistical difference in CCI values between the tinnitus cohort and their matched controls. However, they found a strong negative correlation between the subjective burden of tinnitus (using both the tinnitus visual analog scale and the tinnitus handicap inventory) when compared to CCI. They also found a negative correlation between CCI and the accompanying SNHL (typically at higher frequencies) [40]. This study seems to support Modugno's argument regarding the proximity of the carotid causing long term inner hair cell damage. It will be difficult to fully evaluate this relationship between CCI, SNHL and tinnitus without more data.

Treatment

Because of the involvement of the carotid artery, this defect is a high-risk location without an easy solution. In general, each case report of CCD has described conservative management and observation. Therefore, there is little supporting data for surgical intervention. In the case of secondary CCD by cholesteatoma erosion (where the CCI may have initially been normal), meticulous removal of matrix may leave a void in the otic capsule and allow a space for bone cement application to reconstitute the capsule, but this is speculative. Additionally, intravascular techniques may be an option but may come with significant risks [41]. See Chap. 16 for a discussion of endovascular therapy of TMWS.

Posterior Semicircular Canal Dehiscence (PSCD)

History

Although posterior semicircular canal dehiscences (PSCD) are uncommon, they have been linked to third window-like symptoms since the 1980s. In 1986, Wadin et al. were the first to describe four possible PSCD cases in their examination of the effects of high jugular fossae in over 100 CT temporal bones. They correlated CT findings with symptoms and proposed the mechanism of a high jugular bulb inducing PSCD as a cause of hearing loss. One of these patients was found to have sudden SNHL, tinnitus and Hennebert's sign [1]. Since that time, many case reports have been published regarding PSCD and some of its unique variations. In 2008, a study followed a pediatric patient with profound mixed hearing loss [42]. Two different reports described symptomatic patients with simultaneous PSCD and SSCD, creating what they described as a fourth window [43, 44].

Prevalence

There have been several large radiographic studies examining the prevalence of PSCD, with values varying from 0.3% to 4.5%, depending on age as well as whether subjects were symptomatic or not. In 2003, a German study reviewed all their department CT scans across a 2-year span, finding an overall prevalence of 4.5% in 507 patients. Of these patients, approximately 60% had bilateral PSCD and 35% had combined PSCD and SSCD. In a separate cohort of patients having no symptoms related to the inner ear, only 0.5% had PSCD [45, 46]. A prospective study in Turkey sought to determine the prevalence of PSCD in asymptomatic ears. Excluding any patient with vertigo, perceived hearing loss, or tinnitus, they examined 410 consecutive patients with multislice CT scans of 0.3 mm slice thickness. They identified a prevalence of 1.2%; bilateral PSCD was found in three of the five identified patients [47]. None of these asymptomatic patients revealed abnormal audiovestibular testing. A 2013 study of 850 consecutive temporal bone CT scans of patients with various otologic complaints demonstrated a prevalence of 13 PSCD cases (0.8%) in 1700 ears [48]. In 2014, Russo et al. determined a PSCD prevalence of 1.2% (five cases out of 412 CT scans reviewed, with a slice thickness of 0.625 mm). All five cases were male, ranging from 16 to 73 years old, and three of the five cases also had at least one SSCD [49]. A smaller study in 2009 examined 131 temporal bone CT scans in pediatric patients 3–21 years old, finding approximately 4% (5/131) with PSCD [50].

Pathogenesis and Relationship with Other Otologic Pathology

The etiology of the PSCD is currently unclear. The presence of PSCD in the pediatric literature might suggest that there is a congenital component. However, if developmental failures in the ossification matrix were the main cause, then greater prevalence rates would be predicted for lateral and posterior semicircular canal dehiscences, to mimic rates closer to those seen in SSCD. For this reason, many authors theorize that despite congenital predisposition, symptoms do not typically begin until adulthood, when a near-dehiscence may fracture due to trauma, exposing the PSC to pressures from the posterior cranial fossa. This creates a more susceptible environment for symptomatic dehiscences, especially for the superior and posterior canals which have a closer relationship to the dura, the middle and posterior cranial fossae respectively. Unsurprisingly, it is these surfaces nearest to the dura that result in the most dehiscences. This corresponds to the posterior aspect of the canal for the posterior semicircular canal as the anterior is protected by petrous bone

[51]. The close relationship of the jugular bulb is an important mechanism for the development of PSCD. In 7 of 12 PSCD cases reported by Gopen et al., a high riding bulb was associated, which contributed to the bias of PSCD to the right side in their series [52]. In a systematic review yielding 47 cases in the literature, the most commonly associated abnormality was a high riding jugular bulb [53]. Symptomatic PSCD can also result from iatrogenic thinning of the otic capsule of the PSC, during skull base surgical approaches or as a consequence of PSC plugging for intractable BPPV [54]. In addition, multiple pathologic conditions have been associated with PCSD, with new symptom onset in pregnancy, fibrous dysplasia, apex cholesteatoma, iatrogenic, Hallermann-Streiff Syndrome, and following endolymphatic sac surgery [55–59]. An additional association was observed with Chiari Malformation type 1 in one study in which they found five of six (83%) patients had PSCD [60]. It is important to recognize that PSCD may involve the vestibular aqueduct, in either normal sized ducts or LVA. In the latter case, it may be difficult to differentiate which TWS entity leads to clinical symptomology or if a combination effect of the two TWS entities exists (Gianoli, personal communication).

Although limited in power, a study in 2015 examined 228 CT scans (456 ears) in children younger than seven years old, to simultaneously identify the prevalence of PSCD and SSCD in the following age strata: (1) less than 6 months, (2) 6–11 months, (3) 12–35 months, and (4) 3–7 years. A total of ten cases of radiographic PSCD were found, with seven found in the <6-month age group. Hearing losses ranging from mild to severe SNHL or even mixed HL were associated with PSCD, but normal hearing was also documented, and the usual outcome was stable hearing. The PSCD prevalence was 16.7%, 2.4%, 1.4%, and 0% in these age groups, respectively, with the youngest group prevalence statistically greater than the other age groups, and these prevalence rates fell to adult rates by age three. There was a corresponding significant increase in bone thickness over the posterior canal with increasing age, (with greater posterior canal bone thickness compared to the superior canal, across age groups older than one year), consistent with the known continuation of otic capsule ossification into early childhood. In fact, some dehiscence cases demonstrated hearing improvement as the otic capsule matured. They also examined histology of 58 temporal bones specimens (from 33 individuals, all less than seven years old) but found no cases of PSCD. Therefore, the authors generally cautioned against viewing radiographic PSCD in children as a pathologic entity. Altogether, their data agreed with the concept of PSCD as a consequence of congenitally thin bone breached by a secondary insult [61].

Radiology

In order to determine if PSCD or SSCD influenced the contralateral canal bone thickness, investigators in Spain examined CT scans of 318 patients from three centers, finding a corresponding thinning of bone of the contralateral superior SCC when an SSCD was discovered (n = 16) but no apparent influence on the bone thickness of the contralateral posterior SCC when a PSCD was present ($n = 2$). Interestingly, neither PSCD case was considered symptomatic. The mean bone thickness separating the posterior SCC from the posterior cranial fossa was 1.9 mm [62]. Using this data set, the same investigators categorized patients into five radiographic patterns of bone thickness of the posterior SCC: thin (≤1.2 mm), normal (0.9–2.5 mm), thick (≥2.6 mm), pneumatized, and dehiscent. Again, only two PSCD cases were identified, one directly to the posterior cranial fossa and the other to the jugular bulb [63]. Another potential category or radiographic pattern is the entity of intracranially protruding posterior SCC. Kundaragi et al. reported a patient with BPPV and a positive Dix-Hallpike bilaterally who also exhibited Tullio phenomenon and a positive Hennebert sign. MRI and CT imaging demonstrated bilateral PSCD with bilateral protrusion of the posterior SCC into the posterior fossa [64].

Symptoms

PSCD can present with classic TWS symptoms, including pulsatile or nonpulsatile tinnitus, autophony, disequilibrium, vertigo, as well as Tullio and Hennebert's phenomenon. In contrast, many patients with PSCD may be asymptomatic or, in the case of pediatric patients, may simply be unable to articulate their symptoms. PSCD symptoms can also overlap with other clinical entities, making the diagnosis challenging in some settings. Krombach et al. reviewed 507 temporal bone CT scans with 1 mm slice thickness over a 2-year period, dividing the scans into three groups: (1) patients presenting with vertigo, (2) patients presenting with other inner ear symptoms such as SNHL or tinnitus, and (3) patients with symptoms unrelated to the inner ear, such as trauma, tumors, or inflammatory disease. They identified 44 patients with canal dehiscences: 23 had PSCD (with eight of those 23 having both PSCD and SSCD), and the remaining 21 had SSCD alone. Of the 23 PSCD cases, 14 were bilateral and nine were unilateral, with a mean defect size of 2.3 mm. In these 23 cases, 86% presented with vertigo, 9% with hearing loss or tinnitus, and 5% with symptoms unrelated to the inner ear, and this difference was statistically significant [46]. Gopen et al. from Children's Hospital Boston reported the first case series of 12 patients with symptomatic PSCD, with an age range from 2 to 67 years, including seven pediatric patients. After obtaining a suspicious clinical history, the diagnosis was made on high-resolution CT and confirmed with VEMP testing (patients with CT findings suspicious for PSCD but normal VEMP testing were excluded). Interestingly, all non-iatrogenic cases were on the right side, due to a high riding jugular bulb, which the authors attributed to right-sided dominance of venous drainage. Two cases were iatrogenic, after vestibular schwannoma resection and mastoidectomy. Of the pediatric cases, two were too young to provide symptoms, but the remaining five reported vertigo with sounds, sporadic vertigo, chronic disequilibrium, or no vestibular symptoms. Of the five adults, all had aural fullness, two had autophony, and the remaining three had pulsatile tinnitus. All adults reported chronic disequilibrium except the one who underwent vestibular nerve sacrifice as part of the tumor resection [52]. In the five PSCD cases reported by Russo et al., tinnitus and aural fullness were the most common symptoms, with none reporting pulsatile tinnitus [49].

Lee et al. presented a series of five PSCD cases and did a systematic literature review, identifying 47 additional cases. Of their five cases, four had no TWS but one patient had sound- and pressure-induced vertigo. Of the 47 cases in the literature, five (10.6%) had bilateral PSCD, seven (14.9%) had concomitant SSCD, and seven (14.9%) were iatrogenic. The most common associated anatomic abnormality was a high riding jugular bulb. In the analysis of symptoms, the most common symptoms were sound-induced vertigo (38.3%), mixed hearing loss (36.2%), tinnitus (34%), aural fullness (29.8%), autophony (27.7%), SNHL (23.4%), disequilibrium (21.3%), conductive hearing loss (19.1%), and pressure-induced vertigo (19.1%) [53]. Another series of five PSCD cases from the Massachusetts Eye and Ear Infirmary demonstrated pulsatile tinnitus in 4/5 (80%), hearing loss in 3/5 (60%), and autophony in 2/5 (40%), with vertigo in 2/5 (40%) [6].

The TWS symptoms associated with PSCD can clinically overlap with common causes of vertigo such as BPPV or Ménière's Disease. Peress et al. reported an illustrative case of a 65-year-old woman diagnosed 25 years earlier with Ménière's Disease on the basis of right hearing loss, bilateral aural fullness, dizziness and nausea with head turning. Her initial audiogram demonstrated SNHL but over the years, a conductive component developed in the right ear, prompting a CT scan which revealed PSCD due to a high riding jugular bulb. Her vertigo had resolved over the years and no treatment other than amplification was recommended [65].

Audiometry, VEMP, and Other Test Findings

In a meta-analysis of PSCD cases, Bear et al. quantified the hearing loss from eight articles containing quality audiograms of 21 patients, comparing air-conduction thresholds from PSCD ears to the contralateral ears as well as normative air-conduction (AC) data. Again, the most common etiology for PSCD was a high riding jugular bulb (12/21 cases). One pediatric patient was excluded since the hearing thresholds were at the limits of the audiometer, leaving 21 cases. They concluded that PSCD patients have significantly worsened AC thresholds at and below 2000 Hz as well as at 4000 and 8000 Hz, compared to their contralateral ears [66]. When comparison was made to age-matched normative data, PSCD patients showed highly significantly worsened AC thresholds at all frequencies from 3000 Hz and below, as well as a highly significant worsening when comparing pure tone average. These results were consistent with the conductive hearing loss seen in SSCD, since a similar third window causes shunting of acoustic energy away from the cochlea. However, since the epidemiologic data only contained AC thresholds, a more complete analysis of the degree of conductive hearing loss could not be performed. The authors also acknowledged that normative data were only available for age groups >48 years, while the average age of the PSCD cases was 27.5 [66].

In the Children's Hospital Boston case series, 8 of 12 PSCD cases had mixed hearing loss (67%) with half of those demonstrating a downsloping pattern, three had conductive hearing loss (25%), and one had profound SNHL (8%). However, since hearing loss was an inclusion criterion, potential PSCD cases without hearing loss had been excluded. Positive VEMP testing with characteristic elevated amplitudes and reduced thresholds was documented in 10 of the 12 cases, although this was expected, since a positive VEMP was a key inclusion criterion [48, 52].

Kubota et al. documented the transition from what appeared to be a mixed but predominantly SNHL into a low-frequency CHL in a 14-year-old girl with PSCD. Her left hearing loss had been discovered at age six during a screening examination and was diagnosed as SNHL at another institution at age 13. She had no dizziness complaints, and a prior brain MRI was normal. ABR testing confirmed the left hearing loss. Her initial CT scan showed a high riding jugular bulb on the left side, which in retrospect demonstrated an intact bony wall between the jugular bulb and the posterior SCC. She was closely followed with audiograms every six months for eight years, and by the eighth year, the bone conduction (BC) thresholds had improved and reached a near normal level, without much change in the air conduction (AC). Based on these air-bone gaps (ABGs), otosclerosis was considered, even though her stapedial reflexes were present. An exploratory tympanotomy failed to reveal any ossicular cause for CHL. However, a repeat CT scan showed a PSCD due to the high riding jugular bulb, and a VEMP test was positive, with an abnormally low threshold and an amplitude more than twice that of the right side [67]. The authors emphasized the dual mechanisms for apparent ABGs in TWS: (1) hypersensitivity of BC hearing and (2) loss of stapes-delivered AC acoustic energy. If the 1st mechanism were dominant, then surgical repair might eliminate the hypersensitivity for BC but not improve the patient's hearing; if the 2nd mechanism were dominant, then surgical repair could improve hearing performance.

Treatment

Currently, very few papers have demonstrated effective surgical treatment of PSCD; management of most reported cases has consisted of observation or use of hearing aids. However, Mikulec and Poe reported successful transmastoid plugging of the PSC in a 34-year-old woman with an inaccessible PSCD on the medial surface, due to a high riding jugular bulb. She had previously been treated with a right stapedectomy for CHL, with three revisions for persistent hearing loss and vestibular symptoms. Her classic TWS presentation included right CHL, autophony, a positive fistula test, Tullio's sign, a VEMP response at 75 dB, and a CT suggestive of a SSCD. However, surgical exploration showed only a blue line of the SSC, and a repair with bone wax and a split calvarial graft did not provide benefit. Following the transmastoid plugging of the PSC, her symptoms were subjectively "70%" improved and her CHL improved, but her VEMP threshold remained at 75 dB, suggesting incomplete occlusion of the defect [68]. Dang et al. reported an unusual case of bilateral combined SSCD and PSCD adjacent to the common crus, with 2–3 mm dehiscences on the right side. The patient reported autophony and right-sided hyperacusis limiting his participation in choir and family activities. Using a right transmastoid approach, both dehiscences were controlled with temporalis fascia plugs followed by small bone chips and bone pate, with significant improvement in his hyperacusis and improvement in his preoperative low frequency hearing loss, allowing him to resume all choir activities. Interestingly, he developed right BPPV and imbalance with head motion postoperatively, adequately treated with the Epley maneuver and vestibular rehabilitation [69]. A third example of PSCD plugging was reported in 2019 with comparable results to the first two cases [70].

As an alternative to plugging, some authors have described a direct repair of PSCD. Lim et al. reported the case of a 66-year-old man with impulsive sound-induced disequilibrium and vertigo of a two-month duration. He noted exacerbation of vertigo when lowering his head forward to tie his shoes, with simultaneous brief pulsatile tinnitus and right aural fullness. His vertigo and pulsatile tinnitus could also be induced by the Valsalva maneuver. His audiogram showed bilateral downsloping SNHL, with an ABG in the right ear, only at 250 Hz. His ocular VEMP thresholds were 65 and 80 dB on the right and left side, respectively. Release of positive pressure applied to the right EAC induced counter-clockwise, down-beating nystagmus. CT imaging demonstrated a diverticulum of the right jugular bulb causing a dehiscence of the inferior aspect of the PSC. Surgical repair was performed through a transmastoid approach, with careful separation of the diverticulum from a 2 mm dehiscence of the PSC just posterior to the ampulla. A construct of bone pate/fascia/conchal cartilage covered by fibrin glue was utilized, and at three months postoperatively, the patient noted resolution of his sound- and position-induced vertigo. His VEMP threshold increased to 85 dB [71]. The same approach was used to treat a high riding jugular bulb causing broad dehiscence of the inferior aspect of the PSC and was described by Gubbels et al. A 20-year-old man presented with noise-induced vertigo and right pulsatile tinnitus following a left otic capsule-sparing temporal bone fracture caused by a ground-level fall four months earlier. His examination revealed Hennebert's sign and a Tullio phenomenon as well as a right cVEMP threshold of 67 dB, compared to a 92 dB on the left. His audiogram showed a symmetric mild to moderately severe SNHL with 96% discrimination bilaterally. Because his noise-induced vertigo interfered with his work around heavy machinery, surgery was offered. They utilized a transmastoid approach to reduce the jugular bulb and repair the dehiscence directly with a layered fascia/bone pate/cortical bone graft. Two months postoperatively, he noted resolution of his vertigo and improvement of his pulsatile tinnitus, and his right cVEMP threshold normalized. Interestingly, a new right 20–40 dB CHL across all frequencies appeared, which resolved by 20 months postoperatively. Late onset mild disequilibrium resolved with vestibular rehabilitation therapy [72].

Cochlear-Jugular Bulb Dehiscence (CJB)

History/Pathogenesis and Relationship with Other Otologic Pathology

In the previous section, jugular bulb dehiscences were described as a frequent cause of PSCD. There is a growing body of literature regarding other jugular bulb related inner ear dehiscences (JBID), most notably involving the vestibular aqueduct (JVAD) and to a lesser degree, the cochlear aqueduct (JCAD). In all types of dehiscences, a large high jugular bulb (HJB) or a jugular bulb diverticulum (JBD) are frequently cited as a correlating factor. JBD are defined as an irregular outpouching of jugular bulb. There is not a consensus of what constitutes a high riding jugular bulb. A jugular bulb may be considered high riding if it reaches the level of the basal turn of the cochlea, it extends above inferior portion of the tympanic annulus or it reaches within 2 mm of the floor of the internal auditory canal [73–75]. Some studies use an additional marker of the lateral semicircular canal to categorize severity HJB. More elaborate categorizations have been proposed classifying HJB into five types with additional divisions into subtypes [76]. In the original radiologic study of 700 temporal bones, Atilla et al. found 20% to be consider HJB. In both Wadin and Atilla's early studies, there were higher percentages of HJB in the right temporal bones, which as mentioned earlier, is consistent with majority of patients having right dominant venous systems [2, 73]. The jugular bulb does not form until after birth. It is initially a thin narrowing junction between the sigmoid sinus and the internal jugular vein. Presumably, a compilation of factors including the temporal bone beginning to pneumatize and the constant back pressure from the heart lend to the jugular bulb taking its shape after two years of age and stabilizing into adulthood. However, characteristic of veins and sinuses, there is much variability in the formation of the jugular bulb [77]. For example, studies have investigated the JB taking a more medial position (MHJB) and affecting inner ear physiology. One study observed that patients with MHJB may have a resulting pressure influence and compression of the endolymphatic sac which may decrease endolymph absorption. In four of the five subjects with MHJB, bony defects were found between the jugular fossa and vestibular aqueduct [78].

Demographics and Prevalence/Radiology

Speculation of HJB association with the cochlear and vestibular aqueduct is documented as early as 1986 in a study conducted by Wadin using temporal bone casting. Of the 58 temporal bone castings categorized as having a HJB, they identified nine JVAD and three JCAD [1]. A noteworthy histological examination of over 1500 temporal bone specimens reported HJB in 8.2% of temporal bones. The found prevalence increased with age and stabilized in the fourth decade of life. Additionally, they found JBID in 2.8% of cases. Of the 44 reported inner ear dehiscences, 41 involved the vestibular aqueduct [79]. A large South Korean study looking at nearly 2300 cases found 9.5% to have HJB. Some of the pertinent exclusion criteria include age less than 10, congenital anomalies, and operated ears. Similar to what has been reported for PSCD, this study found a right side predominance (right: left ratio of 1.88:1) [80]. A radiologic study that divided patients into cohorts based on symptoms identified 14/176 patient with JVAD and one patient with both JVAD and JCAD. Interestingly, over one-third of the recurrent vertigo cohort was found to have JVAD on imaging [81]. Park et al. divided HJB into type-1 reaching above inferior part of round window and type-2 defined as dome of JB higher than the inferior edge of IAC. Consistent with prior studies, around 90% of the JBID involved JVAD. When comparing type-1 HJB to the more severe category of type-2, type-2 had a higher percentage of JVAD by a factor of three (15.9% compared 2.9%) [82].

Symptoms/Audiometry, VEMP, and Other Test Finding

As with other TWS described, JBID clinical presentation can vary in type and quantity. Interestingly, the literature on topic has been conflicting with several small case studies discussing associated TWS, however, several larger studies have not found statistical differences between specific symptoms and/or hearing loss with JBVAD. Friedman et al. reported nine patients with JVAD. Half of the tested patients had VEMP testing indicative of TWS. Tinnitus was reported in most patients. Several patients had CHL and several SNHL. One theory for this finding is SNHL results from hair cell degeneration from the hemodynamic changes caused the jugular dehiscences [74]. In another study by Friedman et al., they combined a study of temporal bone microscopy and a review of 30 patients with identified JBID. Similar to ratios presented in other studies, a majority of the dehiscences involved vestibular aqueduct. Of the 1500 specimens analyzed, the study found that JVAD was infrequently associated with endolymphatic hydrops. Of the two identified, only one had clinical symptoms of Ménière's disease [83]. In a study of 200 temporal bone images of patients with Ménière's disease, no difference was found between JBID and Ménière's disease but there was a correlation between JBID and medial position HJB [84]. Although there has not been an association between Ménière's disease and JBID, Friedman et al. found a small but greater than predicted association with otosclerosis, hinting at a possible predisposing underlying pathophysiologic mechanism. In nearly half the JBID, patients were asymptomatic. The authors discussed several factors including overdiagnosis of JBID on imaging studies or that these dehiscences could generally be well tolerated [83]. In 2015, a study of over 8000 temporal bone CT scans identified 46 patients with JVAD. Half presented with SNHL while only 6% had tinnitus and 4.3% had vertigo, however, none of these numbers were statically significant [85]. Similarly, Kupfer et al. investigated 900 pediatric patients with an overall JVAD prevalence of 8.6%. They did not find a statically significant relationship between JVAD and hearing loss of any type [86]. A Turkish study in 2017 correlating 1500 temporal bones with symptoms identified a similar JVAD prevalence of 8.2%. This study similarly did not find an association of JVAD with tinnitus or vertigo. However, in the group of patients with pathology limited to dehiscence on CT imaging, 60% were found to have hearing loss on audiometry and had a statically higher level of median air-bone conduction values. Interestingly, 18 patients were found to have near-dehiscence of JVAD. In this group, six were found to have unilateral hearing loss (two with CHL and three with SNHL) [87]. Thus, occasionally JVAD may result in third window symptomology. However, it is often asymptomatic and a clear correlation with tinnitus or vertigo has not been established. Current literature does not support a strong correlation with hearing loss but in symptomatic patients, there may be a CHL contribution. To this date, symptomology of cochlear aqueduct dehiscence has not been well published because it is a rare entity. It may appear similarly to JAVD in which it is often silent but occasionally causes TWS.

Treatment

In the literature, these cases have typically been treated conservatively due to low prevalence and are frequently asymptomatic. However, a study based in northern France describes treating symptomatic patients with JVAD using endovascular techniques to resolve vertigo and pulsatile tinnitus. They describe the use of coils filling the jugular bulb abnormality. All patients had resolution of symptoms and one year postoperatively, had no documented thromboembolic or hemorrhagic complication [88]. Additional surgical treatments may include ligation or embolization of the jugular vein or even reconstructing the bony labyrinth and lowering the jugular bulb. A study by Couloigner et al. looked at 13 patients with disabling vertigo attacks and pulsatile tinnitus attributed to Ménière's disease with associated high jugular bulb. Surgical intervention for each patient included exposing the lateral and posterior walls of the jugular bulb using subfacial and infralabyrinthine approaches. The high jugular bulb was then progressively lowered using large pieces of surgical wax surrounded by Surgicel, to avoid potential embolism in the event of jugular bulb injury. In several cases, the endolymphatic sac was exposed and incised. After several months postoperatively, they reported a decrease in tinnitus in 31% of patients and a complete disappearance in 23%. Vertigo disappeared in 54% of patients and decreased in intensity in 38%. There was no change in postoperative mean pure-tone auditory thresholds [89]. With JBD often involving the vestibular aqueduct, one could postulate that an endolymphatic sac-jugular bulb decompression might provide benefit. A study by Gianoli et al. investigated a modified endolymphatic sac decompression surgery to include wide decompression of the sigmoid sinus, posterior cranial fossa dura, and endolymphatic sac, in a group of 35 patients who had previously failed medical treatment for Ménière's disease. Bone was removed from the sinodural angle to the jugular bulb. At two years post-surgery,

92% of vestibular symptoms were resolved or mild. This study did not look in detail at changes in symptoms of tinnitus [90]. Although both studies did not investigate these surgical interventions as it relates to third window entities, these surgical interventions showed symptomatic improvements and may be beneficial in specific patient populations, such as JVAD patients who may also have endolymphatic hydrops; however, further studies are needed. In summary, this third window entity is infrequently severe enough to warrant surgery. However, when necessary, there are various surgical interventions that may be considered, including those listed above.

Large Vestibular Aqueduct

History

There is extensive literature discussing the relationship of large vestibular aqueduct (LVA) with SNHL. This section will focus on LVA in context of being a third window entity. The vestibular aqueduct is a “J”-shaped bony canal connecting the vestibule of the bony labyrinth with the posterior cranial fossa. Although the otic labyrinth reaches near adult dimensions by mid-term, the posterior fossa continues to develop and grow causing a downward traction on the distal vestibular duct causing the characteristic shape. The temporal bone continues to develop until adult size is reached by three years old. According to a study by Pyle et al., the LVA is not a result of arrested development or failure of narrowing early in embryogenesis but rather, a continued aberrant growth [91–94].

In the 1970s, Valvassori and Clemis described the VA as approximately 10 mm long. They further categorized the VA as able to be divided into a proximal segment that is around 1.5 mm in length and 0.3 mm in diameter, and a distal section which is distinctly triangular shape with it base towards the posterior cranial fossa. The apex of this distal section increases from 0.5 mm, where it connects with the proximal segment, until it expands to over 5.0 mm at the most distal portion where it ends at the endolymphatic sac. This distal segment is approximately 8.5 mm long [95–97]. LVA was first reported in 1967 by Valvassori and Clemis who later went to expand on “Ménière’s-like disturbances” with associated radiographical findings of vestibular aqueduct abnormalities. The most common radiographic criteria for diagnosis of LVA is the Valvassori criteria, defined as an axial diameter of greater than 1.5 mm at the midpoint of the distal segment. Another LVA measurement gaining traction is the Cincinnati criteria which defines LVA as an axial width ≥2 mm at the operculum and/or ≥1 mm at the midpoint in children with nonsyndromic SNHL

[98–100]. LVA is often bilateral. In a study based in Japan, 91% (346/380) of reported cases were bilateral [101].

Audiometry, VEMP, and Other Test Findings

LVA has been shown to be in isolation or various congenital disorders such as Pendred syndrome, CHARGE syndrome, and branchiootorenal syndromes [102–104]. There have been numerous pathogenic mutations identified that correlate with LVA, most notably mutations in the SLCD26A4 gene [105]. Head trauma has also been described to be a significant risk factor for developing symptomatic LVA [101]. A LVA is the most commonly identified radiographic abnormality in children presenting with SNHL. In the SNHL population, LVA literature has varied in terms of the criteria used for measurements. As a result, the reported incidence figures have varied greatly too, at times as high as 15% in pediatric patients with SNHL [106]. A histological study of 1600 temporal bones (850 cases) found a LVA temporal bone rate of 3.9% (63/1608) [103]. As early as 1999, a pattern of CHL and mixed hearing loss had begun to emerge. In fact, Govaerts et al. reported mixed or CHL in 90% of cases, stating that the conductive component is a pure cochlea conductive loss and may be misinterpreted for middle ear disease such as ventilation or ossicular chain pathology [107]. One year later, a study compared patients with sudden SNHL compared with SNHL combined with LVA. They found that the air-bone gap in patients with LVA was always larger than the idiopathic group [108]. In other studies, the modiolar area and level of deficiency, as well as the volume of both endolymphatic sac and/or duct, did not correlate with the severity of hearing loss [106, 109, 110]. However, one of these studies reported a relationship between the VA morphology and thickness with the degree of hearing loss. Realization that a LVA may be a distinct third window entity began to formalize. A short study by Sheykholeslami published cVEMPs values on three patients with LVA. Two of the three showed significant decreased thresholds consistent with TWS. The remaining patient had normal cVEMP but a large air-bone gap [111]. To further investigate the absence of middle ear contribution to the low frequency CHL with air-bone gap found in LVA, Merchant et al. observed eight patients with LVA under a battery of measurements including the umbo velocity by laser Doppler vibrometery, tympanometry, acoustic reflex testing, distortion product otoacoustic emission testing, VEMP, and even middle ear exploration in some of the patients. Their data showed that the CHL findings in LVA were not consistent with middle ear pathology [112]. Another study evaluating middle ear pathology was conducted by Mimura et al. in 2005. This group performed the Bing test on a group of nine patients. This test is based on the principle that occlusion of the external auditory canal improves perception of bone-conducted sounds unless there is a conductive hearing loss impairment. The patients' perceptions did not change with the Bing test, giving support to the third window contribution [113].

Pathogenesis and Relationship with Other Otologic Pathology

By this time, it was hypothesized that the SNHL is a result from possible associated cochleovestibular malformations manifesting at higher frequencies while the CHL is a result of a third window component in which a LVA causes dissipation of sound energy. According to the teaching file at Massachusetts Eye and Ear Infirmary, 36% (60/165) of the ears evaluated demonstrated cochleovestibular malformations [6]. Zhou et al. reported 43% of patients had coinciding cochlear malformations such Mondini dysplasia [114]. Although there are many associated syndromes with LVA, a definitive explanation of what causes cochleovestibular malformations has not been established. A recent study based in Switzerland proposed disturbances in epithelial ion transport as a mechanism. Previously established in LVA mouse models, they investigated this theory in postmortem temporal bones of two individuals with symptomatic LVA. They have found that the enlarged endolymphatic sac had epithelium that was overall atypical in differentiation and lacked certain key ion transport proteins [115]. It appears much more literature is needed to further analyze the SNHL component of LVA. Pang et al. looked at acoustic models, investigating the effect of LVA on CHL. From a patient population size of 16, they measured various aspects of the LVA and compared predicted CHL using a simulated lumped-parameter model with actual measured values. Their results did not suggest a significant correlation between the extent of dilation and measured CHL levels. The simulated model values were able to predict an overall trend at lower frequencies but there were high degrees of patient variability. Suggesting manipulation of the simulation may assist better predictive values or that a pathologic third window effect may not be the only influence in determining the CHL component for LVA patients [96].

Radiology

Currently, it is unclear which imaging modality is best when assessing for LVA. Historically, CT imaging has been the preferred choice. A study in 2017 looked at 141 patients who were diagnosed with LVA and had both an available high-resolution CT and high-resolution MRI of the temporal bone. Three double blinded neuroradiologists were asked to evaluate for LVA with 2:1 age-matched controls. This study showed excellent inter-rater reliability and a concordance rate for both image modalities diagnosing LVA of 88%. Fifteen ears had LVA on CT imaging but not MRI, while two ears had LVA on MRI but on CT [116]. They concluded that both imaging modalities were comparable. Another study in 2019 compared imaging modalities of 58 patients with both available images and compared them with the two standard criteria of measuring LVA, the Valvassori and the Cincinnati criteria. The concordance rate with 93%. The MRI alone diagnosed 2/58 patients using the Valvassori criteria while the CT alone diagnosed 2/58 using the Valvassori and the 4/58 using the Cincinnati criteria. The study discussed the theoretical benefit of MRI for situations in which there may be clearly dilated extra-osseous endolymphatic sac seen on MRI, and yet the intra-osseous components are within normal limits and would appear normal on CT [99].

Symptoms

The clinical presentation of the LVA is diverse but hearing loss appears to be the dominant feature. In a Japanese Survey published in 2017, nearly 90% (341/380) had hearing loss and about 9% (34/380) reported vertiginous symptoms. Notably, 52% showed profound hearing loss and 48% showed asymmetric hearing loss (>10 dB) [101]. In the teaching file at Massachusetts Eye and Ear infirmary, 98 patients with LVA were included. They described 68% (67/98) with hearing loss and 6% (6/98) with vertigo [6]. In a study by Zhou et al. examining 54 patients, all patients had hearing loss to a varying degree. Air-bone gaps were seen in 80% of patients, who had either CHL or mixed hearing loss. This study highlighted the importance of having complete audiologic exams as they encountered some patients diagnosed with SNHL who lacked proper bone conduction thresholds, resulting in a missed conductive component [114]. A study in 2012 followed patient audiograms over an eight-year period. At the beginning of the study, 61% were in the mild and moderate hearing loss range, after eight years, that percentage only changed to 64%. In fact, although they did observe air-conduction differences at several frequencies, there was not a statistical change in bone conduction or air-bone gap at the conclusion of the study [94]. Kwesi et al. investigated the audiometry results of patients with LVA with and without HJB. They found that concurrent HJB resulted in higher air conduction thresholds at multiple frequencies and higher bone conduction thresholds at 250 and 500 Hz. They found no difference in air-bone gap between the two groups [117]. In 2021, a study of 221 pediatric patients with hearing loss found that across all types of hearing loss, the most common third window abnormality was LVA (41/402 ears). Additionally, they reported the CHL group showed a significant relationship between LVA and superior semicircular malformations [118].

LVA can also affect the vestibular system. A study in 2020 looked at 23 children and six adults with LVA and analyzed the cVEMP and oVEMP testing. Interestingly, when compared to match controls, the children's vestibular testing was not found to be significantly different. However, in the adult patient group, amplitudes of the oVEMP were significantly higher and amplitudes of cVEMP were significantly lower for patients with LVA compared to the healthy control group. This could be a result of small sample size or that children are often more resilient to vestibular diseases. This may also indicate a disease progression of the otolithic organs [119]. However, an earlier study had contrasting data. In 2011, an analysis of 25 pediatric cases, ages three to 20 found abnormally low VEMP thresholds in 92% (34/37) of the ears with LVA [120]. In a study of 41 cases of confirmed LVA, about half of the patients reported vertiginous symptoms, with half of these describing recurrent attacks. However, no differences in aqueduct size, hearing thresholds, or age at visit were found between the vertiginous and non-vertiginous groups [21, 22].

Treatment

Currently, cochlear implantation is the mainstay for pediatric patients with progressive SNHL although various surgical interventions have been attempted. In 1997, a small case series of seven patients underwent endolymphatic sac obliteration. The argument for such a procedure at the time was theorizing the SNHL from LVA is a result of possible hydraulic forces transmitted from the endolymphatic sac into the cochlea or possibly reflux of hyperosmolar fluids into the cochlea. Six of the seven patients had no change in postoperative hearing while one continued to have progressive SNHL [121]. However, as understanding of LVA has grown, these types of operations have fallen out of favor. As mentioned earlier, cochlear implantation is a common intervention for the well selected patient. In a retrospective intuitional study looking at 18 years of clinical practice, 103 patients were identified with symptomatic LVA. Forty-one patients had bilateral implants while 52 had unilateral implants. They found the average age of CI surgery was 8.6 years old [122]. Another study found excellent results when analyzing CI outcomes in 176 patients with symptomatic LVA. By analyzing postoperative speech perception testing, they found the median Bamford-Kowal Bench sentence test score was 93% with a lower quartile score of 85% [123]. This study argues that patients with symptomatic LVA may be among the best candidates for CI.

Other Dehiscences

There are many other possible third window abnormalities. A few notable examples such as the influences of otosclerosis and perilymphatic fistulas will be discussed in depth in other chapters. Rare case reports of TWS have been published. A case report in 2004 elaborated on a subarcuate venous malformation in proximity to the SSC causing symptoms of autophony, sound and pressure induced nystagmus, and CHL. Of note, there was no dehiscence at the apex of the SSC in proximity to the tegmen [124]. Another uncommon dehiscence is that of cochlear-internal auditory canal dehiscence (CIACD). A 2019 study looked at 134 subjects with otosclerosis which found 14 ears with an involved IAC [125]. Another case report in 2018 described a woman with low-frequency mixed hearing loss associated with episodic vertigo found to have both CFD and CIACD [29]. Similar to the concept of an LVA, it has been postulated that enlarged IAC may cause TWS. However, current literature has been incompatible with this theory. In one such study of an analysis 247 children, McClay et al. found no difference in the prevalence of SNHL between patients with and without a large IAC [126]. Although not extensively described as a TWS, modiolar dysplasia has been proposed as a possible etiology of TWS in relationship to possible modiolar-IAC dehiscences. The modiolus is a cone-shaped central bony axis with a spiral canal of osseous cochlea winding approximately two and a half turns. At the junction of the IAC and the modiolus, the lamina cribrosa and habenula perforata transmit to the cochlear nerve and blood vessels via a central normal bony defect at the base of modiolus [127]. Zheng et al. helped to classify three groups of Mondini malformations based on Mondini's original descriptions and the Phelps classification. All three types have less than the established normal 2.5 cochlear turns. Of note, one of these groups of malformations are the Mondini-like dysplasias, in which type B consists of 1.5 to 2 turns of cochlea with hypoplasia or absence of the bony wall at the base of modiolus, with or without a communication between the IAC and the cochlea [128]. A case report by Karlberg et al. in 2003 describes a 17-year-old female presenting with significant air-bone gap at 250 Hz. Initially thought to have otosclerosis, CT imaging was consistent with Mondini-like dysplasias type B without evidence of SSCD or otosclerosis [129]. Although a plausible cause of TWS, more research will be needed to further understand this lesser known TWS.

In a novel paper published in 2020, Gadre et al. published a newly described TWS based on a subset of head trauma patients who developed various TWS symptomology including intermittent vertigo or dizziness, and hyperacusis. These patients largely had been diagnosed with "post-concussive syndrome" [130]. After extensive workup of 28 patients over an 11-year period, membranous or hypermobile stapes footplates were identified. All these patients had reported normal otic capsule on CT imaging; however, diagnosis was assisted using the gray-scale invert function to evaluate the stapes footplate. All patients were found to have either Hennebert or Tullio signs. cVEMP demonstrated 76% of patients had subnormal thresholds preoperatively. Audiometric data were variable without a consistent pattern. All patients underwent surgical interventions in which the mucosa around the oval and round window niches were denuded and fat grafts packed in the round window niche, under the arch of the stapes and anterior and posterior to the stapes crurae. During surgery, 65% had identifiable bony defects in the stapes footplates which appeared to be covered by a translucent membrane. Only 22% had evidence of true perilymph leakage and the remaining ears were found to have either small cracks in the footplate or no defect noted. In this latter group of patients, they were considered to have probable hypermobile stapes footplates. Impressively, 85.7% of patients showed complete ameliorations of symptoms and no cases of hearing deterioration. This group theorizes that rapid acceleration/deceleration of the temporal bone may cause subluxation of the stapes footplate, devascularizing the blood supply leading to bony necrosis over time and development of delayed TWS [130].

Bony dyscrasias of the inner ear may present with TWS. Richard and Linthicum described a case report of a cavity in an osteosclerotic focus communicating with the SCD. This patient exhibited an air-bone gap and Tullio phenomenon. This patient underwent CI with good postoperative results [131]. In addition to otosclerosis, the abnormal local bony remodeling seen in Paget's disease is thought to cause a "distributive" TWS. Loss of bone density may result in microfistulae of the inner ear. This in turn results in enhanced conduction of low-frequency sound energy by the pagetic bone, dissipating sound energy transmitted through the stapes footplate away from the cochlea consequently developing an air-bone gap [4, 132, 133].

It is important to be aware of subsets of patients who present with symptomatic TWS with either radiologically identified thin but not frankly dehiscent bones, or patients with TWS but absence of any clinically identifiable TWS etiology. Ward et al. evaluated ten patients in which 64% were found to have thin SCC apexes but not complete dehiscence. Each patient presented with autophony or sound and/or pressure induced vertigo. Each showed low-frequency air-bone gaps. These patients underwent surgical plugging with a middle cranial fossa approach with significant decrease in air-bone gaps and symptoms [134]. An interesting study by Wackym et al. [30] compared six patients with symptomatic TWS with radiographic evidence of SSCD with six symptomatic patients without evidence of SSCD. These two patient populations were identical in symptomology preoperatively. The six patients with SSCD underwent middle cranial fossa approach with canal plugging procedures, while the six without evidence of dehiscence underwent round window reinforcement surgeries. In both groups, resolution of symptoms occurred for all patients [30]. Of note, both patient groups had a high prevalence of previous trauma. It is possible that the non-dehiscent group may in fact suffer from lesser known TWS entities such as hypermobile stapes footplate which is associated with prior trauma. Regardless, the highlighted improvement of symptoms for all patients in this subgroup following round window reinforcement surgeries suggests this option as a viable treatment for patients suffering from clinical TWS without clearly identifiable third window pathologies.

Conclusion

In summary, this wide array of other otic capsule dehiscences can be predicted based on the anatomic proximity of other structures adjacent to the labyrinth. The clinician should remain vigilant for these dehiscences when patients present with

TWS symptoms yet do not display classic CT evidence for SSCD. Knowledge of the existence of the more obscure forms of dehiscence, as well as a thorough familiarity with temporal bone imaging in multiple planes, will be invaluable for the accurate diagnosis and potential treatment of these elusive conditions. Much more research is needed, and future efforts could be directed towards development of a standardized reporting framework for any given otic capsule dehiscence, as well as artificial intelligence-aided inspection of otic capsule integrity on temporal bone CT scans.

References

1. Wadin K, Thomander L, Wilbrand H. Effects of a high jugular fossa and jugular bulb diverticulum on the inner ear. A clinical and radiologic investigation. Acta Radiol Diagn. 1986;27(6):629–36. https://doi.org/10.1177/028418518602700603.
2. Wadin K, Wilbrand H. The topographic relations of the high jugular fossa to the inner ear. A radioanatomic investigation. Acta Radiol Diagn. 1986;27(3):315–24. https://doi.org/10.1177/028418518602700312.
3. Minor LB, Solomon D, Zinreich JS, Zee DS. Sound- and/or pressure-induced vertigo due to bone dehiscence of the superior semicircular canal. Arch Otolaryngol Head Neck Surg. 1998;124(3):249–58. https://doi.org/10.1001/archotol.124.3.249.
4. Merchant SN, Rosowski JJ. Conductive hearing loss caused by third-window lesions of the inner ear. Otol Neurotol. 2008;29(3):282–9. https://doi.org/10.1097/mao.0b013e318161ab24.
5. Attias J, Preis M, Shemesh R, Hadar T, Nageris BI. Animal model of cochlear third window in the scala vestibuli or scala tympani. Otol Neurotol. 2010;31(6):985–90. https://doi.org/10.1097/MAO.0b013e3181e3d49a.
6. Ho ML, Moonis G, Halpin CF, Curtin HD. Spectrum of third window abnormalities: semicircular canal dehiscence and beyond. AJNR Am J Neuroradiol. 2017;38(1):2–9. https://doi.org/10.3174/ajnr.A4922.
7. Bigelow DC, Kay DJ, Rafter KO, Montes M, Knox GW, Yousem DM. Facial nerve stimulation from cochlear implants. Am J Otol. 1998;19(2):163–9. Retrieved from https://www.ncbi.nlm.nih.gov/pubmed/9520052
8. Blake DM, Tomovic S, Vazquez A, Lee HJ, Jyung RW. Cochlear-facial dehiscence–a newly described entity. Laryngoscope. 2014;124(1):283–9. https://doi.org/10.1002/lary.24223.
9. Koroulakis DJ, Reilly BK, Whitehead MT. Cochlear-facial dehiscence in a pediatric patient. Pediatr Radiol. 2020;50(5):750–2. https://doi.org/10.1007/s00247-019-04600-4.
10. Fang CH, Chung SY, Blake DM, Vazquez A, Li C, Carey JP, Jyung RW. Prevalence of cochlear-facial dehiscence in a study of 1,020 temporal bone specimens. Otol Neurotol. 2016;37(7):967–72. https://doi.org/10.1097/MAO.0000000000001057.
11. Schart-Moren N, Larsson S, Rask-Andersen H, Li H. Anatomical characteristics of facial nerve and cochlea interaction. Audiol Neurootol. 2017;22(1):41–9. https://doi.org/10.1159/000475876.
12. Marquet J. Congenital malformations and middle ear surgery. J R Soc Med. 1981;74(2):119–28. Retrieved from https://www.ncbi.nlm.nih.gov/pubmed/7205846
13. Declau F, Jacob W, Montoro S, Marquet J. Dehiscence of the facial canal: developmental aspects. Int J Pediatr Otorhinolaryngol. 1991;21(1):21–32. https://doi.org/10.1016/0165-5876(91)90056-h.

14. Crovetto MA, Whyte J, Rodriguez OM, Lecumberri I, Martinez C, Fernandez C, Vrotsou K. Influence of aging and menopause in the origin of the superior semicircular canal dehiscence. Otol Neurotol. 2012;33(4):681–4. https://doi.org/10.1097/MAO.0b013e31824f9969.
15. Redleaf MI, Blough RR. Distance from the labyrinthine portion of the facial nerve to the basal turn of the cochlea. Temporal bone histopathologic study. Ann Otol Rhinol Laryngol. 1996;105(4):323–6. https://doi.org/10.1177/000348949610500416.
16. Zellhuber N, Helbig R, James P, Bloching M, Lyutenski S. Multi-mode grounding and monophasic passive discharge stimulation avoid aberrant facial nerve stimulation following cochlear implantation. Clin Case Rep. 2022;10(2):e05360. https://doi.org/10.1002/ccr3.5360.
17. Chung SY, Kim DI, Lee BH, Yoon PH, Jeon P, Chung TS. Facial nerve schwannomas: CT and MR findings. Yonsei Med J. 1998;39(2):148–53. https://doi.org/10.3349/ymj.1998.39.2.148.
18. Loos E, Wuyts L, Puls T, Foer B, Casselman JW, Bernaerts A, Somers T. Cochlear erosion due to a facial nerve schwannoma. J Int Adv Otol. 2019;15(2):330–2. https://doi.org/10.5152/iao.2019.5304.
19. Remenschneider AK, Gaudin R, Kozin ED, Ishai R, Quatela O, Hadlock TA, McKenna MJ. Is the cause of sensorineural hearing loss in patients with facial schwannomas multifactorial? Laryngoscope. 2017;127(7):1676–82. https://doi.org/10.1002/lary.26327.
20. Weitzmann MN, Ofotokun I, Titanji K, Sharma A, Yin MT. Bone loss among women living with HIV. Curr HIV/AIDS Rep. 2016;13(6):367–73. https://doi.org/10.1007/s11904-016-0336-6.
21. Song JJ, Hong SK, Lee SY, Park SJ, Kang SI, An YH, Koo JW. Vestibular manifestations in subjects with enlarged vestibular aqueduct. Otol Neurotol. 2018;39(6):e461–7. https://doi.org/10.1097/MAO.0000000000001817.
22. Song Y, Alyono JC, Bartholomew RA, Vaisbuch Y, Corrales CE, Blevins NH. Prevalence of radiographic cochlear-facial nerve dehiscence. Otol Neurotol. 2018;39(10):1319–25. https://doi.org/10.1097/MAO.0000000000002015.
23. Wackym PA, Balaban CD, Zhang P, Siker DA, Hundal JS. Third window syndrome: surgical management of cochlea-facial nerve dehiscence. Front Neurol. 2019;10:1281. https://doi.org/10.3389/fneur.2019.01281.
24. Shayman CS, Middaugh JL, Hullar TE. Taste disturbance due to cochlear implant stimulation. Otol Neurotol. 2016;37(8):1036–9. https://doi.org/10.1097/mao.0000000000001143.
25. Fang CH, Chung SY, Mady LJ, Raia N, Lee H-J, Ying Y-LM, Jyung RW. Facial nerve stimulation outcomes after cochlear implantation with cochlear-facial dehiscence. Otolaryngol Case Rep. 2017;3:12–4. https://doi.org/10.1016/j.xocr.2017.04.003.
26. Kaufman AC, Naples JG, Bigelow DC, Eliades SJ, Brant JA, Kaufman HS, Ruckenstein MJ. Lateral wall electrodes increase the rate of postactivation nonauditory percepts. Otol Neurotol. 2020;41(5):e575–9. https://doi.org/10.1097/mao.0000000000002610.
27. Camerin GR, Passos UL, da Costa SS, Gebrim E, Cruz OLM. Cochlear-facial dehiscence detected after cochlear implant. Otol Neurotol. 2020;41(2):e293–4. https://doi.org/10.1097/MAO.0000000000002536.
28. Chen J, Chen B, Zhang L, Li Y. Severe and persistent facial nerve stimulation after cochlear implantation in a patient with cochlear–facial dehiscence: a case report. J Int Med Res. 2021;49(11):03000605211057823. https://doi.org/10.1177/03000605211057823.
29. Garaycochea O, Dominguez PD, Manrique M, Manrique-Huarte R. Cochlear-internal canal and cochlear-facial dehiscence: a novel entity. J Int Adv Otol. 2018;14(2):334–6. https://doi.org/10.5152/iao.2018.5089.
30. Wackym PA, Wood SJ, Siker DA, Carter DM. Otic capsule dehiscence syndrome: superior semicircular canal dehiscence syndrome with no radiographically visible dehiscence. Ear Nose Throat J. 2015;94(8):E8–E24. https://doi.org/10.1177/014556131509400802.
31. Modugno GC, Brandolini C, Cappello I, Pirodda A. Bilateral dehiscence of the bony cochlear basal turn. Arch Otolaryngol Head Neck Surg. 2004;130(12):1427–9. https://doi.org/10.1001/archotol.130.12.1427.

32. Young RJ, Shatzkes DR, Babb JS, Lalwani AK. The cochlear-carotid interval: anatomic variation and potential clinical implications. AJNR Am J Neuroradiol. 2006;27(7):1486–90. Retrieved from https://www.ncbi.nlm.nih.gov/pubmed/16908564
33. Gunbey HP, Aydin H, Cetin H, Gunbey E, Karaoglanoglu M, Cay N, Alhan A. MDCT assessment of the cochlear-carotid interval. Neuroradiol J. 2011;24(3):439–43. https://doi.org/10.1177/197140091102400315.
34. Shoman NM, Samy RN, Pensak ML. Contemporary neuroradiographic assessment of the cochleo-carotid partition. ORL J Otorhinolaryngol Relat Spec. 2016;78(4):193–8. https://doi.org/10.1159/000369622.
35. Kim HH, Wilson DF. A third mobile window at the cochlear apex. Otolaryngol Head Neck Surg. 2006;135(6):965–6. https://doi.org/10.1016/j.otohns.2005.04.006.
36. Neyt P, Govaere F, Forton GE. Simultaneous true stapes fixation and bilateral bony dehiscence between the internal carotid artery and the apex of the cochlea: the ultimate pitfall. Otol Neurotol. 2011;32(6):909–13. https://doi.org/10.1097/MAO.0b013e318225573f.
37. Young L, Isaacson B. Cochlear and petrous carotid canal erosion secondary to cholesteatoma. Otol Neurotol. 2010;31(4):697–8. https://doi.org/10.1097/MAO.0b013e31819bd803.
38. Oliver JR, Chen DS, Pearl MS, Carey JP, Sun DQ. Carotid artery-cochlear dehiscence. Otol Neurotol. 2020;41(2):e290–2. https://doi.org/10.1097/MAO.0000000000002494.
39. Cetin MA, Hatipoglu HG, Ikinciogullari A, Koseoglu S, Ozcan KM, Yuksel E, Dere H. The importance of carotid-cochlear interval in the etiology of hearing loss. Indian J Otolaryngol Head Neck Surg. 2013;65(4):345–9. https://doi.org/10.1007/s12070-013-0643-9.
40. Gunbey HP, Gunbey E, Sayit AT, Aslan K, Unal A, Incesu L. The impact of the cochlear-carotid interval on tinnitus perception. Surg Radiol Anat. 2016;38(5):551–6. https://doi.org/10.1007/s00276-015-1607-4.
41. Lund AD, Palacios SD. Carotid artery-cochlear dehiscence: a review. Laryngoscope. 2011;121(12):2658–60. https://doi.org/10.1002/lary.22391.
42. Paladin AM, Phillips GS, Raske ME, Sie KC. Labyrinthine dehiscence in a child. Pediatr Radiol. 2008;38(3):348–50. https://doi.org/10.1007/s00247-007-0696-6.
43. Manzari L. Multiple dehiscences of bony labyrinthine capsule. A rare case report and review of the literature. Acta Otorhinolaryngol Ital. 2010;30(6):317–20. Retrieved from https://www.ncbi.nlm.nih.gov/pubmed/21808455
44. Manzari L, Modugno GC. Bilateral dehiscence of both superior and posterior semicircular canals. Otol Neurotol. 2009;30(3):423–5. https://doi.org/10.1097/MAO.0b013e3181684048.
45. Crovetto M, Whyte J, Rodriguez OM, Lecumberri I, Martinez C, Eléxpuru J. Anatomo-radiological study of the superior semicircular canal dehiscence radiological considerations of superior and posterior semicircular canals. Eur J Radiol. 2010;76(2):167–72. https://doi.org/10.1016/j.ejrad.2009.05.038.
46. Krombach GA, DiMartino E, Schmitz-Rode T, Prescher A, Haage P, Kinzel S, Gunther RW. Posterior semicircular canal dehiscence: a morphologic cause of vertigo similar to superior semicircular canal dehiscence. Eur Radiol. 2003;13(6):1444–50. https://doi.org/10.1007/s00330-003-1828-5.
47. Erdogan N, Songu M, Akay E, Mete BD, Uluc E, Onal K, Oyar O. Posterior semicircular canal dehiscence in asymptomatic ears. Acta Otolaryngol. 2011;131(1):4–8. https://doi.org/10.3109/00016489.2010.502184.
48. Elmali M, Polat AV, Kucuk H, Atmaca S, Aksoy A. Semicircular canal dehiscence: frequency and distribution on temporal bone CT and its relationship with the clinical outcomes. Eur J Radiol. 2013;82(10):e606–9. https://doi.org/10.1016/j.ejrad.2013.06.022.
49. Russo JE, Crowson MG, DeAngelo EJ, Belden CJ, Saunders JE. Posterior semicircular canal dehiscence: CT prevalence and clinical symptoms. Otol Neurotol. 2014;35(2):310–4. https://doi.org/10.1097/MAO.0000000000000183.
50. Chen EY, Paladin A, Phillips G, Raske M, Vega L, Peterson D, Sie KC. Semicircular canal dehiscence in the pediatric population. Int J Pediatr Otorhinolaryngol. 2009;73(2):321–7. https://doi.org/10.1016/j.ijporl.2008.10.027.

51. Di Lella F, Falcioni M, Piazza P. Dehiscence of posterior semicircular canal. Otol Neurotol. 2007;28(2):280–1. https://doi.org/10.1097/01.mao.0000231592.64972.5b.
52. Gopen Q, Zhou G, Poe D, Kenna M, Jones D. Posterior semicircular canal dehiscence: first reported case series. Otol Neurotol. 2010;31(2):339–44. https://doi.org/10.1097/MAO.0b013e3181be65a4.
53. Lee JA, Liu YF, Nguyen SA, McRackan TR, Meyer TA, Rizk HG. Posterior semicircular canal dehiscence: case series and systematic review. Otol Neurotol. 2020;41(4):511–21. https://doi.org/10.1097/MAO.0000000000002576.
54. Cremer PD, Migliaccio AA, Pohl DV, Curthoys IS, Davies L, Yavor RA, Halmagyi GM. Posterior semicircular canal nystagmus is conjugate and its axis is parallel to that of the canal. Neurology. 2000;54(10):2016–20. https://doi.org/10.1212/wnl.54.10.2016.
55. Brantberg K, Bagger-Sjoback D, Mathiesen T, Witt H, Pansell T. Posterior canal dehiscence syndrome caused by an apex cholesteatoma. Otol Neurotol. 2006;27(4):531–4. https://doi.org/10.1097/01.mao.0000201433.50122.62.
56. Goddard JC, Oliver ER, Meyer TA. Bilateral posterior semicircular canal dehiscence in the setting of Hallermann-Streiff syndrome. Ear Nose Throat J. 2012;91(9):362–3. Retrieved from https://www.ncbi.nlm.nih.gov/pubmed/22996707
57. Kiumehr S, Mahboubi H, Djalilian HR. Posterior semicircular canal dehiscence following endolymphatic sac surgery. Laryngoscope. 2012;122(9):2079–81. https://doi.org/10.1002/lary.23474.
58. McCall AA, Curtin HD, McKenna MJ. Posterior semicircular canal dehiscence arising from temporal bone fibrous dysplasia. Otol Neurotol. 2010;31(9):1516–7. https://doi.org/10.1097/MAO.0b013e3181be6b12.
59. Meehan T, Nogueira C, Rajenderkumar D, Shah J, Stephens D, Dyer K. Dehiscence of the posterior and superior semicircular canal presenting in pregnancy. B-ENT. 2013;9(2):165–8. Retrieved from https://www.ncbi.nlm.nih.gov/pubmed/23909125
60. Kuhn JJ, Clenney T. The association between semicircular canal dehiscence and Chiari type I malformation. Arch Otolaryngol Head Neck Surg. 2010;136(10):1009–14. https://doi.org/10.1001/archoto.2010.169.
61. Meiklejohn DA, Corrales CE, Boldt BM, Sharon JD, Yeom KW, Carey JP, Blevins NH. Pediatric semicircular canal dehiscence: radiographic and histologic prevalence, with clinical correlation. Otol Neurotol. 2015;36(8):1383–9. https://doi.org/10.1097/MAO.0000000000000811.
62. Gracia-Tello B, Cisneros A, Crovetto R, Martinez C, Rodriguez O, Lecumberri I, Whyte J. Effect of semicircular canal dehiscence on contralateral canal bone thickness. Acta Otorrinolaringol Esp. 2013;64(2):97–101. https://doi.org/10.1016/j.otorri.2012.10.004.
63. Cisneros AI, Whyte J, Martinez C, Gracia-Tello B, Whyte A, Obon J, Crovetto MA. Radiological patterns of the posterior semicircular canal. Surg Radiol Anat. 2014;36(2):137–40. https://doi.org/10.1007/s00276-013-1155-8.
64. Kundaragi NG, Mudali S, Karpagam B, Priya R. Intracranially protruded bilateral posterior and superior SCCs with multiple dehiscences in a patient with positional vertigo: CT and MR imaging findings and review of literature. Indian J Radiol Imaging. 2014;24(4):406–9. https://doi.org/10.4103/0971-3026.143904.
65. Peress L, Telian SA, Srinivasan A. Dehiscence of the posterior semicircular canal. Am J Otolaryngol. 2015;36(1):77–9. https://doi.org/10.1016/j.amjoto.2014.08.012.
66. Bear ZW, McEvoy TP, Mikulec AA. Quantification of hearing loss in patients with posterior semicircular canal dehiscence. Acta Otolaryngol. 2015;135(10):974–7. https://doi.org/10.3109/00016489.2015.1060630.
67. Kubota M, Kubo K, Yasui T, Matsumoto N, Komune S. Development of conductive hearing loss due to posterior semicircular canal dehiscence. Auris Nasus Larynx. 2015;42(3):245–8. https://doi.org/10.1016/j.anl.2014.10.014.
68. Mikulec AA, Poe DS. Operative management of a posterior semicircular canal dehiscence. Laryngoscope. 2006;116(3):375–8. https://doi.org/10.1097/01.mlg.0000200358.93385.5c.

69. Dang PT, Kennedy TA, Gubbels SP. Simultaneous, unilateral plugging of superior and posterior semicircular canal dehiscences to treat debilitating hyperacusis. J Laryngol Otol. 2014;128(2):174–8. https://doi.org/10.1017/S0022215113003605.
70. Philip A, Mammen MD, Lepcha A, Alex A. Posterior semicircular canal dehiscence: a diagnostic and surgical conundrum. BMJ Case Rep. 2019;12(7):e229573. https://doi.org/10.1136/bcr-2019-229573.
71. Lim HW, Park HJ, Jung JH, Chung JW. Surgical treatment of posterior semicircular canal dehiscence syndrome caused by jugular diverticulum. J Laryngol Otol. 2012;126(9):928–31. https://doi.org/10.1017/S0022215112001570.
72. Gubbels SP, Zhang Q, Lenkowski PW, Hansen MR. Repair of posterior semicircular canal dehiscence from a high jugular bulb. Ann Otol Rhinol Laryngol. 2013;122(4):269–72. https://doi.org/10.1177/000348941312200409.
73. Atilla S, Akpek S, Uslu S, Ilgit ET, Isik S. Computed tomographic evaluation of surgically significant vascular variations related with the temporal bone. Eur J Radiol. 1995;20(1):52–6. https://doi.org/10.1016/0720-048x(95)00619-2.
74. Friedmann DR, Le BT, Pramanik BK, Lalwani AK. Clinical spectrum of patients with erosion of the inner ear by jugular bulb abnormalities. Laryngoscope. 2010;120(2):365–72. https://doi.org/10.1002/lary.20699.
75. Shao KN, Tatagiba M, Samii M. Surgical management of high jugular bulb in acoustic neurinoma via retrosigmoid approach. Neurosurgery. 1993;32(1):32–6. https://doi.org/10.1227/00006123-199301000-00005.
76. Manjila S, Bazil T, Kay M, Udayasankar UK, Semaan M. Jugular bulb and skull base pathologies: proposal for a novel classification system for jugular bulb positions and microsurgical implications. Neurosurg Focus. 2018;45(1):E5. https://doi.org/10.3171/2018.5.FOCUS18106.
77. Friedmann DR, Eubig J, McGill M, Babb JS, Pramanik BK, Lalwani AK. Development of the jugular bulb: a radiologic study. Otol Neurotol. 2011;32(8):1389–95. https://doi.org/10.1097/MAO.0b013e31822e5b8d.
78. Haginomori S, Sando I, Miura M, Orita Y, Hirsch BE. Medial high jugular bulb. Otol Neurotol. 2001;22(3):423–5. https://doi.org/10.1097/00129492-200105000-00034.
79. Friedmann DR, Eubig J, Winata LS, Pramanik BK, Merchant SN, Lalwani AK. Prevalence of jugular bulb abnormalities and resultant inner ear dehiscence: a histopathologic and radiologic study. Otolaryngol Head Neck Surg. 2012;147(4):750–6. https://doi.org/10.1177/0194599812448615.
80. Woo CK, Wie CE, Park SH, Kong SK, Lee IW, Goh EK. Radiologic analysis of high jugular bulb by computed tomography. Otol Neurotol. 2012;33(7):1283–7. https://doi.org/10.1097/MAO.0b013e318259b6e7.
81. Maiolo V, Savastio G, Modugno GC, Barozzi L. Relationship between multidetector CT imaging of the vestibular aqueduct and inner ear pathologies. Neuroradiol J. 2013;26(6):683–92. https://doi.org/10.1177/197140091302600612.
82. Park JJ, Shen A, Loberg C, Westhofen M. The relationship between jugular bulb position and jugular bulb related inner ear dehiscence: a retrospective analysis. Am J Otolaryngol. 2015;36(3):347–51. https://doi.org/10.1016/j.amjoto.2014.12.006.
83. Friedmann DR, Eubig J, Winata LS, Pramanik BK, Merchant SN, Lalwani AK. A clinical and histopathologic study of jugular bulb abnormalities. Arch Otolaryngol Head Neck Surg. 2012;138(1):66–71. https://doi.org/10.1001/archoto.2011.231.
84. Park JJ, Shen A, Keil S, Kuhl C, Westhofen M. Jugular bulb abnormalities in patients with Meniere's disease using high-resolution computed tomography. Eur Arch Otorhinolaryngol. 2015;272(8):1879–84. https://doi.org/10.1007/s00405-014-2996-4.
85. Li S, Shen N, Cheng Y, Sha Y, Wang Z. The effect of jugular bulb-vestibular aqueduct dehiscence on hearing and balance. Acta Otolaryngol. 2015;135(11):1103–7. https://doi.org/10.3109/00016489.2015.1062141.

86. Kupfer RA, Hoesli RC, Green GE, Thorne MC. The relationship between jugular bulb-vestibular aqueduct dehiscence and hearing loss in pediatric patients. Otolaryngol Head Neck Surg. 2012;146(3):473–7. https://doi.org/10.1177/0194599811430045.
87. Tanrivermis Sayit A, Elmali M, Kemal O, Terzi Y. Radiological, clinical and audiological evaluation of jugular bulb-vestibular aqueduct dehiscence. Acta Otolaryngol. 2017;137(12):1221–5. https://doi.org/10.1080/00016489.2017.1360516.
88. Thenint MA, Barbier C, Hitier M, Patron V, Saleme S, Courtheoux P. Endovascular treatment of symptomatic vestibular aqueduct dehiscence as a result of jugular bulb abnormalities. J Vasc Interv Radiol. 2014;25(11):1816–20. https://doi.org/10.1016/j.jvir.2014.07.013.
89. Couloigner V, Grayeli AB, Bouccara D, Julien N, Sterkers O. Surgical treatment of the high jugular bulb in patients with Meniere's disease and pulsatile tinnitus. Eur Arch Otorhinolaryngol. 1999;256(5):224–9. https://doi.org/10.1007/s004050050146.
90. Gianoli GJ, Larouere MJ, Kartush JM, Wayman J. Sac-vein decompression for intractable Meniere's disease: two-year treatment results. Otolaryngol Head Neck Surg. 1998;118(1):22–9. https://doi.org/10.1016/s0194-5998(98)70370-5.
91. Arenberg IK. Abnormalities, congenital anomalies, and unusual anatomic variations of the endolymphatic sac and vestibular aqueduct: clinical, surgical, and radiographic correlations. Group 3, 4, and 5 abnormalities. Am J Otol. 1982;3(3):221–40. Retrieved from https://www.ncbi.nlm.nih.gov/pubmed/7055236
92. Fujita S, Sando I. Postnatal development of the vestibular aqueduct in relation to the internal auditory canal. Computer-aided three-dimensional reconstruction and measurement study. Ann Otol Rhinol Laryngol. 1994;103(9):719–22. https://doi.org/10.1177/000348949410300910.
93. Pyle GM. Embryological development and large vestibular aqueduct syndrome. Laryngoscope. 2000;110(11):1837–42. https://doi.org/10.1097/00005537-200011000-00014.
94. Saliba I, Gingras-Charland ME, St-Cyr K, Decarie JC. Coronal CT scan measurements and hearing evolution in enlarged vestibular aqueduct syndrome. Int J Pediatr Otorhinolaryngol. 2012;76(4):492–9. https://doi.org/10.1016/j.ijporl.2012.01.004.
95. Emmett JR. The large vestibular aqueduct syndrome. Am J Otol. 1985;6(5):387–415. Retrieved from https://www.ncbi.nlm.nih.gov/pubmed/3876777
96. Pang J, Wang Y, Cheng Y, Chi F, Li Y, Ni G, Ren D. Conductive hearing loss in large vestibular aqueduct syndrome -clinical observations and proof-of-concept predictive modeling by a biomechanical approach. Int J Pediatr Otorhinolaryngol. 2021;146:110752. https://doi.org/10.1016/j.ijporl.2021.110752.
97. Valvassori GE, Clemis JD. The large vestibular aqueduct syndrome. Laryngoscope. 1978;88(5):723–8. https://doi.org/10.1002/lary.1978.88.5.723.
98. Boston M, Halsted M, Meinzen-Derr J, Bean J, Vijayasekaran S, Arjmand E, Greinwald J. The large vestibular aqueduct: a new definition based on audiologic and computed tomography correlation. Otolaryngol Head Neck Surg. 2007;136(6):972–7. https://doi.org/10.1016/j.otohns.2006.12.011.
99. Connor SEJ, Dudau C, Pai I, Gaganasiou M. Is CT or MRI the optimal imaging investigation for the diagnosis of large vestibular aqueduct syndrome and large endolymphatic sac anomaly? Eur Arch Otorhinolaryngol. 2019;276(3):693–702. https://doi.org/10.1007/s00405-019-05279-x.
100. Vijayasekaran S, Halsted MJ, Boston M, Meinzen-Derr J, Bardo DM, Greinwald J, Benton C. When is the vestibular aqueduct enlarged? A statistical analysis of the normative distribution of vestibular aqueduct size. AJNR Am J Neuroradiol. 2007;28(6):1133–8. https://doi.org/10.3174/ajnr.A0495.
101. Noguchi Y, Fukuda S, Fukushima K, Gyo K, Hara A, Nakashima T, Kitamura K. A nationwide study on enlargement of the vestibular aqueduct in Japan. Auris Nasus Larynx. 2017;44(1):33–9. https://doi.org/10.1016/j.anl.2016.04.012.

102. Berrettini S, Forli F, Bogazzi F, Neri E, Salvatori L, Casani AP, Franceschini SS. Large vestibular aqueduct syndrome: audiological, radiological, clinical, and genetic features. Am J Otolaryngol. 2005;26(6):363–71. https://doi.org/10.1016/j.amjoto.2005.02.013.
103. Hirai S, Cureoglu S, Schachern PA, Hayashi H, Paparella MM, Harada T. Large vestibular aqueduct syndrome: a human temporal bone study. Laryngoscope. 2006;116(11):2007–11. https://doi.org/10.1097/01.mlg.0000237673.94781.0a.
104. Phelps PD, Coffey RA, Trembath RC, Luxon LM, Grossman AB, Britton KE, Reardon W. Radiological malformations of the ear in Pendred syndrome. Clin Radiol. 1998;53(4):268–73. https://doi.org/10.1016/s0009-9260(98)80125-6.
105. Li Y, Zhu B, Su J, Yin Y, Yu F. Identification of SLC26A4 mutations p.L582LfsX4, p.I188T and p.E704K in a Chinese family with large vestibular aqueduct syndrome (LVAS). Int J Pediatr Otorhinolaryngol. 2016;91:1–5. https://doi.org/10.1016/j.ijporl.2016.08.026.
106. Antonelli PJ, Nall AV, Lemmerling MM, Mancuso AA, Kubilis PS. Hearing loss with cochlear modiolar defects and large vestibular aqueducts. Am J Otol. 1998;19(3):306–12. Retrieved from https://www.ncbi.nlm.nih.gov/pubmed/9596180
107. Govaerts PJ, Casselman J, Daemers K, De Ceulaer G, Somers T, Offeciers FE. Audiological findings in large vestibular aqueduct syndrome. Int J Pediatr Otorhinolaryngol. 1999;51(3):157–64. https://doi.org/10.1016/s0165-5876(99)00268-2.
108. Nakashima T, Ueda H, Furuhashi A, Sato E, Asahi K, Naganawa S, Beppu R. Air-bone gap and resonant frequency in large vestibular aqueduct syndrome. Am J Otol. 2000;21(5):671–4. Retrieved from https://www.ncbi.nlm.nih.gov/pubmed/10993456
109. Lemmerling MM, Mancuso AA, Antonelli PJ, Kubilis PS. Normal modiolus: CT appearance in patients with a large vestibular aqueduct. Radiology. 1997;204(1):213–9. https://doi.org/10.1148/radiology.204.1.9205250.
110. Naganawa S, Koshikawa T, Iwayama E, Fukatsu H, Ishiguchi T, Ishigaki T, Ichinose N. MR imaging of the enlarged endolymphatic duct and sac syndrome by use of a 3D fast asymmetric spin-echo sequence: volume and signal-intensity measurement of the endolymphatic duct and sac and area measurement of the cochlear modiolus. AJNR Am J Neuroradiol. 2000;21(9):1664–9. Retrieved from https://www.ncbi.nlm.nih.gov/pubmed/11039347
111. Sheykholeslami K, Schmerber S, Habiby Kermany M, Kaga K. Vestibular-evoked myogenic potentials in three patients with large vestibular aqueduct. Hear Res. 2004;190(1-2):161–8. https://doi.org/10.1016/S0378-5955(04)00018-8.
112. Merchant SN, Nakajima HH, Halpin C, Nadol JB Jr, Lee DJ, Innis WP, Rosowski JJ. Clinical investigation and mechanism of air-bone gaps in large vestibular aqueduct syndrome. Ann Otol Rhinol Laryngol. 2007;116(7):532–41. https://doi.org/10.1177/000348940711600709.
113. Mimura T, Sato E, Sugiura M, Yoshino T, Naganawa S, Nakashima T. Hearing loss in patients with enlarged vestibular aqueduct: air-bone gap and audiological Bing test. Int J Audiol. 2005;44(8):466–9. https://doi.org/10.1080/14992020500057665.
114. Zhou G, Gopen Q, Kenna MA. Delineating the hearing loss in children with enlarged vestibular aqueduct. Laryngoscope. 2008;118(11):2062–6. https://doi.org/10.1097/MLG.0b013e31818208ad.
115. Eckhard AH, Bachinger D, Nadol JB Jr. Absence of endolymphatic sac ion transport proteins in large vestibular aqueduct syndrome-a human temporal bone study. Otol Neurotol. 2020;41(10):e1256–63. https://doi.org/10.1097/MAO.0000000000002832.
116. Deep NL, Carlson ML, Weindling SM, Barrs DM, Driscoll CLW, Lohse CM, Hoxworth JM. Diagnosing large vestibular aqueduct: radiological review of high-resolution CT versus high-resolution volumetric MRI. Otol Neurotol. 2017;38(7):948–55. https://doi.org/10.1097/MAO.0000000000001482.
117. Kwesi AB, Yu J, Wang C, Wang Y, Chuang F, Yan X, Sun Y. Effect of high jugular bulb on the hearing loss characteristics in patients with LVAS: a pilot study. Front Cell Dev Biol. 2021;9:743463. https://doi.org/10.3389/fcell.2021.743463.

118. Sarioglu FC, Pekcevik Y, Guleryuz H, Cakir Cetin A, Guneri EA. The relationship between the third window abnormalities and inner ear malformations in children with hearing loss. J Int Adv Otol. 2021;17(5):387–92. https://doi.org/10.5152/iao.2021.9482.
119. Zhang Y, Chen Z, Zhang Y, Hu J, Wang J, Xu M, Zhang Q. Vestibular-evoked myogenic potentials in patients with large vestibular aqueduct syndrome. Acta Otolaryngol. 2020;140(1):40–5. https://doi.org/10.1080/00016489.2019.1687937.
120. Zhou G, Gopen Q. Characteristics of vestibular evoked myogenic potentials in children with enlarged vestibular aqueduct. Laryngoscope. 2011;121(1):220–5. https://doi.org/10.1002/lary.21184.
121. Wilson DF, Hodgson RS, Talbot JM. Endolymphatic sac obliteration for large vestibular aqueduct syndrome. Am J Otol. 1997;18(1):101–6. Retrieved from https://www.ncbi.nlm.nih.gov/pubmed/8989959
122. Hura N, Stewart M, Walsh J. Progression of hearing loss and cochlear implantation in large vestibular aqueduct syndrome. Int J Pediatr Otorhinolaryngol. 2020;135:110133. https://doi.org/10.1016/j.ijporl.2020.110133.
123. Hall AC, Kenway B, Sanli H, Birman CS. Cochlear implant outcomes in large vestibular aqueduct syndrome-should we provide cochlear implants earlier? Otol Neurotol. 2019;40(8):e769–73. https://doi.org/10.1097/MAO.0000000000002314.
124. Brantberg K, Greitz D, Pansell T. Subarcuate venous malformation causing audiovestibular symptoms similar to those in superior canal dehiscence syndrome. Otol Neurotol. 2004;25(6):993–7. https://doi.org/10.1097/00129492-200411000-00022.
125. Shim YJ, Bae YJ, An GS, Lee K, Kim Y, Lee SY, Song JJ. Involvement of the internal auditory canal in subjects with cochlear otosclerosis: a less acknowledged third window that affects surgical outcome. Otol Neurotol. 2019;40(3):e186–90. https://doi.org/10.1097/MAO.0000000000002144.
126. McClay JE, Tandy R, Grundfast K, Choi S, Vezina G, Zalzal G, Willner A. Major and minor temporal bone abnormalities in children with and without congenital sensorineural hearing loss. Arch Otolaryngol Head Neck Surg. 2002;128(6):664–71. https://doi.org/10.1001/archotol.128.6.664.
127. Kendi TK, Arikan OK, Koc C. Magnetic resonance imaging of cochlear modiolus: determination of mid-modiolar area and modiolar volume. J Laryngol Otol. 2004;118(7):496–9. https://doi.org/10.1258/0022215041615236.
128. Zheng Y, Schachern PA, Cureoglu S, Mutlu C, Dijalilian H, Paparella MM. The shortened cochlea: its classification and histopathologic features. Int J Pediatr Otorhinolaryngol. 2002;63(1):29–39. https://doi.org/10.1016/s0165-5876(01)00642-5.
129. Karlberg M, Annertz M, Magnusson M. Mondini-like malformation mimicking otosclerosis and superior semicircular canal dehiscence. J Laryngol Otol. 2006;120(5):419–22. https://doi.org/10.1017/S0022215106000934.
130. Gadre AK, Edwards IR, Baker VM, Roof CR. Membranous or hypermobile stapes footplate: a new anatomic site resulting in third window syndrome. Front Neurol. 2020;11:871. https://doi.org/10.3389/fneur.2020.00871.
131. Richard C, Linthicum FH Jr. An unexpected third window in a case of advanced cavitating otosclerosis. Otol Neurotol. 2012;33(6):e47–8. https://doi.org/10.1097/MAO.0b013e318245cb3b.
132. Monsell EM. The mechanism of hearing loss in Paget's disease of bone. Laryngoscope. 2004;114(4):598–606. https://doi.org/10.1097/00005537-200404000-00002.
133. Ota I, Sakagami M, Kitahara T. The third mobile window effects in otology/neurotology. J Int Adv Otol. 2021;17(2):156–61. https://doi.org/10.5152/JIAO.2021.8632.
134. Ward BK, Wenzel A, Ritzl EK, Gutierrez-Hernandez S, Della Santina CC, Minor LB, Carey JP. Near-dehiscence: clinical findings in patients with thin bone over the superior semicircular canal. Otol Neurotol. 2013;34(8):1421–8. https://doi.org/10.1097/MAO.0b013e318287efe6.

Chapter 8
Perilymphatic Fistula

P. J. Valigorsky III, Gerard J. Gianoli, and Dennis Fitzgerald

Introduction and Definition

Broadly defined, a perilymphatic fistula (PLF) is any communication between the inner ear/perilymphatic space and outside the otic capsule. This definition would encompass essentially all third mobile window disorders (TMWD), including superior semicircular canal dehiscence (SSCD) and temporal bone fractures inclusive of the otic capsule. However, more specifically, PLF has come to define an abnormal opening in the areas of the oval or round window between the inner ear and middle ear space. The diagnosis of a PLF has been controversial since its initial reports as a complication from stapedectomy surgery. There is no controversy about the existence of PLF as a clinical entity after stapes surgery or trauma. The controversy surrounds its diagnosis, particularly in suspect cases that had not undergone stapedectomy or trauma, otherwise known as "spontaneous perilymphatic fistula." This term, "spontaneous perilymphatic fistula," is actually a misnomer. More appropriately, the term should be, "PLF without a known cause." An analogy would be the development of an inguinal hernia. Some hernias occur from a particular activity and others develop without a known activity. To a lesser extent, controversies surround appropriate treatment and its relative frequency.

In the era prior to awareness of TMWD, almost certainly, patients had been diagnosed with PLF who had other types of TMWD, such as SSCD. We have witnessed patients like this in our own practice—initially diagnosed with PLF, only to be later

P. J. Valigorsky III
American University of Antigua College of Medicine, Osbourn, Antigua and Barbuda

G. J. Gianoli (✉)
Ear and Balance Institute, Covington, LA, USA

D. Fitzgerald
Otolaryngology Head and Neck Surgery, Jefferson Hospital, Philadelphia, PA, USA

G. J. Gianoli, P. Thomson (eds.), *Third Mobile Window Syndrome of the Inner Ear*, https://doi.org/10.1007/978-3-031-16586-3_8

identified as having SSCD. However, the traditional surgical treatment of PLF has included reinforcement of the areas of the oval window (OW) and round windows (RW), which has often alleviated symptoms in patients with other TMWD.

The current thinking is that the pathophysiology of TMWD (see Chap. 3) is based on the simple presence of a bony defect in the otic capsule producing abnormal fluid dynamics of the inner ear, thus producing TMWD symptoms. However, this theory does not explain the presence of asymptomatic bony defects, progressive hearing loss in TMWD cases, sensorineural hearing loss in TMWD, vertigo spells that last longer than the duration of the known triggers of sound or straining (i.e., vertigo spells lasting hours) or a Ménière's type presentation. Another aspect of the pathophysiology could stem from individual anatomy with relatively direct connection between the cerebrospinal fluid space and the perilymphatic space. These patients would have a higher fluid pressure in the inner ear, known as perilymphatic hypertension. These exceptions to the current theory raise the question as to whether PLF may play a role in the pathophysiology of TMWD.

One notable case early in our career raised this question:

In October 1996, a 39-year-old female presented with sudden right-sided profound hearing loss (only hearing ear pre-injury) and vertigo which occurred after a grand mal seizure with head injury. She had normal premorbid hearing in the right ear and profound loss in the left ear. This episode left her profoundly deaf bilaterally. She had an uncontrolled seizure disorder with a history of multiple head injuries from grand mal seizures. The hearing loss and vertigo failed to respond to bedrest and high-dose prednisone. She was referred to us for further evaluation and treatment nine days out from her event. Her vertigo spells were provoked by straining and typically lasted 15 min per episode, occurring 1–3 times a day. Her physical exam demonstrated a left-beating spontaneous nystagmus, and the office fistula test was subjectively abnormal in the right ear, although it was difficult to interpret objectively due to the ongoing spontaneous nystagmus. A middle ear exploration was performed with reinforcement of the oval and round windows, and an endolymphatic sac decompression was performed on the following day. Postoperatively the patient had immediate relief from episodic vertigo although disequilibrium persisted and concomitant BPPV was treated later. More impressive was a dramatic improvement in the hearing in the operative ear—to a mild loss (30 db) in the low frequencies, sloping to a profound loss in the high frequencies. She was vertigo free and had stable hearing until March 2000 despite repeated seizures with head injuries. After another head injury, she again developed profound right hearing loss and episodic vertigo. A CT scan at that time demonstrated bilateral SSCD. (Our first SSCD repair was done in January 1998.) A right-sided middle fossa SSCD repair (capping) with oval and round window reinforcement was performed. Postoperatively, the episodic vertigo resolved but there was minimal improvement in hearing. She remained free of vertigo until she passed away nine months later from a presumed intracranial hemorrhage. Did this patient have a PLF and the SSCD was incidental, or vice versa? Was PLF part of the SSCD pathophysiology causing her strain-induced vertigo? Without the seizures and head injuries, would she have remained asymptomatic? Was the prior left profound hearing loss related to the left SSCD or some other subtle congenital defect that was undetectable at that time, e.g. modiolar defect?

Wackym et al. [1] proposed the entity of a CT negative otic capsule dehiscence in which the patients present with similar clinical findings and test findings as other TMWD but have no identifiable bony defect on CT scan. Presumably, these patients represent either patients who had a bony defect not yet identified or have PLF. Gadre et al. [2] reported on membranous and hypermobile stapes cases successfully treated with OW reinforcement. These were identified on preoperative high-resolution CT scan using gray-scale inverse windowing technique. Recently, Gianoli et al. [3] reported an as yet identified labyrinthine dehiscence of the horizontal semicircular canal where the tympanic segment of the facial nerve crosses near its ampullated end, adjacent to the oval window. See Fig. 8.1. This anatomic defect was linked to TMWD presentation with abnormal fistula testing and cVEMP testing. These patients would have been considered PLF patients in the past and would have undergone OW/RW reinforcement with likely similar outcomes. Given these above findings, we propose the clinical definition of PLF should be as noted in Fig. 8.2.

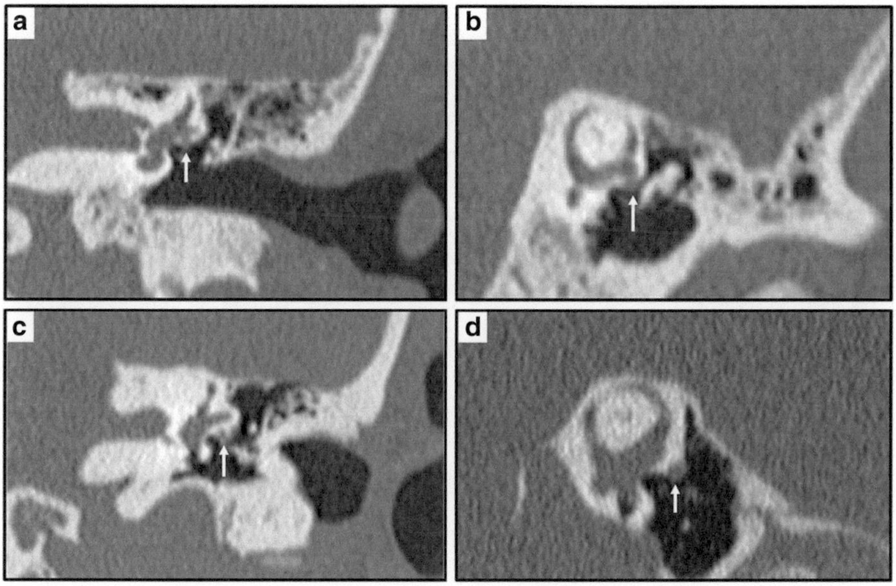

Fig. 8.1 CT scan demonstrating (**a**) HSC-FND on coronal imaging, (**b**) HSC-FND on Poschl imaging, (**c**) normal HSC and facial nerve anatomy on coronal imaging, and (**d**) normal HSC and facial canal on Poschl imaging

Clinical Definition of Perilymphatic Fistula:

1. History and physical findings consistent with TMWD
2. Objective Testing consistent with TMWD
3. CT scan that does not demonstrate a bony defect of the otic capsule

Fig. 8.2 Clinical definition of PLF

The presence of a bony defect would imply the bony defect is integral in the pathophysiology for the patients' disorder but does not preclude the possibility of PLF being part of the pathophysiologic process. However, the inability to identify a bony defect/dehiscence does not exclude the presence of a yet unidentified otic capsule lesion. Several anomalies of the otic capsule have been reported that could be the source for such patients and there may be more yet to be identified. Subtle defects identified include membranous or hypermobile stapes, abnormal Internal Auditory Canal-Cochlear patency, Modiolar defects, horizontal semicircular canal-facial nerve dehiscence, an enlarged internal auditory canal, and cochlear-facial dehiscence. Kohut et al. [4] proposed microfissures of the fissula ante fenestram and the floor of the round window as areas for a possible PLF source. Figure 8.3 demonstrates an

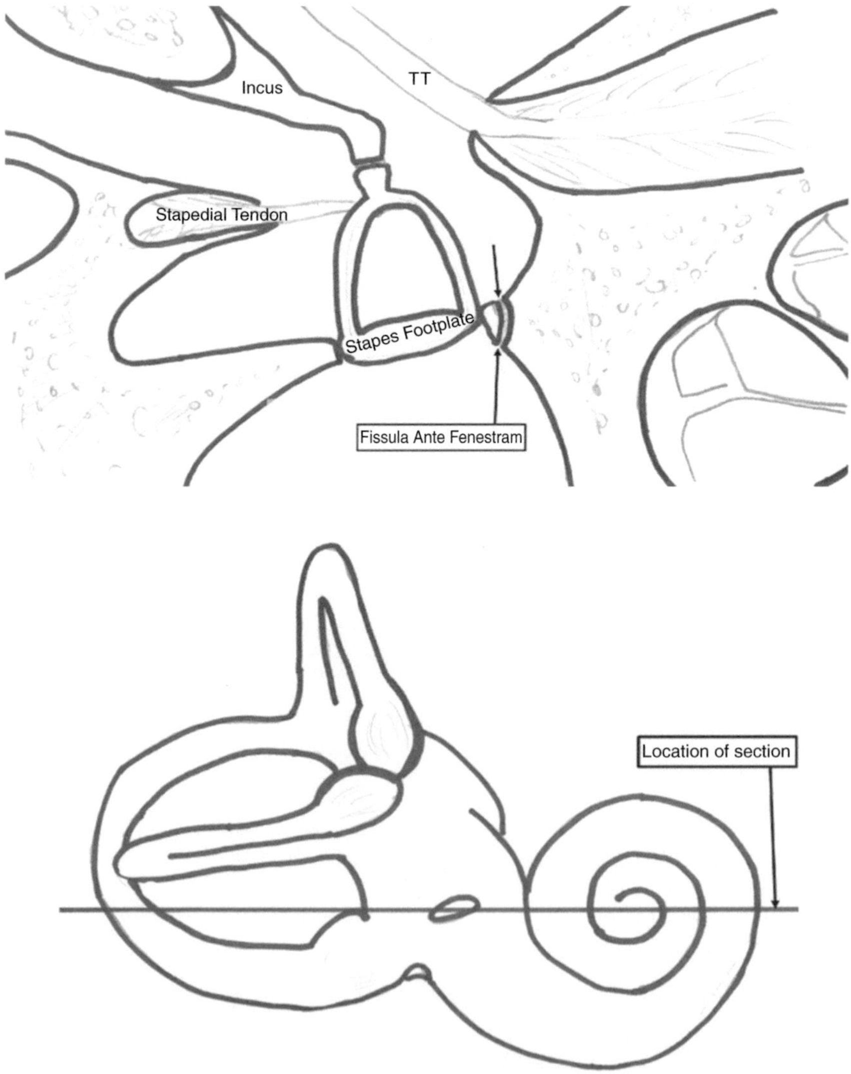

Fig. 8.3 Fissula Ante Fenestram—anatomic diagram. Adapted [4]

artist's rendition of the fissula ante fenestram, located anterior to the oval window. It projects from the junction of the vestibule and scala vestibuli that extends to the periosteum of the middle ear just beneath the cochleariform process, where the tendon of the tensor tympani muscle turns laterally toward the malleus. The fissula ante fenestram is typically not visible on CT scan but, due to its location, can be a source for what would otherwise be presumed to be an oval window PLF. A histologic section of the fissula ante fenestram can be seen on the Mass Eye and Ear Otopathology website, L-181: https://tinyurl.com/56cy3naw

Etiology

The etiology of PLF can be categorized as either resulting from an identified cause (post-stapedectomy, trauma) or an unidentified cause ("spontaneous") [5] (Fig. 8.4). The first case of PLF was reported in 1959 following a stapedectomy; it was found that the polyethylene prosthesis used in the procedure was displaced inferiorly, which resulted in a lack of contact to the incus and PLF [6]. More recently, Ashman and Jyung [7] reported a case of a 50-year-old female where they discovered a pseudomeningocele-like presentation following a stapedectomy. They used a Nitinol prosthesis secured to the incus and followed with a circumferential tragal perichondral graft with Gelfoam packing. This resulted in an improvement of symptoms. Post-stapedectomy PLF has become a well-recognized complication of stapes surgery, with its frequency less common with tissue seals and small fenestra approaches rather than total footplate removal.

Trauma is also a well-recognized cause for PLF, including both implosive and explosive trauma. Goodhill described explosive trauma as increased subarachnoid space and central pressure that transmits through a pre-existing defect to the inner ear [8, 9]. He described the implosive route of trauma as increased middle ear pressure or direct tympanic membrane pressure causing the oval or round window to rupture. Activities such as weightlifting and vaginal delivery cause sustained bouts of increased intracranial pressure and have been implicated as a source for explosive

Fig. 8.4 Etiology of PLF

Etiology of Perilymphatic Fistula:

- Post-Stapes surgery
- Trauma
  - o Implosive
  - o Explosive
- "Spontaneous"
  - o Idiopathic Intracranial Hypertension
  - o Anatomic otic capsule defects
  - o Forgotten trauma or inciting event

trauma. Patients with pseudotumor cerebri may be more susceptible due to their already elevated intracranial pressure.

In contrast, the underlying etiology for implosive trauma involves inadequate pressure equalization between the middle ear and pressure external to the body. Increases in ambient pressure occur when a person moves from a low to a high pressure such as scuba diving or air travel [10]. Increased ambient pressure can also result from direct trauma to the external auditory canal, such as a slap to the ear or an explosion. In a case presented by Sheridan et al. [11], a 28-year-old male had resurfaced after SCUBA diving 35 feet under water, with complaints of hearing loss, nausea, and imbalance. His audiogram revealed sensorineural hearing loss and he was managed conservatively. Subsequently his symptoms had returned and he underwent exploratory tympanotomy. Middle ear exploration discovered an oval window perilymph leak. The window was patched using temporalis fascia.

Direct trauma has also been associated with PLF, including direct penetrating trauma and general head trauma. The mechanism for penetrating trauma is a simple direct breach usually at the oval window. This has been reported in Q-tip trauma and even due to intratympanic steroid perfusion [12]. The mechanism for blunt head trauma resulting in PLF is presumed to be due to a traveling wave of pressure from the intracranial space through the inner ear resulting in a window breach, which represents another type of an explosive event.

The so-called spontaneous PLF is one where there is no obvious provocateur for the pathology—no trauma, stapes surgery, implosive event, or explosive event. In this case, some patients, especially if the symptoms are of long duration, may have forgotten the antecedent event. An alternative explanation is an anatomic anomaly that allows for increased pressure transmission from intracranially to the inner ear, making the round or oval window more susceptible to breach. There have been several anatomic anomalies that could fulfill this distinction and includes most of the TMWD identified in this textbook.

The last etiology to consider is erosive processes. Infectious erosive processes such as otosyphilis and mass lesions eroding into the otic capsule must also be included in the spectrum of disorders presenting with TMWS. In the past, these have been referred to as labyrinthine fistulas and were described as presenting similar to how a PLF would present. Now, they would more likely be referred to as a part of the spectrum of TMWD. Cholesteatoma is the most common of erosive processes that we encounter. These can be acquired or congenital in origin, but the TMWS may be delayed until a critical amount of erosion has occurred. Patients typically present in a comparable manner with strain-induced dizziness, ear fullness, and conductive or mixed hearing loss, but will also typically have otorrhea.

Pathophysiology

The cochlear aqueduct can be defined as a bony channel, which contains the fibrous periotic duct and connects the perilymphatic space with the subarachnoid space

[13]. It is suggested that the cochlear aqueduct provides a direct connection between CSF and perilymph fluid in both a normal labyrinth and in malformations [14]. The length and patency of the cochlear aqueduct varies between subjects. With age the cochlear aqueduct grows in length and the arachnoid tissue contained in the aqueduct becomes denser. Thus, explaining the varying patency of the cochlear aqueduct among different age groups [15, 16].

The round and oval windows are separated by the rigid osseous spiral lamina and basilar membrane. Other than the neurovascular bundles, the remainder of the labyrinth is encased in bone. When pressure is applied to the stapes it travels through the scala vestibuli, eventually reaching the elastic membrane of the round window. The interaction of the flexible basilar and tectorial membrane induces shearing of the cochlear inner hair cells. Vestibular hair cells are enclosed in the bony labyrinth and are protected from sound induced movement of perilymph [17].

Activities that increase intracranial pressures can transmit pressure through a patent cochlear aqueduct to the inner ear. An additional possible connection is through the internal auditory canal (IAC) and in fact has been demonstrated to occur with CSF contrasted CT scan. Increases in hydrostatic pressure of perilymph are released by the opening of the otic capsule or a breach of the oval or round windows. CSF pressure leads to an efflux of perilymph from CSF entering the scala tympani through the cochlear aqueduct [18]. This suggests that perilymph flow is the direct result of increased intracranial pressure forcing CSF through the cochlear aqueduct.

Space occupied by CSF is part of a dynamic pressure system, which determines intracranial pressure. The normal physiologic pressure of CSF is 3–4 mmHg (4–5.4 cm H_2O) before the age of one, and in adults pressure ranges from 10 to 15 mmHg (13–20 cm H_2O) [19]. As we age, the middle and inner ear becomes more adaptive to intracranial pressure changes. The length of the cochlear aqueduct increases and the density of arachnoid in the lumen increases. These adaptations are suggested to dampen the effects of sudden pressure changes in the subarachnoid space thus protecting the inner ear from rapid changes in pressure [15]. If pressure is transmitted to the vestibular organs, it must do so without causing endolymph to flow. When endolymph is caused to flow, vestibular stimulation results [17]. The complete enclosure of perilymph ensures that pressure is equally distributed and aids in the prevention of inappropriate pressure being transmitted to the vestibular sensors.

Inner ear trauma occurs when rapid pressure changes are transmitted to the inner ear from either the middle ear space or the cerebral spinal fluid [10]. This can result in a tear of the basilar membrane, perilymphatic fistula or hemorrhage. Thus, the explosive route suggests that sudden increases in CSF pressure are transmitted through the cochlear aqueduct, the IAC, or some other otic capsule defect to the scala tympani, leading to rupture of the round window or basilar membrane [8]. The implosive route is the result of sudden increases in tubotympanic pressure with round window or oval window ligament rupture. There may also be disruption of internal labyrinthine membranes that would result in hearing loss, vertigo, and tinnitus [8].

Vestibular symptoms can be divided into either intermittent or persistent. Like other TMWS, there can be quite a variation in the description of vestibular symptoms, but a common feature is exacerbation or provocation of vestibular symptoms with activities that raise intracranial pressure. It is also not unusual for PLF patients to have concomitant BPPV as a secondary pathology, making positional exacerbation of vestibular symptoms another feature. In these cases, presumably the pressure effects that caused breach in the oval or round window areas also caused a dislodgement of otoconia from the utricle.

Third window syndromes, including perilymphatic fistulas, can occur as a consequence of traumatic head injury. This is commonly mistaken for a traumatic brain injury or a post-concussive syndrome [2]. Head trauma has been proposed as one of the "second events" that provokes the onset of TMWS in patients with anatomic dehiscence present since childhood. Similarly, head trauma has been identified as a mechanism by which PLF may occur. The proposed theory is the traveling wave theory of pressure transmitted from intracranially through the inner ear, resulting in labyrinthine concussion, intralabyrinthine hemorrhage, endolymphatic hydrops, and PLF.

Clinical Presentation

Patients with suspected PLF can present with sudden or fluctuating sensorineural hearing loss, tinnitus, aural fullness, rotational vertigo, lightheadedness, disequilibrium, and motion intolerance. A patient can present with complaints of purely auditory, vestibular or a combination of both. Seltzer and McCabe [20] collected data on 91 patients with a confirmed diagnosis of PLF and found that 82% had auditory symptoms and 8% had auditory symptoms as the sole complaint. Eighty one percent of the patients had vestibular symptoms and 12% complained of only vestibular symptoms. The audiologic and vestibular symptoms were widely variable. The typical vestibular symptoms are chronic disequilibrium with episodes of vertigo provoked by straining. The chronic disequilibrium is akin to what is seen with an uncompensated vestibular loss.

Post-stapedectomy PLF symptoms can occur in as little as a week or can present years after surgery [21]. A diagnosis of PLF should be suspected in a patient presenting with sensorineural hearing loss and dizziness following a stapedectomy. The diagnosis can be commonly mistaken for Ménière's disease, with a similar presentation of vertigo and sensorineural hearing loss. In some cases, a CT scan may show fluid in the middle ear and/or pneumolabyrinth [22]. CT scan is the preferred method of imaging since it will also help rule out otic capsule defects. However, the finding of pneumolabyrinth is a rare but specific finding strongly suggestive of a breach in the labyrinth. In the absence of a bony defect, a window breach is presumed.

The variable signs and symptoms of PLF, and their similarities to other pathologies, contribute to the controversy surrounding the missed or misdiagnosed PLF. A thorough history and physical exam are pertinent for an accurate diagnosis. One should maintain a high index of suspicion for PLF among patients who present with sudden sensorineural hearing loss and/or vestibular symptoms following explosive trauma (Valsalva maneuver, weightlifting), implosive trauma (bomb explosions, hand slap to the ear canal) or barotrauma (deep-sea diving, air travel). Hearing loss associated with trauma is often sudden, progressive/fluctuant but can have a delayed presentation.

There is a strong association between barotrauma and the production of perilymphatic fistulas. Patients with a history of deep-sea diving or recent airline travel presenting with sensorineural hearing loss should be suspected of having a perilymphatic fistula. Pullen [23] found 48 cases of PLF out of 62 patients who had experienced barotrauma from deep-sea diving. The results corroborated previous findings. The majority of the cases were found to have a round window PLF.

After an inciting event that has produced a PLF, the patient will usually experience hearing loss and vertigo. Nausea and vomiting are usually associated with vertigo. Audiometric examination may reveal a sensorineural hearing loss. Fluctuating symptoms can be reproducible or exacerbated by performing the Valsalva maneuver, which increases intracranial and intralabyrinthine pressure. A preferential leaning to one side has also been noted. Between vertigo spells, the patients often report chronic disequilibrium as would be reported by those experiencing an uncompensated vestibulopathy.

While symptoms presenting immediately after a traumatic event make for a more confident diagnosis, most cases are not so straightforward. The onset of symptoms can occur weeks to months or even years after an inciting event and the symptoms experienced by the patient can fluctuate. This makes it difficult for the patient to precisely recall an event that may have caused the trauma. The fluctuation of symptoms may be difficult for the patient to explain to the physician. Trigger avoidance also changes the clinical presentation, with patients either consciously or unconsciously avoiding straining, masking the most classic symptoms.

Symptoms associated with PLF are remarkably similar to other TMWD, such that physicians should assess for other TMWD such as superior SSCD, cochlear-facial dehiscence (CFD), and horizontal semicircular canal erosion by cholesteatoma or other mass lesions. These syndromes can present with similar symptoms to PLF and can present concomitantly with PLF. SSCD and other TMWD typically present with hearing loss, strain-induced vertigo, and autophony [24, 25]. The presence of sound and pressure induced vertigo along with autophony should raise the clinician's suspicion of a TMWD [25]. Some have argued the presence of Tullio phenomenon would favor an otic capsule dehiscence over PLF, but others have reported Tullio phenomenon among PLF patients as well, making this distinction more difficult [25–27].

Diagnosis

The controversy surrounding the diagnosis of PLF stems from non-specific symptoms, a lack of trauma or surgery in many cases, no definitive preoperative diagnostic test, and no good gold standard for diagnosis. The symptoms are similar to more common conditions such as Vestibular Migraine, Ménière's disease, and Vestibular Neuritis. For this reason, without knowledge of an antecedent event to the onset of symptoms, PLF can be commonly misdiagnosed. Unfortunately, the preoperative tests proposed for diagnosis of PLF, are also frequently abnormal in other TMWD further complicating the picture.

The gold standard for diagnosis of PLF, to which other preoperative testing is compared, has been intraoperative identification of clear fluid emanating from the round or oval window areas. However, this has been problematic. The volume of perilymphatic fluid in the inner ear is estimated to be 75 μl. Consequently, the amount of fluid potentially seen would be even smaller, maybe 2–5 μl of clear fluid. This gold standard is compromised by subjective qualifications that can vary tremendously from one surgeon to another. The fluid seen at the time of middle ear exploration may represent transudate or local anesthetic that had been injected preoperatively, which could lead to a false positive diagnosis. Furthermore, an intermittent PLF may not leak at the time of middle ear exploration leading to a false negative diagnosis. There have been no universally accepted means of getting around this problem. Consequently, using intraoperative identification as the gold standard (fluid identification), upon which preoperative testing has been compared, is less than ideal [28, 29].

The primary concern following a traumatic head injury is to rule out possible intracerebral hemorrhage with a non-contrast CT scan of the head. While this type of scan is quick in determining the presence of intracranial hemorrhage, it is not an acceptable means for assessing temporal bone pathologies [30]. A high-resolution CT scan is needed to visualize the subtleties of the inner ear and temporal bone fractures following a traumatic head injury, as well as identifying concomitant labyrinthine dehiscences. Venkatasamy et al. [31] proposed that a combination of CT and MRI is a fast and reliable method for the accurate diagnosis of round and oval window fistulas, with a sensitivity of 80%. Of the 17 participants that were enrolled in the study, the most common sign on imaging was fluid filling the round or oval window area. This seems to be a unique idea since it is difficult to imagine any imaging technique seeing a few microliters of perilymph. However, the presence of pneumolabyrinth on CT is highly suggestive of a Perilymphatic Fistula [31].

Audiometric testing and tuning fork testing may show a unilateral sensorineural hearing loss. The ear that is affected is typically the side where the fistula is located. However, PLF can present with conductive, sensorineural hearing loss or mixed losses [30]. Hearing loss alone, however, is a non-specific finding for PLF.

Platform posturography pressure test (PPT) demonstrated a high sensitivity (97%) in the diagnosis of PLF and a 93% specificity by one group [32]. Pressure is applied to the auditory canal while standing on the posturography platform under sensory organization test 5 (eyes closed and sway referenced surface). The pressure is applied to the external ear canal rapidly from 0 to +400 mm H20. If a fistula is present the changes in pressure are transmitted to the inner ear causing vestibular stimulation. If the postural sway has an amplitude of greater than two standard deviations in any direction from the base, the test is considered positive [30]—representing saccular stimulation and a vestibulospinal reflex. However, Sheppard et al. [33] used platform posturography to test patients with suspected PLF and other balance disorders. Their data concluded a 56% diagnostic specificity for a confirmed PLF, but using identification of perilymph fluid in the inner ear. Experienced surgeons have questioned the identification of perilymph fluid intraoperatively as "proof" of a PLF as discussed earlier in the chapter [30]. Anecdotally, we have found that other TMWD such as SSCD often have abnormal results on PPT, but this tends to be more specific than sensitive.

Videonystagmography (VNG) is frequently performed for PLF patients. Abnormal results of caloric testing and spontaneous nystagmus have a low sensitivity or specificity in identifying PLF. However, tests such as fistula testing, Valsalva testing or Tullio testing during VNG have a reasonably higher sensitivity. These are not part of most VNG protocols but could be easily incorporated. These tests would objectively support the subjective complaints of patients with sound or strain-induced dizziness. Keep in mind, however, these tests are also frequently abnormal in other TMWD.

The fistula test is usually performed at bedside but can be performed during VNG recording. The typical VNG fistula test entails using a tympanometer to pressurize the ear canals while recording eye movements, looking for nystagmus. A positive test (presence of nystagmus) is suggestive of a fistula, but the lack of nystagmus does not rule out the presence of a fistula. Hain and Ostrowski [34] found that little nystagmus was produced during fistula testing when a window fistula was present using this method. An alternative method we advocate is the use of a handheld Bruening Otoscope with alternating positive and negative pressure application to the tympanic membrane under direct visualization, while watching concomitant eye movement with infrared video oculography. Phase-locked movement of the eyes (a positive Hennebert's sign) or the patient feeling a shifting sensation or nausea is considered a positive Hennebert's symptom. A positive Hennebert's symptom has about the same sensitivity, 60%, as a positive PPT [30]. The identification of nystagmus is considerably less sensitive.

Performing the Valsalva maneuver causes changes in perilymph pressure. This test can be positive when a fistula is present. This can be performed with a closed glottis (i.e., Glottic Valsalva) or with insufflation (Nasal Valsalva). Resulting nystagmus is considered a positive result. However, this can also be abnormal in other TMWD and in Chiari malformation [35].

The Tullio phenomenon refers to disequilibrium/vertigo induced by sound [36]. Tullio demonstrated that loud sounds produced nystagmus and head movement in dogs and pigeons with surgically fenestrated superior canals [37]. While the Tullio test has been used for the diagnosis of SCD, it has shown diagnostic potential for PLF. However, a positive Tullio test can also be positive in normal subjects. Pyykko [38] conducted testing using low-frequency sound stimulation on fifty-seven control subjects, seven with suspected PLF and seven with other inner ear pathologies, while postural stability was measured on a balance platform. All the patients with PLF exhibited altered postural stability. The controls with a purely sensorineural hearing loss did not exhibit instability. This phenomenon suggests a saccular vestibulospinal stimulation in response to sound. Similarly, the Tullio test can be performed with infrared video observation to enhance identification of concomitant nystagmus.

The Vibration-Induced Nystagmus test (VINT) is a test that is sensitive to vestibular asymmetry with an abnormal result (i.e., nystagmus) being non-specific to the underlying cause of the asymmetry. However, VINT has also been advocated as a means to detect SSCD by means of the character of the induced nystagmus. Typically, in SSCD, the VINT will produce an upbeat torsional nystagmus, whereas with other pathologies horizontal nystagmus is more commonly encountered. Therefore, although an "abnormal result" does not specifically denote SSCD, an abnormal result with characteristic upbeat torsional nystagmus does correlate with SSCD. One study reported that the combination of VINT with upbeat torsional nystagmus and the presence of high frequency oVEMP (4 kHz) combined, resulted in a high probability of detecting SSCD on CT [39]. A source for potential false positive results we have witnessed is the concomitant existence of SSCD and a unilateral vestibular loss. It must also be pointed out that a positive result indicating SSCD does not in itself exclude the possibility of a concomitant PLF.

VEMP has been proposed for detection of SCD. However, abnormally responsive VEMP responses have been reported in PLF. It is yet to be seen whether this can distinguish between these two entities [40].

Electrocochleography (ECOG) has been used in the identification of Ménière's disease (endolymphatic hydrops) and PLF. An increase in summating potential and the action potential ratio is suggestive of Ménière's and PLF [15]. Some authors have suggested that all PLFs have increased endolymphatic hydrops, the histopathologic finding in Ménière's disease [30]. However, ECOG is also frequently abnormal in SSCD and other TMWD which has been demonstrated to return to normal with successful repair of SSCD [41].

Biomarkers have been proposed for diagnosis of PLF intraoperatively. Cochlintomoprotein (CTP) exists only in the perilymph and is not found in blood, saliva, or CSF [42]. Its detection intraoperatively can be useful for confirmation at the time of middle ear exploration. However, it is not helpful for preoperative identification which limits its benefits.

Another biomarker proposed for the detection of PLF was beta-2 transferrin. It is found in CSF and perilymph. Buchman et al. took samples of perilymph from 20 patients and compared them with negative controls. The results showed that only 5% of the known perilymph samples and none of the control samples were positive for beta-2 transferrin [43]. These results suggest the beta-2 transferrin biomarker may not be a reliable test for the diagnosis of PLF.

Treatment

The treatment for PLF can be divided into two categories: conservative or surgical. The decision on which treatment plan to pursue is influenced by several factors including: the etiology of the fistula, severity of symptoms, and whether the patient is a good surgical candidate. Typically, surgical intervention is the treatment of choice for trauma induced fistulas [44]. A perilymph fistula of idiopathic origin or with no known recollection of trauma may be managed conservatively. Conservative therapy entails bed rest and avoiding activities that can increase intracranial pressure. Maitland [44] suggests that patients on bed rest elevate their heads to a 30-degree angle. Patients are to avoid strenuous activities and are given laxatives to avoid straining when defecating. Gotto et al. [45] looked at 44 cases of PLF and found that 50% were associated with nose blowing, strenuous lifting and air travel. Patients' symptoms are monitored for a few weeks while on conservative therapy and, if there is a lack of improvement, surgical intervention can be considered [25]. While the benefits of conservative therapy have not been well analyzed, the gold standard for the management and treatment of PLF involves selecting good surgical candidates and early surgical repair for the best possible outcomes [46].

Depending on the surgical procedure used to repair a PLF, it can be done in-office or in the operating room. There are a variety of techniques and materials that can be used with the goal of sealing the fistula. Most experienced surgeons use tissue grafts in both the areas of the oval and round window niches [30]. Traditionally the use of temporalis fascia has been the gold standard of grafting material for PLF [47]. The tissue seals need to be applied to areas in the oval and round windows that have been scarified to allow for a permanent scar to form.

Sarna et al. found that in cases where excessive tissue graft was used, conductive hearing loss was a side effect and advocated the use of Gelfoam to seal around the fascia and oval window [25]. However, Gelfoam dissolves over a brief period of time and it has been argued would be a poor choice for a permanent closure. Garj et al. [48] proposed the use of intratympanic blood injections due to feasibility, low cost, and its minimally invasive nature. The procedure involves the application of local anesthetic to the tympanic membrane, then injecting 0.5 mL of blood into the middle ear. Patients are then placed in a semi-recumbent position for 20 min to allow for blood to adequately reach the oval and round windows. Their results showed that two of the three patients had complete resolution of symptoms the very next day. However, this is a limited number of subjects, and blood seals would seem to be as equally temporary seals as Gelfoam.

While conservative and surgical therapies are both viable options, most studies have concluded that if conservative therapy is pursued, for many patients surgical intervention may still be necessary. The timing of surgery after the incident has been shown to be crucial in optimal resolution of symptoms.

Outcome

Many prior studies on the outcome from PLF surgery are almost certainly contaminated by the presence of unrecognized labyrinthine dehiscences that would more than likely be addressed separately in current neurotologic practice. These prior studies need to be evaluated in that context, while newer studies are much less likely to have such contamination. Furthermore, it is likely that many of the successes of PLF surgery in patients with concomitant dehiscences are integral as to the etiology of recurrent PLF syndrome, much as we have seen with recurrent TMWS after window reinforcement surgery.

Success from PLF surgery has a dichotomous outcome with vestibular symptom resolution much higher than hearing outcomes. The range of successful improvement of vestibular complaints is 85–90%, whereas hearing improvement ranges from 20 to 49% [20, 45, 49]. Controversy regarding the timing of surgery revolves around the question of hearing improvement. Some have argued for immediate surgical intervention with the concern of delay causing further hearing deterioration. While others have argued that the low success in hearing improvement mitigates the need for early surgical intervention, since vestibular symptom resolution does not appear to be so time sensitive.

Complications from PLF surgery are relatively low compared to surgical intervention for direct repair of labyrinthine dehiscences such as SSCD. Some may have residual conductive hearing loss from scarring due to window reinforcement but this can be minimized by using tiny pieces of grafting material. Aside from this, complications are what would be expected from a typical middle ear exploration—infection, perforation, etc. [49].

Conclusion

In summary, we define PLF as a patient who has TMWS (including symptoms and test findings consistent with TMWD) yet has no evidence of a bony dehiscence of the otic capsule. These patients may have an identical presentation as other TMWD. There is a significant question as to whether PLF can be distinguished on physiologic testing from other TMWD, with PLF patients frequently having abnormal fistula testing, Valsalva testing, Tullio testing, ECOG, and VEMP testing. Audiometric testing may demonstrate similar low-frequency conductive gaps, mixed loss, or sensorineural loss, making audiometry unhelpful in distinguishing PLF from other TMWD. Some have looked for a test that differentiates PLF from other TMWD, but there only appears to be one test that differentiates the two entities: a CT scan that demonstrates the presence or absence of an otic capsule defect. Future research may help delineate an anatomic or physiologic basis that defines PLF and distinguishes it from other more recently identified TMWD. The question as to whether PLF plays a part in the pathophysiology of other TMWD is an open one that future research hopefully resolves. Treatment is similar to other TMWD with trigger avoidance being the prime mode of non-surgical management, and window reinforcement as the surgical treatment of choice.

References

1. Wackym PA, Wood SJ, Siker DA, Carter DM. Otic capsule dehiscence syndrome: superior semicircular canal dehiscence syndrome with no radiographically visible dehiscence. Ear Nose Throat J. 2015;94(8):E8–E24. https://doi.org/10.1177/014556131509400802.
2. Gadre AK, Edwards IR, Baker VM, Roof CR. Membranous or hypermobile stapes footplate: a new anatomic site resulting in third window syndrome. Front Neurol. 2020;11:871. https://doi.org/10.3389/fneur.2020.00871. PMID: 32973657; PMCID: PMC7468399.
3. Gianoli G, Soileau J, Shore B. Description of a New Labyrinthine Dehiscence: Horizontal Semicircular Canal Dehiscence at the Tympanic Segment of the Facial Nerve. Front Neurol. 2022;13:879149. https://doi.org/10.3389/fneur.2022.879149. PMID: 35832172; PMCID: PMC9271764.
4. Kohut RI, Hinojosa R, Thompson JN, Ryu JH. Idiopathic perilymphatic fistulas. A temporal bone histopathologic study with clinical, surgical, and histopathologic correlations. Arch Otolaryngol Head Neck Surg. 1995;121(4):412–20. https://doi.org/10.1001/archotol.1995.01890040036006. Erratum in: Arch Otolaryngol Head Neck Surg 1995;121(12):1436.
5. Weber PC, Perez BA, Bluestone CD. Congenital perilymphatic fistula and associated middle ear abnormalities. Laryngoscope. 1993;103(2):160–4. https://doi.org/10.1002/lary.5541030207.
6. Steffen TN, House HP, Sheehy JL. The slipped strut problem. A review of 52 cases. Ann Otol Rhinol Laryngol. 1963;72:191–205. https://doi.org/10.1177/000348946307200116.
7. Ashman PE, Jyung RW. Perilymphatic fistula manifesting as a pseudomeningocele-like presentation following stapedectomy. Ear Nose Throat J. 2020;101(6):232–4. https://doi.org/10.1177/0145561320965200.
8. Goodhill V. Labyrinthine membrane ruptures in sudden sensorineural hearing loss. Proc R Soc Med. 1976;69(8):565–72. PMID: 981244; PMCID: PMC1864538.
9. Singleton GT, Goodhill V. "Sudden deafness and round window rupture." (Laryngoscope 1971;81(9):1462-74). Laryngoscope. 1997;107(5):577–9. https://doi.org/10.1097/00005537-199705000-00002.
10. O'Neill OJ, Brett K, Frank AJ. Middle ear barotrauma. In: StatPearls. Treasure Island: StatPearls Publishing; 2022.
11. Sheridan MF, Hetherington HH, Hull JJ. Inner ear barotrauma from scuba diving. Ear Nose Throat J. 1999;78(3):181, 184, 186-7 passim.
12. Qureshi HA, Zeitler DM. Intratympanic steroid injection complicated by iatrogenic perilymphatic fistula: a cautionary tale. Laryngoscope. 2021;131(9):2088–90. https://doi.org/10.1002/lary.29613. Epub 2021 May 11. PMID: 33973652.
13. Bachor E, Byahatti S, Karmody CS. The cochlear aqueduct in pediatric temporal bones. Eur Arch Otorhinolaryngol. 1997;254(1):34–8. https://doi.org/10.1007/BF02439718. PMID: 9065622.
14. Palmieri A, Ettorre GC. Cochlear and vestibular acqueducts. Radiol Med. 2004;107(5-6):541–53; quiz 554-5. English, Italian. PMID: 15195017.
15. Kutz JW. Perilymphatic fistula: practice essentials, history of the procedure, problem. Medscape. 2021. https://emedicine.medscape.com/article/856806-overview#:%7E:text=Perilymphatic%20fistula%20(PLF)%20occurs%20when,of%20inner%20ear%20fluid%20imbalance. Accessed 18 April 2022.
16. Włodyka J. Studies on cochlear aqueduct patency. Ann Otol Rhinol Laryngol. 1978;87(1):22–8. https://doi.org/10.1177/000348947808700105. PMID: 623414.
17. Carey J, Amin N. Evolutionary changes in the cochlea and labyrinth: Solving the problem of sound transmission to the balance organs of the inner ear. Anat Rec A Discov Mol Cell Evol Biol. 2006;288(4):482–9. https://doi.org/10.1002/ar.a.20306. PMID: 16552774.

18. Salt AN, Hirose K. Communication pathways to and from the inner ear and their contributions to drug delivery. Hear Res. 2018;362:25–37. https://doi.org/10.1016/j.heares.2017.12.010. Epub 2017 Dec 19. PMID: 29277248; PMCID: PMC5911243.
19. Sakka L, Coll G, Chazal J. Anatomy and physiology of cerebrospinal fluid. Eur Ann Otorhinolaryngol Head Neck Dis. 2011;128(6):309–16. https://doi.org/10.1016/j.anorl.2011.03.002. Epub 2011 Nov 18. PMID: 22100360.
20. Seltzer S, McCabe BF. Perilymph fistula: the Iowa experience. Laryngoscope. 1986;96(1):37–49. https://doi.org/10.1288/00005537-198601000-00007. PMID: 3941579.
21. Harrison WH, Shambaugh GE Jr, Derlacki EL, Clemis JD. Perilymph fistula in stapes surgery. Laryngoscope. 1967;77(5):836–49. https://doi.org/10.1288/00005537-196705000-00011. PMID: 6026276.
22. Prisman E, Ramsden JD, Blaser S, Papsin B. Traumatic perilymphatic fistula with pneumolabyrinth: diagnosis and management. Laryngoscope. 2011;121(4):856–9. https://doi.org/10.1002/lary.21439. Epub 2011 Feb 8. PMID: 21305555.
23. Pullen FW. Perilymphatic fistula induced by barotrauma. Am J Otol. 1992;13(3):270–2. PMID: 1609857.
24. Minor LB, Solomon D, Zinreich JS, Zee DS. Sound- and/or pressure- induced vertigo due to bone dehiscence of the superior semicircular canal. Arch Otolaryngol Head Neck Surg. 1998;124:249–58. https://doi.org/10.1001/archotol.124.3.249.
25. Sarna B, Abouzari M, Merna C, Jamshidi S, Saber T, Djalilian HR. Perilymphatic fistula: a review of classification, etiology, diagnosis, and treatment. Front Neurol. 2020;11:1046. https://doi.org/10.3389/fneur.2020.01046. PMID: 33041986; PMCID: PMC7522398.
26. Blake DM, Tomovic S, Vazquez A, Lee HJ, Jyung RW. Cochlear-facial dehiscence–a newly described entity. Laryngoscope. 2014;124(1):283–9. https://doi.org/10.1002/lary.24223. PMID: 23712934.
27. Suzuki M, Okamoto T, Ushio M, Ota Y. Two cases of Tullio phenomenon in which oval and round window reinforcement surgery was effective. Auris Nasus Larynx. 2019;46(4):636–40. https://doi.org/10.1016/j.anl.2018.10.022. PMID: 30573214.
28. Matsuda H, Sakamoto K, Matsumura T, Saito S, Shindo S, Fukushima K, Nishio SY, Kitoh R, Shibasaki O, Ito A, Araki R, Usami SI, Suzuki M, Ogawa K, Hasegawa T, Hagiwara Y, Kase Y, Ikezono T. A nationwide multicenter study of the Cochlin tomo-protein detection test: clinical characteristics of perilymphatic fistula cases. Acta Otolaryngol. 2017;137(565):53–9. https://doi.org/10.1080/00016489.2017.1300940. Epub 2017 Apr 3. PMID: 28368720.
29. Hornibrook J. Perilymph fistula: fifty years of controversy. ISRN Otolaryngol. 2012;2012:281248. https://doi.org/10.5402/2012/281248. PMID: 23724269; PMCID: PMC3658483.
30. Fitzgerald DC. Persistent dizziness following head trauma and perilymphatic fistula. Arch Phys Med Rehabil. 1995;76(11):1017–20. https://doi.org/10.1016/s0003-9993(95)81041-2. PMID: 7487449.
31. Venkatasamy A, Al Ohraini Z, Karol A, Karch-Georges A, Riehm S, Rohmer D, Charpiot A, Veillon F. CT and MRI for the diagnosis of perilymphatic fistula: a study of 17 surgically confirmed patients. Eur Arch Otorhinolaryngol. 2020;277(4):1045–51. https://doi.org/10.1007/s00405-020-05820-3. Epub 2020 Feb 10. PMID: 32040717.
32. Black FO, Lilly DJ, Peterka RJ, Shupert C, Hemenway WG, Pesznecker SC. The dynamic posturographic pressure test for the presumptive diagnosis of perilymph fistulas. Neurol Clin. 1990;8(2):361–74. PMID: 2359383.
33. Shepard NT, Telian SA, Niparko JK, Kemink JL, Fujita S. Platform pressure test in identification of perilymphatic fistula. Am J Otol. 1992;13(1):49–54. PMID: 1598986.
34. Hain TC, Ostrowski VB. Limits of normal for pressure sensitivity in the fistula test. Audiol Neurootol. 1997;2(6):384–90. https://doi.org/10.1159/000259263. PMID: 9390842.
35. Hoppes CW, Lambert KH, Zalewski C, Pinto R, Burrows H, McCaslin D. The supine superior semicircular canal dehiscence test. Am J Audiol. 2021;30(3):475–80. https://doi.org/10.1044/2021_AJA-21-00011. PMID: 34153201; PMCID: PMC8642096.

36. Kaski D, Davies R, Luxon L, Bronstein AM, Rudge P. The Tullio phenomenon: a neurologically neglected presentation. J Neurol. 2012;259(1):4–21. https://doi.org/10.1007/s00415-011-6130-x. Epub 2011 Jul 9. PMID: 21743992.
37. Tullio P. Das Ohr und die Entstehung der Sprache und Schrift. Berlin: Urban and Schwarzenberg; 1929.
38. Pyykkö I, Ishizaki H, Aalto H, Starck J. Relevance of the Tullio phenomenon in assessing perilymphatic leak in vertiginous patients. Am J Otol. 1992;13(4):339–42. PMID: 1415497.
39. Batuecas-Caletrío Á, Jara A, Suarez-Vega VM, Marcos-Alonso S, Sánchez-Gómez H, Pérez-Fernández N. Skull vibration-induced nystagmus and high frequency ocular vestibular-evoked myogenic potentials in superior canal dehiscence. Audiol Res. 2022;12(2):202–11. https://doi.org/10.3390/audiolres12020023. PMID: 35447743; PMCID: PMC9030186.
40. Modugno GC, Magnani G, Brandolini C, Savastio G, Pirodda A. Could vestibular evoked myogenic potentials (VEMPs) also be useful in the diagnosis of perilymphatic fistula? Eur Arch Otorhinolaryngol. 2006;263(6):552–5. https://doi.org/10.1007/s00405-006-0008-z. Epub 2006 Feb 16. PMID: 16482456.
41. Arts HA, Adams ME, Telian SA, El-Kashlan H, Kileny PR. Reversible electrocochleographic abnormalities in superior canal dehiscence. Otol Neurotol. 2009;30(1):79–86. https://doi.org/10.1097/MAO.0b013e31818d1b51. PMID: 19092559.
42. Lee K, Ochi N, Yamahara K, Makino K, Ikezono T. A case of perilymphatic fistula with inner ear anomaly diagnosed preoperatively by the cochlin-tomoprotein detection test. Case Rep Otolaryngol. 2020;2020:9476915. https://doi.org/10.1155/2020/9476915.
43. Buchman CA, Luxford WM, Hirsch BE, Fucci MJ, Kelly RH. Beta-2 transferrin assay in the identification of perilymph. Am J Otol. 1999;20(2):174–8. PMID: 10100518.
44. Maitland CG. Perilymphatic fistula. Curr Neurol Neurosci Rep. 2001;1(5):486–91. https://doi.org/10.1007/s11910-001-0111-x. PMID: 11898560.
45. Goto F, Ogawa K, Kunihiro T, Kurashima K, Kobayashi H, Kanzaki J. Perilymph fistula–45 case analysis. Auris Nasus Larynx. 2001;28(1):29–33. https://doi.org/10.1016/s0385-8146(00)00089-4. PMID: 11137360.
46. Comacchio F, Mion M. Sneezing and perilymphatic fistula of the round window: case report and systematic review of the literature. J Int Adv Otol. 2018;14(1):106–11. https://doi.org/10.5152/iao.2018.4336. PMID: 29764784; PMCID: PMC6354484.
47. Vartiainen E. What is the best method of treatment for labyrinthine fistulae caused by cholesteatoma? Clin Otolaryngol Allied Sci. 1992;17(3):258–60. https://doi.org/10.1111/j.1365-2273.1992.tb01839.x. PMID: 1505095.
48. Garg R, Djalilian HR. Intratympanic injection of autologous blood for traumatic perilymphatic fistulas. Otolaryngol Head Neck Surg. 2009;141(2):294–5. https://doi.org/10.1016/j.otohns.2009.05.024. PMID: 19643271.
49. Fitzgerald DC, Getson P, Brasseux CO. Perilymphatic fistula: a Washington, DC, experience. Ann Otol Rhinol Laryngol. 1997;106:830–7. https://doi.org/10.1177/000348949710601005.

Part II
Diagnosis

Gerard J. Gianoli

Introduction

The burden of disease inflicted by TMWD has been underestimated and we are just coming to grips with that. It has been hard to measure its impact on the individual and society. However, the patient suffering from vestibular disorders goes beyond vertigo, hearing loss, tinnitus, and other physical ramifications. There is a psychological toll inflicted by a disorder that has no outward manifestations to demonstrate to those around you and can lead to the suspicion of feigned illness. Fortunately, we now have the capacity to objectively diagnose these disorders that have slipped through clinicians' fingers in the past. The triad for diagnosis has been established for some time now and includes:

1. History compatible with TMWD
2. Diagnostic testing that objectively supports TMWD
3. High-resolution CT findings identifying an otic capsule defect

The one exception to the above is the patient who fulfills criteria in the history and diagnostic testing but has a normal CT scan. We believe this group of patients represent one of the following:

1. A bony dehiscence that has yet to be identified
2. A so-called near-dehiscence
3. A round or oval window perilymphatic fistula

The following section will extensively review the means to diagnose TMWD, highlighting the above three pillars of diagnosis.

Chapter 9
Vestibular Symptoms and Magnitude of Disease Burden

Alan Desmond, Brady Workman, and Pedrom Sioshansi

Much has changed in the world of vestibular management since the first reported cases of Superior Canal Dehiscence by Lloyd Minor in 1998. New test techniques such as Video Head Impulse Test (vHIT) and Vestibular Evoked Myogenic Potential (VEMP) tests now allow evaluation of all five vestibular end organs in each labyrinth. Subsequent studies have uncovered additional third mobile window syndromes (TMWS) that can be identified with appropriate imaging protocols. These techniques are slowly growing in awareness and utilization, but the majority of patients do not have ready access. There is also a lack of awareness of TMWS by many practitioners, drastically increasing the risk of misdiagnosis. There is generally a delay between the establishment of convincing clinical evidence, and the widespread use of modern procedures. A well-known quote from Max Planck, Nobel Prize winner in 1918, eloquently sums up the challenge in changing practitioners' protocols to evolve with scientific breakthroughs: "*A new scientific truth does not triumph by convincing its opponents and making them see the light, but rather because its opponents eventually died, and a new generation grows up that is familiar with it.*" While this quote doesn't hold true for all practitioners, it does elucidate the difficulties encountered in changing management trends. This chapter reviews the frequency, impact, and presentation of vestibular disorders in general, and reviews inefficiencies and obstacles patients and practitioners must overcome to obtain or provide effective care to this patient population.

Dizziness is one of the most commonly reported symptoms across all clinical settings with 15% of adults reporting dizziness annually, and 15–35% of adults seeking medical care due to dizziness during their lifetime [1–3]. Dizziness was the primary reporting symptom for 4% of all visits to the emergency department in the

A. Desmond (✉) · B. Workman · P. Sioshansi
Wake Forest University Baptist Medical Center, Otolaryngology Head & Neck Surgery, Winston Salem, NC, USA
e-mail: adesmond@wakehealth.edu; bsworkma@wakehealth.edu; psioshan@wakehealth.edu

G. J. Gianoli, P. Thomson (eds.), *Third Mobile Window Syndrome of the Inner Ear*, https://doi.org/10.1007/978-3-031-16586-3_9

USA and the primary complaint of "vestibular symptoms" accounted for nearly 7% of all patients evaluated in an emergency department in Switzerland [4, 5]. These data likely underestimate the true number of emergency department patients being seen for dizziness, as they don't account for those cases where dizziness is part of a symptom cluster. Despite these staggering numbers, the actual incidence of dizziness is likely much higher, as population based studies have shown that only half of participants that are dizzy seek medical care [2].

The general term "dizziness" can be caused by a multitude of pathologies, including but not limited to: otologic, neurologic, cardiovascular, orthopedic, psychiatric, metabolic, and ophthalmologic disorders, as well as medication side effects. Often the cause is multifactorial with multiple abnormalities accounting for the general complaint of dizziness. Numerous studies find that, regardless of practice setting, vestibular disorders are the most likely cause of the complaint of "dizziness." Vestibular disorders, including vestibular migraine, account for between 32% and 46% of patients seen clinically with a reporting symptom of dizziness followed by orthostatic hypotension, affecting between 10% and 15% of individuals reporting dizziness. Life threatening causes for dizziness, including cardiovascular and cerebrovascular conditions, account for less than 15% of patients in all clinical settings [1, 5–9].

Refining the Complaint of "Dizziness"

Patients may use the term "dizziness" to describe sensations such as rotary vertigo, light-headedness and pre-syncope, disorientation, and gait instability or imbalance. A survey of primary care and specialist providers found 20 different descriptors of symptoms that would fall under the vague heading of "dizziness" [10]. These are very different complaints with a multitude of possible causes. Additional details about one's dizziness symptoms are required in order to determine the source.

The majority of patients complaining of dizziness are seen in the primary care setting, with only 23% being evaluated by specialists in otolaryngology or neurology [11]. A 2008 review of clinical practice indicates that generalists are less likely to seek additional details regarding the patient's complaints of dizziness, while specialists such as otolaryngologists, neurologists, and audiologists are far more likely to seek more specific detailed history information regarding the patient's complaint [12]. Primary care physicians may be limited due to time, training or test facilities as 70–80% of patients complaining of dizziness in primary care received a diagnosis of "unspecified dizziness" following initial examination [13]. Changes in the delivery of health care have affected available face-to-face time between physician and patient. The advent of Electronic Medical Records (EMR), changes in insurance reimbursement, and unaddressed inflation have resulted in the average patient visit face-to-face time decreasing from 45 minutes in the 1970s and 1980s, to 15 minutes in 2004 [14, 15].

Patients experiencing acute vertigo are more likely to seek evaluation at an emergency department (ED). Acute vestibular syndrome (AVS) accounts for over two million visits to the ED annually in the USA. The primary role of the ED is to identify and treat life-threatening conditions, so the focus of the exam is largely around determining if an acute neurologic or cardiac emergency, such as stroke or cardiac arrest, is the cause. As recently as 2008, in the emergency department the most common tests ordered for a patient complaining of dizziness or vertigo are blood tests, pulse oximetry, chest X-ray, urinalysis, cardiac monitoring and computed tomography (CT) [16]. Tests that may uncover vestibular dysfunction are rarely performed.

As noted previously, the primary focus in evaluating a patient with complaints of acute vertigo in the emergency department is to identify or rule out life-threatening conditions such as cerebrovascular accident or myocardial infarction. Despite this being the focus of the exam in this setting, the efficiency of diagnostic strategies used in the emergency room to identify or rule out stroke has been studied with disturbing results. While the following studies are focused primarily on the identification or misidentification of CVA, they portray a pattern of narrowly focused testing that is unlikely to identify TMWS patients. One can argue that diagnosis of vestibular disorders is not within the scope of emergency medicine; however, opportunities exist for development of clinical guidelines and clinical pathway recommendations for undiagnosed dizziness and vertigo in the emergency department.

David Newman-Toker [17] points out that the cost of dizziness presentations to the emergency department accounted for over $10 billion per year as of 2013, primarily the result of hospital admission in nearly 20% and neuro imaging obtained in approximately 40%. Costs can be presumed to be increasing, as there has been an increase in the rate of neuro imaging patients in the ED over the past decade. CT scanning is the most frequently used imaging technique in patients presenting with dizziness at the ED and has been found to be insensitive and frequently incorrect in identifying or ruling out ischemic brainstem stroke. Zwergal and Dietrich [5] state "likely reasons for this deplorable situation are an overreliance on chief complaint (e.g., vertigo, dizziness) for differentiation of peripheral and central causes, inadequate knowledge or application of bedside oculomotor examinations, and a high level of confidence in the imaging results, which may be often false negative for stroke in the acute situation." A 2018 study exploring emergency department physician reasons for ordering CT scans (not restricted to CT scans just of the head or just for the complaint of vertigo/dizziness) found that the concerns regarding misdiagnosis, medico-legal risk, risk of contrast, patient wishes, and "what colleagues would do" were primary influencers in the decision process [18].

Neuroradiology literature, in discussing appropriate imaging for the complaint of dizziness, reports that unless there are specific neurological features suggesting "central" involvement, imaging yields relevant information in only 1.5% of patients, with less than 1% of imaging studies leading to a change in management [19].

Alternative strategies for assessment of acute vertigo in the ED have been proposed with limited acceptance and application. The HINTS protocol for evaluation of AVS (acute vestibular syndrome) is an established and sensitive technique that can reliably distinguish between peripheral vertigo such as vestibular neuritis/labyrinthitis, and more worrisome conditions such as posterior fossa stroke. The HINTS protocol is gaining slow acceptance [20], and is used infrequently and sometimes incorrectly in the ED [21]. A recent study determined that sensitivity and accuracy of the HINTS protocol is significantly higher when performed by neurology specialists when compared to ED physicians. Frustratingly, the conclusion of the study was that the HINTS protocol might not be suitable for the ED, rather than a call for additional training to obtain adequate skills [22].

Further evidence of the need for additional training includes findings that when the HINTS protocol is performed in the ED, the outcome does not significantly change the course of treatment, primarily because the examiners did not correctly identify patients with AVS versus patients with episodic vertigo [23].

Another proposed approach is to offer more specific specialty examination through remote telehealth using emergency department based video-oculography equipment [24]. This approach can significantly improve diagnostic accuracy and reduction in unnecessary imaging studies. The diagnosis of "nonspecific dizziness" was reduced by more than 50% and the number of CT scans ordered on this group of patients was reduced from the current national average of approximately 40%, down to less than 3% [25].

These studies indicate a clear opportunity for substantial cost savings and improved patient care with improvements in training, equipment, and referral patterns when managing patients complaining of dizziness in the acute care setting [25]. There is currently no clinical practice guideline available for acute vestibular syndrome, despite studies indicating that adult onset acute vertigo is a primary concern for clinical guidance in the emergency department [26]. For a thorough review of the assessment of acute vertigo, the reader is referred to *Acute Dizziness, Vertigo, and Unsteadiness* [27].

Vestibular Disorders

Vestibular disorders are a common cause for dizziness in any clinical setting and most vestibular disorders can be diagnosed and effectively treated. The most common vestibular disorder is benign paroxysmal positional vertigo (BPPV) [28]. Symptoms associated with BPPV are recurrent episodes of brief vertigo, lasting less than one minute in duration, following head movement and position change. Some of the more common provoking movements include: lying supine, sitting up from a supine position, rolling over in bed, head tilt forward or backward. This condition occurs when otoconia migrate into one or more of the semicircular canals of the vestibular labyrinth, resulting in nystagmus and vertigo associated with head movement. BPPV accounts for 17–42% of all patients with a symptom of vertigo [29]. Canalith repositioning maneuvers, such as the Epley maneuver, have been shown effective at resolving the symptoms of BPPV by removing the otoconia from the affected canal through a series of timed head movements [29].

Vestibular migraine frequently presents as recurrent episodes of spontaneous dizziness lasting for minutes up to days in duration, often with associated migraine features such as headache, photophobia, and phonophobia. Inter-ictal symptoms often include increased sensitivity to self-motion and external visual motion [30]. Vestibular migraine is thought to be a migraine variant that affects the central vestibular structures leading to dizziness symptoms. Vestibular migraine accounts for 6–10% of patients across clinical settings, yet emerging data show that vestibular migraine is likely much more prevalent and is under diagnosed [7, 31–33]. Vestibular migraine is the most frequent cause for dizziness in children and adolescents [7, 34]. Individuals with vestibular migraine often have a prior history or family history of traditional migraine. Vestibular migraine is often managed through a combination of dietary modifications, supplementation, and/or medications.

Vestibular neuritis or labyrinthitis most often refers to a viral inflammatory process of the labyrinth and/or the vestibulocochlear nerve. Vestibular neuritis presents as an acute episode of spontaneous vertigo lasting for hours to days in duration. Many individuals experience diaphoresis, nausea, and vomiting associated with the prolonged vertigo. If the insult affects the entirety of the labyrinth, as in the case of labyrinthitis, then there is often associated change in hearing, tinnitus, or aural fullness in the affected ear. Vestibular neuritis/labyrinthitis is thought to be the third most common vestibular disorder [35]. Studies show that vestibular neuritis/labyrinthitis accounts for between 3 and 10% of dizziness in outpatient clinics [3, 7, 36]. At initial onset, treatments are often focused on managing the acute symptoms and may include anti-emetic and vestibular suppressants. Oral steroids are also frequently prescribed, although there is conflicting evidence on whether this leads to better outcomes [37–39]. Many individuals affected by vestibular neuritis recover while others are left with variable degrees of permanent dysfunction. In general, those with greater degrees of dysfunction will experience more residual symptoms of dizziness and imbalance. Living with chronic vestibular dysfunction can cause symptoms of head movement induced dizziness and disequilibrium that is exacerbated when ambulating in scenarios with poor lighting or uneven ground. Vestibular rehabilitation can assist in central vestibular compensation and can reduce the symptoms associated with chronic vestibular dysfunction [40, 41].

Ménière's disease presents as recurrent episodes of spontaneous vertigo that persist for minutes to hours in duration with associated fluctuating hearing, tinnitus, and aural fullness in the affected ear. There are multiple theories for the etiology of Ménière's disease; however, the condition remains poorly understood to date. It is generally agreed upon that endolymphatic hydrops is associated with the condition [42–45]. Ménière's disease accounts for 3–11% of patients seen in dizziness clinics [3, 7]. The prevalence of Ménière's disease is thought to be 190/100,000 individuals [46]. For most individuals the episodes of vertigo reduce in intensity and frequency within 5–10 years from initial symptom onset, however, the hearing loss associated with the condition is often permanent [47]. Treatments for Ménière's disease are variable, likely due to the poor understanding for the cause of the disorder. Common first line treatments can include dietary modifications such as reducing the intake of sodium, caffeine, alcohol, and tobacco. If there is limited response to dietary modifications, additional medical treatments can also include diuretics and medications such as betahistine. Intratympanic treatments can vary from the use of steroids for a therapeutic effect to aminoglycosides that have an ototoxic effect on the vestibular labyrinth. Additionally, there are surgical procedures including, but not limited to, endolymphatic sac decompression and vestibular nerve section [48].

Vestibular schwannoma can cause symptoms of progressive dizziness, imbalance, hearing loss, and tinnitus due to the tumor growth on the vestibulocochlear nerve. Vestibular schwannoma is a benign mass that arises from the Schwann cells of the vestibulocochlear nerve. It is an intracranial neoplasm with an incidence of 0.6/100,000 to 0.8/100,000 person-years [49, 50]. These are most often extremely slow growing tumors and the symptoms may be present for years before identification of the tumor. Treatments typically consist of gamma knife radiation or surgical resection [51, 52].

Prevalence and Symptoms of Various Third Mobile Window Syndrome Variants

A third mobile window syndrome (TMWS) refers to a third area of mobility within the labyrinth, which alters the hydrodynamics of the system. This can lead to a plethora of symptoms including but not limited to: Tullio phenomenon, Hennebert sign, autophony, pulsatile tinnitus, and conductive hyperacusis. TMWSs are a relatively recent discovery with the specific condition of superior canal dehiscence syndrome (SCDS) first reported in the literature in 1998 [53]. SCDS is the most commonly recognized TMWS with a prevalence of 2–10% on CT temporal bone [54, 55]. Temporal bone studies indicate prevalence of 0.5% dehiscence and near dehiscence in 1.4% [56]. SCDS is felt to be congenital in most cases but may also be associated with temporal bone fracture or even idiopathic intracranial hypertension [57–59]. SCDS can be repaired surgically through resurfacing or minimally invasive procedures such as round window reinforcement [59].

Lateral semicircular canal fistulas are most commonly associated with cholesteatoma or iatrogenic injury; therefore, the presentation will largely be dependent on the etiology. The incidence of labyrinthine fistula in patients with cholesteatoma has been estimated between 2.7% and 12%, and 90% of these fistulas involve the lateral canal [60]. Similar to other forms of perilymphatic fistulas, patients may note pressure, or acoustic stimuli elicit vertigo. In cases of chronic otitis media, patients may develop acute symptoms of labyrinthitis due to translocation of infectious or inflammatory mediators into the labyrinth.

Posterior semicircular canal fistulas are much rarer than fistulas of the superior and lateral canal and may present differently. These most commonly present with sound-induced vertigo followed by mixed-hearing loss and tinnitus, while pressure-induced vertigo is less common [61]. The incidence of PSCD is estimated to be 0.38% in ears and 2.16% in patients, and may be associated with a high riding jugular bulb [62]. The incidence in children ranges from 1.3 to 43%, significantly higher than in adults, as the rates reportedly decrease with age [61]. This may be due to bone mineralization that occurs around the posterior semicircular canal and posterior fossa during development [63].

Perilymphatic fistula (PLF) describes any abnormal communication between the perilymph containing spaces of the labyrinth with the middle ear, mastoid, or intracranial cavity, but the term is most commonly used to refer to compromise at the level of the oval or round window. This most typically occurs following trauma, iatrogenic injury, or may occur idiopathically [64]. The estimated incidence is 1.5/100,000, although they may occur more commonly in children with other congenital anomalies of the ear [65]. PLFs characteristically present with acute onset of unilateral hearing loss, tinnitus, vertigo, aural fullness, and disequilibrium. Symptoms often fluctuate and may be associated with straining rather than be sound or pressure induced, as is common in other third window syndromes [64].

Cochlear-facial nerve dehiscence (CFD) is a relatively newly described entity, first described in 2014. It occurs when there is a bony dehiscence between the basal turn of the cochlear and the labyrinthine segment of the facial nerve, creating an effective third window which results in pseudo-conductive hearing loss, autophony, and pulsatile tinnitus [66]. The radiographic prevalence of CFD has been reported at 5.4% [67], however, the true prevalence is likely closer to 0.59% based on a histologic study of 1020 temporal bone specimens [68]. Given the location of the bony partition between the cochlea and facial nerve, this process is less likely to be influenced by acquired external factors such as cholesteatoma or elevated intracranial pressure. There is negative correlation of the cochlear-facial bony partition width with increasing age, while male sex and non-Caucasian race were positive predictors of bony partition width.

Cochlear carotid dehiscence is a rare entity with only sporadic case reports throughout the literature. The true prevalence of cochlear carotid dehiscence is unknown, although histologic studies have shown up to 7.7% of temporal bones may demonstrate a bony dehiscence somewhere along the course of the carotid canal [69]. Cochlear carotid dehiscence tends to occur between the basal turn of the cochlea and the genu of the vertical and horizontal segments of the petrous carotid and has been proposed as a mimic of various otologic pathologies, however, the most commonly reported symptoms are pulsatile tinnitus, conductive hearing loss, or a mid-to-high frequency SNHL [70]. The conductive loss and pulsatile tinnitus are thought to be due to the third mobile window, while the SNHL has been proposed to result from chronic pressure induced damage from internal carotid artery pulsation on cochlear hair cells within the basal turn [71].

Enlarged vestibular aqueduct syndrome (EVAS) is one of the most common malformations of the inner ear and is caused by a pathologic enlargement of the connection between the vestibular aqueduct and the vestibule, which effectively acts as a third window by transmitting acoustic energy through the aqueduct to the dura [72, 73]. This often occurs bilaterally, has a slight female preponderance, and may be found as an isolated abnormality or associated with various congenital conditions such as CHARGE syndrome, Pendred syndrome, or branchio-oto-renal syndrome [55]. The majority of patients present with sensorineural hearing loss, although a subset will have a conductive component in the low frequencies due to the third-window effect, while vertigo is less common [74]. Early diagnosis is important due to the progressive nature of hearing loss and risk of sudden loss following head trauma. Hearing loss may be congenital, or may be progressive and sudden onset following head trauma [75].

The Impact of TMWS and Dizziness

Most dizziness symptoms are transient and resolve with time or treatment; however, for 1/3rd of all individuals dealing with dizziness, the condition becomes chronic [76]. Factors that may lead to condition chronicity include misdiagnosis and incorrect treatment, a history of prior psychological disorders including pre-existing anxiety traits, or the etiology of one's dizziness. Those individuals that fall into these categories may even develop secondary conditions such as persistent postural perceptual dizziness (PPPD), which can be found in up to 25% of individuals after suffering from vestibular symptoms [77]. Living with chronic dizziness can impact all facets of one's life resulting in a myriad of secondary complications. Those living with dizziness have been found to have impaired physical and mental health related quality of life measures, and even abnormal sleep duration when compared to their non-dizzy peers [78, 79]. On clinical examination, patients living with dizziness often report difficulty concentrating or mental fog. One study showed an eight-fold increased odds of difficulties with concentrating or remembering in patients experiencing vestibular vertigo [80].

Dizziness can have many economic and societal impacts. Patients that have undiagnosed vestibular symptoms have been shown to have higher resource consumption in both physician workload and radiology resources in the emergency department [4]. For working individuals that suffer from dizziness, around 50% felt that their work productivity decreased or they had to work less due to their dizziness, 25% had to change jobs, and between 12 and 21% had to quit working altogether [81, 82]. Dizziness accounts for the highest attributable cause for disability in individuals over the age of 65 [83]. The estimated lifetime economic burden per person dealing with dizziness is $69,929 USD or a total lifetime societal burden of 227 billion USD for those over 60 years of age [81].

Vestibular disorders can also have a large psychological impact on those affected. Nearly 30% of those dealing with dizziness report at least one anxiety disorder and those dealing with vestibular vertigo are three times more likely to experience anxiety, depression or panic disorder [80, 84]. Those with a prior history of psychiatric conditions are at a significantly higher risk of developing psychiatric conditions after suffering from a vestibular disorder [85, 86]. Depression and anxiety symptoms seem to be quite common for those dealing with vestibular migraine and Ménière's disease but it is worth noting that TMWS conditions were not included in this study [87].

Dizziness can increase one's risk of falling. Approximately 34% of patients suffering from dizziness fall, while only 9% of non-dizzy adults fall [88]. Falls can lead to serious injury and have been shown to be the leading cause of both fatal and non-fatal injuries among patients over the age of 65 [89]. Injuries related to falls can result in: longer duration stays in the hospital, higher healthcare cost, loss of independence, social isolation and depression [90–92]. With advancements in medical care, our population is aging. It is estimated that there will be one billion individuals over the age of 65 by the year 2030 [93]. Dizziness and falls are enormous societal problems that are only going to increase with the aging of our populations. Appropriate identification and management of dizziness could reduce fall related burdens.

Due to the recent discovery of TMWS as a diagnostic entity there are limited data reflecting the full extent of the impacts associated with living with a TMWS. What is known is that patients suffering from TMWS are likely to be misdiagnosed or endure a longer period of time to receive a correct diagnosis [94–96]. This likely leads to higher rates of condition chronicity and greater social, psychological, and economic impacts than if the condition was identified correctly in an expedient manner. This is disconcerting as 95% of individuals that received surgical correction for TMWS, particularly those with SCDS, would recommend surgical correction to others [94]. Barriers to appropriate diagnosis are likely related to a lack of awareness by front line providers and the over-reliance on traditional vestibular function testing such as videonystagmography by specialty physicians. Those studies that do exist show that patients with TMWS have adverse effects in nearly all facets of life including: lower health related quality of life measures than their age matched peers, restrictions on their social, physical and work lives, mental fatigue, as well as cognitive deficits associated with the condition [95, 97, 98].

Most vestibular disorders can be treated or managed effectively; however, current assessment and management trends often lead to incorrect, missed, or delayed diagnoses [99]. This is unfortunate given the multitude of life altering symptoms and secondary complications associated with chronic dizziness. TMWS are no exception to these poor assessment and management trends and due to the higher rates of misdiagnosis and the longer duration to receive a diagnosis, one can extrapolate that the psychological, monetary, physical, and societal impacts of living with a TMWS are likely quite high. Appropriate identification and treatment of patients dealing with dizziness is essential to allow for a better quality of life for those affected and to reduce the ever growing healthcare expenses associated with their care.

Evolution of Vestibular Management Strategies

Diagnostic and treatment options for patients complaining of dizziness or vertigo have improved dramatically in the past three decades. Unfortunately, these improvements are not widely or consistently used. There is also significant variability among diagnostic protocols, not only between primary care and specialty centers, but also a "comprehensive vestibular evaluation" at one specialty clinic may vary dramatically from a similarly advertised evaluation in another [100].

Past Approaches to the Complaint

In 1972, Drachman and Hart proposed an algorithm for diagnosing the general complaint of dizziness, which included the recommendation for the practitioner to ask for more specific details in the form of the question, "What do you mean by "dizziness""? They suggested that patients' complaints be grouped into four categories: (1) Vertigo, (2) Pre-Syncope, (3) Disequilibrium, (4) Lightheadedness (other), attributing each complaint with a likely etiology. A sample of various pathologies that may present as vertigo, pre-syncope, or disequilibrium makes it clear that etiology cannot be reliably determined by the nature or category of a subjective complaint.

Vertigo
BPPV, Ménière's, Vestibular Neuritis/Labyrinthitis, Vestibular Migraine, Posterior Fossa Infarct, Multiple Sclerosis, Orthostatic Hypotension, TMWS.
Pre-Syncope
Cardiac and non-cardiac issues including worrisome conditions such as aortic stenosis and cardiomyopathy, and more benign conditions such as hypovolemia, dehydration, and hypotension.
Disequilibrium
Peripheral Neuropathy, Orthopedic issues, Cardiovascular issues, Vestibular hypofunction, TMWS, CNS medications, Cerebellar dysfunction.
Lightheadedness (other)
Anxiety, Migraine, Concussion/TBI.

A 1994 historical review of management strategies employed in primary care indicated that the most common tests ordered were "laboratory testing (33.6%), advanced testing (11.4%), referral to a specialist (9.3%), medication (61.3%), observation (71.8%), reassurance (41.6%), and behavioral recommendations (15%)." The advanced testing group consisted primarily of imaging studies [101]. Past reviews of referral patterns to specialists from around that same time, in both Europe and USA, indicated only 3–10% of patients complaining of dizziness at the primary care level were referred on for specialty consultation [102, 103].

A more recent review [104] of management strategies employed for patients complaining of dizziness in primary care revealed that referrals to specialists had increased to 24% and the prescription of medications had decreased to 23%.

Similarly, current primary care literature advocates a very different approach proposing the use of validated diagnostic protocols [105]. Validated diagnostic protocols include the performance of the Dix-Hallpike test for the complaint of positional vertigo, as BPPV is the most common vestibular pathology. The first Clinical Practice Guideline (CPG) for BPPV was published in 2008 with an update in 2017 strongly recommending a Dix-Hallpike test prior to making a diagnosis or recommending treatment for BPPV, and recommending against the use of meclizine (Antivert) as a treatment option. Unfortunately, these protocols are used inconsistently [29].

Current primary care literature also advocates a targeted approach with complaints of dizziness using the novel diagnostic approach of using timing of symptoms, triggers that provoke symptoms, and targeted examination. This protocol is known as TiTraTe. The HINTS protocol, which is used for the complaint of acute vertigo, is a quick and sensitive technique for separating peripheral disorders from brainstem pathology as a source for acute vertigo without necessarily arriving at a diagnosis. The TiTraTe approach is intended to arrive at a diagnosis regarding cause of the patient's complaint of dizziness [106].

Availability of Vestibular Function Testing

Not unlike many medical procedures in the USA, vestibular testing has suffered from dramatic reductions in reimbursement while at the same time clinics and practitioners are faced with increases in equipment and operating expense. Reimbursement for the standard VNG battery has decreased by 57% over the past 20 years. Adding the roughly 50% decrease in dollar value due to inflation, reimbursement for basic vestibular testing (the most widely available videonystagmography (VNG) battery) has decreased in actual value by close to 75% [107]. This has impacted the availability and utilization of vestibular function testing in USA. Countries with Healthcare Services not directly related to fee for service may have different obstacles to overcome.

The VNG test battery, aside from improvements in recording techniques, has not changed since it was introduced 60–80 years ago. This battery of tests is very limited in scope and detection of vestibular disorders. A VNG test battery includes examination for spontaneous and gaze nystagmus, ocular motility, positional nystagmus, and asymmetries in response to caloric irrigation. None of these tests would evoke nystagmus associated with TMWS, and would likely be considered normal in TMWS patients.

Abnormalities related to TMWS can be recorded with VNG equipment, but the standard battery of tests would need to be expanded to include introduction of vibration, loud sound (Tullio phenomenon), and introduction of middle ear pressure (insufflation, Valsalva or Toynbee) to document triggered nystagmus [108].

Both cervical and ocular VEMPs are considered to be helpful in identifying semicircular canal dehiscence [109, 110]. VEMP testing is not a part of routine vestibular function tests in most specialty offices in the USA and it requires additional equipment than what is utilized for VNG. Precise utilization data are not available, as Medicare has only recently assigned a billing code, procedure descriptor, and reimbursement for VEMP testing.

Summary

Vestibular disorders, both historically and currently, suffer from frequent misdiagnosis and ineffective treatments. These inefficiencies lead to reduced quality of life, increased healthcare costs, and increased incidence of injurious falls. There are many barriers confronted by patients suffering from vestibular disorders and especially those with lesser-known vestibular disorders like TMWS. Increased awareness and education both on the part of the patient and physician are critical steps in providing effective care for this population.

References

1. Molnar A, McGee S. Diagnosing and treating dizziness. Med Clin North Am. 2014;98(3):583–96. https://doi.org/10.1016/j.mcna.2014.01.014.
2. Neuhauser HK. The epidemiology of dizziness and vertigo. Handb Clin Neurol. 2016;137:67–82. https://doi.org/10.1016/B978-0-444-63437-5.00005-4.
3. Neuhauser HK, Lempert T. Vertigo: epidemiologic aspects. Semin Neurol. 2009;29(5):473–81. https://doi.org/10.1055/s-0029-1241043.
4. Müller M, Goeldlin MB, Gaschen J, Sauter TC, Stock S, Wagner F, Exadaktylos AK, Fischer U, Kalla R, Mantokoudis G. Characteristics and resource needs in patients with vestibular symptoms: a comparison of patients with symptoms of unknown versus determined origin. BMC Emerg Med. 2020;20(1):70. https://doi.org/10.1186/s12873-020-00361-8.
5. Zwergal A, Dieterich M. Vertigo and dizziness in the emergency room. Curr Opin Neurol. 2020;33(1):117–25. https://doi.org/10.1097/WCO.0000000000000769.
6. Bösner S, Schwarm S, Grevenrath P, Schmidt L, Hörner K, Beidatsch D, Bergmann M, Viniol A, Becker A, Haasenritter J. Prevalence, aetiologies and prognosis of the symptom dizziness in primary care—a systematic review. BMC Fam Pract. 2018;19:33. https://doi.org/10.1186/s12875-017-0695-0.
7. Kim H-J, Lee J-O, Choi J-Y, Kim J-S. Etiologic distribution of dizziness and vertigo in a referral-based dizziness clinic in South Korea. J Neurol. 2020;267(8):2252–9. https://doi.org/10.1007/s00415-020-09831-2.
8. Kroenke K, Hoffman RM, Einstadter D. How common are various causes of dizziness? A critical review. South Med J. 2000;93(2):160–7; quiz 168.
9. Newman-Toker DE, Hsieh Y-H, Camargo CA, Pelletier AJ, Butchy GT, Edlow JA. Spectrum of dizziness visits to US emergency departments: cross-sectional analysis from a nationally representative sample. Mayo Clin Proc. 2008;83(7):765–75. https://doi.org/10.4065/83.7.765.
10. Sommerfeldt JM, Fischer JL, Morrison DA, McCoul ED, Riley CA, Tolisano AM. A dizzying complaint: investigating the intended meaning of dizziness among patients and providers. Laryngoscope. 2021;131(5):E1443–9.
11. Dunlap PM, Khoja SS, Whitney SL, Freburger JK. Assessment of health care utilization for dizziness in ambulatory care settings in the United States. Otol Neurotol. 2019;40(9):e918–24. https://doi.org/10.1097/MAO.0000000000002359.
12. Polensek SH, Sterk CE, Tusa RJ. Screening for vestibular disorders: a study of clinicians' compliance with recommended practices. Med Sci Monitor. 2008;14(5):CR238–242.
13. Geser R, Straumann D. Referral and final diagnoses of patients assessed in an academic vertigo center. Front Neurol. 2012;3:169. https://doi.org/10.3389/fneur.2012.00169.
14. Drossman DA, Ruddy J. Improving patient-provider relationships to improve health care. Clin Gastroenterol Hepatol. 2020;18(7):1417–26. https://doi.org/10.1016/j.cgh.2019.12.007.

15. Coffron MR, Zlatos C. Medicare physician payment on the decline: it's not your imagination. The Bulletin. 2019. https://bulletin.facs.org/2019/09/medicare-physician-payment-on-the-decline-its-not-your-imagination/.
16. Kerber KA, Meurer WJ, West BT, Fendrick AM. Dizziness presentations in U.S. emergency departments, 1995–2004. Acad Emerg Med. 2008;15(8):744–50.
17. Newman-Toker DE. Missed stroke in acute vertigo and dizziness: it is time for action, not debate. Ann Neurol. 2016;79(1):27–31. https://doi.org/10.1002/ana.24532.
18. Kadhim-Saleh A, Worrall JC, Taljaard M, Gatien M, Perry JJ. Self-awareness of computed tomography ordering in the emergency department. CJEM. 2018;20(2):275–83. https://doi.org/10.1017/cem.2017.45.
19. Connor SEJ, Sriskandan N. Imaging of dizziness. Clin Radiol. 2014;69(2):111–22. https://doi.org/10.1016/j.crad.2013.10.013.
20. Quimby AE, Kwok ESH, Lelli D, Johns P, Tse D. Usage of the HINTS exam and neuroimaging in the assessment of peripheral vertigo in the emergency department. J Otolaryngol Head Neck Surg. 2018;47(1):54. https://doi.org/10.1186/s40463-018-0305-8.
21. Regis A, LePage R, Bodunde O, Turgeon Z, Ohle R. P106: the HINTS exam: an often misused but potentially accurate diagnostic tool for central causes of dizziness. Can J Emerg Med. 2019;21(S1):S102. https://doi.org/10.1017/cem.2019.297.
22. Ohle R, Montpellier R-A, Marchadier V, Wharton A, McIsaac S, Anderson M, Savage D. Can emergency physicians accurately rule out a central cause of vertigo using the HINTS examination? A systematic review and meta-analysis. Acad Emerg Med. 2020;27(9):887–96. https://doi.org/10.1111/acem.13960.
23. Dmitriew C, Regis A, Bodunde O, Lepage R, Turgeon Z, McIsaac S, Ohle R. Diagnostic accuracy of the HINTS exam in an emergency department: a retrospective chart review. Acad Emerg Med. 2021;28(4):387–93. https://doi.org/10.1111/acem.14171.
24. Shaikh AG, Bronstein A, Carmona S, Cha Y-H, Cho C, Ghasia FF, Gold D, Green KE, Helmchen C, Ibitoye RT, Kattah J, Kim J-S, Kothari S, Manto M, Seemungal BM, Straumann D, Strupp M, Szmulewicz D, Tarnutzer A, et al. Consensus on virtual management of vestibular disorders: urgent versus expedited care. Cerebellum. 2020;1–5:4. https://doi.org/10.1007/s12311-020-01178-8.
25. Zee D, Newman-Toker D, Tourkevich R, Brune A, Green K, Peterson S, Fanai M, Otero-Millan J, Gold D. Diagnostic impact of a device-enabled remote "tele-dizzy" consultation service (58). Neurology. 2020;94(15 Suppl) https://n.neurology.org/content/94/15_Supplement/58
26. Eagles D, Stiell IG, Clement CM, Brehaut J, Kelly A-M, Mason S, Kellermann A, Perry JJ. International survey of emergency physicians' priorities for clinical decision rules. Acad Emerg Med. 2008;15(2):177–82. https://doi.org/10.1111/j.1553-2712.2008.00035.x.
27. Voetsch B, Sehgal S. Acute dizziness, vertigo, and unsteadiness. Neurol Clin. 2021;39(2):373–89. https://doi.org/10.1016/j.ncl.2021.01.008.
28. Lüscher M, Theilgaard S, Edholm B. Prevalence and characteristics of diagnostic groups amongst 1034 patients seen in ENT practices for dizziness. J Laryngol Otol. 2014;128(2):128–33. https://doi.org/10.1017/S0022215114000188.
29. Bhattacharyya N, Gubbels SP, Schwartz SR, Edlow JA, El-Kashlan H, Fife T, Holmberg JM, Mahoney K, Hollingsworth DB, Roberts R, Seidman MD, Steiner RWP, Do BT, Voelker CCJ, Waguespack RW, Corrigan MD. Clinical practice guideline: benign paroxysmal positional vertigo (update). Otolaryngology Head Neck Surg. 2017;156(3_Suppl):S1–S47. https://doi.org/10.1177/0194599816689667.
30. Bednarczuk NF, Bonsu A, Ortega MC, Fluri A-S, Chan J, Rust H, de Melo F, Sharif M, Seemungal BM, Golding JF, Kaski D, Bronstein AM, Arshad Q. Abnormal visuo-vestibular interactions in vestibular migraine: a cross sectional study. Brain. 2019;142(3):606–16. https://doi.org/10.1093/brain/awy355.
31. Agrawal Y, Ward BK, Minor LB. Vestibular dysfunction: prevalence, impact and need for targeted treatment. J Vestib Res. 2013;23(3):113–7. https://doi.org/10.3233/VES-130498.
32. Lempert T, Neuhauser H. Epidemiology of vertigo, migraine and vestibular migraine. J Neurol. 2009;256(3):333–8. https://doi.org/10.1007/s00415-009-0149-2.

33. Nowaczewska M. Vestibular migraine—an underdiagnosed cause of vertigo. Diagnosis and treatment. Neurol Neurochir Pol. 2020;54(2):106–15. https://doi.org/10.5603/PJNNS.a2020.0031.
34. Wiener-Vacher SR. Vestibular disorders in children. Int J Audiol. 2008;47(9):578–83. https://doi.org/10.1080/14992020802334358.
35. Strupp M, Brandt T. Vestibular neuritis. Semin Neurol. 2009;29(5):509–19. https://doi.org/10.1055/s-0029-1241040.
36. Sekitani T, Imate Y, Noguchi T, Inokuma T. Vestibular neuronitis: epidemiological survey by questionnaire in Japan. Acta Otolaryngol Suppl. 1993;503:9–12. https://doi.org/10.3109/00016489309128061.
37. Sjögren J, Magnusson M, Tjernström F, Karlberg M. Steroids for acute vestibular neuronitis—the earlier the treatment, the better the outcome? Otol Neurotol. 2019;40(3):372–4. https://doi.org/10.1097/MAO.0000000000002106.
38. Wegner I, van Benthem PPG, Aarts MCJ, Bruintjes TD, Grolman W, van der Heijden GJMG. Insufficient evidence for the effect of corticosteroid treatment on recovery of vestibular neuritis. Otolaryngol Head Neck Surg. 2012;147(5):826–31. https://doi.org/10.1177/0194599812457557.
39. Yoo MH, Yang CJ, Kim SA, Park MJ, Ahn JH, Chung JW, Park HJ. Efficacy of steroid therapy based on symptomatic and functional improvement in patients with vestibular neuritis: a prospective randomized controlled trial. Eur Arch Otorhinolaryngol. 2017;274(6):2443–51. https://doi.org/10.1007/s00405-017-4556-1.
40. Sulway S, Whitney SL. Advances in vestibular rehabilitation. Adv Otorhinolaryngol. 2019;82:164–9. https://doi.org/10.1159/000490285.
41. Tokle G, Mørkved S, Bråthen G, Goplen FK, Salvesen Ø, Arnesen H, Holmeslet B, Nordahl SHG, Wilhelmsen KT. Efficacy of vestibular rehabilitation following acute vestibular neuritis: a randomized controlled trial. Otol Neurotol. 2020;41(1):78–85. https://doi.org/10.1097/MAO.0000000000002443.
42. Cureoglu S, da Costa Monsanto R, Paparella MM. Histopathology of Meniere's disease. Oper Tech Otolaryngol Head Neck Surg. 2016;27(4):194–204. https://doi.org/10.1016/j.otot.2016.10.003.
43. Luryi AL, Morse E, Michaelides E. Pathophysiology and diagnosis of Meniere's disease. In: Babu S, Schutt CA, Bojrab DI, editors. Diagnosis and treatment of vestibular disorders. Cham: Springer International Publishing; 2019. p. 165–88. https://doi.org/10.1007/978-3-319-97858-1_13.
44. Merchant SN, Adams JC, Nadol JB. Pathophysiology of Meniere's syndrome: are symptoms caused by endolymphatic hydrops? Otol Neurotol. 2005;26(1):74–81. https://doi.org/10.1097/00129492-200501000-00013.
45. Yamane H, Sunami K, Iguchi H, Sakamoto H, Imoto T, Rask-Andersen H. Assessment of Meniere's disease from a radiological aspect – saccular otoconia as a cause of Meniere's disease? Acta Otolaryngol. 2012;132(10):1054–60. https://doi.org/10.3109/00016489.2012.680980.
46. Harris JP, Alexander TH. Current-day prevalence of Ménière's syndrome. Audiol Neurootol. 2010;15(5):318–22. https://doi.org/10.1159/000286213.
47. Huppert D, Strupp M, Brandt T. Long-term course of Menière's disease revisited. Acta Otolaryngol. 2010;130(6):644–51.
48. Magnan J, Özgirgin ON, Trabalzini F, Lacour M, Escamez AL, Magnusson M, Güneri EA, Guyot JP, Nuti D, Mandalà M. European position statement on diagnosis, and treatment of Meniere's disease. J Int Adv Otol. 2018;14(2):317–21. https://doi.org/10.5152/iao.2018.140818.
49. Propp JM, McCarthy BJ, Davis FG, Preston-Martin S. Descriptive epidemiology of vestibular schwannomas. Neuro Oncol. 2006;8(1):1–11. https://doi.org/10.1215/S1522851704001097.
50. Thompson TL, Amedee R. Vertigo: a review of common peripheral and central vestibular disorders. Ochsner J. 2009;9(1):20–6.

51. Chamoun R, MacDonald J, Shelton C, Couldwell WT. Surgical approaches for resection of vestibular schwannomas: translabyrinthine, retrosigmoid, and middle fossa approaches. Neurosurg Focus. 2012;33(3):E9. https://doi.org/10.3171/2012.6.FOCUS12190.
52. Fu VX, Verheul JB, Beute GN, Leenstra S, Kunst HPM, Mulder JJS, Hanssens PEJ. Retreatment of vestibular schwannoma with gamma knife radiosurgery: clinical outcome, tumor control, and review of literature. J Neurosurg. 2017;129(1):137–45. https://doi.org/10.3171/2017.3.JNS162033.
53. Minor LB, Solomon D, Zinreich JS, Zee DS. Sound- and/or pressure-induced vertigo due to bone dehiscence of the superior semicircular canal. Arch Otolaryngol Head Neck Surg. 1998;124(3):249–58. https://doi.org/10.1001/archotol.124.3.249.
54. Berning AW, Arani K, Branstetter BF. Prevalence of superior semicircular canal dehiscence on high-resolution CT imaging in patients without vestibular or auditory abnormalities. Am J Neuroradiol. 2019;40(4):709–12. https://doi.org/10.3174/ajnr.A5999.
55. Ho M-L, Moonis G, Halpin CF, Curtin HD. Spectrum of third window abnormalities: semicircular canal dehiscence and beyond. Am J Neuroradiol. 2017;38(1):2–9. https://doi.org/10.3174/ajnr.A4922.
56. Carey JP, Minor LB, Nager GT. Dehiscence or thinning of bone overlying the superior semicircular canal in a temporal bone survey. Arch Otolaryngol Head Neck Surg. 2000;126(2):137–47. https://doi.org/10.1001/archotol.126.2.137.
57. Berkiten G, Gürbüz D, Akan O, Tutar B, Tunç MK, Karaketir S, Bircan HS, Berkiten E, Sarı H, Atar Y, Uyar Y. Dehiscence or thinning of bone overlying the superior semicircular canal in idiopathic intracranial hypertension. Eur Arch Otorhinolaryngol. 2021;279(6):2899–904. https://doi.org/10.1007/s00405-021-07020-z.
58. Peng KA, Ahmed S, Yang I, Gopen Q. Temporal bone fracture causing superior semicircular canal dehiscence. Case Rep Otolaryngol. 2014;2014:817291. https://doi.org/10.1155/2014/817291.
59. Ward BK, Carey JP, Minor LB. Superior Canal dehiscence syndrome: lessons from the first 20 years. Front Neurol. 2017;8:177. https://doi.org/10.3389/fneur.2017.00177.
60. Zwierz A, Masna K, Burduk P. Middle-ear cholesteatoma co-existing with labyrinthine fistula and vestibular schwannoma. Eur Arch Otorhinolaryngol. 2020;277(4):999–1003. https://doi.org/10.1007/s00405-020-05796-0.
61. Lee JA, Liu YF, Nguyen SA, McRackan TR, Meyer TA, Rizk HG. Posterior semicircular canal dehiscence: case series and systematic review. Otol Neurotol. 2020;41(4):511–21. https://doi.org/10.1097/MAO.0000000000002576.
62. Spasic M, Trang A, Chung LK, Ung N, Thill K, Zarinkhou G, Gopen QS, Yang I. Clinical characteristics of posterior and lateral semicircular canal dehiscence. J Neurol Surg B Skull Base. 2015;76(6):421–5. https://doi.org/10.1055/s-0035-1551667.
63. Meiklejohn DA, Corrales CE, Boldt BM, Sharon JD, Yeom KW, Carey JP, Blevins NH. Pediatric semicircular canal dehiscence: radiographic and histologic prevalence, with clinical correlation. Otol Neurotol. 2015;36(8):1383–9. https://doi.org/10.1097/MAO.0000000000000811.
64. Sarna B, Abouzari M, Merna C, Jamshidi S, Saber T, Djalilian HR. Perilymphatic fistula: a review of classification, etiology, diagnosis, and treatment. Front Neurol. 2020;11:1046. https://doi.org/10.3389/fneur.2020.01046.
65. Weber PC, Perez BA, Bluestone CD. Congenital perilymphatic fistula and associated middle ear abnormalities. Laryngoscope. 1993;103(2):160–4. https://doi.org/10.1002/lary.5541030207.
66. Blake DM, Tomovic S, Vazquez A, Lee H-J, Jyung RW. Cochlear-facial dehiscence—a newly described entity. Laryngoscope. 2014;124(1):283–9. https://doi.org/10.1002/lary.24223.
67. Song Y, Alyono JC, Bartholomew RA, Vaisbuch Y, Corrales CE, Blevins NH. Prevalence of radiographic cochlear–facial nerve dehiscence. Otol Neurotol. 2018;39(10):1319–25. https://doi.org/10.1097/MAO.0000000000002015.
68. Fang CH, Chung SY, Blake DM, Vazquez A, Li C, Carey JP, Francis HW, Jyung RW. Prevalence of cochlear-facial dehiscence in a study of 1,020 temporal bone specimens. Otol Neurotol. 2016;37(7):967–72. https://doi.org/10.1097/MAO.0000000000001057.

69. Moreano EH, Paparella MM, Zelterman D, Goycoolea MV. Prevalence of carotid canal dehiscence in the human middle ear: a report of 1000 temporal bones. Laryngoscope. 1994;104(5 Pt 1):612–8. https://doi.org/10.1002/lary.5541040515.
70. Gunbey HP, Gunbey E, Sayit AT, Aslan K, Unal A, Incesu L. The impact of the cochlear-carotid interval on tinnitus perception. Surg Radiol Anat. 2016;38(5):551–6. https://doi.org/10.1007/s00276-015-1607-4.
71. Young RJ, Shatzkes DR, Babb JS, Lalwani AK. The cochlear-carotid interval: anatomic variation and potential clinical implications. Am J Neuroradiol. 2006;27(7):1486–90.
72. Merchant SN, Rosowski JJ. Conductive hearing loss caused by third-window lesions of the inner ear. Otol Neurotol. 2008;29(3):282–9. https://doi.org/10.1097/mao.0b013e318161ab24.
73. Valvassori GE, Clemis JD. The large vestibular aqueduct syndrome. Laryngoscope. 1978;88(5):723–8. https://doi.org/10.1002/lary.1978.88.5.723.
74. Noguchi Y, Fukuda S, Fukushima K, Gyo K, Hara A, Nakashima T, Ogawa K, Okamoto M, Sato H, Usami S-I, Yamasoba T, Yokoyama T, Kitamura K. A nationwide study on enlargement of the vestibular aqueduct in Japan. Auris Nasus Larynx. 2017;44(1):33–9. https://doi.org/10.1016/j.anl.2016.04.012.
75. Alemi AS, Chan DK. Progressive hearing loss and head trauma in enlarged vestibular aqueduct: a systematic review and meta-analysis. Otolaryngol Head Neck Surg. 2015;153(4):512–7. https://doi.org/10.1177/0194599815596343.
76. Nazareth I, Yardley L, Owen N. Outcome of symptoms of dizziness in a general practice community sample. Fam Pract. 2000;16:616–8.
77. Staab JP, Eckhardt-Henn A, Horii A, Jacob R, Strupp M, Brandt T, Bronstein A. Diagnostic criteria for persistent postural-perceptual dizziness (PPPD): consensus document of the committee for the classification of vestibular disorders of the Bárány Society. J Vestib Res. 2017;27(4):191–208. https://doi.org/10.3233/VES-170622.
78. Albathi M, Agrawal Y. Vestibular vertigo is associated with abnormal sleep duration. J Vestib Res. 2017;27(2–3):127–35. https://doi.org/10.3233/VES-170617.
79. Weidt S, Bruehl AB, Straumann D, Hegemann SCA, Krautstrunk G, Rufer M. Health-related quality of life and emotional distress in patients with dizziness: a cross-sectional approach to disentangle their relationship. BMC Health Serv Res. 2014;14:317. https://doi.org/10.1186/1472-6963-14-317.
80. Bigelow RT, Semenov YR, du Lac S, Hoffman HJ, Agrawal Y. Vestibular vertigo and comorbid cognitive and psychiatric impairment: the 2008 National Health Interview Survey. J Neurol Neurosurg Psychiatry. 2016;87(4):367–72. https://doi.org/10.1136/jnnp-2015-310319.
81. Kovacs E, Wang X, Grill E. Economic burden of vertigo: a systematic review. Heal Econ Rev. 2019;9(1):37. https://doi.org/10.1186/s13561-019-0258-2.
82. van der Zaag-Loonen HJ, van Leeuwen RB. Dizziness causes absence from work. Acta Neurol Belg. 2015;115(3):345–9. https://doi.org/10.1007/s13760-014-0404-x.
83. Mueller M, Strobl R, Jahn K, Linkohr B, Peters A, Grill E. Burden of disability attributable to vertigo and dizziness in the aged: results from the KORA-age study. Eur J Pub Health. 2014;24(5):802–7. https://doi.org/10.1093/eurpub/ckt171.
84. Wiltink J, Tschan R, Michal M, Subic-Wrana C, Eckhardt-Henn A, Dieterich M, Beutel ME. Dizziness: anxiety, health care utilization and health behavior--results from a representative German community survey. J Psychosom Res. 2009;66(5):417–24. https://doi.org/10.1016/j.jpsychores.2008.09.012.
85. Best C, Eckhardt-Henn A, Tschan R, Dieterich M. Psychiatric morbidity and comorbidity in different vestibular vertigo syndromes. Results of a prospective longitudinal study over one year. J Neurol. 2009;256(1):58–65. https://doi.org/10.1007/s00415-009-0038-8.
86. Staab JP, Ruckenstein MJ. Expanding the differential diagnosis of chronic dizziness. Arch Otolaryngol Head Neck Surg. 2007;133(2):170–6. https://doi.org/10.1001/archotol.133.2.170.
87. Eckhardt-Henn A, Best C, Bense S, Breuer P, Diener G, Tschan R, Dieterich M. Psychiatric comorbidity in different organic vertigo syndromes. J Neurol. 2008;255(3):420–8. https://doi.org/10.1007/s00415-008-0697-x.

88. Lin HW, Bhattacharyya N. Impact of dizziness and obesity on the prevalence of falls and fall-related injuries. Laryngoscope. 2014;124(12):2797–801. https://doi.org/10.1002/lary.24806.
89. Bergen G, Stevens MR, Burns ER. Falls and fall injuries among adults aged ≥65 years—United States, 2014. MMWR Morb Mortal Wkly Rep. 2016;65(37):993–8. https://doi.org/10.15585/mmwr.mm6537a2.
90. Baris VK, Intepeler SS, Yeginboy EY. The cost of serious patient fall-related injuries at hospitals in Turkey: a matched case-control study. Clin Nurs Res. 2018;27(2):162–79. https://doi.org/10.1177/1054773816671521.
91. Khow KSF, Visvanathan R. Falls in the aging population. Clin Geriatr Med. 2017;33(3):357–68. https://doi.org/10.1016/j.cger.2017.03.002.
92. Peng K, Tian M, Andersen M, Zhang J, Liu Y, Wang Q, Lindley R, Ivers R. Incidence, risk factors and economic burden of fall-related injuries in older Chinese people: a systematic review. Inj Prev. 2019;25(1):4–12. https://doi.org/10.1136/injuryprev-2018-042982.
93. Roberts AW, Ogunwole SU, Blakeslee L, Rabe MA. The population 65 years and older in the United States: 2016; 2018.
94. Alkhafaji MS, Varma S, Pross SE, Sharon JD, Nellis JC, Santina CCD, Minor LB, Carey JP. Long-term patient-reported outcomes after surgery for superior canal dehiscence syndrome. Otol Neurotol. 2017;38(9):1319–26. https://doi.org/10.1097/MAO.0000000000001550.
95. Öhman J, Forssén A, Sörlin A, Tano K. Patients' experiences of living with superior canal dehiscence syndrome. Int J Audiol. 2018;57(11):825–30. https://doi.org/10.1080/14992027.2018.1487086.
96. Thomson P. A hole in my life: battling chronic dizziness. Los Gatos: Smashwords; 2017.
97. Ocak I, Topsakal V, Van de Heyning P, Van Haesendonck G, Jorissen C, van de Berg R, Vanderveken OM, Van Rompaey V. Impact of superior canal dehiscence syndrome on health utility values: a prospective case-control study. Front Neurol. 2020;11:552495. https://doi.org/10.3389/fneur.2020.552495.
98. Wackym PA, Balaban CD, Mackay HT, Wood SJ, Lundell CJ, Carter DM, Siker DA. Longitudinal cognitive and neurobehavioral functional outcomes before and after repairing otic capsule dehiscence. Otol Neurotol. 2016;37(1):70–82. https://doi.org/10.1097/MAO.0000000000000928.
99. Kerber KA, Newman-Toker DE. Misdiagnosing dizzy patients: common pitfalls in clinical practice. Neurol Clin. 2015;33(3):565–75. https://doi.org/10.1016/j.ncl.2015.04.009.
100. Strupp M, Grimberg J, Teufel J, Laurell G, Kingma H, Grill E. Worldwide survey on laboratory testing of vestibular function. Neurol Clin Pract. 2020;10(5):379–87. https://doi.org/10.1212/CPJ.0000000000000744.
101. Sloane PD, Dallara J, Roach C, Bailey KE, Mitchell M, McNutt R. Management of dizziness in primary care. J Am Board Fam Pract. 1994;7(1):1–8.
102. Maarsingh OR, Dros J, Schellevis FG, van Weert HC, van der Windt DA, ter Riet G, van der Horst HE. Causes of persistent dizziness in elderly patients in primary care. Ann Fam Med. 2010;8(3):196–205. https://doi.org/10.1370/afm.1116.
103. Sloane PD. Dizziness in primary care. Results from the National Ambulatory Medical Care Survey. J Fam Pract. 1989;29(1):33–8.
104. Dunlap PM, Khoja SS, Whitney SL, Freburger JK. Assessment of physician adherence to guidelines for the diagnosis and treatment of benign paroxysmal positional vertigo in ambulatory care settings. JAMA Otolaryngol Head Neck Surg. 2018;144(9):845–6. https://doi.org/10.1001/jamaoto.2018.1859.
105. Muncie HL, Sirmans SM, James E. Dizziness: approach to evaluation and management. Am Fam Physician. 2017;95(3):154–62.
106. Newman-Toker DE, Edlow JA. TiTrATE: a novel, evidence-based approach to diagnosing acute dizziness and vertigo. Neurol Clin. 2015;33(3):577–99, viii. https://doi.org/10.1016/j.ncl.2015.04.011.
107. Desmond A. The state of vestibular testing for dizzy patients. Dizziness depot. 2018. https://hearinghealthmatters.org/dizzinessdepot/2018/the-state-of-vestibular-testing/.

108. Cremer PD, Minor LB, Carey JP, Della Santina CC. Eye movements in patients with superior canal dehiscence syndrome align with the abnormal canal. Neurology. 2000;55(12):1833–41. https://doi.org/10.1212/wnl.55.12.1833.
109. Fife TD, Satya-Murti S, Burkard RF, Carey JP. Vestibular evoked myogenic potential testing. Neurol Clin Pract. 2018;8(2):129–34. https://doi.org/10.1212/CPJ.0000000000000430.
110. Fife TD, Colebatch JG, Kerber KA, Brantberg K, Strupp M, Lee H, Walker MF, Ashman E, Fletcher J, Callaghan B, Gloss DS. Practice guideline: cervical and ocular vestibular evoked myogenic potential testing: report of the guideline development, dissemination, and implementation subcommittee of the American Academy of Neurology. Neurology. 2017;89(22):2288–96. https://doi.org/10.1212/WNL.0000000000004690.

Chapter 10
Taking the Patient History

Arun Pajaniappane and Paul Radomskij

Detailed patient history is the single most important aspect in the diagnosis and management of vestibular disorders. It requires time, a keen clinician, and patience. However, it can be an area which is often neglected in the assessment, resulting in misdiagnosis.

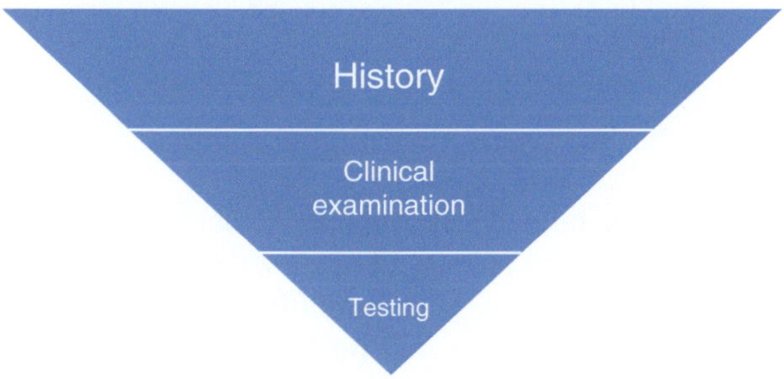

History taking from the vestibular patient requires an adapted approach to ensure that pertinent aspects are adequately covered, whilst retaining the wider scope and

A. Pajaniappane (✉)
Department of Audiovestibular Medicine and Audiology, St George's University Hospitals NHS Foundation Trust, London, UK

Harley Street Audiovestibular Clinic, London, UK
e-mail: arun.pajaniappane@stgeorges.nhs.uk

P. Radomskij
Department of Audiovestibular Medicine and Audiology, St George's University Hospitals NHS Foundation Trust, London, UK

UCL Ear Institute, London, UK
e-mail: p.radomskij@ucl.ac.uk

G. J. Gianoli, P. Thomson (eds.), *Third Mobile Window Syndrome of the Inner Ear*, https://doi.org/10.1007/978-3-031-16586-3_10

structure of the traditional medical history. The vestibular history will cover aspects of acute episodes, as well as the more chronic symptoms patients may experience.

Patient history should routinely cover audiological, vestibular, and relevant neurological symptoms. Past medical history, otological history, and history of migraine all offer clues to the underlying pathophysiology of patient symptoms. Systems review would help in recognition of other systemic causes of dizziness. Various useful acronyms have been coined to guide clinicians in taking an adequate vestibular history and are explored further below.

Newman-Toker and Edlow [1] proposed a novel paradigm with the acronym TitrATE to aid clinicians in diagnosing acute dizziness and vertigo (Box 10.1).

Box 10.1 Acute Dizziness and Vertigo

Timing: Classification of the dizziness into acute, episodic, or chronic.

Triggers: Identification of an obvious trigger such as head position or trauma.

And

Targeted ***E***xam: Utilisation of specific bedside clinical tests and eye movement examination to help differentiate central vs. peripheral causes.

As part of the diagnostic process, they proposed classification of four disparate vestibular syndromes as outlined below:

Acute Vestibular Syndrome (AVS) is defined as acute onset persistent, continuous vestibular symptoms lasting at least 24 h, sometimes in conjunction with other features such as nausea, vomiting, gait instability, head motion intolerance, and nystagmus. It can be further divided into **post-exposure AVS** whereby the acute vertigo is directly from an insult such as trauma or drug exposure, or **spontaneous AVS**.

Episodic Vestibular Syndrome (EVS) is used to describe discrete episodic attacks of vestibular symptoms which can be seconds, minutes or several hours. It can be separated into episodes which are triggered by an action or event such as head movement or postural change known as **Triggered EVS**, or **Spontaneous EVS** which occurs without any preceding triggers.

Symptoms in many cases of Third Mobile Window Disorders (TMWD) are usually of insidious and gradual onset. However, some may present more acutely following an insult such as head trauma or straining. Recognition of such symptoms and the possibility of TMWD at an early stage enables appropriate prompt re-direction to specialist services for earlier diagnosis and management.

TMWD can also present as classical Triggered EVS. It then becomes important for the clinician to clearly define triggers, time frames, and exacerbating factors to guide the diagnosis.

Acronyms such as SO STONED [2] and DISCOHAT [3] have been proposed to aid the clinician in taking an appropriate history from the vestibular patient. These cover some of the key aspects of the history that require to be addressed to help formulate a diagnosis, and can be useful particularly to the inexperienced clinician.

The letters of the acronym SO STONED are useful to describe any acute attacks and are outlined in Box 10.2.

Box 10.2 SO STONED

Symptoms: the type of vestibular symptom such as vertigo, imbalance, light-headedness, etc.

Often: the frequency of vestibular symptoms or if it is more continuous.

Since: the trigger to the onset of symptoms.

Trigger: the trigger to each specific attack such as head movement, loud sounds, etc.

Otology: associated auditory symptoms such as hearing loss, aural fullness, hyperacusis, autophony.

Neurology: associated neurological symptoms such as headaches, weakness, tingling, visual symptoms, etc.

Evolution: the natural history and progression of each episode/attack.

Duration: the duration of each attack/episode.

Another proposed acronym to aid history taking is DISCOHAT (Box 10.3), which can be useful as an adjunct to the above when symptoms are more chronic in nature.

Box 10.3 DISCOHAT

Darkness: symptomatic exacerbation in darkness and uneven surfaces.

Imbalance: unsteadiness on mobilisation.

Supermarket: visual sensitivity such as in crowded areas or with fast moving objects.

Cognitive: memory and concentration difficulties.

Oscillopsia: illusion of movement.

Head motion intolerance: intolerance of quick head movements in any direction.

Autonomic: postural dizziness, tachy- or bradycardia, sweating and pallor.

Tiredness.

TMWD such as superior semicircular canal dehiscence (SSCD) can be found incidentally in the absence of any symptoms. 1.4% of cadaveric temporal bones [4] and 3–10% on high resolution computerised tomography (HRCT) [5, 6] have been found to have SSCD. History is the only reliable way to correlate imaging findings to symptoms of TMWD.

Patients with TMWD can manifest with a range of audiological and vestibular symptoms. In this chapter, we aim to structure the history taking of the vestibular patient with a focus on TMWD symptoms.

Presenting Complaint and History (Symptoms)

The main symptom(s) of the patient should be clearly identified and defined at the outset. This will not only help in the diagnostic process, but will serve to identify and address aspects of the condition that the patient finds most intrusive and disabling.

Patients with vestibular disorders can generally present with one or more symptoms. However, this is even more relevant in TMWD patients who can present with a disparate range of symptoms, both audiological and vestibular, either in isolation or in combination. In a study by Pfammatter et al. [7] of 27 patients with SSCD, 78% of patients presented with cochleovestibular symptoms, whilst 15% with cochlear symptoms in isolation and 7% with vestibular symptoms in isolation.

Descriptive terms in the patient history can be very variable as audiovestibular symptoms can be difficult to describe. Clinicians should be aware of the variety of terminology used by patients to describe symptoms and be able to guide the history to elicit further pertinent details. A range of open and closed questions should be employed to tease out the relevant history without the risk of clinician bias.

Vestibular symptoms encompass a range of patient descriptors including vertigo, dizziness, unsteadiness, and imbalance. It is a common and potentially disabling complaint. Expert consensus on the definition of different terms [8] have been agreed upon as outlined in Box 10.4.

Box 10.4 Expert Consensus on Definition of Terminology for Vestibular Symptoms

Dizziness (also otherwise referred to as giddiness, light-headedness, or non-specific dizziness): A sensation of disordered spatial orientation without a sense of motion.

Vertigo is defined as the illusion of movement or distorted self-motion when there is no movement of the patient or head.

Presyncope (otherwise also referred to as near syncope of feeling faint): A sensation of imminent loss of consciousness. Light-headedness can be pre-syncope, dizziness or both.

Syncope: Transient, rapid onset loss of consciousness resulting in fall, followed by complete and spontaneous recovery without residual neurological dysfunction. Patients with presyncope or syncope would require careful consideration of a potential cardiovascular etiology.

Unsteadiness (also disequilibrium or imbalance): A sensation of instability to no particular direction, either when still or on mobilisation.

Patients with TMWD can present with either episodic vestibular symptoms, chronic imbalance [9, 10], or both. Episodic vestibular symptoms can be spontaneous [11] or can be provoked by various triggers including pressure and sound [10] further described below. If chronic unsteadiness or imbalance is a feature, it typically tends to get worse with triggering activity.

In TMWD, auditory features can be the main presenting complaint and can present in isolation without vestibular symptoms. Patients may report hearing loss due to increased sensitivity of bone conduction thresholds which results in a (pseudo) conductive hearing loss on audiometry [12]. Hearing loss tends to be stable, although progression has also previously been reported [13].

However, increased bone conduction sensitivity can also result in hyperacusis, as well as enhanced perception of sounds such as autophony of own voice, chewing, neck movements, eyeballs moving, and hearing one's own footsteps [14]. Autophony of vascular flow can also present as pulsatile tinnitus [15] particularly when TMWD are associated with the superior petrosal sinus [16]. However, patients generally do not tend to report autophony of breathing which tends to be more a feature in patulous Eustachian tube [9, 17].

Trigger

In EVS, trigger identification to the provocation of symptoms is crucial in differentiating between vestibular disorders. Many vestibular symptoms may only occur when triggered by a stimulus, such as head position in BPPV, or dietary factors in vestibular migraine.

In TWMD, vestibular symptoms can be variable and follow no set patterns. They can be triggered by loud sounds in up to 90% of patients [14]. As a result, patients may experience and describe nystagmus [18]. This is known as the Tullio phenomenon and was first described in animals by Professor Tullio in 1929.

Otherwise, activities which raise middle ear and/or intracranial pressure such as the Valsalva manoeuvre, nose blowing, lifting, straining and coughing can also provoke vestibular symptoms, and have been reported in up to 73% of patients [14]. In practice, this can be triggered on clinical examination by applying pressure to the external auditory meatus provoking the Hennebert sign.

Audiological symptom trigger tends to be related to autophony and hence may be provoked by the triggering movement or activity such as neck turning, eyeballs moving, walking, etc.

Barometric pressure changes have also been shown to provoke symptoms in a range of vestibular conditions. Activation of the vestibular nucleus has been shown in relation to barometric changes in mice [19]. It can be a feature in many patients with TMWD disorders, and would require to be elicited on detailed history taking [20].

Frequency and Duration of Symptoms

Frequency and duration of symptoms are another key part of the history to be explored, as different vestibular disorders typically present over differing time scales.

Vestibular and audiological symptoms in TMWD can present variably but generally tend to be transient and temporally related to the duration of the stimulus.

Patients may also report spontaneous attacks or a background of chronic disequilibrium with trigger related episodic exacerbation [10]. Hence, a detailed history identifying and differentiating different types and duration of dizziness which can co-exist in the same patient is key to the diagnostic process.

Associated Symptoms

Many vestibular disorders typically present with associated symptoms which aid in the differentiation of underlying pathology. Hence it is important to specifically enquire with regard to these as part of the patient history. Symptoms include auditory features such as tinnitus, hyperacusis, aural fullness, and hearing loss. Headaches and photosensitivity can be a feature in migraine related vestibular disorders. Sweating, pallor, heat intolerance, and palpitations can be a feature of dizziness related to dysautonomia.

Audiological symptoms as described earlier can be present in TMWD, either in isolation or in association with vestibular symptoms.

Systemic symptoms can be present in many vestibular disorders and hence may not have particular diagnostic significance. Provocation of autonomic symptoms and drop attacks [21] have previously been described in cases of TMWD.

Peripheral vestibular disorders typically do not present with any associated neurological features such as headaches, neuropathy, or weakness, compared to central vestibular disorders. However, involuntary head movement when exposed to loud sounds has been reported in TMWD [22]. Patients with a range of vestibular disorders including TMWD may also report brain fog, disorientation or discombobulation [9].

Causative Mechanism

The trigger to the onset of symptoms is useful to determine the mechanism of development of the vestibular disorder, which in turn can help guide diagnosis and management. Hence enquiring specifically regarding the trigger to the onset of symptoms, with open and closed questions as well as pertinent examples, is useful to guide the patient during history.

Many vestibular disorders can be triggered by acute vertigo secondary to labyrinthitis or vestibular neuritis. Other trigger mechanisms include head trauma, exposure to ototoxic medications or substances, and migraine disorder amongst many others.

TMWD disorders can be congenital but are also commonly acquired. Proposed mechanisms include thinning of the bone overlying bone of superior semicircular canal which can either be congenital or age-related deterioration. In certain cases, it can be further compromised provoking a third window effect because of other triggers such as head trauma [23]. Barotrauma [17] such as with scuba or skydiving, and other activities that rapidly alter middle ear/intracranial pressure can also potentially act as triggers. This includes excessive straining, blowing the nose forcefully, and lifting amongst others. Development of TMWD with the effort of childbirth has also been reported [24].

Past Medical History

The prevalence of Chiari I malformation has been found to be substantially higher in patients with SSCD (23%) [25]. Pathogenesis is thought to be secondary to raised intracranial pressures. Hence previously diagnosed Chiari malformation may help guide diagnosis.

Migraine can be a common comorbidity with TMWD which can act as a migraine trigger [9]. Hence patients with this overlap do need to be identified and treated appropriately with migraine prophylaxis. Migraine related audiovestibular symptoms can overlap with TMWD symptoms, and only detailed history will help to delineate the different conditions.

General review of other medical comorbidities and drug history are useful for surgical planning should the patient be considered for surgery, or to assess for drug interactions should pharmacotherapy be considered.

Past otological, surgical, and particularly neurosurgical history will help identify patients who may be at risk of having developed iatrogenic post-surgical TMWD.

Patients with TWMD typically tend to have seen multiple clinicians with no firm diagnosis. Defining the patient journey to this point, as well as exploring previous investigations and treatments including medical, surgical and physiotherapy among others, will help to guide the diagnostic process as well as provide insight into the potential treatment options available going forward.

Family History

Genetic susceptibility has also been implicated within family groups with SSCD and TMWD [26]. Hence enquiring about family members with similar symptoms or diagnoses is also a worthwhile endeavour.

Psycho-social Comorbidity

There are well recognised links between vestibular disorders and anxiety. Patients with dizziness can also be impaired in their ability to work due to symptoms. Audiovestibular symptoms can hence have a significant impact on daily functioning, social and work life [27]. Enquiring on the impact of the vestibular disorder on the patient's life can be useful in building rapport and a holistic picture. More focused questions using DISCOHAT or similar can help identify and address specific scenarios.

Psychological interventions [28] such as CBT have been shown to be effective in reducing the symptom burden in vestibular patients. Hence recognition of the psycho-social impact in the history, and addressing this as part of overall management at an early stage, is vital to the holistic management of vestibular patients. This is even more important in patients presenting with TMWD disorders who may have had a protracted patient journey prior to diagnosis, with cumulative accumulation of psychological comorbidity.

Paediatric Patients

There are limited data and experience of TMWD in paediatric patients. Whilst radiological evidence of TMWD and SSCD can commonly be incidentally identified in paediatric populations, clinical manifestation is much rarer. Paediatric patients are also likely to present much later due to the difficulties in accurately describing the disparate range of presentations on history. The clinician therefore requires a high degree of perseverance, insight, and patience to elicit an accurate history, employing specific and closed questioning at appropriate times to enquire about such symptoms.

Neurodevelopmental disorders including autistic spectrum disorder, cerebral palsy, and Down syndrome can be a co-existent finding (11.5%) in TMWD and worth enquiring on history. Chiari I malformation, craniofacial abnormalities, enlarged vestibular aqueduct, and other otological problems have also been found in association [29, 30].

Auditory symptoms such as hearing loss, hyperacusis, tinnitus, and autophony appear to be much more common than vestibular symptoms in the paediatric cohort. Hearing loss was by far the most common feature affecting 50.8% on systematic review of the published literature [29, 30].

Summary

At the end of the "patient conversation", time should be made available to summarise the information that the patient has provided to allow for any necessary clarification or rectification. The aim is to develop a shared understanding between the clinician and the patient. Any explanation by the clinician should be part of the shared decision-making process of "what is going to happen next". The next steps and plan of action should aim to meet the patient's medical needs, and match their expectations with what is potentially achievable.

Conclusion

History taking in the vestibular patient can be complex and time consuming but ultimately rewarding, having the most impact on eventual diagnosis and management. History taking is not a one-off process and may be part of an ongoing conversation with the patient to establish the details of symptoms. Patients may recall crucial aspects of their history at a later stage. TMWD such as SSCD have previously been described as the "great otological mimicker" [31] further emphasising the importance of detailed patient history to identify consistent symptoms and help differentiate from other vestibular disorders. The Bárány Society have recently published a consensus document on proposed diagnostic criteria to help with the diagnostic process in SSCD [32].

TMWD are a group of conditions which present variably, atypically, and often get misdiagnosed, resulting in protracted patient journeys and prolonged potentially disabling symptoms. Often this can be due to a cursory history and missed details of the presenting complaint. Consequently, patients may be labelled with alternate diagnosis and remain poorly responsive to treatment. Hence, revisiting the history at every opportune moment and reviewing existing diagnosis is never wasted effort, particularly in such cases.

References

1. Newman-Toker DE, Edlow JA. TiTrATE. Neurol Clin. 2015;33(3):577–99. https://doi.org/10.1016/j.ncl.2015.04.011.
2. Wuyts FL, Van Rompaey V, Maes LK. "SO STONED": common sense approach of the dizzy patient. Front Surg. 2016;3:32. https://doi.org/10.3389/fsurg.2016.00032.
3. Paredis S, van Stiphout L, Remmen E, et al. DISCOHAT: an acronym to describe the spectrum of symptoms related to bilateral vestibulopathy. Front Neurol. 2021;12:771650. https://doi.org/10.3389/fneur.2021.771650.
4. Carey JP, Minor LB, Nager GT. Dehiscence or thinning of bone overlying the superior semicircular canal in a temporal bone survey. Arch Otolaryngol Head Neck Surg. 2000;126(2):137–47. https://doi.org/10.1001/archotol.126.2.137.

5. Masaki Y. The prevalence of superior canal dehiscence syndrome as assessed by temporal bone computed tomography imaging. Acta Otolaryngol. 2011;131(3):258–62. https://doi.org/10.3109/00016489.2010.526145.
6. Cloutier JF, Bélair M, Saliba I. Superior semicircular canal dehiscence: positive predictive value of high-resolution CT scanning. Eur Arch Otorhinolaryngol. 2008;265(12):1455–60. https://doi.org/10.1007/s00405-008-0672-2.
7. Pfammatter A, Darrouzet V, Gartner M, Somers T, Dinther JV, Trabalzini F. A superior semicircular canal dehiscence syndrome multicenter study: is there an association between size and symptoms? Otol Neurotol. 2010;31(3):447–54.
8. Bisdorff A, Von Brevern M, Lempert T, Newman-Toker DE. Classification of vestibular symptoms: towards an international classification of vestibular disorders. J Vestib Res. 2009;19(1–2):1–13. https://doi.org/10.3233/VES-2009-0343.
9. Ward BK, Carey JP, Minor LB. Superior canal dehiscence syndrome: lessons from the first 20 years. Front Neurol. 2017;8:177. https://doi.org/10.3389/fneur.2017.00177.
10. Minor LB, Solomon D, Zinreich JS, Zee DS. Sound- and/or pressure-induced vertigo due to bone dehiscence of the superior semicircular canal. Arch Otolaryngol Head Neck Surg. 1998;124(3):249. https://doi.org/10.1001/archotol.124.3.249.
11. Naert L, Berg R, Heyning P, et al. Aggregating the symptoms of superior semicircular canal dehiscence syndrome. Laryngoscope. 2018;128(8):1932–8. https://doi.org/10.1002/lary.27062.
12. Merchant SN, Rosowski JJ. Conductive hearing loss caused by third-window lesions of the inner ear. Otol Neurotol. 2008;29(3):282–9. https://doi.org/10.1097/MAO.0b013e318161ab24.
13. Patel NS, Hunter JB, O'Connell BP, Bertrand NM, Wanna GB, Carlson ML. Risk of progressive hearing loss in untreated superior semicircular canal dehiscence. Laryngoscope. 2017;127(5):1181–6. https://doi.org/10.1002/lary.26322.
14. Minor LB. Clinical manifestations of superior semicircular canal dehiscence. Laryngoscope. 2005;115(10):1717–27. https://doi.org/10.1097/01.mlg.0000178324.55729.b7.
15. Liu Z, Bi W, Li J, et al. Superior semicircular canal dehiscence in relation to the superior petrosal sinus: a potential cause of pulsatile tinnitus. Clin Radiol. 2015;70(9):943–7. https://doi.org/10.1016/j.crad.2015.04.017.
16. Aw GE, Parker GD, Halmagyi GM, Saxby AJ. Pulsatile tinnitus in superior semicircular canal dehiscence cured by endovascular coil occlusion of the superior petrosal sinus. Otol Neurotol. 2021;42(5):e629–30. https://doi.org/10.1097/MAO.0000000000003012.
17. Bi WL, Brewster R, Poe D, et al. Superior semicircular canal dehiscence syndrome. J Neurosurg. 2017;127(6):1268–76. https://doi.org/10.3171/2016.9.JNS16503.
18. Watson SR, Halmagyi GM, Colebatch JG. Vestibular hypersensitivity to sound (Tullio phenomenon): structural and functional assessment. Neurology. 2000;54(3):722–8. https://doi.org/10.1212/wnl.54.3.722.
19. Sato J, Inagaki H, Kusui M, Yokosuka M, Ushida T. Lowering barometric pressure induces neuronal activation in the superior vestibular nucleus in mice. PLoS One. 2019;14(1):e0211297. https://doi.org/10.1371/journal.pone.0211297.
20. Gadre AK, Edwards IR, Baker VM, Roof CR. Membranous or hypermobile stapes footplate: a new anatomic site resulting in third window syndrome. Front Neurol. 2020;11:871. https://doi.org/10.3389/fneur.2020.00871.
21. Brantberg K, Ishiyama A, Baloh RW. Drop attacks secondary to superior canal dehiscence syndrome. Neurology. 2005;64(12):2126–8. https://doi.org/10.1212/01.WNL.0000165953.48914.B0.
22. Cremer PD, Minor LB, Carey JP, Della Santina CC. Eye movements in patients with superior canal dehiscence syndrome align with the abnormal canal. Neurology. 2000;55(12):1833–41. https://doi.org/10.1212/wnl.55.12.1833.
23. McCrary HC, Babajanian E, Patel N, et al. Superior semicircular canal dehiscence syndrome following head trauma: a multi-institutional review. Laryngoscope. 2021;131(11):E2810. https://doi.org/10.1002/lary.29751.

24. Watters KF, Rosowski JJ, Sauter T, Lee DJ. Superior semicircular canal dehiscence presenting as postpartum vertigo. Otol Neurotol. 2006;27(6):756–68. https://doi.org/10.1097/01.mao.0000227894.27291.9f.
25. Kuhn JJ, Clenney T. The association between semicircular canal dehiscence and Chiari type I malformation. Arch Otolaryngol Head Neck Surg. 2010;136(10):1009. https://doi.org/10.1001/archoto.2010.169.
26. Niesten MEF, Lookabaugh S, Curtin H, et al. Familial superior canal dehiscence syndrome. JAMA Otolaryngol Head Neck Surg. 2014;140(4):363–8. https://doi.org/10.1001/jamaoto.2013.6718.
27. Bronstein AM, Golding JF, Gresty MA, et al. The social impact of dizziness in London and Siena. J Neurol. 2010;257(2):183–90. https://doi.org/10.1007/s00415-009-5287-z.
28. Schmid G, Henningsen P, Dieterich M, Sattel H, Lahmann C. Psychotherapy in dizziness: a systematic review. J Neurol Neurosurg Psychiatry. 2011;82(6):601–6. https://doi.org/10.1136/jnnp.2010.237388.
29. Lee GS, Zhou G, Poe D, et al. Clinical experience in diagnosis and management of superior semicircular canal dehiscence in children. Laryngoscope. 2011;121(10):2256–61. https://doi.org/10.1002/lary.22134.
30. Lagman C, Ong V, Chung LK, et al. Pediatric superior semicircular canal dehiscence: illustrative case and systematic review. J Neurosurg Pediatr. 2017;20(2):196–203. https://doi.org/10.3171/2017.3.PEDS1734.
31. Zhou G, Gopen Q, Poe DS. Clinical and diagnostic characterization of canal dehiscence syndrome: a great otologic mimicker. Otol Neurotol. 2007;28(7):920–6.
32. Ward BK, van de Berg R, van Rompaey V, et al. Superior semicircular canal dehiscence syndrome: diagnostic criteria consensus document of the committee for the classification of vestibular disorders of the Bárány Society. J Vestib Res. 2021;31(3):131–41. https://doi.org/10.3233/VES-200004.

Chapter 11
Diagnostic Testing of Third Mobile Window Disorders

Surangi Mendis, Jay Patel, and Nehzat Koohi

Introduction

When a semicircular canal dehiscence (SSCD) syndrome is suspected, the clinician must have a clear diagnostic pathway in place for the work up of third mobile window disorders (TMWD). The presenting symptoms of TMWD can potentially be non-specific. SSCD syndrome was first described only in 1998 [1]. As such, individual neuro-otology departments may not have the most up-to-date evidenced-based guidance to inform the creation of a unit-specific diagnostic criteria for investigation of TMWD, particularly as this area is continually evolving. Furthermore, investigations to evaluate patients presenting with a suspected third-window condition require specific clinical expertise in order to perform and

S. Mendis (✉)
Department of Neuro-Otology, Royal National ENT and Eastman Dental Hospitals, UCLH, London, UK

Department of Audiovestibular Medicine, St Ann's Hospital, Whittington Health NHS Trust, London, UK
e-mail: surangi.mendis@nhs.net

J. Patel
Department of Neuro-Otology, Royal National ENT and Eastman Dental Hospitals, UCLH, London, UK
e-mail: jay.patel18@nhs.net

N. Koohi
Centre for Vestibular and Behavioural Neurosciences, Department of Clinical and Movement Neurosciences, UCL Institute of Neurology, University College London, London, UK

Stroke Services, National Hospital for Neurology and Neurosurgery, University College London Hospitals, London, UK

The UCL Ear Institute, University College London, London, UK
e-mail: n.koohi@ucl.ac.uk

G. J. Gianoli, P. Thomson (eds.), *Third Mobile Window Syndrome of the Inner Ear*, https://doi.org/10.1007/978-3-031-16586-3_11

interpret both the radiological and audiovestibular test findings, and these investigations can be costly, potentially restricting their availability to tertiary or quaternary centres. All ENT, audiovestibular and neuro-otological clinicians worldwide, no matter the setting, should therefore be familiar with the presenting symptoms and clinical examination findings in various TMWD and have an established clinical pathway to refer onwards to a specialist centre for full diagnostic work up and management if required. Similarly, awareness of the condition in general should be raised, worldwide, across a range of healthcare settings such that patients, who may initially present to family-practice or the emergency room, can similarly be referred onwards for appropriate investigation in a timely manner.

The presenting symptoms of SSCD can include pressure- and sound-induced vertigo, autophony, aural fullness, hyperacusis, pulsatile or non-pulsatile tinnitus [2, 3], due to increased sensitivity towards bone conducted sound. This resultant bone conduction hyperacusis forms the premise of the diagnostic testing of TMWD. Subjects may also present with chronic disequilibrium and cognitive difficulties [4–6], possibly related to vestibular effects on visuospatial ability, attention and executive function. Because the treatment of SSCD can be surgical, it is crucial to accurately confirm the diagnosis to identify the correct candidates for treatment and also avoid unnecessary, potentially complex, intracranial surgery for those in whom there is an alternative diagnosis. Additionally, even if surgical treatment is not opted for, the diagnosis should of course be correct to enable the patient and clinician to explore the appropriate treatment avenues, for example, trigger avoidance or physiotherapy-based vestibular rehabilitation. Vestibular symptoms are notorious for being poorly investigated and managed in some settings [7–10], particularly if no dedicated neuro-otology or audiovestibular service exists where provision is patchy. Therefore simply formulating a diagnosis with the purpose of being able to confidently counsel the patient with regard to their treatment options, but also reassure the patient that there is a defined cause for their symptoms, which are sometimes perceived to be ‘unusual’ (e.g., autophony), can be hugely therapeutic.

There is no single gold standard test or biomarker in relation to SSCD. Therefore a combination of symptomatology, clinical examination findings, audiovestibular function tests and imaging techniques are typically employed as a diagnostic test battery. As such, testing for SSCD can be complex, costly and is limited to centres with the available facilities and expertise to provide such assessments and investigations. However, as previously alluded to, the most basic clinical examination and assessment require little to no expertise or equipment and thus we argue that performing this basic bedside or office assessment in all patients presenting with autophony, pressure- or noise-induced dizziness and/or pulsatile tinnitus, and those in whom low frequency conductive hearing loss is found on audiometric testing, is essential. Positive findings using these initial screening tools should prompt the clinician to consider further targeted testing.

The authors herein take the opportunity to present a range of diagnostic means, providing details of the sensitivity and specificity of each of the tests, with the aim of encouraging individual clinicians and departments to create, refine or adapt their own diagnostic pathways for investigation of TMWD. Although the availability of diagnostic equipment and clinical expertise will determine which specific tests can be employed in each centre, we hope that this will streamline the diagnostic process for TMWD, as at present significant variability exists with regard to the diagnostic processes involved, meaning that it is difficult to compare diagnostic and treatment options between various centres, potentially complicating and hindering further research in this area. We summarise this chapter by proposing our own diagnostic framework incorporating some of the tests and investigations outlined. Emphasis is deliberately placed upon the importance of eliciting and obtaining objective evidence of pressure- and sound-induced nystagmus, given that these tests are easily performed with basic test equipment available in most neuro-otological clinical settings, thus allowing the diagnosis to be suspected in the first place, particularly given that the incidence of TMWD and SSCD syndrome is likely to be formally under-reported and the true prevalence and incidence unknown, as these tests are currently underutilized.

Basic Audiovestibular Physiology Relevant to Diagnostic Testing for SSCD

In the presence of normal bony covering of the superior semicircular canal (SSC), an air conducted acoustic stimulus results in the movement of the stapes footplate and oval window, and a subsequent pressure wave across the basilar membrane in the cochlea and an equal outward movement of the round window. In the presence of a dehiscence, the energy created by stapes footplate and oval window motion is shunted away from its usual route and toward the third window (Fig. 11.1). As a result, the pressure difference across the basilar membrane in the cochlea decreases and energy transmission to the vestibular sense organs increases. Obtaining objective evidence of these variations in pressure differences form the basis of the diagnostic tests used to formulate the diagnosis of TMWD and refute other pathologies, such as Ménière's disease or otosclerosis, that may present similarly.

In all TMWD, the underlying principle is that the mobile window exists on the scala vestibuli side of the cochlear partition [12]. It has the effect of artificially improving the bone conduction thresholds and worsens the air conduction thresholds, due to shunting of energy away from the cochlea and towards the labyrinth via a dehiscent pathway. Such pathways may be anatomically discrete or diffuse [11]. Examples of discrete TMWD pathways include those situated in the semicircular canals (SSCD or lateral or posterior canal dehiscence), the bony encasement of vestibule (enlarged vestibular aqueduct, modiolus malformation of the inner ear) or the cochlea (x-linked stapes gusher, carotid-cochlear dehiscence).

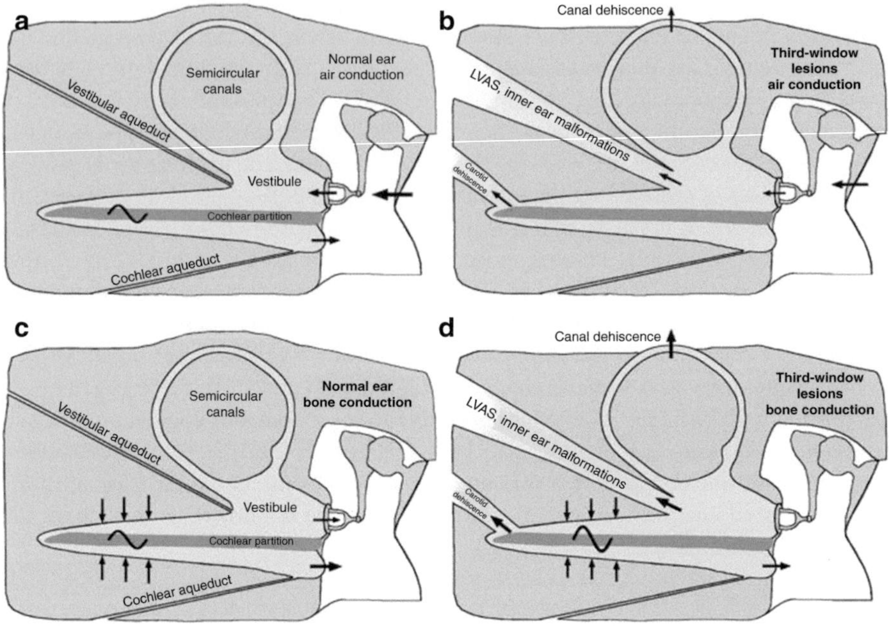

Fig. 11.1 Adapted with permission from [11]. (**a**) Normal ear, air conduction. Air conducted sound stimuli enters the vestibule via movement of the stapes in the oval window. The pressure difference between the scala vestibuli and scala tympani causes onward movement of the cochlear partition. The volume velocities of the oval and round windows are equal in magnitude but opposite in phase. (**b**) Third-window lesions, air conduction. It is hypothesised that a third window (in one of the canals, the vestibule or the scala vestibuli) allows a portion of the acoustic energy entering the vestibule through motion of the stapes to be shunted away from the cochlea. The shunting occurs primarily at low frequencies, resulting in a hearing loss by air conduction. (**c**) Normal ear, bone conduction. Compression of inner ear fluid by bone conducted sound results in a hearing percept because of an inequality in the impedance between the scala vestibuli side and the scala tympani side of the cochlear partition. This inequality is primarily due to a difference in the impedance between the oval and windows. As a result, there is a pressure difference across the cochlear partition, resulting in motion of the basilar membrane that leads to perception of bone conducted sound. (**d**) Third-window lesions, bone conduction. A third window increases the difference between the impedance on the scala vestibuli side and the scala tympani side of the cochlear partition by lowering the impedance on the vestibuli side, thereby improving the cochlear response to bone conduction. In patients with healthy cochleae as in SCD, supranormal bone conduction thresholds may be evident

Historical Aspects

In as early as the 1890s, experiments conducted by Ewald on pigeons with surgically fenestrated semicircular canals showed the presence of nystagmus when pressure was applied in the same plane (Hennebert's sign) [13]. In 1929 Tullio showed that loud noise could induce nystagmus in surgically fenestrated superior canals of dogs (Tullio's phenomenon) [14].

The first cohort of patients with SSCD was described over 20 years ago in 1998 by Lloyd Minor and colleagues [1]. These eight subjects all had pressure- and sound-induced dizziness, seven of the eight had eye movement abnormalities in the plane of the SSC objectively recorded using video-oculography or scleral search coil, and all had evidence of SSCD on temporal bone imaging undertaken in the axial and coronal planes.

The earliest descriptions of SSCD dubbed the condition as 'the great otological mimicker' given the non-specificity of the reported symptoms and their overlap with those described by subjects with proven otosclerosis, Ménière's disease, patulous eustachian tube dysfunction and perilymph fistulae [15, 16]. Subsequent literature went on to describe the valuable clinical examination and investigation findings characteristic of a TMWD, and these test findings in combination with radiological evidence of dehiscence, led to the triad of signs and symptoms, audiovestibular results and imaging becoming the cornerstone for reaching the diagnosis in those suspected to have the syndrome.

Over time, accuracy of the individual test components has improved and the value of additional testing was recognised, thus significantly improving the overall diagnostic process and allowing the exclusion of other differential diagnoses that may present similarly or with a 'third-window effect', such as posterior or lateral semicircular canal dehiscence, perilymph fistulae, cochlea-facial nerve dehiscence (CFD) or carotid-canal dehiscence (CCD).

Early diagnostic criteria were developed on the basis of the symptoms seen initially in patients with suspected SSCD, diagnosed when symptoms corresponded with reduced VEMP thresholds, a low frequency air-bone gap on audiometric testing and radiological findings, who went on to improve subjectively and on objective testing following plugging or resurfacing of the superior semicircular canal as intervention [17–19]. However symptoms, as previously mentioned, can be non-specific and also notoriously difficult to describe; patients may not actually associate their vertigo with sound or environmental pressure changes as a trigger. Some examination findings can also be suggestive of *any* third-window syndrome without this being specific to SSCD. And the CT finding of a thinning or dehiscence of the superior semicircular canal is not necessarily specific to SSCD; radiological dehiscence of the superior canal was identified on multiplanar ultra-high-resolution computerised tomography on 5.8% of routine CT temporal bone scans (in 17 of 191 subjects) but only 2 of the 17 subjects were found to have symptoms compatible with SSCDs (0.5% prevalence) [20]. Many studies quote higher figures for radiological prevalence depending on the CT slice thickness used [21–24]. This implies that the mere presence of the dehiscence of the superior semicircular canal is insufficient to create symptoms in all subjects and that CT imaging may overestimate the incidence of dehiscence. Furthermore, the presence of the dehiscence alone may be insufficient to truly create the third window effect as the overlying dura may be sufficiently noncompliant or stiff to ensure that pressure is not transmitted easily, or the third-window effect might only ensue following a secondary event, such as head injury, following damage to the overlying dura. However, whilst this is theoretical, for the third mobile window syndrome to be symptomatic, one requires the same degree of compliance from the round/oval windows. This is the basis for window reinforcement procedures, essentially increasing the compliance of the windows, ideally to pre-symptom status, to reduce the third mobile window effect.

It was previously noted that when a dehiscence is present, sound energy entering at the oval window is shunted away from the cochlear and towards the area of absent or thin bone. Bone conducted sounds are also conducted more readily via the dehiscence resulting in multiple investigative findings such as:

- Eye movements in the plane of the affected semicircular canal that can be induced by either increased pressure or sound within the ear canal, e.g. via the valsalva manoeuvre.
- Low-frequency conductive hearing loss.
- Unusually low or negative bone conduction thresholds on audiometry.
- Low cervical vestibular evoked myogenic potentials (cVEMP) threshold, with raised amplitude.

As with any relatively new condition, it is of paramount importance to have clearly defined diagnostic criteria, as this will not only facilitate greater understanding of the condition and a higher diagnostic pick up rate, but patient recruitment to research trials also becomes standardised. This is crucial if progress is to be made in terms of understanding the pathophysiology and evidence-based treatment strategies for this otolaryngological condition. Having a clear diagnostic route also allows the clinician to communicate the epidemiology, typical presenting features and expected progression to the patient. Given that surgery for SSCD can improve the patient's quality of life and reverse the audiovestibular test finding abnormalities in refractory cases or where symptoms are particularly disabling, having a clear route to reaching an accurate diagnosis when faced with a patient with a potential TMWD is of paramount importance.

Over time, imaging techniques have improved such that increased resolution CT scanning is now available and advances have been made with regards to the sensitivity and specificity of the audiological and vestibular function tests available, particularly VEMP testing.

Making the Diagnosis of SSCD and Other TMWD

In 2021, as part of the International Classification of Vestibular Disorders developed by The Bárány Society, a sub-committee of international experts in SSCD proposed the following criteria [2] based on the best available evidence at the time of writing:

All of the following must be present to make the diagnosis of SSCD:

1. At least one of the following symptoms consistent with the presence of a 'third mobile window' in the inner ear:

   (a) Bone conduction hyperacusis.
   (b) Sound-induced vertigo and/or oscillopsia time-locked to the stimulus.
   (c) Pressure-induced vertigo and/or oscillopsia time-locked to the stimulus.
   (d) Pulsatile tinnitus.

2. At least one of the following signs or diagnostic tests indicating a 'third mobile window' in the inner ear:

    (a) Nystagmus characteristic of excitation or inhibition of the affected superior semicircular canal evoked by sound, or by changes in middle ear pressure or intracranial pressure.
    (b) Low-frequency negative bone conduction thresholds on pure tone audiometry.
    (c) Enhanced VEMP responses (low cervical VEMP thresholds or high ocular VEMP amplitudes).

3. High-resolution temporal bone CT imaging with multiplanar reconstruction demonstrating dehiscence of the superior semicircular canal.
4. Not better accounted for by another vestibular disease or disorder.

Pictorially represented (Fig. 11.2), the diagnosis of TMWD should be made with a combination of:

(a) **Symptomatology** compatible with TMWD.

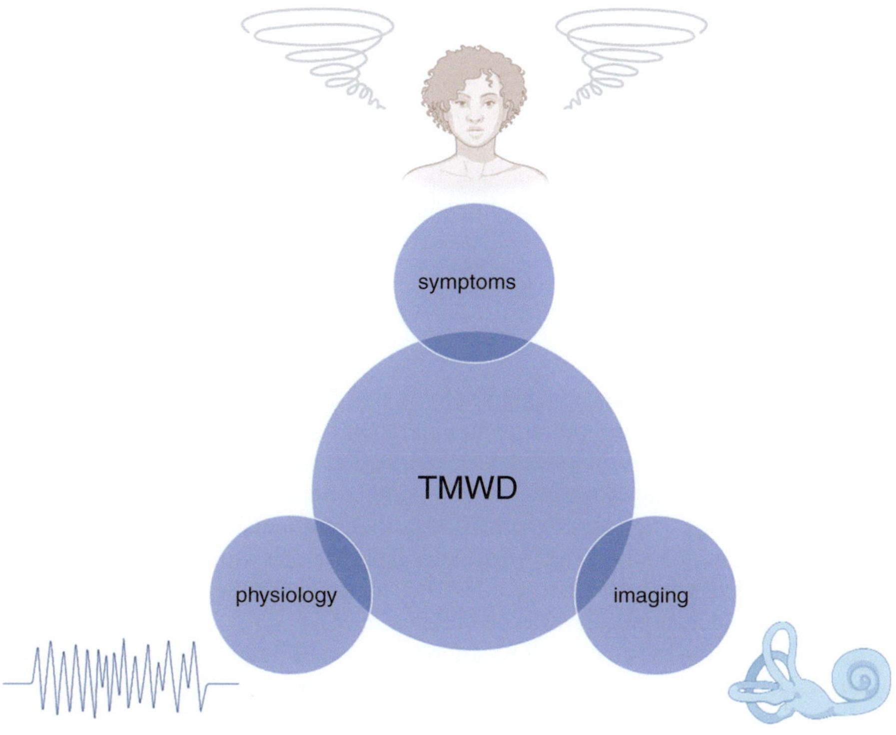

Fig. 11.2 Pictorial representation of the diagnosis of TMWD. A combination of symptomatology, imaging and physiological findings should be used to conclude that a subject has a TMWD. In cases of no-identified otic capsule dehiscence (no-iOCD), the diagnosis may be reached in subjects without radiological evidence of TMWD but who have suggestive symptoms and physiological test findings

(b) **Radiological** evidence of dehiscence or another anatomical defect consistent with a third mobile window.
(c) **Physiological** evidence of a TMWD abnormality (VEMP, audiometric, video-nystagmography [VNG] for oculographic recording of nystagmus induced by pressure changes or sound) or other objective evidence compatible with a TMWD.

The exception to this representation would be cases of SSCD syndrome with no radiological evidence of dehiscence, the so-called no-identified otic capsule dehiscence (no-iOCD) [5]. Such patients are symptomatic, and the presence of these symptoms are supported by physiological evidence of a TMWD, but without imaging findings compatible with dehiscence. Resolution or improvement in both symptoms and the electrophysiological abnormalities have been reported following surgical intervention, suggesting that radiological confirmation of dehiscence, whilst desirable, should not completely exclude the diagnosis of TWMD in a patient who displays symptoms.

The referenced Bárány Society paper [2] concludes that of all the physiological tests available, low frequency conductive hearing loss and increased ocular vestibular evoked myogenic potentials (oVEMP) amplitude have been shown to be the strongest predictive factors for making a diagnosis of SSCD and for choosing surgical repair. The authors have already argued that whilst the audiometry and VEMP test findings are hugely important, the absence of either conductive hearing loss or the characteristic VEMP results does not necessarily exclude a TMWD. If symptoms, examination findings and pressure- or sound-induced nystagmus can be elicited and TMWD is strongly suspected, if imaging reveals a dehiscent superior semicircular canal, for example, the diagnosis certainly can still be met.

Symptoms

TMWD symptoms are touched upon briefly in this diagnostics chapter given that if the symptoms of autophony, pulsatile tinnitus, sound- or pressure-induced dizziness are reported, this should prompt bedside examination and subsequent objective testing to confirm the presence of sound- or pressure-induced nystagmus. The ability to elicit these findings using oculography is essential, particularly given that they can be reproduced with limited equipment and expertise and would be sufficient, as minimum physiological evidence of a TMWD, to prompt further radiological investigation to obtain anatomical evidence of dehiscence.

Bone conduction hyperacusis (i.e., autophony), sound-induced vertigo, pressure-induced vertigo and pulsatile tinnitus are the four symptoms that most commonly prompt clinicians to further investigate for a TMWD. These four symptoms form the basis of the relevant physiological tests which should be undertaken to help formulate the diagnosis:

- Tullio phenomenon (can this be objectively measured by applying noise to the ear canal to generate and record nystagmus?)
- Pressure- or strain-induced vertigo (can this be replicated with Valsalva testing?)
- Autophony and pulsatile tinnitus (is there evidence of abnormal shunting of sound energy away from the conventional pathway via the cochlear and towards the area of dehiscence manifesting as raised air conduction thresholds and artificially lowered or negative bone conduction thresholds on audiometry, or lower thresholds and raised amplitudes on cVEMP testing?)

Autophony is thought to be the most common presenting symptom of SSCD [15, 25]. A recent study suggests that less than half of patients with SSCD syndrome experience pressure- and/or sound-induced vertigo [26].

Consequences of bone conduction hyperacusis can include:

- Autophony; hearing one's voice loudly, or in a distorted fashion, in the affected ear.
- Abnormally loud perception of one's own body sounds, such as 'hearing' the eyes blink, hearing the footsteps in the affected ear, etc.
- Pulsatile tinnitus, as sound associated with normal vascular flow through the vessels of the inner ear is transmitted more readily via the third-window to the dehiscence.

Sound-induced dizziness, vertigo or oscillopsia (Tullio phenomenon) is typically reported. Oscillopsia may manifest as blurring or 'bouncing' of vision in response to loud sounds. The crucial feature is that the onset of the typically low-frequency, loud environmental sound is time-locked with the onset of the vestibular symptom(s) due to pressure being transmitted via the oval window toward the dehiscence and across the sensory epithelia of the labyrinth.

Pressure-induced dizziness, vertigo or oscillopsia (Hennebert's sign) and/or a subjective sense of imbalance can be triggered either by a valsalva manoeuvre (attempting to exhale with the nostrils and mouth, or the glottis, closed to increase pressure in the middle ear and the chest) or by pressure applied to the tragus. By the same token, any source of raised intracranial pressure such as heavy lifting, straining, sneezing or coughing, can result in dizziness in the presence of TMWD. Symptoms of TMWD can arise following labour during childbirth [27, 28]. The onset of the stimulus is again time-locked to the onset of the vertigo or nystagmus, occurring either at the application of the stimulus, during its presence or at the point it is removed.

Head rotation-induced tinnitus and autophony have been reported as the only presenting symptoms in a patient later diagnosed with SSCD (with supportive electrophysiological and radiological evidence) [29]. Head rotation in the plane of the right semicircular canal with an angular velocity exceeding 600°/s repeatedly induced a 'cricket' sound in the patient's right ear.

All of the above-described bone conduction hyperacusis descriptions occur due to the low impedance caused by the mobile third window effect.

The source of the pulsatile tinnitus may be one of the following, or a combination of:

- Transmitted pulsations of the dura.
- Changes in intracranial pressure.
- Turbulent flow through the intracranial venous sinuses—usually the superior petrosal sinus [30].

Symptoms may be purely audiological or vestibular, as opposed to a combination of both. Patients are expected to have at least one, or a combination of, the above symptoms in order to meet the diagnostic criteria for SSCD syndrome.

Numerous additional symptoms are also described by SSCD patients; these include cognitive dysfunction, aural fullness, headaches including migraine, chronic imbalance, spatial disorientation and anxiety [4–6]. Although these symptoms are less likely to be voluntarily reported without prompting, it is crucial that the clinician actively explores these with the patient as, given the complex connections that exist between the cortical vestibular and limbic pathways, they are commonly present and can have a profound effect on the patient's quality of life [31]. These symptoms are theoretically not due to a third window effect, although may still occur secondary to the dehiscent SSC and can improve with standard surgical intervention, although with less improvement reported compared to the standard, more frequently arising bone conduction hyperacusis effects.

Summary of symptoms reported in SSCD syndrome and TMWDs (this list is not exhaustive):

Most common:
- Hearing loss
- Autophony
- Pulsatile tinnitus
- Sound-induced dizziness
- Pressure- or strain-induced dizziness
- Chronic imbalance

Common but may not be actively reported by patients:
- Cognitive dysfunction
- Aural fullness
- Headaches including migraine
- Spatial disorientation
- Anxiety
- Low mood

Less commonly reported:
- Head rotation induced tinnitus

Perceived precipitating factors could include:
- Head injury
- Intracranial or previous otological surgery

Clinical Examination

Clinical examination may increase the suspicion of a third-window phenomenon, even in the absence of specialist audiometric and vestibular function test availability.

The examination should begin with routine otoscopy to exclude clinically apparent middle ear disease. Tuning fork tests with a 512 Hz fork may provide evidence of a conductive impairment; with Weber test lateralising to the affected ear based on the reported side of subjectively reduced hearing, autophony, pulsatile tinnitus or other symptoms, and Rinne test resulting in abnormally better bone conduction of sound with the tuning fork placed over the mastoid compared to air conducted sound. When vibration in the 125–1000 Hz frequency range has been presented to three different stimulation sites in SSCD and controls, the SSCD patients showed an enhanced sensitivity for lower stimulus frequencies [32], suggesting testing with 128 or 256 Hz tuning forks may be preferable.

Close observation of the eye movements and a detailed oculomotor examination should be undertaken, including assessment of spontaneous- and gaze-evoked nystagmus in the horizontal and vertical planes, saccades, smooth pursuit and the clinical VOR via head thrust testing, all of which would likely be normal in suspected SSCD.

Eliciting Hennebert's Sign

Hennebert's sign is defined as eye movements provoked by pressure changes within the external auditory canal. Ideally performed with the aid of Frenzel goggles to remove visual fixation, pressure can be applied by firmly placing the clinician's index finger over the tragus of the SSCD-suspected and the contralateral ear separately. A Politzer bulb may be used to achieve the same effect. In the presence of a third window, positive pressure would be expected to evoke a conjugate vertical-torsional deviation with the eyes rotating upwards and away from the affected ear (Fig. 11.3) [16]. These eye movements align in the plane of the affected superior semicircular canal. Nystagmus may be elicited by increasing intracranial or middle ear pressure via a Valsalva manoeuvre against a closed glottis or with a plugged or pinched nose. Of note, nystagmus elicited via nasal versus glottic Valsalva usually produces nystagmus in opposing directions. Tympanometry equipment may also elicit nystagmus briefly and the patient will likely complain of dizziness during the assessment—this forms the basis of the fistula test, outlined in further detail below, again raising the suspicion of a positive pressure-induced finding characteristic of third-window pathology.

Hennebert's sign is best observed with the head in the plane of the superior semicircular canal and is accentuated when the pupil is aligned with the plane of the superior semicircular canal. For example, vertical eye movements are seen when the eyes are turned towards the affected side, i.e. asking the patient to look right during assessment of the right ear [2].

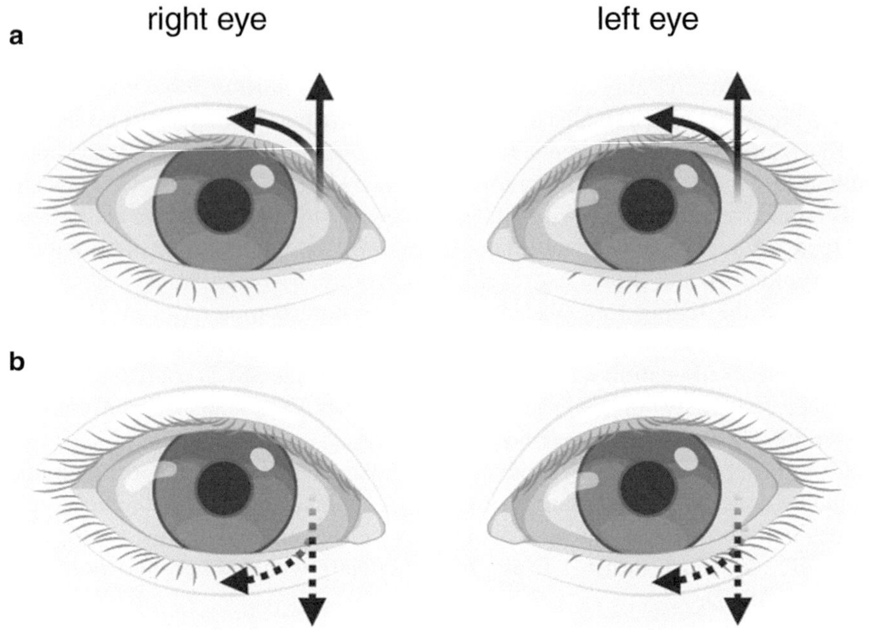

Fig. 11.3 Demonstration of Hennebert's sign. Hennebert's sign associated with left superior semicircular canal dehiscence. Positive pressure in the left ear results in a conjugate vertical-torsional ocular deviation with the eyes rotating up and away from the left ear (solid arrows, **a**). This reverses with negative pressure (dashed arrows, **b**)

Hennebert's sign is not specific to SSCD; dizziness and vertigo induced by pressure changes occur in various other TMWDs and other inner ear disorders including otosyphilis [33], Ménière's disease [34, 35] and perilymphatic fistula [36, 37]. In the case of SSCD syndrome, when present this results in nystagmus specifically occurring in the plane of the SSC, suggestive of the site of lesion. The dehiscence creates a third mobile window, which, in the case of positive pressure being applied to the external auditory canal or loud noise or a Valsalva manoeuvre against pinched nostrils, permits an extra, abnormal transmission route of pressure preferentially shunting endolymph through the affected SSC. The resultant ampullofugal endolymph flow in the SSC creates afferent nerve stimulation resulting in nystagmus with the slow phase rotating up and away from the affected ear. In the case of left SCC stimulation, the brain perceives this as movement of the head down and rolling towards the left, so the VOR attempts to compensate by creating a slow phase velocity movement upwards and to the right to counteract this, i.e. an upward torsional movement with the superior role rotating away from the affected ear. Conversely, when negative pressure is applied to the external auditory canal or a Valsalva manoeuvre against a closed glottis causing an increase in intracranial pressure results in a downward force at the site of the SSCD. This results in ampullopetal endolymph movement in the SSC, thus inhibiting the corresponding afferents, causing a downward torsional eye movement with the superior pole rotating towards the affected ear.

The prevalence of Hennebert's sign in patients with SSCD syndrome is still unknown and the absence of this sign certainly does not exclude a TWMD. Hennebert's sign can be negative but Tullio's phenomenon is positive in subjects and vice versa.

Fistula Test: The Use of Tympanometry Equipment to Demonstrate Hennebert's Sign

Clinical impedance test equipment should be used in manual mode for this test. The starting pressure can be set to +300 decapascals (daPa). The clinician should then push and hold the manual button for approximately 20–25 s whilst simultaneously observing the eyes for abnormal eye movement. This observation can be done manually or using VNG goggles or Frenzel goggles to remove fixation. The manual button can be used to adjust to deliver more negative or positive pressure as required. Alternatively, a Bruening hand-held insufflator can be used to provide positive and also negative pressure, and look for phase-locked eye movements using the VNG recording. Again, insufflation takes place over 20–25 s with pre- and post-recording.

Observing Tullio Phenomenon

An audiometer can be used to deliver varying frequencies and levels of pure tones. Typically, tones of close to or just above 100 dBHL can be required to induce and record the nystagmus. This level is high and will approach uncomfortable loudness level (ULL) for some subjects, therefore the sound application should be brief (10 s) and increased in a stepwise fashion from quiet to loud to ascertain the threshold for induction of nystagmus and subjective vertigo or dizziness.

When Tullio testing was first undertaken in the early 2000s, every frequency that the audiometers could emit (250 Hz–8 kHz) was tested. Very few patients responded with nystagmus and the report of symptoms beyond 1 kHz, and it was noted that 500 Hz gave the best yield. Therefore testing then changed to pulse-tone 500 Hz over a 10 s time frame. This is useful when the test is positive but nasal valsalva has been shown to be much more sensitive in TMWDs.

Since there are no standard ways of doing these tests, it is fertile ground for future research to see which yield the most sensitive and specific outcomes in the near future.

A summary of the suggested office-based clinical examination is given in Table 11.1:

Table 11.1 Suggested office-based clinical examination

	Assessment	Possible findings in TMWD
Clinical examination	Otoscopy	Normal
	Oculomotor examination	Normal
	Cranial nerve and cerebellar examination	Normal
Office-based tests	Tuning fork tests	Conductive hearing loss
	Assessment for nystagmus with positive pressure testing using:	Vertical-torsional nystagmus in the plane of the SSC
	– The finger of the clinician applying firm pressure to the tragus of the affected ear	
	– Fistula test	
	– Nasal valsalva manoeuvre	
	– Glottic valsalva manoeuvre	
	Assessment for nystagmus with sound-induced testing	Vertical-torsional nystagmus in the plane of the SSC

Investigations

Investigations undertaken in cases of suspected TMWD should include:

(a) Those which demonstrate the patient's normal middle ear status and
(b) Those which provide physiological evidence of a TMWD.

Middle Ear Assessment

Investigation of middle ear function should include tympanometry and stapedial reflect testing as a minimum. Additional tests are outlined including otoacoustic emission testing, laser doppler vibrometry and speech testing.

Immittance Testing

Audiometric findings alone would be insufficient to support a diagnosis of SSCD and should be interpreted in the context of an audiological test battery to establish a set of findings that would be supportive of third-window pathology, including SSCD. Conductive hearing loss can also be seen in any middle or outer ear pathology, but normal tympanometry and stapedial reflex findings should distinguish SSCD and TWMDs from such causes.

Immittance testing provides information of the subjects' middle ear status (presence of tympanic membrane perforation, middle ear effusions, ossicular chain discontinuity, for example). In a mobile third-window syndrome, the tympanometry function is expected to be normal bilaterally. The positive, then negative pressure change and tone of 226 Hz is generated via the tympanometry probe tip, with the

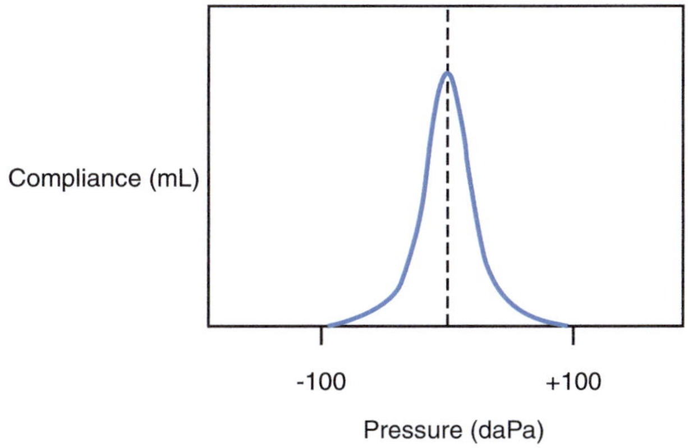

Fig. 11.4 Type A tympanometry trace reflective of normal middle ear function

tympanic membrane responses to sound applied at different pressures. A normal, peaked 'type A' trace is seen when compliance is plotted against varying pressure changes (Fig. 11.4).

Stapedial Reflex Testing

Stapedial reflexes, also known as acoustic reflexes, are expected to be present in TMWD. When assessed in combination with the presence of third window symptomatology, it becomes an effective means of screening patients with conductive hearing loss to exclude a TMWD prior to middle ear exploration. The positive and negative predictive values for ossicular pathology were 89% and 57% when acoustic reflexes were used in isolation but increased to 94% and 71%, respectively, when combined with questioning for TMWD symptoms [38]. Therefore, the presence of even one present reflex or TMWD symptom should prompt further diagnostic testing to prove or refute the presence of a TWMD.

The acoustic reflex is the contraction of the stapedius muscle elicited by the presentation of an acoustically loud sound. When either ear is presented with a loud sound, the stapedius muscles on both sides contract. Contraction of the stapedius muscle tilts the anterior stapes away from the oval window and stiffens the ossicular chain. This results in increased impedance which is measured as a small decrease in compliance by an ear canal probe. The stapedius muscle is innervated by the seventh cranial (facial) nerve (CNVII) [39].

For both pathways, the loud sound travels through the outer, middle and inner ear, then along the vestibulocochlear nerve (CNVIII) to the brainstem arriving at the cochlear nucleus (Fig. 11.5). From here the signal travels to the superior olivary complex and to the CNVII nuclei. The signal is then transmitted via CNVII causing contraction of the stapedius muscle [39].

Acoustic reflexes are expected to be absent ipsilaterally in the case of a middle ear disorder, as such conditions typically prevent the probe from measuring a change in compliance when the stapedius muscle contracts. This is the case in most

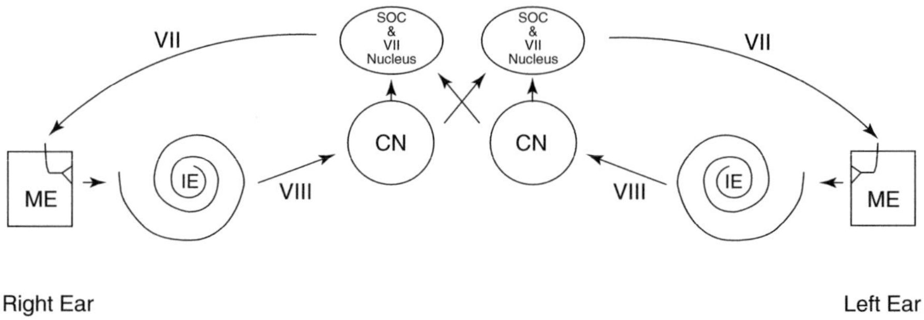

Fig. 11.5 Reproduced with permission by the author and AudiologyOnline [40]. The acoustic reflex pathway. ME, middle ear; IE, inner ear; VIII, vestibulocochlear nerve; CN, cochlear nucleus; SOC, superior olivary complex; VII, facial nerve

Fig. 11.6 (**a**) Normal acoustic reflex thresholds. Cases of SSCD would typically have normal thresholds such as these. (**b**) Typical acoustic reflex thresholds expected in the case of a left-sided conductive hearing loss due to middle or outer ear pathology

a

	Frequency	.5 kHz	1 kHz	2 kHz	4 kHz
Probe R	Stim R (ipsi)	85	85	85	85
	Stim L (contra)	90	90	90	90
Probe L	Stim L (ipsi)	80	80	80	80
	Stim R (contra)	85	85	85	85

b

	Frequency	.5 kHz	1 kHz	2 kHz	4 kHz
Probe R	Stim R (ipsi)	85	85	85	85
	Stim L (contra)	100	100	100	105
Probe L	Stim L (ipsi)	X	X	X	X
	Stim R (contra)	X	X	X	X

conductive hearing losses, but TMWD including SSCD syndrome would be the exception to this rule.

In patients with normal middle ear function, including SSCD cases, stapedial reflexes are expected to be normal (Fig. 11.6a). In contrast, these reflexes would be absent ipsilaterally in the case of conductive hearing loss with abnormal middle ear function (Fig. 11.6b).

Laser Doppler Vibrometry

Although its use is not widespread or mainstream, ear canal reflectance can also be measured via laser doppler vibrometry (LDV) to investigate cases of conductive hearing loss in the absence of middle ear disease. Such a scenario typically arises due to one of three underlying pathologies; (1) ossicular discontinuity, (2) ossicular fixation (most often from a fixed stapes due to otosclerosis), or (3) in the case of a TMWD disorder [39]. The HLV-1000 laser Doppler vibrometer by Polytec Inc. (Waldbronn, Germany) can be used to measure sound-induced umbo velocity [41]. The umbo is the most inferior tip of the malleus. Umbo velocity and ear canal reflectance can be used to distinguish between the three main subsects of conductive hearing loss with normal middle ear function [42].

Taken in combination with audiometric, tympanometry, acoustic reflex and CT findings, this investigation differentiates between the above-described pathologies. With the advent and increasingly widespread use of VEMP testing and also high-resolution CT, its use has fallen out of favour and it is now primarily used as a research tool. Few clinicians have the expertise to perform oto-microscopy and point the laser on to the umbo repeatedly. Gathering and evaluation of the data requires a specific skill set. The test equipment is also costly, although a less expensive device exists, the Mimosa.

To undertake this test, the patient lies supine on an examination couch with the ear facing up. Microscopy is used to observe the umbo throughout the test period, and a sound-coupler, microphone and etymyotic earphone are passed into the ear canal, with an additional laser also focused onto the tympanic membrane using a prism. The light reflected from the tympanic membrane is recorded via the equipment's laser velocity decoder. The frequencies of the transmitted and reflected light allow the sound-induced oscillation of the umbo to be calculated. When comparing umbo-velocity transfer function between patients with SSCD and normal subjects, the air-bone gap on audiometry should be taken into consideration; in general, larger increases in 700 Hz umbo-velocity have been seen in ears with larger air-bone gaps at 500 Hz, and conversely, a large proportion of SSCD ears had LDV findings that were comparable to normal, reflective of the fact that two thirds of the SSCD ears in that sample had normal hearing with no air-bone gap.

The presence of a low-frequency air-bone gap has sometimes mistakenly hinted towards the presence of stapes fixation, resulting in unnecessary middle ear explorative surgery. LDV measurements can help to reduce this risk as, in general (although not always), the umbo velocity is likely to be normal in SSCDs. In a sample of 26 ears with surgically-confirmed SSCD and 57 cases of fixed stapes, this criteria of 0 dB umbo velocity at 700 Hz was found to correctly identify all but one of the 26 SSCD ears but falsely identified four out of 57 cases of stapes fixation [42]. Stapes fixation generally results in lower-than-normal LDV values due to resultant reduced compliance of the ossicular pathway.

Speech Testing

The speech detection threshold, speech recognition threshold and word-recognition scores would typically be normal or may be mildly raised in cases of TMWD, particularly in the case of a sizeable conductive hearing loss.

Otoacoustic Emission Testing

As with immittance and reflex testing, otoacoustic emission (OAE) responses are usually absent in cases of middle ear disease but are present in TMWD. The most commonly utilised OAE test modality is the transient-evoked otoacoustic emission protocol.

Investigations Undertaken to Provide Physiological Evidence of TMWD

Video-Oculography Recordings: Tullio Testing and Eliciting Hennebert's Sign

The previously-described noise and pressure stimulation protocols can be repeated with objective recording via binocular infrared goggle video-oculography in order to increase the sensitivity of the clinical examination. This allows for assessment of nystagmus using positive pressure, negative pressure and sound application, with and without fixation. Recordings should be made before and during application of the individual modes of stimulation.

The authors anecdotally note that some clinicians do not seem to undertake these tests, perhaps given that the literature in relation to their use for investigation of TWMDs appears to be quite minimal. These tests were first described in Minor's original article and they are, in many cases, more sensitive for SSCD syndrome than VEMP testing or other objective investigations which are considered to be conventional means of evaluating a suspected TMWD.

A Suggested Tone-Evoked Nystagmus Protocol

Binocular infrared VNG goggles should be used to observe for nystagmus whilst pure tones are presented monaurally via TDH39 headphones or inserts using a calibrated audiometer. Tones are presented for approximately 1 s at intensities starting at 70 dB HL, increasing in 10 dB increments, up to 110 dB HL from 125 Hz through to 6 kHz.

Nystagmus is representative of SSC stimulation if it consists of vertical and torsional eye movements with SPV directed upward and rolling the superior poles of the eyes to the contralateral side (i.e., excitatory in the plane of the affected canal).

A Suggested Skull Vibration Induced Nystagmus Protocol

Bone conducted vibration has been shown to provoke a skull vibration induced nystagmus (SVIN) in SSCD [43]. This assessment can be likened to a vestibular Weber test to assess asymmetric vestibular function of unilateral TWMD [44].

The frequency of vibration applied will depend on availability of the vibrator within individual departments; in Europe a 100 Hz device is most commonly used. The subject should be sitting upright and the device is applied perpendicularly to the skull, directly on to the left and then right mastoid and also the vertex [45]. Vibration results in instant stimulation of all labyrinthine structures bilaterally and, in the case of SSCD, torsional and horizontal SVIN is observed beating towards the affected side in 95% when stimulation is applied at the vertex [46]. The slow phase velocity of the ensuing nystagmus has been shown to be significantly higher on vertex stimulation at 100 Hz and 300 Hz ($P = 0.04$) than via the mastoids [46]. Again, recordings should be made before and during vibration using video-oculography.

In summary, SVIN demonstrates instantaneous torsional and horizontal nystagmus towards the affected side in unilateral SSCD syndrome with a greater sensitivity on vertex stimulation.

Pure Tone Audiometry

Audiometry should be undertaken in all patients suspected to have SSCD. Even if the air conduction (AC) thresholds are normal, it is necessary to obtain the bone conduction (BC) thresholds if a TMWD is suspected. If the difference between AC and unmasked BC thresholds is >10 dB, the BC thresholds should be masked to assess the left and right ear separately. The air-bone gap (ABG) is calculated by subtracting the bone conduction threshold from the air conduction threshold. The mean of 500, 1000, 2000 and 4000 Hz frequencies measures the 4-frequency ABG. The closure of ABG can be calculated as the preoperative ABG minus the postoperative ABG.

Many, but not all, patients with SSCDS have a low frequency (≤ 2000 kHz) air-bone gap, with no gap or only a small gap seen at higher frequencies. Characteristically the largest AB gap is seen at 250 Hz. The low frequency (<2000 Hz) bone conduction thresholds are sometimes at supranormal levels, 0 to −20 dB or better [46]. Normal hearing thresholds may also be seen. Another potential finding is that of negative bone conduction thresholds. The negative threshold implies that those are better than the majority of the population. However, sensorineural hearing loss may also co-exist, for various reasons including secondary to presbyacusis in older subjects, and therefore the bone conduction thresholds may well be within normal range, although most characteristically, an air-bone gap exists. For this reason, even if the AC thresholds are within normal range, the BC thresholds should be documented in all patients reporting autophony, sound-induced dizziness and pulsatile tinnitus.

Yuen et al. have previously demonstrated that a low frequency ABG is seen in patients with SSCD of size ≥3 mm and that the size of the ABG may correlate with the size of the dehiscence [47].

If Uncomfortable Loudness Levels (ULLs) are established and loud-noise was noted to be tolerable, pure tones of 500, 1000 and 2000 Hz presented at 100–120 dB HL presented in the affected ear may provoke symptoms of imbalance, vertigo and/or result in vertical torsional nystagmus.

ABGs in conductive or mixed hearing loss will be seen in a wide variety of other inner ear pathology including Ménière's disease, widened vestibular aqueduct, gusher syndrome, cochlear dehiscence and Paget's disease as well as cerebral vascular anomalies such as dural arteriovenous fistula [48]. Therefore, audiometric findings should form part of a wider audiovestibular diagnostic work up in a patient suspected to have TMWD.

Vestibular-Evoked Myogenic Potentials Testing

Vestibular-evoked myogenic potentials (VEMPs) testing has evolved to become a cost-effective screening tool in the diagnosis of TMWD. It is the most widely used method to provide objective evidence of a physiological TMWD.

VEMPs are electromyographic reflex tests that represent the function of the saccule (cervical VEMP) or utricle (ocular VEMP). cVEMP testing utilizes an inhibitory reflex pathway from the saccule to the ipsilateral sternocleidomastoid muscle. The oVEMP uses an excitatory pathway from the utricle to the contralateral inferior oblique muscle [49]. In SSCD, the VEMP tests are often abnormal, as the auditory stimuli used to evoke these myogenic potentials are transmitted in an enhanced fashion in the affected inner ear resulting in abnormal activation of the vestibulo-ocular and vestibulocollic pathways [49]. Patients with SSCD typically have:

- Reduced cVEMP thresholds in response to click or tone-burst stimuli and raised cVEMP amplitudes.
- Reduced oVEMP thresholds and raised oVEMP amplitudes.

'Textbook' VEMP findings seen in various vestibular conditions are given in summary in Table 11.2.

VEMP testing is therefore an essential diagnostic test in the audiovestibular test battery when evaluating a patient with a suspected TMWD. However, they cannot be relied upon as a sole or gold standard diagnostic tool, as the absence of an expected VEMP finding does not completely exclude a TMWD. As previously discussed, some patients with normal imaging, or normal VEMP findings may still have a clinically-treatable TMWD, if alternative evidence of TMWD-compatible physiology can be obtained.

Table 11.2 cVEMP and oVEMP findings in vestibular conditions affecting the inner ear and/or central vestibular pathways. In all cases, these are classical or 'textbook' findings but absence of these findings specifically does not exclude the condition

Condition	cVEMP findings	oVEMP findings
SSCD	Reduced threshold	Reduced threshold
	Increased amplitude	Increased amplitude
Ménière's disease	The inter-aural amplitude difference ratio of the VEMP may correlate with the stage of Ménière's disease [49, 50]	Increased amplitude
Vestibular neuritis	Reduced amplitude on affected side	Absent
Vestibular migraine	Normal	Normal

Basic Principles of VEMP Testing

Tullio et al. first described sound- and pressure-induced activation of the vestibulo-ocular and vestibulocollic pathways in the presence of iatrogenically fenestrated third windows in pigeons [13]. It is on this premise that VEMP testing is useful in SSCD assessment as objective measurement of this observation is achieved.

The cVEMP assesses saccular and inferior vestibular nerve function via function of the vestibulocollic reflex through ipsilateral inhibition of the sternocleidomastoid muscle.

The oVEMP provides a measure of utricular and superior vestibular nerve function via vestibulo-ocular projections through contralateral excitation of the inferior oblique eye muscle.

The saccule and utricle are primarily responsible for detection of linear acceleration and gravity detection in the horizontal and vertical plane, respectively, but these two otolith organs are also sensitive to sound; this is the basis of the vestibular evoked myogenic potential [49].

Acoustic or vibration stimulation can be utilised during testing whilst responses are recorded from either the contracted ipsilateral sternocleidomastoid muscle or the contralateral inferior ocular musculature in upgaze. In general, the most widely used stimulus is the 500 Hz tone burst [49].

Figure 11.7 illustrates the basic VEMP circuitry.

However, in cases of third-window syndromes such as SSCD, where the semicircular canals are sensitized to sound, the pathway is disrupted via abnormal activation of the vestibulo-ocular and vestibulocollic pathways, such that the VEMP amplitude is increased and the threshold is decreased. This was first proven in 1994 by Colebatch et al. when a subject who described sound-induced dizziness was found to have low cVEMP thresholds and enlarged cVEMP amplitude compared with healthy controls and local normative data [52]. The 500 Hz threshold was originally the one that best differentiated between SSCD patients and healthy controls.

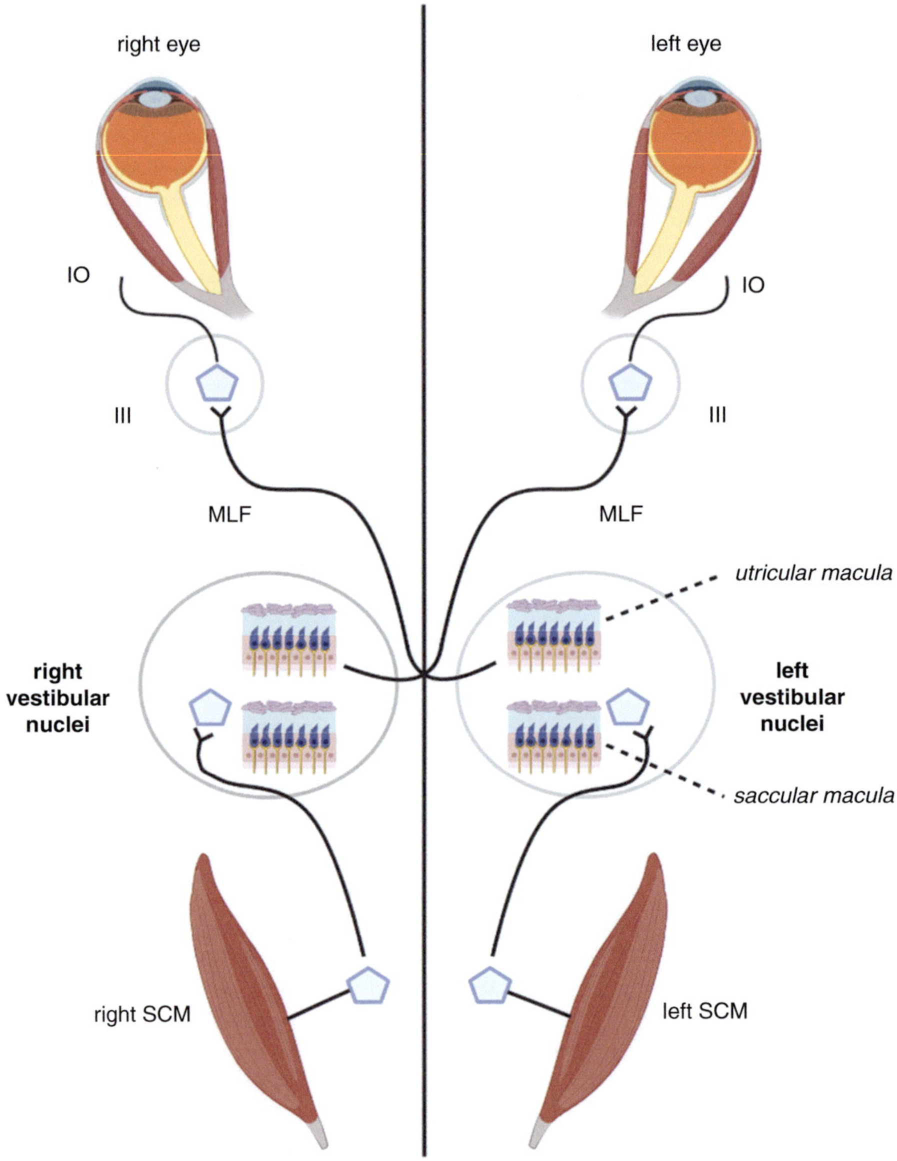

Fig. 11.7 cVEMP and oVEMP circuitry [51]. cVEMP; sound stimulates the saccule, which in turn activates the inferior vestibular nerve, lateral vestibular nucleus, 11th cranial nerve nucleus and then the sternocleidomastoid muscle, mostly ipsilaterally. oVEMP; utricular excitatory inputs protrude to the superior oblique, superior rectus and medial rectus eye muscles ipsilaterally and the inferior oblique and inferior rectus muscles on the contralateral side via the medial longitudinal fasciculus and vestibular nuclei

Note that caution should be exercised as VEMP amplitudes can be reduced, or thresholds increased, in the context of middle ear disease [53–55] as well as age (the response decreases dramatically after the age of 60) [56, 57] and so these results must be interpreted in the context of a complete test battery.

cVEMP vs. oVEMP Testing

The original VEMP abnormality reported in SSCD was the cVEMP [52, 58], and thus this is the most widespread VEMP diagnostic test employed when investigating a TMWD. In normal subjects, cVEMP thresholds ~100 dB are considered normal. Low cVEMP thresholds, typically <85 dB, may be suggestive of SSCD [59]. The classical finding in the context of SSCD is of low threshold, abnormally large, sound-induced cVEMP [49]. However, data from 2012 from 29 patients highlighted that oVEMPs actually had lower thresholds and increased amplitudes to a greater extent when compared to cVEMP responses, making oVEMP amplitudes more sensitive and specific for the diagnosis of SSCD than cVEMP thresholds [60]. cVEMP amplitudes showed a twofold increase in response to 500 Hz tone bursts compared with controls, whereas oVEMP amplitudes showed a tenfold increase [60]. Peak-to-peak amplitudes for both click-evoked (cut off value $\geq$9.9 μV) and tone-burst evoked (cut off value $\geq$17.1 μV) oVEMPs had specificity >98% and sensitivity of 100% for SSCD, whereas the click-evoked cVEMP threshold $\leq$85 dB nHL in the same cohort had a sensitivity of 86% and sensitivity of 90% for the diagnosis of SSCD [61]. Thus it was demonstrated that oVEMP amplitudes were superior to cVEMP thresholds in the diagnosis of SSCD. oVEMPs can therefore potentially be utilized as an effective screening tool for SCDS, in combination with other electrophysiological measures if required, before or alongside CT imaging.

Other groups have also reported that the 4 kHz oVEMP amplitude can improve detection of SSCDs compared to 500 Hz tone burst oVEMPs [61]. In a large cohort of 902 patients (1804 ears), the 4 kHz oVEMP responses had a sensitivity of 86.5% and a specificity of 87.8%, with the specificity increasing to 96.8% when an amplitude cut off of >15 μV was used [62]. A two-step protocol of click air conduction oVEMP amplitudes and 125 Hz bone conduction oVEMP latency measures has been shown to optimize the specificity of VEMP testing in SSCD [63].

Although many institutions record cVEMP thresholds using 500 Hz tone burst stimuli delivered at a high threshold of 90–100 dBHL, higher frequency testing may be of better clinical use. It has been shown that best diagnostic accuracy of cVEMP testing in SSCD patients is achieved with 2000-Hz tone burst stimuli [63]. The 2 and 4 kHz sound stimuli are at the upper edge of the otolith organ tuning curve. Since the saccule is relatively insensitive to high frequency sound stimuli, vestibular stimulation by such a high frequency sound stimulus, such as 2 or 4 kHz, would ordinarily not produce a cVEMP or oVEMP response in healthy subjects. However, in the case of SSCD, the saccule receives a higher energy stimulus due to the third-window shunting, resulting in a repeatable cVEMP response to high frequency stimuli.

A limitation of the studies analysing cVEMP responses in third-window syndrome conditions, and of many diagnostic tests for SSCD, is that the 'gold standard' modality used to clarify the presence of the SSCD is CT imaging. As described previously, CT alone can overestimate the size and presence of a SSCD and also identify a number of asymptomatic dehiscences. It also relies on the radiological expertise of the reporting radiologist and there exists a degree of inter-reporting variability. Therefore the cVEMP and oVEMP data described should be interpreted with this borne in mind. Future studies analysing the 'Third Window Indicator' before and after surgical intervention in a cohort with radiologically and later surgically confirmed SSCD, but also subjective improvement in symptoms following intervention, could be considered to remedy this.

cVEMP and oVEMP testing in thin bony covering of a near dehiscent SSC can be most useful; such cases can be challenging as despite the fact there being no clear dehiscence, via as yet unexplained mechanisms, a large proportion of such patients report having symptoms typical of a full dehiscence. cVEMP and oVEMP amplitudes in these individuals have been shown to be either raised [64] or normal interestingly, as one would perhaps expect with an intact SSC, given that the shunting of acoustic energy from the cochlea to the vestibular apparatus does not occur in such individuals. VEMP testing is therefore considered to be helpful in the case of a radiologically suspected thin SSC. However, a number of patients with normal or borderline VEMP results would be excluded from surgery if it was considered 'crucial', therefore VEMP testing is considered to be complimentary but the results do not solely determine surgical candidacy. However, exactly how and why such patients are so clearly and, in some cases, strongly symptomatic, and the physiological mechanisms underpinning this, is yet to be delineated. In this sense, the optimal treatment strategy for such patients remains unclear.

Combining VEMP and Audiometric Data

The presence of the third window effectively shunts the travelling acoustic wave away from the cochlea and towards the labyrinth resulting in bone conduction-induced hyperacusis and an air-bone gap on audiometric testing but with normal middle ear and stapedial reflex function. Given that this finding is not solely unique to SSCD and third-window phenomena, various groups have sought to increase the sensitivity and specificity for identification of SSCD by combining VEMP and audiometric testing, such that this demonstrates that sound is both shunted away from the cochlea AND towards the vestibule. A cVEMP-based diagnostic tool for SCD patients that seems to be more useful than cVEMP threshold alone is the Third-Window Indicator (TWI) [65]. The TWI combines cVEMP threshold with the audiometric low-frequency air-bone gap (ABG) from the ipsilateral ear and improves the differentiation of SSCD patients from healthy subjects.

When the ABG and cVEMP thresholds are obtained at the same frequency, i.e. the ABG was subtracted from the cVEMP threshold at 250, 500 and 1000 Hz, the positive predictive value of diagnosis of SSCD was increased, with the difference being largest at 250 Hz. It has been shown that subtracting the 250 Hz ABG from the 500 Hz cVEMP threshold (proposed as the 'Third Window Indicator') improved differentiation of SSCD from age-matched healthy controls, with a sensitivity of 82% and a specificity of 100%, versus 46% sensitivity and 100% specificity for the 500 Hz cVEMP threshold alone [64, 66].

The TWI therefore combines information from two inner ear organs, both the saccule and cochlea, to provide evidence of third-window syndrome dysfunction with better sensitivity and specificity than either of the two investigations would be able to provide separately.

VEMP Testing vs. Testing in Other Causes of Otolith Dysfunction

cVEMP testing utilizes stimulation of the saccule (not the SSC) and oVEMP is based upon utricular stimulation (not SSC). The reason these tests are hyper-responsive is due to the increased compliance of the inner ear system with shunting of pressure towards the utricle and saccule specifically, not the SSC. Many symptoms in TMWD are due to indirect stimulation of the otolithic organs but not so commonly tested for, and often incorrectly attributed to the SSC. Additional otolith testing would however be expected to be normal, given that the site of pathology is the SSC itself. Such otolith tests include:

- Subjective visual vertical.
- Subjective visual horizontal.
- Ocular counter roll testing.

These tests, although expected to be normal, would be worth undertaking in cases where diagnostic uncertainty remains. Their use may be underutilized in diagnostic testing for TMWD. Symptoms of otolith dysfunction can be distinguished from those of SSC dysfunction [67]. Symptoms of otolith dysfunction are more subtle and include:

- Ocular torsion and asymmetric vertical stationary eye movements secondary to generation of the VOR originating from the utricle. Unilateral utricular asymmetry can cause blurred vision or diplopia which may alter with head position. (See Chap. 14 for an in-depth discussion.)
- Imbalance or a subjective rocking sensation due to saccular dysfunction which ordinarily are involved in control of the postural muscles via the vestibulospinal reflex.

Example cVEMP and oVEMP Protocols

VEMP testing in general, and in particular its use in assessment of a patient presenting with a third-window syndrome, is an evolving field within audiovestibular diagnostic testing. Various tweaks in the test protocols have been described with the aim of optimizing the specificity of this assessment arm in the SSCD test battery, such that it can be combined with highly sensitive imaging to increase the detection rate of true SSCD.

cVEMP Test Protocol [68]

The thresholds and amplitude norms should be established for each department.

In testing a normal subject, one would typically start at the maximum intensity of 105 dBnHL but in suspected SSCD, testing should commence at a lower level, i.e. 80–90 dBnHL. Clicks are presented in decrements of 10 dBnHL and 5 dB up to locate the threshold. The subject will lie on the examination couch with the torso elevated at 30-degree from horizontal. They are instructed to lift their heads from the head rest by flexing their necks to provide tonic background muscle activity. To ensure adequate SCM activation, the tester should continually monitor to see that the rectified EMG activity is kept at or above 50 μV. The electrode montage (Fig. 11.8) consists of a non-inverting electrode placed at the midpoint of the SCM muscle belly (A1, A2), an inverting electrode placed on the sternoclavicular junction (Cz), and a ground electrode placed on the forehead. The p13 (P1) potential is identified as the first distinctive trough in the waveform, occurring approximately 10–14 ms after stimulus onset, and the n23 (N1) potential is identified as the first negative peak in the waveform, occurring approximately 19–23 ms after stimulus onset (Fig. 11.9).

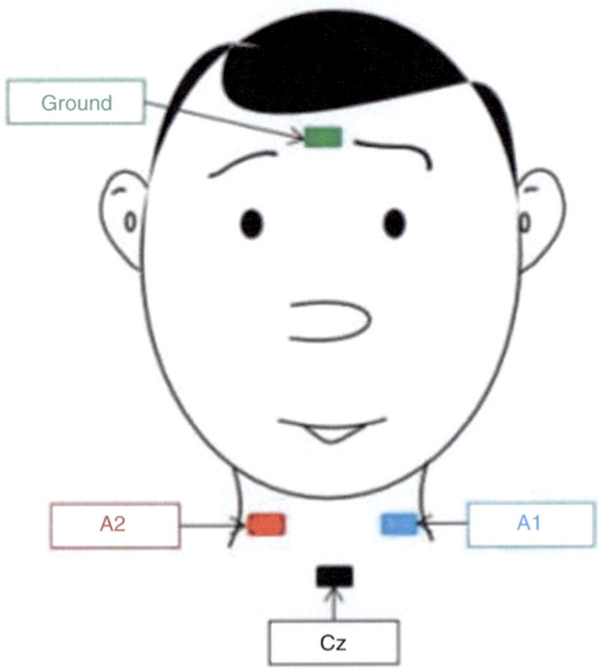

Fig. 11.8 cVEMP electrode montage. Gnd = forehead, Active (A1, A2) = SCM (middle point or upper 1/3 of muscle belly), CREF (Cz) = sternoclavicular junction

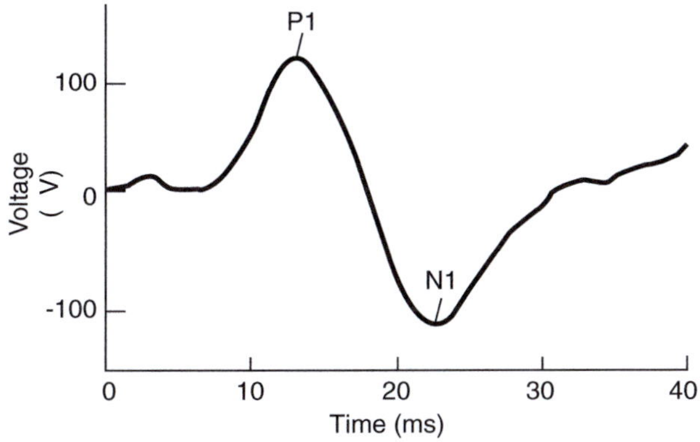

Fig. 11.9 cVEMP trace from a healthy control subject

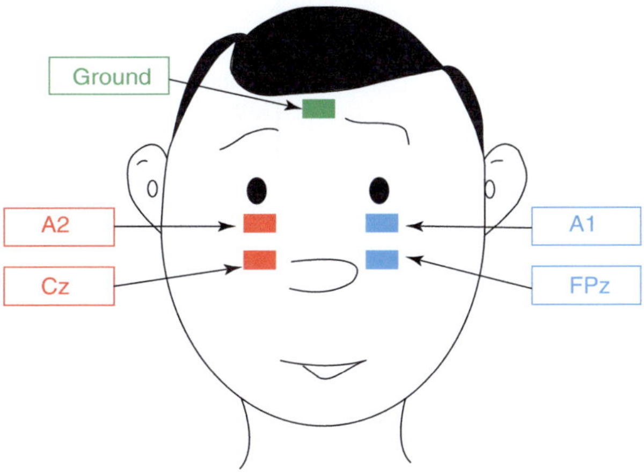

Fig. 11.10 oVEMP electrode montage. Gnd = forehead, Active (A1, A2) = inferior oblique—as close to eye as possible, just below and in the centre, CREF (Fpz, Cz) = directly underneath active electrodes without touching so as to avoid electrical bridge

oVEMP Test Protocol [69]

The subject will lie on the examination couch with the torso elevated at 30-degree from horizontal. Twenty-degree vertical saccades from the line of primary gaze orientation should be performed to ensure that symmetrical signals are recorded from both eyes before recording oVEMP results; if the signal change shows >25% asymmetry the electrodes require re-siting. Subjects are instructed to fix their gaze on a line on the ceiling located 30-degrees up from their primary gaze orientation. A possible electrode montage (Fig. 11.10) should consist of a non-inverting electrode placed on the cheek approximately 5 mm below the eyelid and centred beneath the pupil, an inverting electrode placed 2 cm below the non-inverting electrode, and a ground electrode placed on the forehead.

The n10 potential is identified as the first distinctive negative peak in the waveform occurring 7–11 ms after stimulus onset, and the p16 potential is identified as the first distinctive positive peak in the waveform 12–16 ms after stimulus onset. The n10 amplitude should be calculated as the amplitude from baseline to the peak of the n10 response, and the peak-to-peak amplitude is calculated as the sum of the n10 and p16 amplitudes (Fig. 11.11).

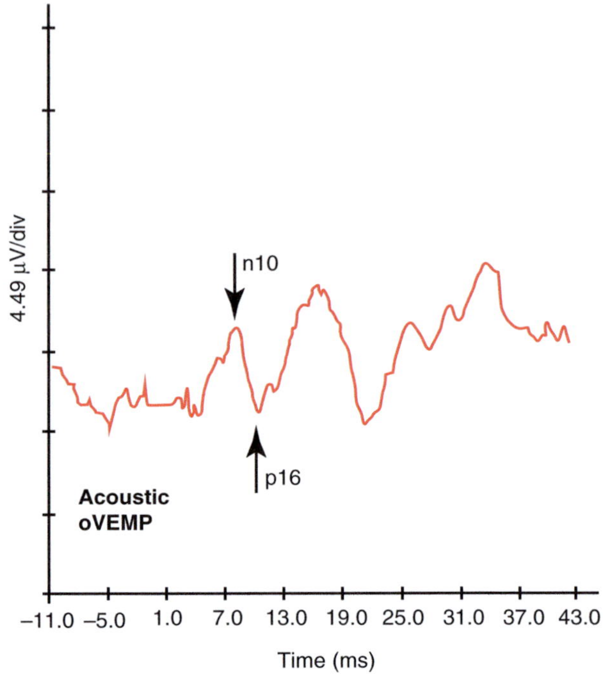

Fig. 11.11 oVEMP trace from a healthy control subject

VEMP Testing: Key Points and Summary

Both cVEMPs and oVEMPs are augmented in SSCD, with high amplitude and low threshold. oVEMP increased amplitude have the best sensitivity and specificity for SSCD. BC VEMPs are still abnormal, yet the threshold reductions are less marked for BC oVEMP and cVEMPs. The best one step screening test for SSCD may be the AC oVEMP which demonstrates enlarged amplitudes in dehiscent ears although only cVEMP thresholds have strong supporting evidence in the literature as to their value in SSCD. cVEMPs, which are inhibitory potentials, require lower than normal stimuli to improve their pick up rates for SCD using amplitude criteria. A high frequency tone-burst at 2000 and 4000 Hz can be particularly effective. Comparison against age-matched normative data is important since VEMP thresholds, amplitudes and tuning characteristics are influenced by age. Successful surgical treatment, e.g. via plugging of the affected SSC has been shown to normalise oVEMP thresholds and amplitudes.

Electrocochleography

Electrocochleography (ECoG) will characteristically show an elevated summating potential (SP) to action potential (AP) ratio in the affected ear and a normal SP/AP value on the unaffected side [70, 71].

Intra-operative electrocochleography used to be employed frequently to test for endolymphatic hydrops associated with Ménière's disease. Arts et al. initially identified that patients with SSCD consistently had a raised SP to AP ratio, and that this abnormality corrects after surgical plugging of the affected canal [72]. These findings have subsequently been observed by other groups. Whilst the results have not been correlated with postoperative hearing outcomes, given that intra-operative testing is invasive and there are other vestibular test modalities available, its clinical utility has largely fallen out of favour. However, pre- and postoperative electrocochleography is still commonly utilized and this can be undertaken in a non-invasive manner.

Quality of Life Measures

Arguably the most important part of the diagnostic process should be establishing the impact of the TMWD on the subject's quality of life. SSCD patients have been found to have significantly lower health utility values than age-matched control groups [73] and poorer quality of life measures which can improve following surgical intervention when indicated [74]. This suggests the negative impact of SSCD and TMWD on generic health-related QoL measures, even when using an instrument that is not designed to be disease-specific but to assess health state in general. Prior to the relatively recent recognition of TMWD amongst healthcare professionals, it should be remembered that a multitude of patients lived with incredibly troublesome, fluctuating symptoms resulting in impact on their ability to work, undertake caring responsibilities or carry out simple daily activities. Until worldwide recognition of this entity becomes commonplace amongst *all* healthcare professionals and also the general public, many people will continue to suffer this plight. Living with symptoms that do not have a readily available diagnostic label has been shown to result in a great level of psychological disability. The medical community and clinicians should remember that given medicine is continually evolving and we increasingly strive to, and are mandated to, practise evidenced-based medicine, one should always be open to exploring a persistently reported abnormality or problematic symptom, even if it does not classically fit with a single diagnostic entity. Lloyd Minor's initial cohort of patients were originally referred to his centre for further otological investigations in patients reporting the then 'bizarre' symptom of autophony, when *psychiatric* evaluation was deemed to be normal. This perception and judgement adds another dimension of psychological disability facing patients who are already living with what was then perceived to be a chronic disability, which we now know to be very treatable. Experts who are able to correctly diagnose and manage neuro-otological symptoms are few and far between and therefore patients may have had multiple, sometimes frustrating, consultations with various other healthcare professionals before they are correctly diagnosed.

In a 2020 study prospectively analysing SSCD patients prior to surgical intervention, the SCCD group had lower health utility values compared to case-matched controls, and one subject with unilateral SSCD had a negative score, indicating a health-state worse than death [74]. The psychiatric morbidity borne by such symptoms should be strongly considered and actively discussed with the patient, and their family or carers if appropriate, when determining surgical candidacy.

As such, the following patient reported outcome measures (PROMs) that are specific to neuro-otology, can be utilized, with full links and details provided in the Appendix:

- DHI; dizziness handicap index.
- SVQ; situational vertigo questionnaire.
- HIT-6; headache-impact test-6.
- PHQ; patient-health questionnaire-9.
- GAD-7; generalised anxiety disorder-7 assessment.

A condition-specific, validated Patient-Reported Outcome Measure (PROM) for TMWD is awaited.

Wackym et al. demonstrated significant improvement in cognitive and neurobehavioural measures in 13 adult and 4 paediatric patients following surgical treatment of SSCD via either plugging of the dehiscence and/or round-window reinforcement, as discussed in further detail in Chap. 6.

Diagnostics: An Illustrative Case of SSCD

A 44-year-old Trombonist was seen in our neuro-otology clinic, having been referred for sub-specialist review from general neurology.

He had a background of extensive dental work since his teenage years, with further surgical interventions more recently. Around 2015, after a season of playing extensively in the theatre, his right ear suddenly felt blocked, with a sense of aural fullness. This persisted with an inability to equalise pressure. At the onset in 2015 he also noticed some slight disequilibrium after walking.

When buzzing on his mouthpiece, he reported the sensation of his whole head vibrating at certain frequencies, with his eye losing focus, and dizziness. He also reported feeling dizzy when he stopped playing. He could sometimes hear his pulse in his head whilst playing. When he undertook target shooting, which he did as a hobby, he also noticed that his pulse sometimes intruded on his aim.

Outside of playing, he also described a constant low level unsteadiness or dizziness. This transiently worsened with straining or changes in posture. He found it difficult to concentrate, and was rather irritable and tired all the time. He described episodes of dysacusis where his hearing appeared to dim over a few seconds as if someone had turned down the volume, and subsequently it would return. He reported being able to hear the movement of his right eye inside his head. He reported feeling clumsy and would trip sometimes, with a tendency to veer off to the right.

Clinical examination from a neuro-otological perspective revealed normal ocular alignment, a full range of eye movements, no spontaneous, or gaze-evoked nystagmus and normal pursuit and saccades. VOR and VOR suppression were normal. Dix-Hallpike and roll test manoeuvres revealed no nystagmus or symptoms. The gait was narrow based and steady, with negative Rombergs. There was no clinical nystagmus with Valsalva or tragal pressure.

A TWMD was suspected from the clinical history. Pure tone audiometry, tympanometry, oVEMP and vHIT testing was requested, as was imaging via CT cone beam of the temporal bones.

Investigation results are given in Fig. 11.12:

Small field-of-view cone beam CT scan of the temporal bone showed a focal dehiscence at the posterior arch of the right superior semicircular canal. He was keen to explore surgical management options and was therefore referred to the surgical (ENT) team for further work up.

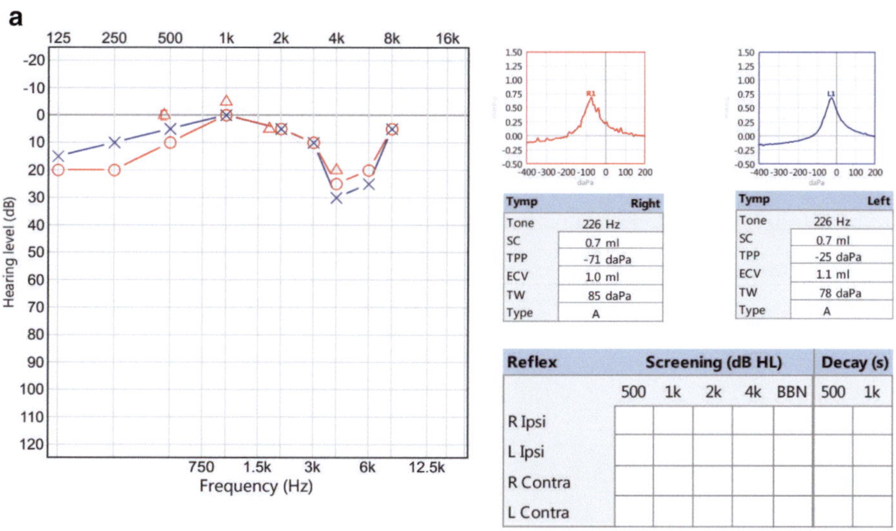

Fig. 11.12 (**a**) oVEMP demonstrates increased oVEMP amplitude on the right, with 78% amplitude asymmetry. The patient was subjectively dizzy when right-sided testing was undertaken at 105 dBnHL. (**b**) Pure tone audiometry showed very mildly raised air conduction (AC) thresholds bilaterally at 4 kHz and at 6 kHz on the left. Although the low frequency AC thresholds are normal, insufficient bone conduction testing had been undertaken as there may well be an air-bone gap. Tympanometry was indicative of normal middle ear function. (**c**) Video head impulse test (vHIT) trace in the same subject; note the presence of covert saccades and borderline low gain in the Right Anterior canal. Whilst the vHIT is subject to lab-defined norms, and this could be defined as normal, the findings are suspicious for Right Anterior (Superior) Canal dysfunction

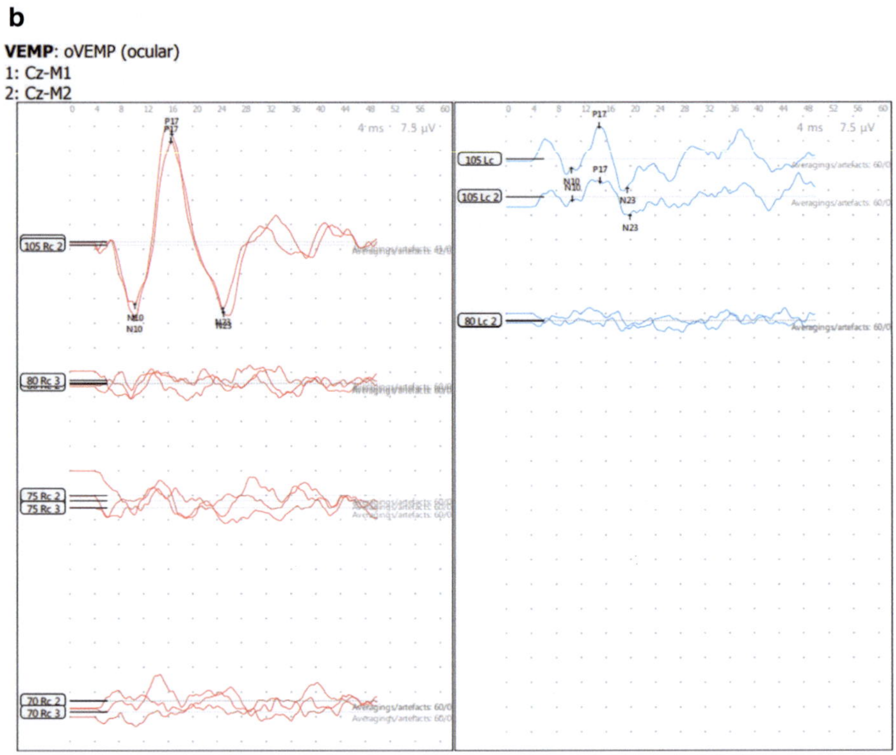

Fig. 11.12 (continued)

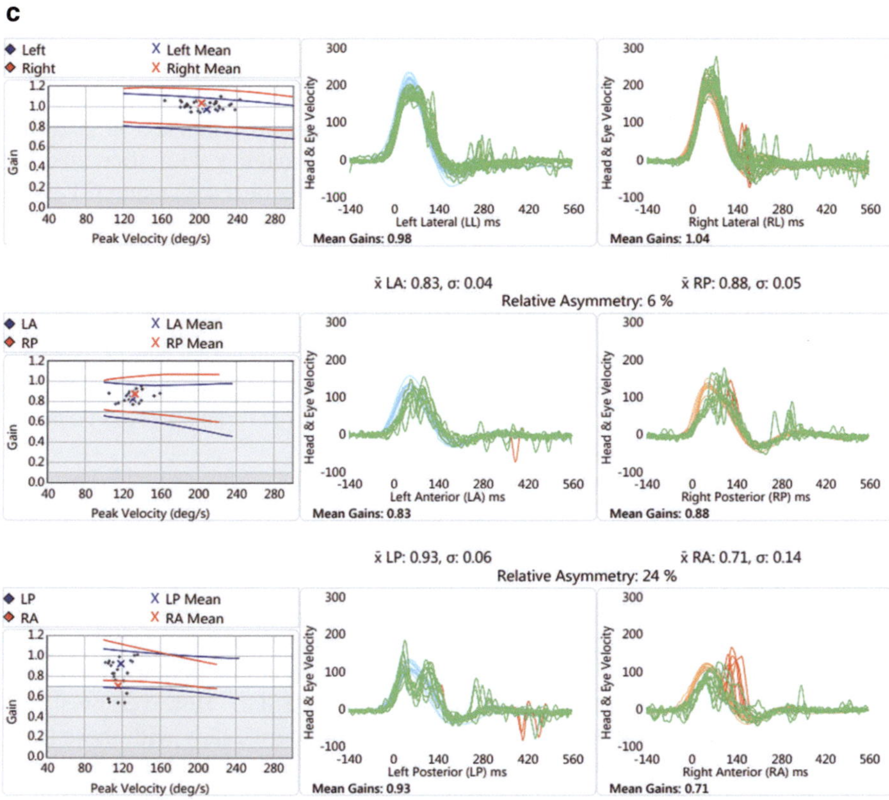

Fig. 11.12 (continued)

From a diagnostics point of view, this case illustrates the following:

- The importance of recording bone conduction thresholds on pure tone audiometry in all cases suspected to have a TWMD.
- It would have been useful to record the specific oVEMP threshold (in addition to the already documented oVEMP amplitude). Additional cVEMP testing is ideally necessary to compare oVEMP and cVEMP data.
- Although it was not possible to elicit nystagmus clinically in the consultation room with tragal pressure or a Valsalva manoeuvre, this testing could have been undertaken with removal of fixation using Frenzel googles. Testing for sound-induced nystagmus could also have been performed. We are inviting the patient back to undertake further diagnostic testing.

What Are Other Physicians and Surgeons Doing When It Comes to Diagnostics?

In a survey of US neuro-otologists and otological surgeons published in 2020, all respondents (n = 54) used ultra-high-resolution CT imaging with slice sizes of 0.625 mm or less to diagnose SSCD (100%), with 11.1% (+ 8.4%) using CT alone as the sole diagnostic method [74]. This latter finding is of concern given the 80% false-positive rate of CT, meaning that this imaging modality should not be used as a screening tool and reserved only if significant suspicion of TMWD is suspected, particularly given the radiation exposure with CT. Several surgeons admitted to seeing SSCD on CT, operating on these patients and finding no actual SSCD, suggesting that imaging findings should **not** be used for diagnosis in isolation and also providing evidence that CT should be undertaken using the thinnest slices possible. A small number used MRI (7.4% + 7.0%) for diagnosis.

To provide electrophysiological evidence of a TMWD, 77.8% (+11.1%) use cervical VEMPs, 38.9% (+13.0%) use ocular VEMPs and 7.4% (+6.9%) use ECOG. 68.5% (+12.4%) use audiometry as part of the diagnostic battery of investigations. Most of those surveyed (83.3%) used a combination of CT imaging and VEMP testing for diagnosis. Most also utilize VEMPs over electrocochleography and audiometry. Specifically, respondents used cervical VEMPs more than ocular VEMPs. However, as previously discussed, studies reveal that ocular VEMPs are more suitable than cervical VEMPs in the diagnosis of SSCD. However, over 20% of respondents do not test the presence of a third mobile window with these tests, suggesting that electrophysiological TMWD testing is underutilized by some US-based clinicians in the diagnostic process. Surveys of the diagnostic algorithms followed by clinicians outside of the US are also warranted as there may be similarly wide variation in practice and this would ultimately go some way towards standardising the pathway.

Other Diagnostic Testing That May Be Helpful for TMWD Diagnosis

Other vestibular function tests which are expected to be normal in TMWD or SSCD:

Video Head Impulse Testing

In contrast to click-evoked VOR, assessment of all six semicircular canals can also be undertaken in the absence of additional external stimuli via video head-impulse testing. A limited number of studies with few subjects have analysed vHIT responses in SSCD patients prior to surgical intervention [75, 76]. It was thought that vHIT could also potentially inform how SSCD affects vestibular function during daily activities and guide rehabilitation for those following a conservative approach in the management of SSCD. However, it has been shown that SSCD can affect the vestibular responses from all three semicircular canals; not necessarily the superior one, with similar responses found in a control group of normal subjects [75]. Although the use of vHIT in the assessment of SSCD is not diagnosis-specific, it can still help with identifying the impact of surgery on all canals prior to any intervention in order to avoid bilateral vestibular failure. Therefore these findings are not disease-specific.

Caloric Testing

Caloric test results are usually unaffected in patients with SSCD; however, when the dehiscence is large (>0.5 mm), unilateral weakness may be demonstrated on the affected side [77].

Rotational Chair Testing

This is also expected to be normal in the majority of TMWD.

Blood Tests

Serological investigations are expected to be normal. However, as part of the diagnostic work up it would be prudent to undertake serology to exclude autoimmune pathology. Example first line screening tests may include:

– FBC, ESR, RF, ANA, complement levels, syphilis testing, lyme disease.

Imaging

Imaging is undertaken in all subjects suspected of having a TWMD. However, it should be noted that imaging only shows anatomical defects but the diagnostic testing demonstrates the physiology of the situation. The two do not always match; some patients with anatomical dehiscence will have normal physiological testing and vice versa. The importance of the imaging is that it illustrates what the baseline anatomy and anatomical defects are, but the testing highlights the physiological impact of that defect. Thus, both sets of findings are crucial and should be utilized in combination to diagnose SSCD.

High-resolution computerised tomography is the imaging modality of choice to visualize possible thinning of the superior semicircular canal or true dehiscence. This should be undertaken via resolution of 0.2 mm or better, and CT images should be evaluated in the planes parallel (Pöschl) and perpendicular (Stenvers) to the plane of the SSC. Although temporal bone CT imaging provides excellent sensitivity for SCD detection, it lacks specificity, meaning it is highly likely to detect any true dehiscence but may also give rise to false positives, suggesting dehiscence when none is there. Furthermore, CT scans can overestimate the presence and size of a dehiscence depending on the slice thickness used. Therefore, for this multitude of reasons, imaging alone cannot be used to guide surgical candidacy for SSCD. MRI imaging may also have a place in the diagnostic work up of TMWD, but mainly as a means to identify other potential pathologies.

Imaging has not been discussed in expansive detail within this chapter given this is covered separately in the dedicated imaging chapter.

Paediatric TMWD

SSCD, posterior SC canal dehiscence (PSCD), enlarged vestibular aqueduct (EVA), X-linked stapes gusher, perilymph fistula (PLF) and bone dyscrasias of the temporal bone comprise the third window abnormalities reported in children [78]. These findings can present with conductive and/or sensorineural hearing loss.

Since SSCD was first reported in 1998, much of the research effort with regard to establishing the most favourable diagnostic and treatment protocols has been concentrated around the adult population. In comparison, little has been published relating to children with TMWD or SSCD specifically. In a UK tertiary neuro-otological centre, of the total 580 children between 5 and 17 years of age assessed in a 30 month period, 13 (2.2%) were found to have radiological evidence of dehiscence, four of which were bilateral [79]. Some of these children had conductive or mixed hearing losses with normal middle ear function, although symptoms consistent with TMWD or disequilibrium were difficult to elicit in many (30.76% and 46.15%, respectively), possibly due to the child's age and difficulty relating to description of complex symptomatology. VEMP testing was not undertaken in this cohort and therefore it remains to be seen whether VEMP testing in the paediatric population will also be of equal importance when creating a diagnostic protocol for TMWD in children.

In the absence of published guidelines for diagnosis, the authors suggest that the adult diagnostic protocols supplied herein be followed as closely as possible, with special emphasis given to the search for objective evidence of sound- or pressure-induced nystagmus, cVEMP and/or oVEMP testing and pure tone audiometry in patients identified as having potential dehiscence on imaging. One would expect that the typical history may not be present but in a child who is completely asymptomatic, in whom a dehiscence is identified incidentally, clinicians should be pragmatic and *not* diagnose a TWMD in such children, as symptoms, of some description at least, should be present even in children to form one of the three crucial diagnostic pillars that should be present in order to reach a full clinical diagnosis.

See Chap. 22 for an in depth discussion of the Paediatric Patient.

Summary

A suggested framework to approach the patient with a suspected third window syndrome:

1. History
   (a) Key questions to identify autophony, sound- or pressure-induced vertigo or dizziness, pulsatile chronic imbalance.
   (b) Specifically enquire about effect of symptoms on mood and quality of life.
2. Examination
   (a) Full oculomotor assessment: expected to be normal.
   (b) **Hennebert's sign:**
      - **Press** on tragus and examine eyes: **vertical or upwards torsional evoked eye movements.**

   (c) **Valsalva** with examination of the eyes: **vertical or upwards torsional evoked eye movements.**
   (d) Positional testing, assessment of gait, romberg test, tandem gait: typically will be normal.
3. Investigations
   (a) **CT** temporal bones: **SSCD** or other TMWD.
   (b) Vestibular function tests: **pressure- and sound-testing** with eye movement recordings: **vertical or upwards torsional evoked eye movements.**
   (c) **Audiometry**: **low frequency conductive hearing loss.**
   (d) VEMP testing.
      - **cVEMP**: **low threshold**, abnormally **large**, sound-induced cVEMP,
      - **oVEMP: low threshold**, abnormally **large**, sound-induced oVEMP,

   (e) Electrocochleography (ECochG):
   (f) Others:
      - Tympanometry—expected to be normal,
      - Acoustic reflexes—expected to be normal.

Concluding Remarks

Despite the increasing reliance and development of sophisticated neurophysiological testing in the diagnostic work up of neuro-otological conditions, the authors surmise that a crucial aspect of the evaluation of those presenting with TMWD is the simple bedside testing to elicit Hennebert's sign or Tullio phenomenon.

Patients with SSCD present with a diverse range of symptoms or no symptoms at all, thus creating a diagnostic and management challenge. Following the proposed diagnostic criteria for SSCD, including at least one symptom consistent with SSCD, CT proof of a dehiscence, and at least one electrophysiologic test supportive of a third mobile window, should be utilized to correctly identify symptomatic cases of SSCD, and avoid over-diagnosis in patients where CT alone is used without any additional testing.

Appendix

Patient reported outcome measures (PROMs).

1. Dizziness Handicap Inventory - DHI https://southampton.stonybrookmedicine.edu/sites/default/files/Dizziness%20Hanicap%20Inventory%20-%20English.pdf
2. SVQ; situational vertigo questionnaire https://neuropt.org/docs/vestibular-sig/situational_vertigo_questionnaireA068B2C6D4D5.pdf?sfvrsn=ef974640_4&sfvrsn=ef974640_4
3. HIT-6; Headache-Impact Test-6 https://bash.org.uk/wp-content/uploads/2012/07/English.pdf
4. PHQ; Patient-Health Questionnaire-9 https://www.med.umich.edu/1info/FHP/practiceguides/depress/phq-9.pdf
5. GAD-7; Generalised Anxiety Disorder-7 Assessment https://adaa.org/sites/default/files/GAD-7_Anxiety-updated_0.pdf
6. Hearing Handicap Inventory for Adults https://www.ummhealth.org/sites/umass-memorial-hospital/files/Documents/Services/Ear_Nose_Throat/Hearing%20Handicap%20Inventory%20For%20Adults.pdf or Speech, Spatial and Qualities of Hearing Scale:
7. Tinnitus Handicap Inventory https://www.ata.org/sites/default/files/Tinnitus_Handicap_Inventory.pdf Measure of auditory disability—autophony, pulsatile tinnitus

References

1. Minor LB, Solomon D, Zinreich JS, Zee DS. Sound- and/or pressure-induced vertigo due to bone dehiscence of the superior semicircular canal. Arch Otolaryngol Head Neck Surg. 1998;124(3):249–58. https://doi.org/10.1001/archotol.124.3.249. PMID: 9525507.
2. Ward BK, van de Berg R, van Rompaey V, Bisdorff A, Hullar TE, Welgampola MS, Carey JP. Superior semicircular canal dehiscence syndrome: diagnostic criteria consensus document of the committee for the classification of vestibular disorders of the Bárány Society. J Vestib Res. 2021;31(3):131–41. https://doi.org/10.3233/VES-200004. PMID: 33522990.
3. Minor LB, Cremer PD, Carey JP, Della Santina CC, Streubel SO, Weg N. Symptoms and signs in superior canal dehiscence syndrome. Ann N Y Acad Sci. 2001;942:259–73. https://doi.org/10.1111/j.1749-6632.2001.tb03751.x. PMID: 11710468.
4. Wackym PA, Mackay-Promitas HT, Demirel S, Gianoli GJ, Gizzi MS, Carter DM, Siker DA. Comorbidities confounding the outcomes of surgery for third window syndrome: outlier analysis. Laryngoscope Investig Otolaryngol. 2017;2(5):225–53. https://doi.org/10.1002/lio2.89. PMID: 29094067; PMCID: PMC5654938.
5. Wackym PA, Wood SJ, Siker DA, Carter DM. Otic capsule dehiscence syndrome: superior semicircular canal dehiscence syndrome with no radiographically visible dehiscence. Ear Nose Throat J. 2015;94(8):E8–E24. https://doi.org/10.1177/014556131509400802. PMID: 26322461.
6. Wackym PA, Balaban CD, Mackay HT, Wood SJ, Lundell CJ, Carter DM, Siker DA. Longitudinal cognitive and neurobehavioral functional outcomes before and after repairing otic capsule dehiscence. Otol Neurotol. 2016;37(1):70–82. https://doi.org/10.1097/MAO.0000000000000928. PMID: 26649608; PMCID: PMC4674143.
7. Hegemann SC, Carey JP. Is superior canal dehiscence congenital or acquired? A case report and review of the literature. Otolaryngol Clin N Am. 2011;44(2):377–82. https://doi.org/10.1016/j.otc.2011.01.009, ix. PMID: 21474012.
8. Wang H, Yu D, Song N, Su K, Yin S. Delayed diagnosis and treatment of benign paroxysmal positional vertigo associated with current practice. Eur Arch Otorhinolaryngol. 2014;271(2):261–4. https://doi.org/10.1007/s00405-012-2333-8. Epub 2013 Mar 2. PMID: 23455578.
9. Newman-Toker DE. Missed stroke in acute vertigo and dizziness: it is time for action, not debate. Ann Neurol. 2016;79(1):27–31. https://doi.org/10.1002/ana.24532. Epub 2015 Dec 12. PMID: 26418192; PMCID: PMC9041814.
10. Atzema CL, Grewal K, Lu H, Kapral MK, Kulkarni G, Austin PC. Outcomes among patients discharged from the emergency department with a diagnosis of peripheral vertigo. Ann Neurol. 2016;79(1):32–41. https://doi.org/10.1002/ana.24521. Epub 2015 Dec 12. PMID: 26385410.
11. Merchant SN, Rosowski JJ. Conductive hearing loss caused by third-window lesions of the inner ear. Otol Neurotol. 2008;29(3):282–9. https://doi.org/10.1097/mao.0b013e318161ab24. PMID: 18223508; PMCID: PMC2577191.
12. Ota I, Sakagami M, Kitahara T. The third mobile window effects in otology/neurotology. J Int Adv Otol. 2021;17(2):156–61. https://doi.org/10.5152/JIAO.2021.8632. PMID: 33893786.
13. Ewald JR. Physiologische Untersuchungen über das Endorgan des Nervus octavus. Wiesbaden: Bergmann; 1892.
14. Tullio P. Das Ohr und die Entstehung der Sprache und Schrift. Berlin: Urban and Schwarzenberg; 1929.

15. Zhou G, Gopen Q, Poe DS. Clinical and diagnostic characterization of canal dehiscence syndrome: a great Otologic mimicker. Otol Neurotol. 2007;28(7):920–6. https://doi.org/10.1097/MAO.0b013e31814b25f2. PMID: 17704722.
16. Shuman AG, Rizvi SS, Pirouet CW, Heidenreich KD. Hennebert's sign in superior semicircular canal dehiscence syndrome: a video case report. Laryngoscope. 2012;122(2):412–4. https://doi.org/10.1002/lary.22413. Epub 2012 Jan 17. PMID: 22252740.
17. Minor LB. Clinical manifestations of superior semicircular canal dehiscence. Laryngoscope. 2005;115(10):1717–27. https://doi.org/10.1097/01.mlg.0000178324.55729.b7. PMID: 16222184.
18. Limb CJ, Carey JP, Srireddy S, Minor LB. Auditory function in patients with surgically treated superior semicircular canal dehiscence. Otol Neurotol. 2006;27(7):969–80. https://doi.org/10.1097/01.mao.0000235376.70492.8e. PMID: 17006348.
19. Carey JP, Migliaccio AA, Minor LB. Semicircular canal function before and after surgery for superior canal dehiscence. Otol Neurotol. 2007;28(3):356–64. https://doi.org/10.1097/01.mao.0000253284.40995.d8. PMID: 17414042.
20. Re M, Gioacchini FM, Salvolini U, Totaro AM, Santarelli A, Mallardi V, Magliulo G. Multislice computed tomography overestimates superior semicircular canal dehiscence syndrome. Ann Otol Rhinol Laryngol. 2013;122(10):625–31. PMID: 24294685.
21. Ceylan N, Bayraktaroglu S, Alper H, Savaş R, Bilgen C, Kirazli T, Güzelmansur I, Ertürk SM. CT imaging of superior semicircular canal dehiscence: added value of reformatted images. Acta Otolaryngol. 2010;130(9):996–1001. https://doi.org/10.3109/00016481003602108. PMID: 20205621.
22. Crovetto M, Whyte J, Rodriguez OM, Lecumberri I, Martinez C, Eléxpuru J. Anatomo-radiological study of the superior semicircular canal dehiscence radiological considerations of superior and posterior semicircular canals. Eur J Radiol. 2010;76(2):167–72. https://doi.org/10.1016/j.ejrad.2009.05.038. Epub 2009 Jun 21. PMID: 19540691.
23. Cloutier JF, Bélair M, Saliba I. Superior semicircular canal dehiscence: positive predictive value of high-resolution CT scanning. Eur Arch Otorhinolaryngol. 2008;265(12):1455–60. https://doi.org/10.1007/s00405-008-0672-2. Epub 2008 Apr 16. PMID: 18415114.
24. Stimmer H, Hamann KF, Zeiter S, Naumann A, Rummeny EJ. Semicircular canal dehiscence in HR multislice computed tomography: distribution, frequency, and clinical relevance. Eur Arch Otorhinolaryngol. 2012;269(2):475–80. https://doi.org/10.1007/s00405-011-1688-6. Epub 2011 Jul 8. PMID: 21739095.
25. Ung N, Chung LK, Lagman C, Bhatt NS, Barnette NE, Ong V, Gopen Q, Yang I. Outcomes of middle fossa craniotomy for the repair of superior semicircular canal dehiscence. J Clin Neurosci. 2017;43:103–7. https://doi.org/10.1016/j.jocn.2017.05.003. Epub 2017 Jun 13. PMID: 28622893.
26. Cozart AC, Kennedy JT III, Seidman MD. A basis for standardizing superior semicircular canal dehiscence management. Ear Nose Throat J. 2021;100(10):NP444–53. https://doi.org/10.1177/0145561320927941. Epub 2020 May 21. PMID: 32436400.
27. Ogutha J, Page NC, Hullar TE. Postpartum vertigo and superior semicircular canal dehiscence syndrome. Obstet Gynecol. 2009;114(2 Pt 2):434–6. https://doi.org/10.1097/AOG.0b013e3181ae8da0. PMID: 19622951; PMCID: PMC2749162.
28. Watters KF, Rosowski JJ, Sauter T, Lee DJ. Superior semicircular canal dehiscence presenting as postpartum vertigo. Otol Neurotol. 2006;27(6):756–68. https://doi.org/10.1097/01.mao.0000227894.27291.9f. PMID: 16936563.
29. Nam EC, Lewis R, Nakajima HH, Merchant SN, Levine RA. Head rotation evoked tinnitus due to superior semicircular canal dehiscence. J Laryngol Otol. 2010;124(3):333–5. https://doi.org/10.1017/S0022215109991241. Epub 2009 Sep 29. PMID: 19785926; PMCID: PMC2822878.
30. Schneiders SMD, Rainsbury JW, Hensen EF, Irving RM. Superior petrosal sinus causing superior canal dehiscence syndrome. J Laryngol Otol. 2017;131(7):593–7. https://doi.org/10.1017/S0022215117001013. Epub 2017 May 15. PMID: 28502274.

31. Öhman J, Forssén A, Sörlin A, Tano K. Patients' experiences of living with superior canal dehiscence syndrome. Int J Audiol. 2018;57(11):825–30. https://doi.org/10.1080/14992027.2018.1487086. Epub 2018 Sep 4. PMID: 30178689.
32. Brantberg K, Verrecchia L, Westin M. Enhanced auditory sensitivity to body vibrations in superior canal dehiscence syndrome. Audiol Neurootol. 2016;21(6):365–71. https://doi.org/10.1159/000450936. Epub 2017 Jan 13. PMID: 28081534.
33. Hennebert C. A new syndrome in hereditary syphilis of the labyrinth. Presse Med Belg Brux. 1911;63:467–70.
34. Nadol JB Jr. Positive "fistula sign" with intact tympanic membrane. Arch Otolaryngol. 1974;100:273–8. https://doi.org/10.1001/archotol.1974.00780040283007.
35. Nadol JB Jr. Positive Hennebert's sign in Ménière's disease. Arch Otolaryngol. 1977;103:524–30. https://doi.org/10.1001/archotol.1977.00780260054005.
36. Minor LB. Labyrinthine fistulae: pathobiology and management. Curr Opin Otolaryngol Head Neck Surg. 2003;11:340–6. https://doi.org/10.1097/00020840-200310000-00006.
37. Sarna B, Abouzari M, Merna C, Jamshidi S, Saber T, Djalilian HR. Perilymphatic fistula: a review of classification, etiology, diagnosis, and treatment. Front Neurol. 2020;11:1046. https://doi.org/10.3389/fneur.2020.01046.
38. Hong RS, Metz CM, Bojrab DI, Babu SC, Zappia J, Sargent EW, Chan EY, Naumann IC, LaRouere MJ. Acoustic reflex screening of conductive hearing loss for third window disorders. Otolaryngol Head Neck Surg. 2016;154(2):343–8. https://doi.org/10.1177/0194599815620162. Epub 2015 Dec 1. PMID: 26626134.
39. Rosowski JJ, Nakajima HH, Merchant SN. Clinical utility of laser-Doppler vibrometer measurements in live normal and pathologic human ears. Ear Hear. 2008;29(1):3–19. https://doi.org/10.1097/AUD.0b013e31815d63a5. PMID: 18091103; PMCID: PMC2572196.
40. Emanuel DC. Acoustic reflex threshold (ART) patterns: an interpretation guide for students and supervisors. AudiologyOnline. 2009; Article 875. www.audiologyonline.com.
41. Nakajima HH, Pisano DV, Roosli C, et al. Comparison of ear-canal reflectance and umbo velocity in patients with conductive hearing loss: a preliminary study. Ear Hear. 2012;33(1):35–43. https://doi.org/10.1097/AUD.0b013e31822ccba0.
42. Merchant GR, Röösli C, Niesten ME, Hamade MA, Lee DJ, McKinnon ML, Ulku CH, Rosowski JJ, Merchant SN, Nakajima HH. Power reflectance as a screening tool for the diagnosis of superior semicircular canal dehiscence. Otol Neurotol. 2015;36(1):172–7. https://doi.org/10.1097/MAO.0000000000000294. PMID: 25076227; PMCID: PMC4267998.
43. Manzari L, Modugno GC, Brandolini C, Pirodda A. Bone vibration-induced nystagmus is useful in diagnosing superior semicircular canal dehiscence. Audiol Neurootol. 2008;13(6):379–87. https://doi.org/10.1159/000148201. Epub 2008 Jul 29. PMID: 18663290.
44. Dumas G, Lion A, Karkas A, Perrin P, Perottino F, Schmerber S. Skull vibration-induced nystagmus test in unilateral superior canal dehiscence and otosclerosis: a vestibular Weber test. Acta Otolaryngol. 2014;134(6):588–600. https://doi.org/10.3109/00016489.2014.888591. Epub 2014 Apr 22. PMID: 24754265.
45. Dumas G, Curthoys IS, Lion A, Perrin P, Schmerber S. The skull vibration-induced nystagmus test of vestibular function—a review. Front Neurol. 2017;8:41. https://doi.org/10.3389/fneur.2017.00041. PMID: 28337171; PMCID: PMC5343042.
46. Dumas G, Tan H, Dumas L, Perrin P, Lion A, Schmerber S. Skull vibration induced nystagmus in patients with superior semicircular canal dehiscence. Eur Ann Otorhinolaryngol Head Neck Dis. 2019;136(4):263–72. https://doi.org/10.1016/j.anorl.2019.04.008. Epub 2019 Apr 25. PMID: 31029487.
47. Yuen HW, Boeddinghaus R, Eikelboom RH, Atlas MD. 15th Yahya Cohen Memorial Lecture—the relationship between the air-bone gap and the size of superior semicircular canal dehiscence. Ann Acad Med Singap. 2011;40(1):59–64. PMID: 21369635.
48. Scarpa A, Ralli M, Cassandro C, Gioacchini FM, Greco A, Di Stadio A, Cavaliere M, Troisi D, de Vincentiis M, Cassandro E. Inner-ear disorders presenting with air-bone gaps: a review.

J Int Adv Otol. 2020;16(1):111–6. https://doi.org/10.5152/iao.2020.7764. PMID: 32401207; PMCID: PMC7224429.
49. Noij KS, Rauch SD. Vestibular evoked myogenic potential (VEMP) testing for diagnosis of superior semicircular canal dehiscence. Front Neurol. 2020;11:695. https://doi.org/10.3389/fneur.2020.00695. PMID: 32793102; PMCID: PMC7385271.
50. Kharkheli E, Japaridze S, Kevanishvili Z, Oz I, Ozluoglu LN. Correlation between vestibular evoked myogenic potentials and disease progression in Ménière's disease. ORL J Otorhinolaryngol Relat Spec. 2019;81(4):193–201. https://doi.org/10.1159/000496088. Epub 2019 Aug 7. PMID: 31390639.
51. Young YH, Huang TW, Cheng PW. Assessing the stage of Meniere's disease using vestibular evoked myogenic potentials. Arch Otolaryngol Head Neck Surg. 2003;129(8):815–8. https://doi.org/10.1001/archotol.129.8.815. PMID: 12925337.
52. Colebatch JG, Rothwell JC, Bronstein A, Ludman H. Click-evoked vestibular activation in the Tullio phenomenon. J Neurol Neurosurg Psychiatry. 1994;57(12):1538–40. https://doi.org/10.1136/jnnp.57.12.1538. PMID: 7798988; PMCID: PMC1073240.
53. Lee JS, Lee SK, Shin IH, Yeo SG, Park MS, Byun JY. Vestibular evoked myogenic potential according to middle ear condition in chronic otitis media with tympanic membrane perforation. Acta Otolaryngol. 2014;134(1):34–40. https://doi.org/10.3109/00016489.2013.836756. Epub 2013 Oct 9. PMID: 24102226.
54. Wang MC, Lee GS. Vestibular evoked myogenic potentials in middle ear effusion. Acta Otolaryngol. 2007;127(7):700–4. https://doi.org/10.1080/00016480601002070. PMID: 17573565.
55. Wang MC, Liu CY, Yu EC, Wu HJ, Lee GS. Vestibular evoked myogenic potentials in chronic otitis media before and after surgery. Acta Otolaryngol. 2009;129(11):1206–11. https://doi.org/10.3109/00016480802620654. PMID: 19863312.
56. Piker EG, Jacobson GP, Burkard RF, McCaslin DL, Hood LJ. Effects of age on the tuning of the cVEMP and oVEMP. Ear Hear. 2013;34(6):e65–73. https://doi.org/10.1097/AUD.0b013e31828fc9f2.
57. Kumar K, Bhat JS, Sequeira NM, Bhojwani KM. Ageing effect on air-conducted ocular vestibular evoked myogenic potential. Audiol Res. 2015;5(2):121. https://doi.org/10.4081/audiores.2015.121. Published 2015 Aug 31.
58. Brantberg K, Bergenius J, Tribukait A. Vestibular-evoked myogenic potentials in patients with dehiscence of the superior semicircular canal. Acta Otolaryngol. 1999;119(6):633–40. https://doi.org/10.1080/00016489950180559. PMID: 10586994.
59. Hunter JB, Patel NS, O'Connell BP, Carlson ML, Shepard NT, McCaslin DL, Wanna GB. Cervical and ocular VEMP testing in diagnosing superior semicircular canal dehiscence. Otolaryngol Head Neck Surg. 2017;156(5):917–23. https://doi.org/10.1177/0194599817690720. Epub 2017 Feb 7. PMID: 28168887.
60. Zuniga MG, Janky KL, Nguyen KD, Welgampola MS, Carey JP. Ocular versus cervical VEMPs in the diagnosis of superior semicircular canal dehiscence syndrome. Otol Neurotol. 2013;34(1):121–6. https://doi.org/10.1097/MAO.0b013e31827136b0.
61. Janky KL, Nguyen KD, Welgampola M, Zuniga MG, Carey JP. Air-conducted oVEMPs provide the best separation between intact and superior canal dehiscent labyrinths. Otol Neurotol. 2013;34(1):127–34. https://doi.org/10.1097/MAO.0b013e318271c32a. PMID: 23151775; PMCID: PMC3621128.
62. Tran ED, Swanson A, Sharon JD, Vaisbuch Y, Blevins NH, Fitzgerald MB, Steenerson KK. Ocular vestibular-evoked myogenic potential amplitudes elicited at 4 kHz optimize detection of superior semicircular canal dehiscence. Front Neurol. 2020;11:879. https://doi.org/10.3389/fneur.2020.00879. PMID: 32982915; PMCID: PMC7477389.
63. Taylor RL, Magnussen JS, Kwok B, et al. Bone-conducted oVEMP latency delays assist in the differential diagnosis of large air-conducted oVEMP amplitudes. Front Neurol. 2020;11:580184. https://doi.org/10.3389/fneur.2020.580184. Published 2020 Oct 29.
64. Noij KS, Herrmann BS, Guinan JJ Jr, Rauch SD. Toward optimizing cVEMP: 2,000-Hz tone bursts improve the detection of superior canal dehiscence. Audiol Neurootol. 2018;23(6):335–44. https://doi.org/10.1159/000493721. Epub 2019 Jan 24. PMID: 30677753; PMCID: PMC6469487.

65. Ward BK, Wenzel A, Ritzl EK, Gutierrez-Hernandez S, Della Santina CC, Minor LB, Carey JP. Near-dehiscence: clinical findings in patients with thin bone over the superior semicircular canal. Otol Neurotol. 2013;34(8):1421–8. https://doi.org/10.1097/MAO.0b013e318287efe6. PMID: 23644303; PMCID: PMC3740012.
66. Noij KS, Duarte MJ, Wong K, Cheng YS, Masud S, Herrmann BS, Curtin HD, Kanumuri VV, Guinan JJ Jr, Kozin ED, Tarabichi O, Jung DH, Lee DJ, Rauch SD. Toward optimizing cervical vestibular evoked myogenic potentials (cVEMP): combining air-bone gap and cVEMP thresholds to improve diagnosis of superior canal dehiscence. Otol Neurotol. 2018;39(2):212–20. https://doi.org/10.1097/MAO.0000000000001655. PMID: 29210947.
67. Gianoli GJ. Post-concussive dizziness: a review and clinical approach to the patient. Front Neurol. 2022;12:718318. https://doi.org/10.3389/fneur.2021.718318. Published 2022 Jan 4.
68. Departmental protocol for cervical vestibular evoked myogenic potentials (cVEMP) test, Royal National Ear Nose and Throat and Eastman Dental Hospitals, June 2020.
69. Departmental protocol for ocular vestibular evoked myogenic potentials (oVEMP) test, Royal National Ear Nose and Throat and Eastman Dental Hospitals, June 2020.
70. Ward BK, Wenzel A, Ritzl EK, Carey JP. Electrocochleography summating potential seen on auditory brainstem response in a case of superior semicircular canal dehiscence. Surg Neurol Int. 2017;8:90. https://doi.org/10.4103/sni.sni_442_15. Published 2017 May 26.
71. Adams ME, Kileny PR, Telian SA, El-Kashlan HK, Heidenreich KD, Mannarelli GR, Arts HA. Electrocochleography as a diagnostic and intraoperative adjunct in superior semicircular canal dehiscence syndrome. Otol Neurotol. 2011;32(9):1506–12. https://doi.org/10.1097/MAO.0b013e3182382a7c. PMID: 22072263.
72. Arts HA, Adams ME, Telian SA, El-Kashlan H, Kileny PR. Reversible electrocochleographic abnormalities in superior canal dehiscence. Otol Neurotol. 2009;30(1):79–86. https://doi.org/10.1097/MAO.0b013e31818d1b51. PMID: 19092559.
73. Ocak I, Topsakal V, Van de Heyning P, Van Haesendonck G, Jorissen C, van de Berg R, Vanderveken OM, Van Rompaey V. Impact of superior canal dehiscence syndrome on health utility values: a prospective case-control study. Front Neurol. 2020;11:552495. https://doi.org/10.3389/fneur.2020.552495. PMID: 33133004; PMCID: PMC7578361.
74. Allsopp T, Kim AH, Robbins AM, Page JC, Dornhoffer JL. Quality of life outcomes after transmastoid plugging of superior semicircular canal dehiscence. Am J Otolaryngol. 2020;41(2):102287. https://doi.org/10.1016/j.amjoto.2019.102287. Epub 2019 Sep 9. PMID: 31761408.
75. Tikka T, Slim MAM, Gaggini M, Kontorinis G. Video head impulse test (vHIT) findings in patients with superior semicircular canal dehiscence: a case-control study. J Int Adv Otol. 2021;17(2):103–8. https://doi.org/10.5152/JIAO.2021.8572. PMID: 33893778.
76. Castellucci A, Piras G, Del Vecchio V, Crocetta FM, Maiolo V, Ferri GG, Ghidini A, Brandolini C. The effect of superior canal dehiscence size and location on audiometric measurements, vestibular-evoked myogenic potentials and video-head impulse testing. Eur Arch Otorhinolaryngol. 2021;278(4):997–1015. https://doi.org/10.1007/s00405-020-06169-3. Epub 2020 Jun 26. PMID: 32592013.
77. Banerjee A, Whyte A, Atlas MD. Superior canal dehiscence: review of a new condition. Clin Otolaryngol. 2005;30(1):9–15. https://doi.org/10.1111/j.1365-2273.2004.00940.x. PMID: 15748182.
78. Sarioglu FC, Pekcevik Y, Guleryuz H, Cakir Cetin A, Guneri EA. The relationship between the third window abnormalities and inner ear malformations in children with hearing loss. J Int Adv Otol. 2021;17(5):387–92. https://doi.org/10.5152/iao.2021.9482.
79. Dasgupta S, Ratnayake SAB. Functional and objective audiovestibular evaluation of children with apparent semicircular canal dehiscence-a case series in a pediatric vestibular center. Front Neurol. 2019;10:306. https://doi.org/10.3389/fneur.2019.00306. PMID: 31001191; PMCID: PMC6454049.

Chapter 12
Imaging of Third Mobile Window Syndromes

Lee M. Bauter, Shweta Kumar, Vince M. Desiato, Gino Mongelluzzo, and Arun K. Gadre

Introduction

Imaging studies play a key role in the evaluation of third window lesions. When a third window lesion is suspected due to a patient's history, physical exam, and audiologic testing, appropriate imaging helps to make the definitive diagnosis [1]. In fact, the most commonly diagnosed third window pathology namely, superior semicircular canal dehiscence (SSCD) was first described in 1998 with computed tomography (CT) findings playing a significant role [2, 3]. Furthermore, most patients with third window lesions will have an unremarkable tympanic membrane and middle ear, making imaging crucial [4].

Technical Considerations

The inner ear is anatomically defined by the bony labyrinth, an endosteum-lined structure within the temporal bone that consists of the cochlear and vestibular organs. Symptoms can result from the enlargement of naturally occurring windows or channels that exist in the bony labyrinth or by the creation of new defects resulting in hydrodynamic third windows [5]. CT scans are most appropriate to visualize

L. M. Bauter · V. M. Desiato · A. K. Gadre (✉)
Department of Otolaryngology-Head and Neck Surgery, Geisinger Medical Center, Danville, PA, USA
e-mail: lmbauter@geisinger.edu; vmdesiato@geisinger.edu; agadre@geisinger.edu

S. Kumar · G. Mongelluzzo
Department of Radiology, Geisinger Medical Center, Danville, PA, USA
e-mail: gjmongelluzzo1@geisinger.edu

G. J. Gianoli, P. Thomson (eds.), *Third Mobile Window Syndrome of the Inner Ear*, https://doi.org/10.1007/978-3-031-16586-3_12

the bony confines of the labyrinth, and are therefore used to assess third window lesion [6]. These lesions are divided into focal or diffuse depending on the extent and location of the bony defect [3]. Patients with these lesions will often have imaging that reveals an unremarkable middle ear anatomy. This helps to differentiate third window pathologies from more common diseases of the middle ear [3]. However, the bony defects and findings associated with many causes of third window pathology are often very subtle, involving structures that are difficult to assess due to their small size and/or orientation [7]. Because of this, specific imaging parameters are best suited for evaluation of this pathology.

As the understanding of third window pathology advances, so too does the understanding of how best to utilize the available resources to make a given diagnosis. When Minor et al. [2] first described SSCD, axial CT slices were acquired with 1 mm slice thickness. Presently, the gold standard for imaging evaluation of third window lesions is high resolution CT scans of the temporal bones with 0.5–1 mm collimation. Isotropic data is acquired with the potential to create three-dimensional multiplanar reformats. Axial, coronal, and sagittal reconstructions are typically provided (Fig. 12.1a, b). The Pöschl and Stenver views (Fig. 12.1c, d), which are dedicated oblique coronal and sagittal reconstructions, are designed to better visualize the superior and posterior semicircular canals, and can improve the localization of third window lesions [6]. Furthermore, digital processing techniques such as gray-scale inversion allow for CT images to be read in finer detail and with increased accuracy [6, 8].

Post-processing filters can also assist in detecting subtle osseous defects. For example, filters can be set to bone edge detection, reducing noise from surrounding structures [9]. Furthermore, utilizing gray-scale inversion (invert function) can provide improved visualization of thin bone or questionable dehiscence [8]. By inverting the image, bone appears dark on the monitor, allowing the clinician to take advantage of the contrast threshold, or the relative luminance increment required to detect a signal. At higher luminance, the contrast threshold is lessened, allowing for better detection of gray-scale between adjacent pixels. As the inversion of the gray-scale causes bone to become dark and other tissues to become bright, the detection of a very thin layer of bone over the semicircular canal or other area of the bony labyrinth becomes easier [8].

In recent years, the use of CT modalities with higher resolutions such as cone beam CT (CBCT) and ultrahigh-resolution CT (UHRCT) has allowed for more accurate localization (slices as thin as 0.15 mm) and diagnosis of third window lesions while decreasing doses of ionizing radiation. These modalities are promising for future care but are not yet available at most institutions [4, 10].

Magnetic resonance imaging (MRI) is less effective at evaluating the bony labyrinth and thus does not usually play a primary role in the evaluation of third window lesions. Small field of view T2-weighted MR imaging can exclude the presence of various third window lesions with high negative predictive value. MRI may also falsely detect lesions if the bony boundary is too thin for assessment, ultimately necessitating the need for CT in cases of equivocal third window pathology [4, 6]. However, much of the utility of MRI lies in its ability to characterize bone marrow

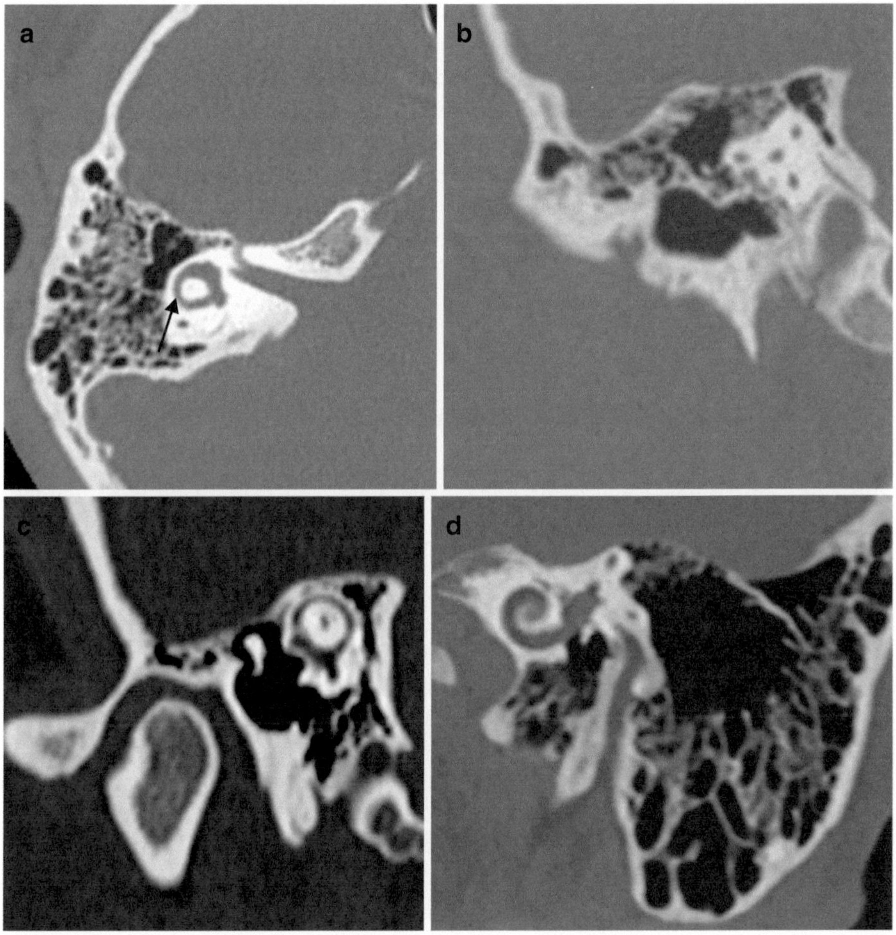

Fig. 12.1 (**a**) Images are in plane with the lateral semicircular canal (arrow). Normal CT scan. (**b**) Coronal image perpendicular to horizontal semicircular canal. (**c**) Pöschl View of the superior semicircular canal. (**d**) Stenver projection

and soft tissue abnormalities, perilymphatic fluid composition (e.g., hemorrhage), and cranial nerve pathology [6]. Additionally, MRI can exclude the presence of intracranial pathology such as temporal encephalocele, vestibular schwannomas, vascular malformations, or lateral skull base meningiomas [11]. These features make MRI helpful in surgical planning. MRI is also invaluable in postoperative evaluation, particularly in patients who are being considered for revision surgery, as the materials used to repair many types of third window lesions are not radiopaque and may not be visualized on CT scans. Thin slice T2-weighted MR imaging is paramount in determining the extent of repair, as well as the location of any residual defect in the bony labyrinth post operatively [11, 12].

The use of imaging in the diagnosis of third window lesions while critical should always be paired with clinical findings when making a diagnosis. Furthermore, many patients with CT evidence of third window lesions are asymptomatic [13, 14]. Therefore, patients who are diagnosed with third window pathology should have symptoms and features of the suspected disease. Due to the subtle nature of the imaging findings, it is to the benefit of the clinician to first suspect the type and location of the defect, and then use imaging to support the diagnosis, allowing for the planning of interventions tailored to the cause. In the following, various types of third window lesions, their associated imaging findings, and related technical aspects are discussed in greater detail.

Superior Semicircular Canal Dehiscence

Superior semicircular canal dehiscence is the most well recognized third window lesion, referring to the extreme thinning or loss of the bony roof (tegmen)of the superior semicircular canal [6]. This leads to a communication between the superior semicircular canal and the middle cranial fossa or the superior petrosal sinus [3, 6]. As mentioned, this condition was first described by Minor et al. in 1998 with the utilization of CT scan aiding in the diagnosis [2]. Since his description, CT scans have been a hallmark diagnostic tool (Fig. 12.2a, b).

SSCD can occur at various locations along the superior semicircular canal. These can be observed and differentiated on CT imaging. A radiologic classification of SSCD has been proposed with the goal of standardizing descriptions and surgical planning. Lookabough et al. [15] classified SSCD by the location of the defect relative to the arcuate eminence. The classification included: lateral upslope defect, arcuate eminence defect, medial downslope defect, superior petrosal sinus related SSCD, and arcuate eminence defect with superior petrosal sinus near-dehiscence. The most common site of dehiscence in this study was along the arcuate eminence(59%), where the bone is the thinnest [6, 15]. The medial downslope was the second most common site (29%), followed by the lateral upslope (8%), and finally the medial downslope associated with the superior petrosal sinus (4%). Less than 1% of cases demonstrated bony dehiscence in two separate locations [15]. Larger bony defects, particularly when greater than 2 mm, and proximity of the defect to the vestibule are considered more likely to be clinically significant [6].

While the detection of an absent bony covering along the superior semicircular canal raises suspicion for the presence of SSCD, it is not a specific finding. CT imaging is imperfect in its ability to capture the physical and spatial features of the anatomy in question. In the absence of appropriate clinical symptoms, CT imaging demonstrating an osseous defect is not sufficient to make a diagnosis [14]. However, if a patient is symptomatic, the accuracy of CT imaging is crucial, as the finding of SSCD on CT may lead to attempted surgical repair [16]. Therefore, various techniques and strategies have been described to maximize the detection of SSCD.

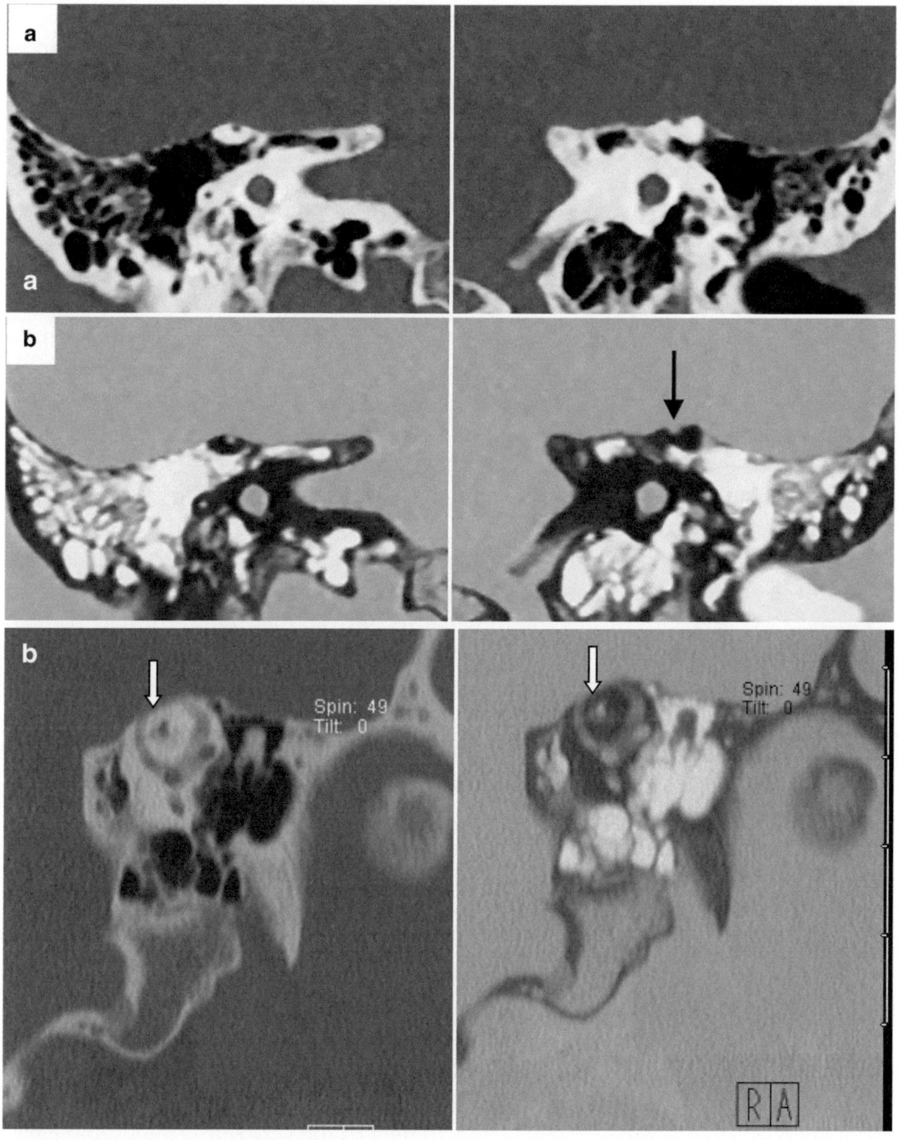

Fig. 12.2 (**a**) SSCD on coronal CT scan: (**a**) standard images suggestive of bilateral SSCD and (**b**) invert function revealing thin bony covering over right superior semicircular canal and left dehiscence (arrow). (Reproduced with permission of Annals of Otology, Rhinology & Laryngology [8]). (**b**) Arrows point to SSCD on Pöschl View using standard images and invert function

The collimation thickness of CT imaging is crucial to its accuracy and utility. When compared to cadaveric studies, CT imaging has been shown to overestimate the true prevalence of SSCD. A review article from 2017 cites the prevalence as 2.1–10.7% on CT scans of the temporal bone but only 0.5–0.6% on cadaveric studies [5]. Furthermore, a cadaveric study of over 1000 CT scans of temporal bones found the rate of SSCD to be 0.5% in temporal bone specimens and 0.7% for individuals (often bilateral) [17]. An additional 1.4% of temporal bone specimens were found to have thin bony boundaries that might appear dehiscent on even the highest resolution CT imaging (≤0.1 mm) [17]. In contrast, a large imaging series from 2003 found that SSCD was observed on 9% of coronal CT images with 1 mm slice thickness. There was a 94% correlation between examiners [18]. Discrepancy between the reported prevalence of SSCD on imaging and in cadavers (and therefore estimated actual prevalence) can most likely be attributed to CT slice thickness. With 1 mm collimation, partial volume averaging can make thin bone appear dehiscent, leading to an inaccurate diagnosis of SSCD. Thinner CT slices (0.5–1 mm) will reduce partial volume averaging effects and subsequently decrease false positive errors [5]. Thinner slices will also allow improved reformatting of images in any plane without distortion. However, as slice thickness decreases, it must be noted that noise will increase, compromising image quality.

Another challenging aspect of imaging the superior semicircular canal is its orientation in relation to the standard planes of CT imaging. The superior semicircular canal lies in a plane approximately 45° divergent from both the sagittal and coronal planes. It is oblique to the standard transverse and coronal planes used in standard CT scans [13]. Because of this, multiplanar reconstructions and reformats parallel to (Pöschl) and perpendicular to (Stenver) the superior semicircular canal are often utilized to evaluate the anatomy [5, 14]. The Pöschl plane displays the superior semicircular canal as a complete ring, highlighting the outer arc. The Stenver plane gives a cross section of the superior cortex of the superior semicircular canal [13]. These orientations allow for better assessment of the overlying bone and any defects therein [9]. Interestingly, a study from 2006 by Branstetter et al. [19] argues that coronal reformations from CT of the temporal bone are sufficient to detect SSCD and that reformations in the plane of Stenver and Pöschl do not routinely aid in diagnosis. However, whether used routinely or only for challenging cases, these two views can be an adjunct in evaluating SSCD.

MRI can play a complementary role in the assessment of primary SSCD. However, it plays a vital role in the post-operative assessment of persistent symptoms [11]. As discussed, MRI is extremely important for ruling out associated intracranial pathology that may affect surgical planning (encephalocele, vestibular schwannoma, vascular malformations, etc.) [11]. Modern MRI has not consistently demonstrated adequate resolution for diagnosing a bony defect of the superior semicircular canal [9]. MRI is able, however, to assess semicircular canal patency on T2-weighted imaging due to the high signal of fluid within the canals [14]. This feature allows MRI to provide high contrast definition between fluid and bone.

High resolution T2-weighted MRI of the temporal bones may demonstrate a hypointense structure between the fluid signal within the semicircular canal and extra axial fluid signal within the overlying middle cranial fossa, consistent with an intact bony roof (Fig. 12.3). This bony covering can be quite thin and is not always visualized. If the roof of the superior semicircular canal is in fact visualized, SSCD

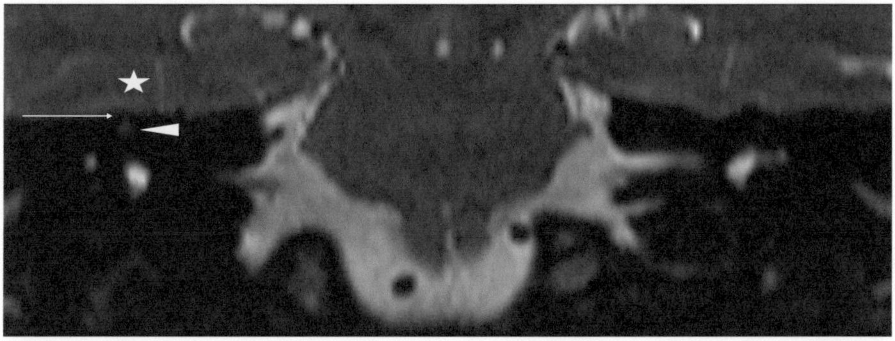

Fig. 12.3 Coronal T2 weighted MRI of the IACs demonstrating a T2 hypointense boundary (arrow) delineating the arcuate eminence of the superior semicircular canal (arrowhead) from the inferior right temporal lobe (star), effectively excluding dehiscence at the arcuate eminence

can safely be excluded. Thus, the negative predictive value of small field of view T2-weighted MRI has been demonstrated as being as high as 100% [20]. However, if an intact roof is not visualized, this should not raise suspicion for or confirm a diagnosis of SSCD. When suspicion of SSCD is raised on MRI, a CT scan of the temporal bones should be acquired to confirm bony dehiscence [6, 20].

MRI is also useful in assessing the adequacy of surgical repair for SSCD. Surgical approaches for repairing SSCD include resurfacing, plugging, or capping of the superior semicircular canal [6]. The goal of these techniques is to create a watertight seal [12]. As most materials for repair of the bony defect are not radio-opaque, post-operative CT provides minimal information regarding the success or extent of the repair [11]. Because MRI is effective at assessing semicircular canal patency, the extent of occlusion postoperatively can be quantified on T2-weighted MRI in the Pöschl reformation [12]. Furthermore, co-registration of CT and MR images has been shown to be useful in determining the location of a residual defect should one be present [12].

SSCD is perhaps the best described third window lesion. Many imaging recommendations, techniques and guidelines have stemmed from our understanding of this pathology. The remaining sections of this chapter will highlight examples of other third window lesions while applying many of the same principles regarding the technical aspects of SSCD imaging to the given pathology.

Posterior Semicircular Canal Dehiscence

As the anatomy of the semicircular canals is similar, evaluation of posterior semicircular canal dehiscence (PSCD) follows the same principles described above (Fig. 12.4).

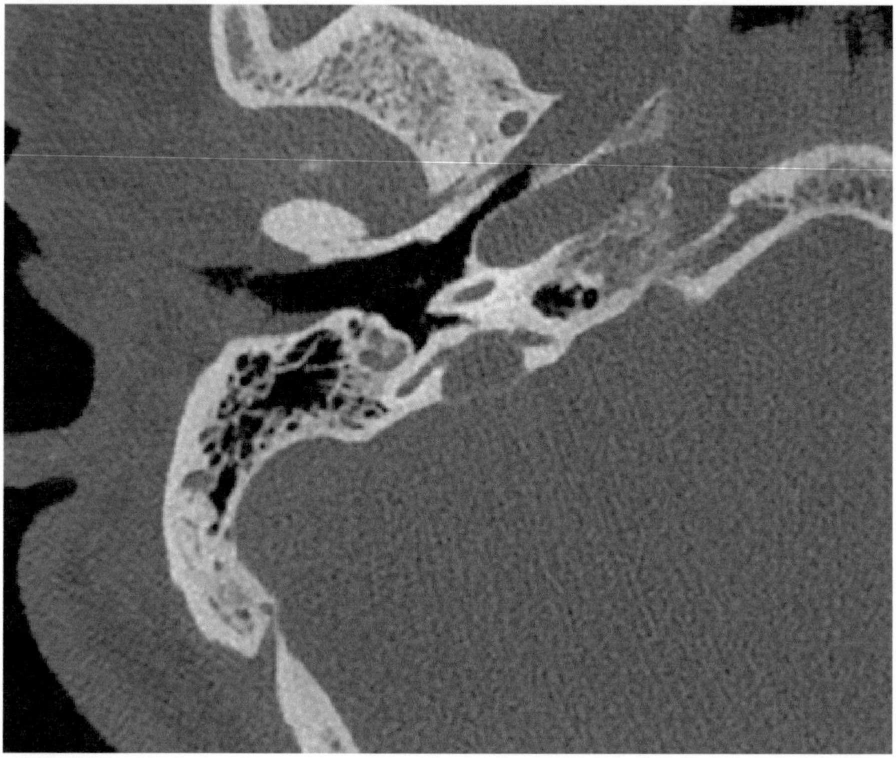

Fig. 12.4 Axial CT scan demonstrating an osseous defect along the posterior wall of the posterior semicircular canal

PSCD is less commonly identified than SSCD. It can be observed in combination with or isolated from SSCD. One study demonstrated that the prevalence of PSCD identified by CT in temporal bones ordered for evaluation of middle ear symptoms was 0.6% or 2/604 cases [21]. Another study found that the prevalence of PSCD was 1.2% in patients undergoing CT scans of temporal bones [22]. In one surgeon's database of patients with third window syndrome, 5 out of 502 syndromic temporal bones demonstrated radiographic evidence of PSCD or approximately 1% [23].

Like SSCD, CT imaging is the investigation of choice for evaluation of PSCD. The posterior semicircular is adjacent to the posterior fossa dura, and may dehisce into this structure via a bony defect or a high riding jugular bulb [6]. With increased prevalence of the right-sided venous system dominance, PSCD occurs more commonly on the right side [24]. PSCD can often be seen on CT scan on axial slices, however, Stenver views parallel to the plane of the canal may be useful in making the diagnosis in assessing for bony dehiscence [15, 24]. Furthermore, like SSCD, MRI has been shown to have a negative predictive value of nearly 100%, and can exclude PSCD from the list of differential diagnoses [20].

Lateral Semicircular Canal Dehiscence and Perilymphatic Fistula

Lateral semicircular canal dehiscence (LSCD) is the least common semicircular canal dehiscence. The lateral semicircular canal is completely covered by the otic capsule which is the densest bone in the body. This makes isolated LSCD extremely rare [6]. Most often a locally destructive process erodes the bony covering of the lateral semicircular canal, causing a perilymphatic fistula [1]. When this erosion involves the semicircular canals (most often the lateral), the vestibule, and/or the scala vestibuli side of the cochlea, third window lesions may result [5]. Erosive processes can be infectious, inflammatory, neoplastic, or vascular (e.g., idiopathic intracranial hypertension) in origin [6]. CT imaging will show erosion into the otic capsule with a dehiscence causing a third window (Fig. 12.5a–c). MRI can help further characterize the erosive process at play including the identification of other complications [6]. Figure 12.6 demonstrates an unusual dehiscence between the tympanic portion of the facial nerve and the horizontal semicircular canal.

Another cause of third window syndrome and related to a perilymph fistula is the recently described membranous or hypermobile stapes footplate syndrome (Fig. 12.7). Several of the clinical features overlap with third window syndromes. By being hypermobile, the stapes can allow the oval window to behave as a third window even in the absence of a true perilymph leak [25]. CT scans aid in assessing this pathology, as small defects in the stapes footplate can be detected on high resolution CT scans. The gray-scale inversion function is especially valuable when assessing for this pathology [8, 25].

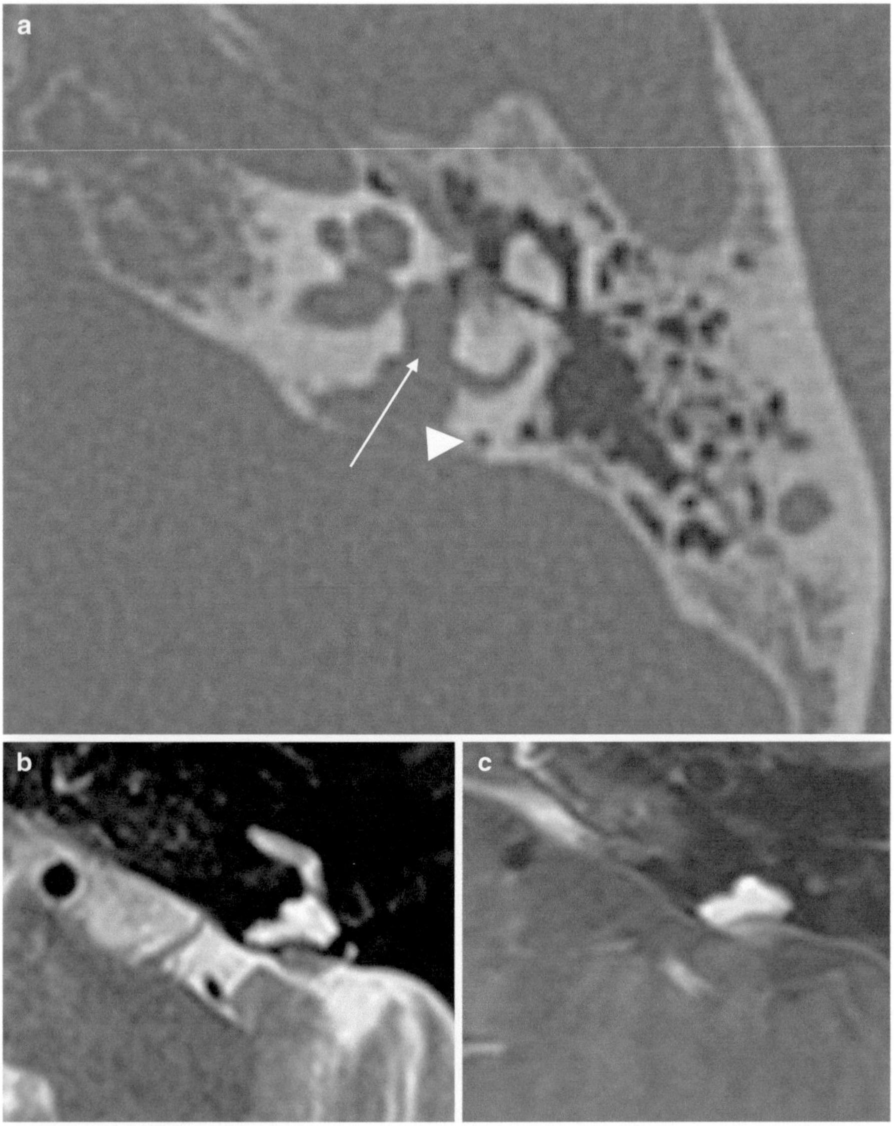

Fig. 12.5 (**a**) Axial non-contrast CT scan of the temporal bone demonstrates a permeative mass compatible with an endolymphatic sac tumor (arrow). The tumor erodes the adjacent bone, dehiscing the posterior semicircular canal (arrowhead) and vestibule (arrow). (**b**) Axial T2 weighted MRI demonstrates a hyperintense enhancing mass of same lesion as in (**a**). (**c**) T1 post-contrast MRI of the same patient demonstrates an enhancing mass

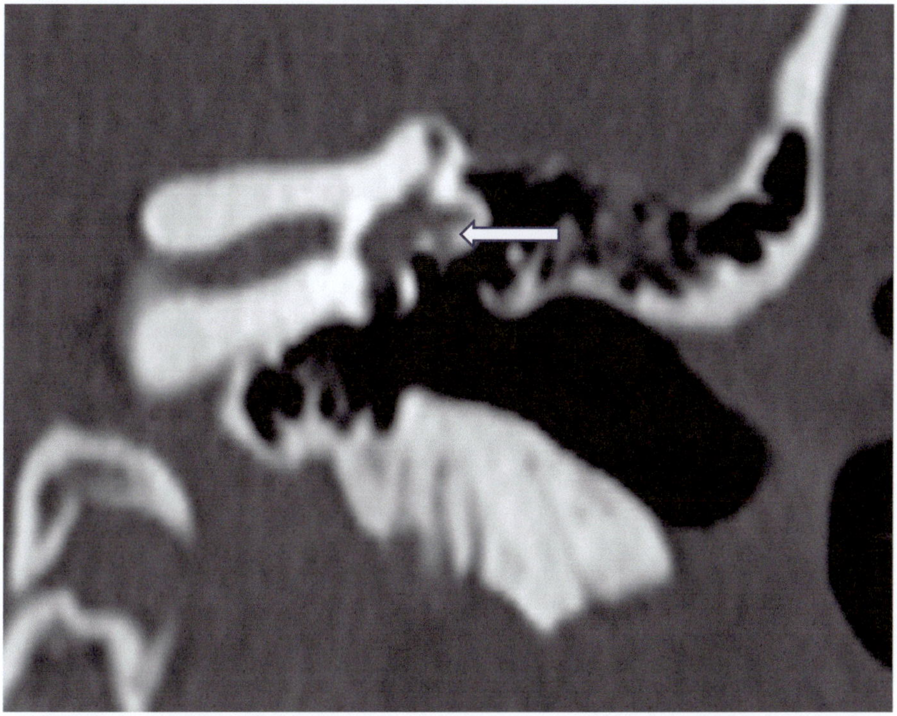

Fig. 12.6 Coronal CT scan demonstrating a defect along the lateral semicircular canal communicating with the facial nerve canal

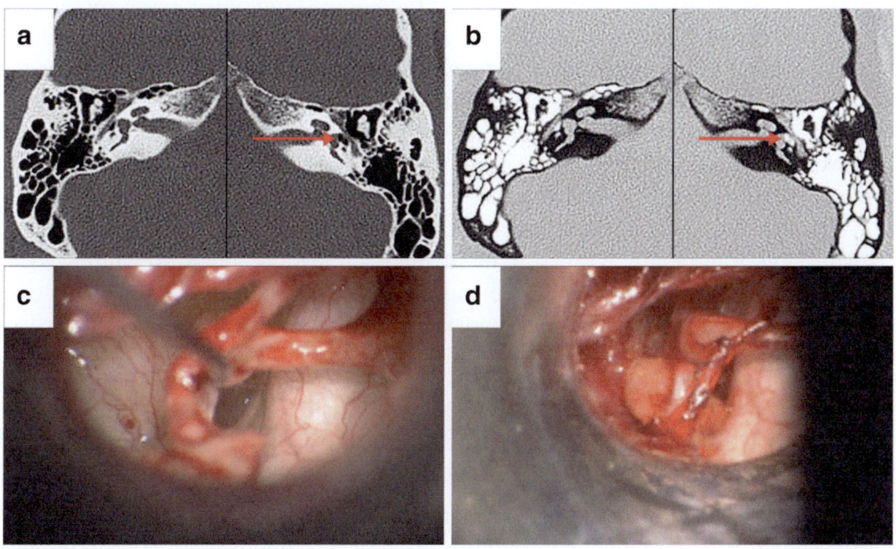

Fig. 12.7 Membranous left stapes footplate (arrows) (**a**) normal axial CT scan. (**b**) Invert function shows membranous stapes footplate clearly. (**c**) Intraoperative view in the same patient. (**d**) Fat grafting. (Reproduced with permission of Annals of Otology, Rhinology & Laryngology [8])

Enlarged Vestibular Aqueduct

Enlarged vestibular aqueduct syndrome (EVA) is a pathologic enlargement of the vestibular aqueduct at the level of the endolymphatic duct. This enlargement may act as a third window due to the transmission of acoustic energy into the posterior cranial fossa [5]. Diagnosis using CT is usually based on the transverse dimension of the vestibular aqueduct. The Cincinnati Criteria established that a width of greater than 2 mm at the operculum, and/or a width greater than 1 mm at the midpoint of the aqueduct is consistent with the diagnosis of an EVA [26]. In practical terms the width of the inferior limb of the posterior semicircular canal can also serve as a reference for ascertaining if an EVA is present. In EVA, the midpoint of the aqueduct is typically larger than that of neighboring posterior semicircular canal [6]. The 45° oblique (Pöschl) view on CT allows for better assessment of the vestibular aqueduct throughout the length of the structure, which is especially useful in cases of borderline enlargement [27]. The vestibular aqueduct may also dehisce into a high riding jugular bulb, with one study reporting a prevalence of 11.5% on CT imaging of the temporal bone [28]. MRI can also be used to assess the EVA, and a study from 2019 demonstrated that there were high levels of diagnostic agreement between CT and MRI evaluation of patients with EVA.

X-Linked Stapes Gusher

Stapes gusher syndrome, also known as X-linked deafness, DFN-3, or Incomplete Partition Type 3 [6], may present with third window symptoms caused by a communication between the internal auditory canal and the scala vestibuli of the cochlea [1]. The typical CT appearance of a stapes gusher morphology consists of a "corkscrew" cochlea with an interscalar septum and an absent modiolus [3]. The internal auditory canal is often bulbous and merges with the cochlea due to an absent lamina cribrosa, the structure that normally separates the basal turn of the cochlea from the internal auditory canal fundus. Absence of this structure allows direct communication between the subarachnoid space and the perilymphatic space, permitting the transmission of intracranial pressure in the inner ear leading to a third window syndrome [6]. Notably, CT from all nine patients with stapes gusher syndrome at one institution demonstrated bilateral temporal bone abnormalities [5].

Cochlear Dehiscence and Bony Dyscrasias

Cochlear dehiscence refers to a focal defect along the bony cover of the cochlea which creates an anomalous communication between the cochlea and the middle ear or nearby vasculature (Fig. 12.8). In a third window syndrome caused by cochlear dehiscence, the scala vestibuli side of the cochlea must be involved [6].

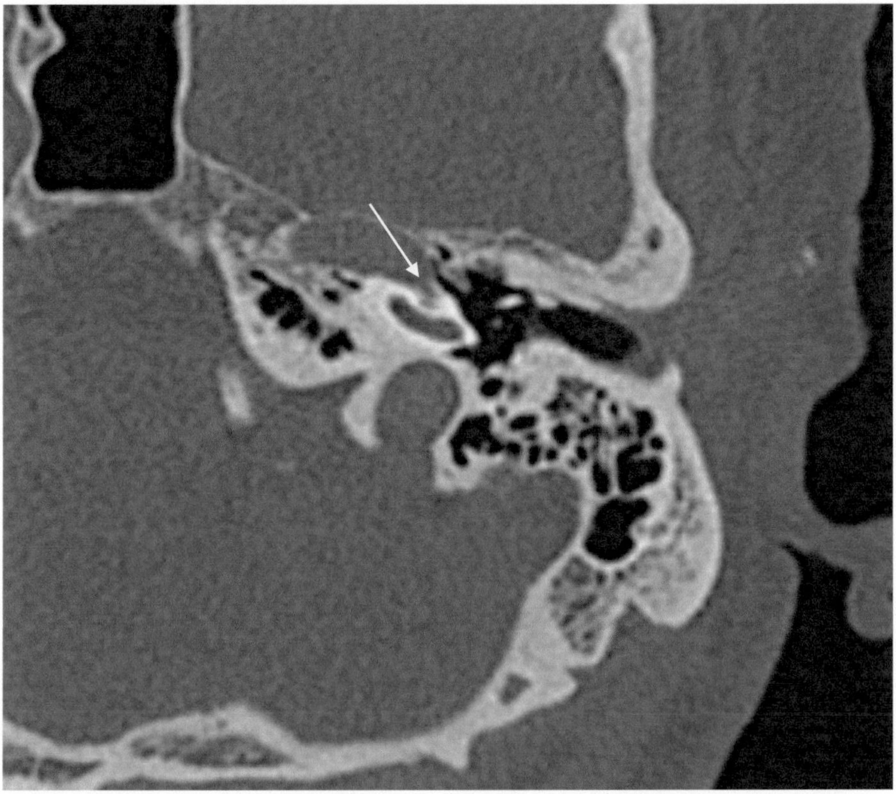

Fig. 12.8 Axial CT scan demonstrating a bony defect along the apical turn of the left cochlea (arrow), creating an anomalous communication with the adjacent left carotid canal

Cochlear-facial nerve dehiscence is a well-known entity, first described in 2014 by Blake et al. [29] This occurs when the bony division between the cochlea and the labyrinthine or tympanic facial nerve segments is eroded or absent, causing a third window syndrome (Fig. 12.9). Another well-described entity is the dehiscence of scala vestibuli side of the cochlea and communication with the internal carotid artery canal [30]. Both of these types of dehiscence can be observed on CT imaging.

In adults, the bony labyrinth is composed of mature avascular endochondral bone, which undergoes no remodeling and is the hardest bone in the body [5, 6]. When the integrity of the bone is compromised by abnormal remodeling, the damaged bone acts as a diffuse defect or a distributed third window lesion [5, 6]. Bony dyscrasias of the otic capsule can also cause a focal third window lesion.

Paget's Disease is a metabolic disorder characterized by diffuse abnormal bony remodeling. In the temporal bone, this can result in numerous microfractures throughout the otic capsule, possibly involving the scala vestibuli side of the cochlear partition [1]. On CT, there is typically diffuse cortical and trabecular thickening of the affected bone with lucent lesions forming earlier in the course of disease and sclerotic lesions forming later on [6].

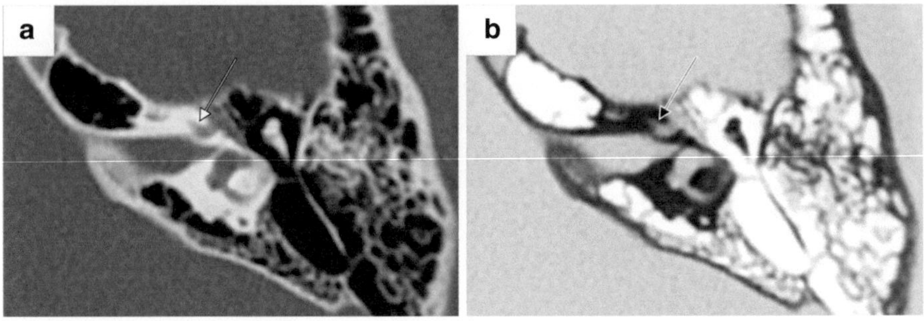

Fig. 12.9 Dehiscence between the labyrinthine segment of the facial nerve and the cochlea (**a**) axial CT scan and (**b**) gray-scale inversion image. (Reproduced with permission of Annals of Otology, Rhinology & Laryngology [8])

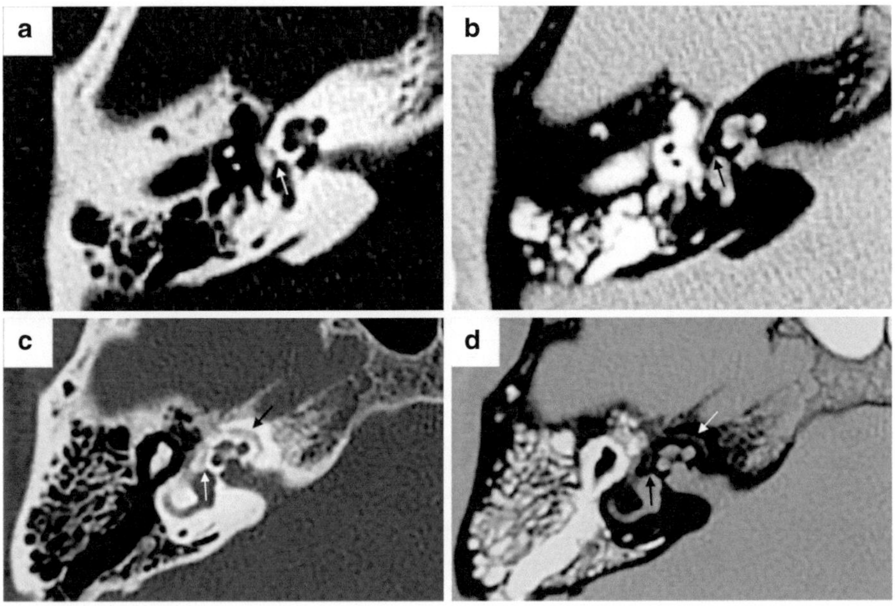

Fig. 12.10 Fenestral Otosclerosis seen in regular and invert-function CT scan (**a**, **b**) and cochlear (retrofenestral) otosclerosis seen in **c**, **d**. (Reproduced with permission of Annals of Otology, Rhinology & Laryngology [8])

Otospongiosis, or otosclerosis, can cause a diffuse third window lesion through abnormal bony remodeling of the endochondral layer of the temporal bone [6]. Fenestral otosclerosis is more common, characterized on CT by the development of lucency (indicating abnormal demineralized bone) at the anterior margin of the oval window in the region of the fissula ante fenestram. In more severe cases, there may be increased proliferation of spongiotic bone, narrowing the oval window and causing ankylosis of the stapes footplate (Fig. 12.10) [31]. MRI is not used for first line evaluation but may demonstrate enhancement in areas of active inflammation. Cochlear or retrofenestral otosclerosis is less common and is often seen concurrently with fenestral otosclerosis [31]. On CT, retrofenestral otosclerosis appears as a ring of demineralized bone surrounding the cochlea. In severe cases of otosclerosis, cavitary plaques can develop. In the chronic setting, there is replacement of the previously seen lucent spongiotic bone on CT with areas of dense sclerotic bone.

Many other conditions that affect bone structure through abnormal remodeling may result in third window lesions, such as hyperparathyroidism. The diffuse demineralization of the otic capsule or a large region of the bony labyrinth may be sufficient to cause a third window syndrome.

Summary

Once a third window syndrome is suspected, CT scans are used to confirm the diagnosis. MRI has negative predictive value, and may have an adjunctive diagnostic role. Imaging studies should not be used in isolation to direct surgical therapy but rather surgical intervention should be directed by the entire clinical, audiological, and electrodiagnostic presentation. The gray-scale inversion techniques on CT scanning have distinct advantages when the radiological diagnosis is in doubt or is questionable.

References

1. Merchant SN, Rosowski JJ. Conductive hearing loss caused by third-window lesions of the inner ear. Otol Neurotol. 2008;29(3):282–9. https://doi.org/10.1097/mao.0b013e318161ab24. PMID: 18223508 PMCID: PMC2577191.
2. Minor LB, Solomon D, Zinreich JS, Zee DS. Sound- and/or pressure-induced vertigo due to bone dehiscence of the superior semicircular canal. Arch Otolaryngol Head Neck Surg. 1998;124(3):249–58. https://doi.org/10.1001/archotol.124.3.249. PMID: 9525507.
3. Moonis G. Imaging of third window lesions of the temporal bone. Semin Roentgenol. 2019;54(3):276–81. https://doi.org/10.1053/j.ro.2019.04.001. PMID: 31376867.
4. Touska P, Connor SEJ. Imaging of the temporal bone. Clin Radiol. 2020;75(9):658–74. https://doi.org/10.1016/j.crad.2020.06.013. PMID: 32690241.
5. Ho ML, Moonis G, Halpin CF, Curtin HD. Spectrum of third window abnormalities: semicircular canal dehiscence and beyond. AJNR Am J Neuroradiol. 2017;38(1):2–9. https://doi.org/10.3174/ajnr.A4922. PMID: 27561833 PMCID: PMC7963676.
6. Ho ML. Third window lesions. Neuroimaging Clin N Am. 2019;29(1):57–92. https://doi.org/10.1016/j.nic.2018.09.005. PMID: 30466645.
7. Casselman JW, Gieraerts K, Volders D, et al. Cone beam CT: non-dental applications. JBR-BTR. 2013;96(6):333–53. https://doi.org/10.5334/jbr-btr.453. PMID: 24617175.
8. Schwartz TR, Lindemann TL, Mongelluzzo G, Wackym PA, Gadre AK. Gray-scale inversion on high resolution computed tomography of the temporal bone: an observational study. Ann Otol Rhinol Laryngol. 2021;130(10):1125–31. https://doi.org/10.1177/0003489421996844. PMID: 33629604.

9. Ward BK, van de Berg R, van Rompaey V, et al. Superior semicircular canal dehiscence syndrome: diagnostic criteria consensus document of the committee for the classification of vestibular disorders of the Barany Society. J Vestib Res. 2021;31(3):131–41. https://doi.org/10.3233/VES-200004. PMID: 33522990.
10. Ohara A, Machida H, Shiga H, Yamamura W, Yokoyama K. Improved image quality of temporal bone CT with an ultrahigh-resolution CT scanner: clinical pilot studies. Jpn J Radiol. 2020;38(9):878–83. https://doi.org/10.1007/s11604-020-00987-5. PMID: 32394364 PMCID: PMC7452920.
11. Eberhard KE, Chari DA, Nakajima HH, Klokker M, Caye-Thomasen P, Lee DJ. Current trends, controversies, and future directions in the evaluation and management of superior canal dehiscence syndrome. Front Neurol. 2021;12:638574. https://doi.org/10.3389/fneur.2021.638574. PMID: 33889125 PMCID: PMC8055857.
12. Chemtob RA, Epprecht L, Reinshagen KL, et al. Utility of postoperative magnetic resonance imaging in patients who fail superior canal dehiscence surgery. Otol Neurotol. 2019;40(1):130–8. https://doi.org/10.1097/MAO.0000000000002051. PMID: 30461526.
13. Curtin HD. Superior semicircular canal dehiscence syndrome and multi-detector row CT. Radiology. 2003;226(2):312–4. https://doi.org/10.1148/radiol.2262021327. PMID: 12563121.
14. Ward BK, Carey JP, Minor LB. Superior canal dehiscence syndrome: lessons from the first 20 years. Front Neurol. 2017;8:177. https://doi.org/10.3389/fneur.2017.00177. PMID: 28503164 PMCID: PMC5408023.
15. Lookabaugh S, Kelly HR, Carter MS, et al. Radiologic classification of superior canal dehiscence: implications for surgical repair. Otol Neurotol. 2015;36(1):118–25. https://doi.org/10.1097/MAO.0000000000000523. PMID: 25122602.
16. Sequeira SM, Whiting BR, Shimony JS, Vo KD, Hullar TE. Accuracy of computed tomography detection of superior canal dehiscence. Otol Neurotol. 2011;32(9):1500–5. https://doi.org/10.1097/MAO.0b013e318238280c. PMID: 22072261.
17. Carey JP, Minor LB, Nager GT. Dehiscence or thinning of bone overlying the superior semicircular canal in a temporal bone survey. Arch Otolaryngol Head Neck Surg. 2000;126(2):137–47. https://doi.org/10.1001/archotol.126.2.137. PMID: 10680863.
18. Williamson RA, Vrabec JT, Coker NJ, Sandlin M. Coronal computed tomography prevalence of superior semicircular canal dehiscence. Otolaryngol Head Neck Surg. 2003;129(5):481–9. https://doi.org/10.1016/s0194-5998(03)01391-3. PMID: 14595270.
19. Branstetter BF, Harrigal C, Escott EJ, Hirsch BE. Superior semicircular canal dehiscence: oblique reformatted CT images for diagnosis. Radiology. 2006;238(3):938–42. https://doi.org/10.1148/radiol.2382042098. PMID: 16424241.
20. Browaeys P, Larson TL, Wong ML, Patel U. Can MRI replace CT in evaluating semicircular canal dehiscence? AJNR Am J Neuroradiol. 2013;34(7):1421–7. https://doi.org/10.3174/ajnr.A3459. PMID: 23518357 PMCID: PMC8051493.
21. Crovetto M, Whyte J, Rodriguez OM, Lecumberri I, Martinez C, Elexpuru J. Anatomo-radiological study of the superior semicircular canal dehiscence radiological considerations of superior and posterior semicircular canals. Eur J Radiol. 2010;76(2):167–72. https://doi.org/10.1016/j.ejrad.2009.05.038. PMID: 19540691.
22. Russo JE, Crowson MG, DeAngelo EJ, Belden CJ, Saunders JE. Posterior semicircular canal dehiscence: CT prevalence and clinical symptoms. Otol Neurotol. 2014;35(2):310–4. https://doi.org/10.1097/MAO.0000000000000183. PMID: 24366470.
23. Wackym PA, Balaban CD, Zhang P, Siker DA, Hundal JS. Third window syndrome: surgical management of cochlea-facial nerve dehiscence. Front Neurol. 2019;10:1281. https://doi.org/10.3389/fneur.2019.01281. PMID: 31920911 PMCID: PMC6923767.
24. Philip A, Mammen MD, Lepcha A, Alex A. Posterior semicircular canal dehiscence: a diagnostic and surgical conundrum. BMJ Case Rep. 2019;12(7):e229573. https://doi.org/10.1136/bcr-2019-229573. PMID: 31270089 PMCID: PMC6613962.

25. Gadre AK, Edwards IR, Baker VM, Roof CR. Membranous or hypermobile stapes footplate: a new anatomic site resulting in third window syndrome. Front Neurol. 2020;11:871. https://doi.org/10.3389/fneur.2020.00871. PMID: 32973657 PMCID: PMC7468399.
26. Boston M, Halsted M, Meinzen-Derr J, et al. The large vestibular aqueduct: a new definition based on audiologic and computed tomography correlation. Otolaryngol Head Neck Surg. 2007;136(6):972–7. https://doi.org/10.1016/j.otohns.2006.12.011. PMID: 17547990.
27. Ozgen B, Cunnane ME, Caruso PA, Curtin HD. Comparison of 45 degrees oblique reformats with axial reformats in CT evaluation of the vestibular aqueduct. AJNR Am J Neuroradiol. 2008;29(1):30–4. https://doi.org/10.3174/ajnr.A0735. PMID: 17947373 PMCID: PMC8119096.
28. Hourani R, Carey J, Yousem DM. Dehiscence of the jugular bulb and vestibular aqueduct: findings on 200 consecutive temporal bone computed tomography scans. J Comput Assist Tomogr. 2005;29(5):657–62. https://doi.org/10.1097/01.rct.0000175499.34213.5d. PMID: 16163038.
29. Blake DM, Tomovic S, Vazquez A, Lee HJ, Jyung RW. Cochlear-facial dehiscence—a newly described entity. Laryngoscope. 2014;124(1):283–9. https://doi.org/10.1002/lary.24223. PMID: 23712934.
30. Kim HH, Wilson DF. A third mobile window at the cochlear apex. Otolaryngol Head Neck Surg. 2006;135(6):965–6. https://doi.org/10.1016/j.otohns.2005.04.006. PMID: 17141096.
31. Andreu-Arasa VC, Sung EK, Fujita A, Saito N, Sakai O. Otosclerosis and dysplasias of the temporal bone. Neuroimaging Clin N Am. 2019;29(1):29–47. https://doi.org/10.1016/j.nic.2018.09.004. PMID: 30466643.

Part III
Treatment

Gerard J. Gianoli

Introduction

When I, Gerard Gianoli, graduated from medical school, the only reasonable option for vestibular schwannoma (VS) treatment was surgical resection. In fact, at that time, it was believed that the earlier the resection the better, since VS represented a progressive disorder that would require surgery when it threatened brainstem compression. So, the sooner it was diagnosed, the smaller it was and the less risk for complications from surgery. Shortly thereafter, stereotactic radiotherapy was introduced as a nonsurgical means for treating VS. This was extremely controversial at the time, but over the years has become another mainstream option for VS patients. As imaging for VS moved from CT scan to MRI scan, smaller tumors were identified. For a variety of reasons, some were managed by observation and serial imaging. This led to the realization that not all VS need any treatment. Consequently, another option available to VS, beyond surgery and stereotactic radiotherapy, is now observation with imaging surveillance.

Similarly, the treatment option for SSCD when initially reported was surgery: a middle fossa craniotomy with occlusion of the superior canal. This then expanded into other surgical options—resurfacing, capping—and other surgical approaches. Then window reinforcement was introduced. Currently, the "mainstream" treatment for TMWD is surgical occlusion repair, or window reinforcement surgery. However, as we learn about the physiology and etiology of TMWD we should expect to see the treatment options expand. In this section, a variety of surgical procedures are discussed, but additional measures to manage TMWD are also presented, including medical therapy, vision-related therapy, and endovascular procedures. Some of these procedures may be supplanted in the future with new options, but if history is our guide, a more likely outcome is an expansion of treatment options to better tailor our approach to the individual patient's needs.

Chapter 13
Medical Therapy

Gerard J. Gianoli and James S. Soileau

There are a multitude of papers detailing surgical treatments for superior semicircular canal dehiscence (SSCD) and other third mobile window disorders (TMWD). However, there is scant mention of medical or non-surgical treatment options, let alone papers dedicated to options/outcomes for medical treatment. There are obvious benefits for successful medical management of TMWD. These include reduced risk, reduced discomfort, and reduced cost. Another potential benefit would be better patient outcomes for some of the symptoms not so well controlled with surgery.

SSCD existed prior to its first report in 1998 [1]. In the pre-1998 days, SSCD patients were typically diagnosed with other otologic conditions. Among these were Ménière's disease, atypical Ménière's disease (vestibular hydrops/cochlear hydrops), perilymph fistula, and vestibular migraine.

One of the first SSCD surgeries in 1998 we performed was a patient with a Ménière's presentation [2]. Two years prior to his presentation, he had been treated with a vestibular nerve section for left-sided aural fullness, hearing fluctuation and episodic vertigo, after a prior unsuccessful endolymphatic sac procedure. He presented to us with similar symptoms on the right side. A CT scan at the time demonstrated bilateral SSCD. A middle fossa craniotomy with repair of the right SSCD resolved his vertigo, right-sided fullness, and hearing fluctuation. Unfortunately for the patient, the left side that had undergone the vestibular nerve section had persistence of hearing fluctuation and fullness.

Similarly, we have witnessed many patients over the past 24 years who had SSCD and had been previously treated for a presumed diagnosis of Ménière's disease. Unlike our patient in 1998, some of these patients did extremely well being managed with conventional Ménière's disease treatment strategies. In 2015, a 75-year-old man presented to us with a 2-year history of right-sided fullness,

G. J. Gianoli (✉) · J. S. Soileau
Ear and Balance Institute, Covington, LA, USA

G. J. Gianoli, P. Thomson (eds.), *Third Mobile Window Syndrome of the Inner Ear*, https://doi.org/10.1007/978-3-031-16586-3_13

hearing fluctuation, and episodic vertigo lasting hours per spell—often precipitated by straining. He had a similar presentation 25 years earlier and was treated with right endolymphatic sac surgery. He requested that we simply "do that same surgery that worked so well 25 years ago." CT scan demonstrated bilateral SSCD and his Valsalva, Fistula, and Tullio tests were abnormal in the right ear. We performed a right SSCD repair via a combined transmastoid-middle fossa approach. He has been free of vertigo since SSCD repair, but he was vertigo free for 23 years after his right endolymphatic sac surgery in 1990. While these examples involve surgery, we have witnessed those who have done extremely well with medical management techniques employed for Ménière's disease as well.

In the management of perilymph fistula (PLF) patients, traditional medical management often involves a period of bedrest and restriction from straining. Again, a considerable number of PLF patients will have had success with such conservative measures. It is interesting to note that many patients previously thought to have PLF, have SSCD and other TMWD.

Many SSCD patients who have successful relief of vertigo and autophony will continue to have persistent symptoms after successful surgical treatment. Of note is the symptom of aural fullness which we and others have found to not be reliably relieved by surgical intervention [3]. An interesting study by Ray et al. [4] looked at 33 ears in 24 patients with SSCD. These patients underwent a 4-h delayed intravenous Gd-enhanced 3D-FLAIR MRI using a compartmental endolymphatic hydrops grading system. They found 27.3% had MRI findings of endolymphatic hydrops. There was no correlation to cVEMP or oVEMP testing, but they did find a greater degree of sensorineural hearing loss in the hydropic patients. Similarly, other MRI studies of SSCD patients have reported 23–80% prevalence of endolymphatic hydrops [4–6]. While it is certainly possible that these may be concomitant Ménière's along with SSCD, this does raise the question as to whether endolymphatic hydrops is part of, or sequela of, SSCD pathophysiology. The corollary is the question of whether traditional medical management of Ménière's would be effective medical management of SSCD.

TMWD is a pressure problem resulting from increased compliance in the inner ear resulting in abnormal cochlear and vestibular stimulation. We propose that anything that reduces the pressure exerted on the inner ear will tend to improve the resulting symptoms from abnormal stimulation. These abnormal pressure influences result from both internal (intracranial) and/or external (middle ear) pressure waves. Surgical repair results in significant reduction in these pressure waves by reducing the inner ear compliance. Medical therapy does not change the inner ear compliance but is aimed at reducing the pressure waves.

These patient experiences led us to reconsider the concept of medical management for SSCD and TMWD in general. We now employ some of these measures before considering surgery in SSCD or TMWD patients. This chapter will detail specifics on medical management of TMWD. We estimate that over half of our patients who would have been considered surgical candidates, respond to a combination of medical measures we describe in this chapter.

One of the biggest challenges facing treatment based on symptoms of TWMD is the variability of symptoms—and their overlap with other disease processes. For some patients, aural fullness or pseudo-conductive hyperacusis is most concerning, whereas others are most bothered by autophony, pulsatile tinnitus, imbalance, or vertigo provoked by sound or pressure. The finding of SSCD on CT scan does not imply causation of symptoms. For instance, we all have seen patients with CT evidence of SSCD and aural fullness, found to have bruxism and temporomandibular joint disorder, which when treated, resolved the aural fullness. Patients also exhibit symptoms related to damage associated with these abnormal pressure waves. These symptoms are treated with supportive care such as antinausea medications and vestibular rehabilitation aimed at expediting central vestibular compensation and treatment of concomitant BPPV. Awareness of these scenarios must also be considered in medical treatment strategies.

Avoidance of Triggers

In a classic scene from a Marx Brothers movie, the patient, as he lifts his arm, says to the doctor, "Doctor, Doctor! It hurts when I do this!" Groucho Marx, who plays the doctor, replies, "Then don't do that." We have all practiced some variation of "Groucho Marx" medicine throughout our careers, and it certainly applies to TMWD. One of the characteristic symptoms of TMWD is strain-induced vertigo/dizziness. Elimination of straining will eliminate many episodes of vertigo for TMWD patients. Many patients know this from prior experience and will avidly avoid such triggers. However, there is a sizeable number of patients who do not understand that this is one of the triggers for their symptoms until it is pointed out by the clinician. While we explain this to patients, we also give them a handout describing things to avoid (Fig. 13.1). We recommend this be strictly followed for six weeks, while other additional medical measures take effect. This is how we have treated PLF patients in the past and is often at least partially successful in resolving the patients' symptoms. Some of the more obvious factors to clinicians, but less so for patients, are weightlifting and other resistance-type exercises. We are assiduous in discussing these restrictions but still find patients who did not understand that abdominal "crunches" (or other core-muscle exercises) will continue to aggravate their condition.

Similarly, we advocate avoidance of activities where the abdomen/chest/head are subjected to major pressure altering conditions. Among these is childbirth by vaginal delivery. We have witnessed many SSCD patients describe their symptoms to occur or worsen after a vaginal delivery. We discuss cesarean section deliveries for our pregnant patients, if medically reasonable. Although anecdotal, we have not seen any exacerbation of TMWD with c-section births.

Another common complaint we have encountered is onset or worsening of TMWD after a non-otologic surgical procedure performed under general anesthesia. When undergoing general anesthesia there are a number of factors that cause large intracranial pressure changes. Patients are pre-hydrated with IV fluids to treat dehydration from an NPO status and to avoid a drop in blood pressure during induction. This fluid loading will cause a rise in intracranial pressure to some degree. After surgery, the patients are often not extubated until fully awake and coughing

EBI Ear& Balance Institute

Gerard J. Gianoli, M.D.
James S. Soileau, M.D.
Kacie S. Harvey, Au.D.

Practice limited to Otology and Neurotology
1401 Ochsner Blvd., Suite A
Covington, Louisiana 70433
985-809-1111
www.earandbalance.net

LABYRINTHINE DEHISCENCE-FISTULA PRECAUTIONS

A labyrinthine dehiscence-fistula is an abnormal opening somewhere around the inner ear. In this condition, the fluid can shift out of the inner ear into another space, such as the middle ear. When this happens, this can tear delicate membranes in the inner ear and cause vertigo/dizziness, tinnitus (ringing in the ear) and hearing loss. Initial treatment of this is geared toward reducing any pressure directed toward the ear. Often, we use dietary methods such as restricting caffeine or salt in the diet to reduce the pressure on the ear. Sometimes a diuretic or fluid pill will be used to reduce fluid pressure as well. In addition, there are a number of activities that you should refrain from in order to reduce pressure on the ear and reduce this from being a problem. Among these are the following:

1.) Avoidance of nose blowing or sneezing through the nose. Sniffing is okay and does not seem to affect the pressure in the inner ear. If you have to sneeze, open your mouth to sneeze. Please do not stifle a sneeze since this is worse than actually sneezing through the nose.

2.) Avoid any strenuous activity. In particular, any activity that increases the pressure in your abdomen or chest will get transmitted to the head and consequently to your inner ears. In general, any activity that requires more effort than lifting 10 pounds should be avoided.

3.) Avoid bending over at the waist. If you need to pick up something off the ground, bend at the knees.

4.) Sexual activity is also restricted since this will place significant pressure on the inner ears as well.

5.) Straining can occur during times of constipation and should be avoided when having a bowel movement. Also, because of this, we recommend a stool softener.

6.) If at all possible, we recommend the period of fistula precautions should begin with 5 days of bed rest with the head elevated above the heart. During this time period you should only get out of bed to go to the bathroom.

7.) If you have a chronic cough or problems with nasal congestion/chronic sneezing, you should contact your physician for aggressive treatment of this since this will make your situation much worse.

8.) Do not use earplugs. You can use cotton with Vaseline to prevent water from getting in the ear.

9.) It is also recommended that you not have any dental work, massages, chiropractic work or physical therapy, during this 6-week period.

The above-mentioned restrictions generally apply for a 6-week period. If you develop any episodes of vertigo during this time period, please note which activities seem to provoke the spell and record them for later consultation. Many patients with perilymphatic fistulas find that this will significantly improve their symptoms. However, if it does not, surgical repair may be required in order to treat your perilymphatic fistula.

NOTE: NOTIFY DOCTOR IMMEDIATELY IF YOU EXPERIENCE LEG PAIN OR SHORTNESS OF BREATH.

Fig. 13.1 Patient handout describing the physical restrictions employed as an initial means to control vertigo triggers. This handout is routinely given to our TMWD patients and is rigidly enforced for the first six weeks of medical therapy, while other medical measures are begun to reduce intracranial pressure (diet and carbonic anhydrase inhibitors or diuretics). After six weeks, the physical restrictions are relaxed but the principle of avoidance of extreme straining remains

with the endotracheal tube in place. This coughing against the endotracheal tube will further cause transient significant increases in intracranial pressure (ICP). Lastly, postoperative nausea and vomiting will add to the pressure increases from above. To minimize the risk to the TMW defect, we make recommendations to the anesthesiologists in Fig. 13.2. Since instituting this strategy, we have not seen any patient with worsening of TMWD after surgery with general anesthesia.

Anesthesia Considerations for Patients with Inner Ear Pathology Undergoing Non-ear Surgery

- Limit the amount of I.V. hydration
- Hyperventilation if possible (CO_2: 26-30)
- Avoid significant intra-thoracic, intra-abdominal or intra-cranial pressure changes
- Consider using an LMA (laryngeal mask airway) if feasible
- Deep extubation if possible (i.e., avoid straining/coughing on endotracheal tube)
- Anti-emetics as indicated – Please consider using high dose Zofran (12 mg IV) preop.

Fig. 13.2 These are the recommendations for anesthesia care of the TMWD patient who is undergoing general anesthesia. The goal is to avoid large changes in intracranial pressure to prevent subsequent exacerbation or recurrence of vestibular symptoms

A very characteristic symptom of TMWD is sound-induced dizziness or Tullio phenomenon. Avoidance of very noisy environments may be possible for some patients but not for others. Where avoidance of noise is not possible, noise-cancelling devices (NCD) offer help. While barrier ear plugs or earmuffs are capable of attenuating high frequency noise (>1 kHz), they are not very useful for attenuating low frequency noise (<1 kHz). Unfortunately, low frequencies are the most inciting sounds for TMWD. Noise-cancelling devices with active sound reduction are aimed at reducing low frequency noise. Noise-cancelling devices employ microphones to measure incoming low frequency sound and have an active output of low frequency sound in the opposite phase (anti-phase) of the incoming sound. This results in the "cancellation" effect [7]. Theoretically, NCDs would significantly reduce both low and high frequency sound-induced vestibular stimulation in sound-sensitive patients who wear them.

Feinberg et al. recently published the "Inverse Tullio Effect" [8]. In this paper, they reported the use of NCDs in TMWD patients resulting in significant resolution of many of their symptoms. However, the most interesting finding was that 40% of the patients treated with NCDs were not aware of any sound sensitivity prior to NCD use. We are bathed in sound and never outside of sound. Even inside a sound-proof booth, noise is present. ANSI (American National Standards Institute) maximum permissible sound levels in audiology sound-proof booths range from 19.5 to 47.5 dB SPL, depending on frequency [9]. It reasons that these patients did not complain of noise sensitivity because they were always exposed to everyday, ambient noise until they went through a trial with an NCD.

Otic barotrauma with eustachian tube dysfunction is a common entity, especially with air travel and scuba diving. Usually this results in nothing worse than otalgia during airplane descent. However, in TMWD patients, otic barotrauma can cause significant exacerbations in vertigo/dizziness and hearing loss [10]. Of course, not all TMWD will have ETD, but for those who do, we advocate proactive measures to prevent otic barotrauma. These measures include nasal decongestants, "Earplanes" and, if these are unsuccessful, myringotomy or ventilation tube placement. Figure 13.3 is the handout we give to patients with TMWD who plan on air travel.

EBI Ear& Balance Institute

Gerard J. Gianoli, M.D., F.A.C.S.
James S. Soileau, M.D.
Kacie S. Harvey, Au.D.
Practice limited to Otology and Neurotology
1401 Ochsner Blvd., Suite A
Covington, Louisiana 70433
985-809-1111

Air flights and the Ear

Airplane flights have been known to aggravate ear problems – both middle ear and inner ear problems. Certain ear problems (**Meniere's syndrome, perilymphatic fistula** and **eustachian tube dysfunction**) have a much higher incidence of worsening during air flights.

If you are planning a trip, flying by plane can certainly aggravate your ear problems. Air travel is always a risk for creating or aggravating inner ear problems. So, the safest thing to do is to avoid air travel and use an alternative transportation – car, bus, train, etc. If you must fly, you should be aware that problems with vertigo may occur and permanent irreversible hearing loss may occur (even if you have never experienced hearing loss as part of your ear problem before). If you must fly, there are several precautions you should take:

1. Use a topical decongestant such as Afrin (if okay with your doctor) before the flight and right before the airplane descends.
2. Do not blow air into your ears to make them "pop" or blow your nose. This can injure your inner ear. Instead chew gum to help open your ears.
3. Do not do anything strenuous during the flight.
4. Avoid caffeine immediately before and during the flight.
5. Never fly with a cold, sinus infection or nasal congestion. Cancel or change your flight if this occurs.
6. If after an air flight you experience hearing loss, tinnitus (ringing in the ear), vertigo, ear pain or a persistent blocked sensation in your ear, you should see an experienced ear doctor immediately.

Fig. 13.3 Patient handout that includes tips on avoidance of problems with air travel. Most TMWD patients do not have significant eustachian tube dysfunction (ETD) and can fly without significant problems, but there is a sizeable portion of TMWD patients who do have ETD. Air travel in this group can provoke significant exacerbation of symptoms. For those with severe ETD, myringotomy and/or ventilation tube placement may be necessary

Upper respiratory tract infections (URI) and allergy flare-ups have been linked to vestibular disorders by multiple studies [11–13]. While multiple theories on the pathophysiology that links URI and allergy with vestibular disorders have been proposed, there is one aspect common to both that has been overlooked. Both URI and allergy are associated with frequent and often vigorous nose-blowing and coughing. Nose-blowing and coughing are known triggers for TMWD. We have employed proactive control of URI and allergy to prevent nose-blowing and coughing to improve the frequency and severity of TMWD symptoms in our patients. We caution our patients against nose-blowing and recommend sniffing, nasal lavage and judicious use of nasal decongestants and cough suppressants during URI. For allergy, we encourage aggressive treatment by their allergy specialists.

Diet

Given the finding of endolymphatic hydrops in SSCD patients mentioned above, it suggests looking at prior medical measures aimed at Ménière's that may be borrowed for use in TMWD. Dietary advice given to our patients include traditional Ménière's diet—avoidance of salt and caffeine [14]. We also discuss the Migraine diet and if there are food triggers for the patient, they are advised to avoid them [15]. We have found a subset of TMWD patients who are sensitive to dietary triggers while others who are not. For this subset, diet is an important aspect of medical therapy.

Medication

Carbonic anhydrase inhibitors have been a mainstay in our medical armamentarium [16]. Acetazolamide is the most prescribed medication of Idiopathic Intracranial Pressure (IIH), and we find it the most useful in TMWD. We suspect the mechanism is the same as in IIH—reduction in ICP. Reduction in ICP will reduce pressure transmission to the TMW and reduce abnormal vestibular stimulation. We find this to be extremely helpful in half of SSCD patients and a higher percent of non-SSCD TMWD patients. The major criticism of acetazolamide is the prevalence of side effects which most commonly include paresthesia, taste disturbance and fatigue. To avoid these side effects, we employ a titration strategy, starting with a low dose and gradually increasing the dose until there is either a resolution of symptoms or the patient cannot tolerate higher doses due to side effects. The range of dosing we have found successful has been very wide—62.5 mg/day to 4000 mg/day—but most patients take 500–1000 mg/day. To limit the side effect of fatigue, we like to use the extended-release version of acetazolamide and have the patient take it at night, prior to bedtime. Patients on carbonic anhydrase inhibitors must be tested initially and monitored periodically with a complete metabolic panel. For patients unable to take acetazolamide due to renal problems or untoward side effects, methazolamide may be substituted.

While we favor carbonic anhydrase inhibitors as our medication of choice, there will be a sizeable portion of patients who cannot use them. For this group, we will employ standard diuretics as we have traditionally used to treat endolymphatic hydrops [16]. While there can certainly be differential dosing to control symptoms, compared to acetazolamide there is less leeway in dosing due to concern of dehydration, hypotension, and diminishing benefits with higher doses of diuretics.

Among medications used in PLF patients are stool softeners to prevent constipation and, hence straining. We find that most patients do not need this, but we discuss this with each patient since they may need this at some point in the future. We have also had a couple of patients with extreme constipation that was integral in the development of TMWD. In those patients, control of their constipation resulted in control of their TMWD symptoms.

Anxiety and panic attacks are found more frequently among patients with vestibular disorders [17] and among TMWD in particular [18]. Control of anxiety and panic attacks will not abate vertigo but can greatly improve the quality of life for these patients. We advocate the use of SSRI for this purpose and have found them helpful controlling these symptoms. We recommend avoidance of long-term (>2 weeks) use of benzodiazepines due to the problems with habituation. There has been a practice of placing patients on daily benzodiazepines—to suppress vestibular function and "prevent" anxiety/panic—which we believe should be highly discouraged. These medications do not resolve the problem of anxiety/panic spells and leads to the additional problem of addiction in the long term. While many clinicians treating vestibular disorders may feel uncomfortable in managing anxiety and panic disorders associated with vertigo, referral to primary care or psychiatry for management would be appropriate.

Migraine has been associated with vertigo, dizziness, and superior canal dehiscence in particular. Migraine has significant symptom overlap with TMWD and has been shown to prolong recovery after SSCD surgery [19]. Given the possibility of overlapping conditions, medical management of migraine prior to planning surgical intervention for TMWD seems prudent, since resolution of migraine may obviate the patient's desire for surgical intervention. Furthermore, given the prolonged recovery noted among migraine patients after SSCD surgery, it would also seem sensible to treat migraine preoperatively. However, it remains to be seen whether preoperative treatment of migraine will improve the longer recovery, and hopefully this will be delineated with future research. Management of migraine entails trigger avoidance, dietary modifications, and medication. For clinicians not comfortable with migraine management, referral to a neurologist is advised.

Other medications we employ are typical of supportive care given to vertiginous patients, including vestibular suppressants and anti-nausea agents. However, we impress upon our patients that these medications are for use only when symptomatic and not for routine use. Routine use of these medications will cause adverse effects on central compensation.

Microprism Lenses

More recently, we have come to recognize that a subset of TMWD patients have visual misalignment. There can be a multitude of symptoms arising from this and these patients can be identified using the binocular vision dysfunction questionnaire [20]. We refer to Neuro-Optometry/Ophthalmology for further evaluation and treatment in these cases. For an in-depth discussion of management of binocular vision dysfunction, see Chap. 14.

Sleep Apnea Evaluation

With the rising incidence of obesity in our society, we have seen a rise in sleep related breathing disorders, such as obstructive sleep apnea (OSA) [21]. OSA has been associated with a higher incidence of peripheral vestibular disorders (particularly Ménière's, BPPV, and sudden hearing loss) than those who do not have OSA [22, 23]. OSA has also been associated with Idiopathic Intracranial Pressure (IIP), transient increases in intracranial pressure, and spontaneous CSF leak [24, 25]. While IIP has been implicated as a possible etiologic role in the development of SSCD (see Chaps. 2 and 19), changes in intracranial pressure (ICP) is one of the main triggers of vertigo in TMWD. Treatment of OSA with CPAP has been demonstrated to improve symptoms and audiometric outcomes in Ménière's [26] as well as non-Ménière's spells of vertigo [27]. Whether OSA and/or IIP have any association with TMWD, however, is immaterial considering the other, far-reaching negative health effects of untreated OSA. Careful assessment of patients at risk for OSA, namely obese patients and those with narrowed airways, should include polysomnography and appropriate referral to a sleep specialist.

Other Medical Problems

The frequent finding of endolymphatic hydrops among SSCD patients suggests that medical measures aimed at its treatment may be reasonably employed. Additionally, control of any associated medical problems would also seem judicious. Many medical problems have been associated with endolymphatic hydrops, including allergy, autoimmune, metabolic, and endocrine (in particular hypothyroidism) disorders [28]. The basic tenant of treating Ménière's disease is to medically optimize treatment of these medical problems prior to considering surgical intervention. We think this same approach is reasonable for TMWD.

Postoperative Medical Therapy

Immediately postoperative, surgeons usually have routine medications dispensed for the expectations of pain, nausea, constipation, etc. In addition to these we prescribe high dose prednisone for 7–10 days with a subsequent taper. The rationale for this is to reduce any inflammatory response which could result in hearing loss and vestibular loss. As to how much, and for how long, we are simply speculating. This would be a good area for future research to help determine (1) are steroids effective for this purpose? (2) if so, are they more beneficial than the potential side effects encountered? (3) and which steroids and for how long? At this point we do not know.

SSCD surgery has been demonstrated to be quite effective for control of vestibular symptoms and autophony but much less so for other symptoms. We have witnessed this in our patients and have found the medical measures detailed above have frequently resulted in resolution or improvement in these symptoms. Again, we are not aware of any detailed analysis of this, but the symptoms that seem most amenable to these medical measures include aural fullness, otalgia, pulsatile tinnitus, hyperacusis, and residual autophony.

Physical Therapy

Vestibular rehabilitation therapy is most successful when treating a fixed peripheral vestibular lesion. By nature, TMWD are fluctuant, due to changes with sound and pressure evoked stimuli. As noted above, many of these patients will have symptom resolution with the medical measures discussed earlier in this chapter. However, in some patients, vestibular loss has occurred, and the patient will exhibit some symptoms attributable to an uncompensated vestibulopathy. If the lesion can be stabilized with medical and/or surgical intervention, vestibular rehabilitation should be employed to complete central vestibular compensation.

Conclusion

As mentioned earlier, there are no controlled trials of non-surgical treatment of TMWD. However, the otologic literature is filled with medical measures employed in the treatment of other vestibular disorders with varying success—and many of the patients in these studies almost certainly had TMWD. Our collective experience with TMWD patients over the past 24 years strongly suggests that medical therapy has a place in the management of TMWD. Especially for patients with mild symptoms and for patients who have persistent symptoms postoperatively, medical management may fill the void that has been present in TMWD.

References

1. Minor LB, Solomon D, Zinreich JS, Zee DS. Sound- and/or pressure-induced vertigo due to bone dehiscence of the superior semicircular canal. Arch Otolaryngol Head Neck Surg. 1998;124(3):249–58. https://doi.org/10.1001/archotol.124.3.249. PMID: 9525507.
2. Smullen JL, Andrist EC, Gianoli GJ. Superior semicircular canal dehiscence: a new cause of vertigo. J La State Med Soc. 1999;151(8):397–400. PMID: 10554474.
3. Ossen ME, Stokroos R, Kingma H, van Tongeren J, Van Rompaey V, Temel Y, van de Berg R. Heterogeneity in reported outcome measures after surgery in superior canal dehiscence syndrome-a systematic literature review. Front Neurol. 2017;8:347. https://doi.org/10.3389/fneur.2017.00347. PMID: 28790965; PMCID: PMC5523725.
4. Ray A, Hautefort C, Guichard JP, Horion J, Herman P, Kania R, Houdart E, Verillaud B, Vitaux H, Attyé A, Eliezer M. MRI contribution for the detection of endolymphatic hydrops in patients with superior canal dehiscence syndrome. Eur Arch Otorhinolaryngol. 2021;278(7):2229–38. https://doi.org/10.1007/s00405-020-06282-3. Epub 2020 Aug 14. PMID: 32797276.
5. Gordon RT, Vining WD. Active noise control: a review of the field. Am Ind Hyg Assoc J. 1992;53(11):721–5. https://doi.org/10.1080/15298669291360427. PMID: 1442563.
6. Sone M, Yoshida T, Morimoto K, Teranishi M, Nakashima T, Naganawa S. Endolymphatic hydrops in superior canal dehiscence and large vestibular aqueduct syndromes. Laryngoscope. 2016;126(6):1446–50. https://doi.org/10.1002/lary.25747. Epub 2015 Nov 3. PMID: 26525170.
7. Johanis M, De Jong R, Miao T, Hwang L, Lum M, Kaur T, Willis S, Arsenault JJ, Duong C, Yang I, Gopen Q. Concurrent superior semicircular canal dehiscence and endolymphatic hydrops: a novel case series. Int J Surg Case Rep. 2021;78:382–6. https://doi.org/10.1016/j.ijscr.2020.12.074. Epub 2020 Dec 26. PMID: 33421957; PMCID: PMC7804363.
8. Feinberg D, Gianoli G, Rosner M. Inverse tullio phenomena: a novel approach to identifying vestibular disorders in patients using a noise cancelling device (NCD) in a binocular vision specialty clinic. Submitted for publication.
9. American National Standards Institute. Maximum permissible ambient noise levels for audiometric test rooms, ANSI S3.1 1991. New York: ANSI; 1991.
10. Kitajima N, Sugita-Kitajima A, Kitajima S. Superior canal dehiscence syndrome associated with scuba diving. Diving Hyperb Med. 2017;47(2):123–6. https://doi.org/10.28920/dhm47.2.123-126. PMID: 28641325; PMCID: PMC6147222.
11. Derebery MJ. Allergic management of Meniere's disease: an outcome study. Otolaryngol Head Neck Surg. 2000;122(2):174–82. https://doi.org/10.1016/S0194-5998(00)70235-X. PMID: 10652386.
12. Jafari Z, Kolb BE, Mohajerani MH. Hearing loss, tinnitus, and dizziness in COVID-19: a systematic review and meta-analysis. Can J Neurol Sci. 2022;49(2):184–95. https://doi.org/10.1017/cjn.2021.63. Epub 2021 Apr 12. PMID: 33843530; PMCID: PMC8267343.
13. Cooper CW. Vestibular neuronitis: a review of a common cause of vertigo in general practice. Br J Gen Pract. 1993;43(369):164–7. PMID: 8323804; PMCID: PMC1372362.
14. Hussain K, Murdin L, Schilder AG. Restriction of salt, caffeine and alcohol intake for the treatment of Ménière's disease or syndrome. Cochrane Database Syst Rev. 2018;12(12):CD012173. https://doi.org/10.1002/14651858.CD012173.pub2.
15. Hindiyeh NA, Zhang N, Farrar M, Banerjee P, Lombard L, Aurora SK. The role of diet and nutrition in migraine triggers and treatment: a systematic literature review. Headache. 2020;60(7):1300–16. https://doi.org/10.1111/head.13836. Epub 2020 May 25. PMID: 32449944; PMCID: PMC7496357.
16. Crowson MG, Patki A, Tucci DL. A systematic review of diuretics in the medical management of Ménière's disease. Otolaryngol Head Neck Surg. 2016;154(5):824–34. https://doi.org/10.1177/0194599816630733. Epub 2016 Mar 1. PMID: 26932948.

17. Beh SC. The neuropsychology of dizziness and related disorders. Otolaryngol Clin N Am. 2021;54(5):989–97. https://doi.org/10.1016/j.otc.2021.05.016. Epub 2021 Jul 20. PMID: 34294432.
18. Wackym PA, Mackay-Promitas HT, Demirel S, Gianoli GJ, Gizzi MS, Carter DM, Siker DA. Comorbidities confounding the outcomes of surgery for third window syndrome: outlier analysis. Laryngosc Investig Otolaryngol. 2017;2(5):225–53. https://doi.org/10.1002/lio2.89. PMID: 29094067; PMCID: PMC5654938.
19. Niesten ME, McKenna MJ, Grolman W, Lee DJ. Clinical factors associated with prolonged recovery after superior canal dehiscence surgery. Otol Neurotol. 2012;33(5):824–31. https://doi.org/10.1097/MAO.0b013e3182544c9e. PMID: 22664897.
20. Feinberg DL, Rosner MS, Rosner AJ. Validation of the binocular vision dysfunction questionnaire (BVDQ). Otol Neurotol. 2021;42(1):e66–74. https://doi.org/10.1097/MAO.0000000000002874. PMID: 33105328.
21. Bibbins-Domingo K, Grossman DC, Curry SJ, Davidson KW, Epling JW Jr, García FA, Herzstein J, Kemper AR, Krist AH, Kurth AE, Landefeld CS, Mangione CM, Phillips WR, Phipps MG, Pignone MP, Silverstein M, Tseng CW, US Preventive Services Task Force. Screening for obstructive sleep apnea in adults: US Preventive Services Task Force recommendation statement. JAMA. 2017;317(4):407–14. https://doi.org/10.1001/jama.2016.20325. PMID: 28118461.
22. Byun H, Chung JH, Jeong JH, Ryu J, Lee SH. Incidence of peripheral vestibular disorders in individuals with obstructive sleep apnea. J Vestib Res. 2022;32(2):155–62. https://doi.org/10.3233/VES-210012. PMID: 34250919.
23. Low WK, Lim EJ. Concomitant obstructive sleep apnoea in patients with Meniere's disease: a case report and literature review. Case Rep Otolaryngol. 2021;2021:5592611. https://doi.org/10.1155/2021/5592611. PMID: 33859856; PMCID: PMC8009700.
24. Rabbani CC, Saltagi MZ, Manchanda SK, Yates CW, Nelson RF. Prevalence of obstructive sleep apnea (OSA) in spontaneous cerebrospinal fluid (CSF) leaks: a prospective cohort study. Otol Neurotol. 2018;39(6):e475–80. https://doi.org/10.1097/MAO.0000000000001805. PMID: 29889790.
25. Sugita Y, Iijima S, Teshima Y, Shimizu T, Nishimura N, Tsutsumi T, Hayashi H, Kaneda H, Hishikawa Y. Marked episodic elevation of cerebrospinal fluid pressure during nocturnal sleep in patients with sleep apnea hypersomnia syndrome. Electroencephalogr Clin Neurophysiol. 1985;60(3):214–9. https://doi.org/10.1016/0013-4694(85)90033-1. PMID: 2578929.
26. Nakayama M, Masuda A, Ando KB, Arima S, Kabaya K, Inagaki A, Nakamura Y, Suzuki M, Brodie H, Diaz RC, Murakami S. A pilot study on the efficacy of continuous positive airway pressure on the manifestations of Ménière's disease in patients with concomitant obstructive sleep apnea syndrome. J Clin Sleep Med. 2015;11(10):1101–7. https://doi.org/10.5664/jcsm.5080. PMID: 26094927. PMCID: PMC4582051.
27. Foster CA, Machala M. The clinical spectrum of dizziness in sleep apnea. Otol Neurotol. 2020;41(10):1419–22. https://doi.org/10.1097/MAO.0000000000002824. PMID: 32740553.
28. Rizk HG, Mehta NK, Qureshi U, Yuen E, Zhang K, Nkrumah Y, Lambert PR, Liu YF, McRackan TR, Nguyen SA, Meyer TA. Pathogenesis and etiology of Ménière disease: a scoping review of a century of evidence. JAMA Otolaryngol Head Neck Surg. 2022;148(4):360–8. https://doi.org/10.1001/jamaoto.2021.4282. PMID: 35142800.

Chapter 14
Visual Manifestations and Treatment: The Intersection of Third Mobile Window Syndrome and Vertical Heterophoria

Debby Feinberg and Mark Rosner

Introduction

The field of optometry has grown significantly from its roots as a specialty concentrating upon the correction of difficulties with visual acuity due to distortions caused by the physical shape of the eye (i.e., nearsightedness, farsightedness, and astigmatism) utilizing corrective lenses. Modern optometry also involves the diagnosis, treatment, and management of diseases and disorders of the eye. They also prescribe medications, perform low vision rehabilitation, practice myopia control, treat glaucoma, prescribe specialty contact lenses, and treat patients with binocular vision conditions or with binocularity. Those working with binocularity include behavioral/developmental optometrists (mainly focused on children with reading/learning difficulties) and neuro-optometrists (treating those with acquired brain injury or ABI). The tools most commonly used for treatment include vision therapy, tints, and focal occlusive techniques (an example would be binasal occlusion).

There currently exists a significant gap in the approach to the treatment of binocular vision dysfunction, which is the ability to consistently and successfully identify and treat very small amounts of vision misalignments known as phorias. Our work, for which we have developed the term "neurovisual medicine," seeks to address this deficiency through the utilization of microprism lenses that aid both in the diagnosis and treatment of phorias.

Supplementary Information The online version contains supplementary material available at [https://doi.org/10.1007/978-3-031-16586-3_14].

D. Feinberg · M. Rosner (✉)
NeuroVisual Medicine Institute, Bloomfield Hills, MI, USA
e-mail: drdebby@nvminstitute.org; drmark@nvminstitute.org

G. J. Gianoli, P. Thomson (eds.), *Third Mobile Window Syndrome of the Inner Ear*, https://doi.org/10.1007/978-3-031-16586-3_14

For several years, our neurovisual medicine practice, while working with patients with vestibular complaints (dizziness, nausea, gait/balance disturbances, and motion sickness), has identified a cohort of patients with third window syndrome (TWS). We have found that noise-cancelling devices (NCDs) are an inexpensive and very safe approach to reduce vestibular symptoms for many patients. Some patients report sufficient symptom improvement that no further treatment is necessary. Others report partial improvement, and are referred to neurotologists for further treatment with medication and/or surgical intervention.

In addition to presenting information about the effectiveness of NCDs, we will describe what we have learned about the underlying causes of these conditions. Our work with patients who benefit from NCDs grew from our discovery that a significant number of patients with severe symptoms, including vestibular dysfunction, reading difficulty, head and neck pain, and anxiety, received significant benefit from lenses that correct for small amounts of vertical heterophoria (VH), a vertical misalignment of the lines of sight in one or both eyes. We will discuss the interaction between visual misalignment and TWS, the impact of sound and hyperacusis on this interaction, the effectiveness of NCDs in the diagnosis and treatment of TWS, and the effectiveness of lenses that correct vertical heterophoria as a treatment for vestibular symptoms of TWS, including dizziness, nausea, and gait/balance disturbances.

Third Window Syndrome and Vertical Heterophoria

TWS is a condition where the seal of the inner ear apparatus is broken by a physical defect, leading to abnormal changes in the fluid pressure of the inner ear. TWS is often associated with Tullio phenomenon, in which patients exposed to sound experience dizziness, vertigo, unstable gait, and nystagmus. Tullio phenomenon is most commonly associated with a dehiscence in the bony surroundings of the vestibular apparatus (frequently the superior semicircular canal) or a perilymph fistula in the round or oval windows [1, 2]. These conditions allow for aberrations to occur to the fluid pressure dynamics and sound wave transmission within the inner ear. In some cases, these abnormalities appear to stimulate the otolith organs, particularly the utricle, in a manner that impacts vertical eye alignment, precipitating VH.

The standard treatment for VH is corrective lenses that include vertical prism which neutralizes the visual misalignment. Optometrists test for VH using two main methods: dissociative techniques that disrupt fusion with one of several tools, including a large diopter prism or a Maddox rod [3, 4] and associative phoria techniques that use dichoptic viewing of a pair of nonius lines, with tests including the Mallett Test, the American Optical (AO) Vectographic Slide, the Wesson Card, the Sheedy Disparometer, and the Saladin Card [5–7].

Diagnosis and Treatment of Vertical Heterophoria

In previous studies, we have found that heterophorias as small as 0.25 diopters (D) can create a wide range of severe symptoms, including dizziness, anxiety, nausea, head and neck pain, and reading issues, which are significantly reduced when patients are treated with vertical microprism correcting for VH (usually between 0.25 and 2.0 D). The authors have published three retrospective studies that show the effect of treatment for VH on symptoms of anxiety, headache and dizziness [8–10]. Participants in the second of these studies generally reported a long history of symptoms and referrals to multiple specialists, including neurology, ENT and ophthalmology, without significant reduction in symptoms. When treated with corrective microprism lenses, they reported dramatic improvement in symptoms in a matter of minutes (Videos 14.1 and 14.2).

After treating thousands of patients, we observed a cohort who continued to experience significant symptoms even after treatment with corrective microprism lenses, and this has led us to develop a hypothesis regarding the underlying processes which points to a link between VH and TWS.

It appears that VH has two different forms with unrelated etiologies. The first type of VH is monocular, and is caused by superior oblique palsy (SOP), which occurs when CN 4 and/or the superior oblique muscle is weak unilaterally, causing supraduction and extorsion of the impacted eye. Monocular VH can be corrected with microprism that corrects vertical misalignment in one eye. While monocular VH interacts with the vestibular system and can cause vestibular symptoms, there does not appear to be any vestibular pathology.

For readers of this chapter, the more significant form of VH is the second type, binocular VH. A patient with binocular VH experiences vertical misalignment in lines of sight in both eyes. We hypothesize that binocular VH is related to a malfunction within the peripheral vestibular apparatus that is mediated through the vestibulo-ocular reflex (VOR), which directs unconscious eye movements that allow a person to maintain visual fixation on a target while their head is in motion. The VOR connects the visual system to parts of the inner-ear vestibular apparatus which affect motion in different axes: the semicircular canals, saccule and utricle. Of these, the utricle is the primary source of automatic vertical eye movement [11].

Pathophysiology of Binocular Vertical Heterophoria

To understand the process by which the binocular vision system and peripheral vestibular system interact, we start with the recognition that the human face is slightly asymmetrical. On a typical face, the eyes are vertically misaligned by 0.5 mm. Misalignments of up to 1 mm are less common, but will appear normal to most observers [12] (Fig. 14.1).

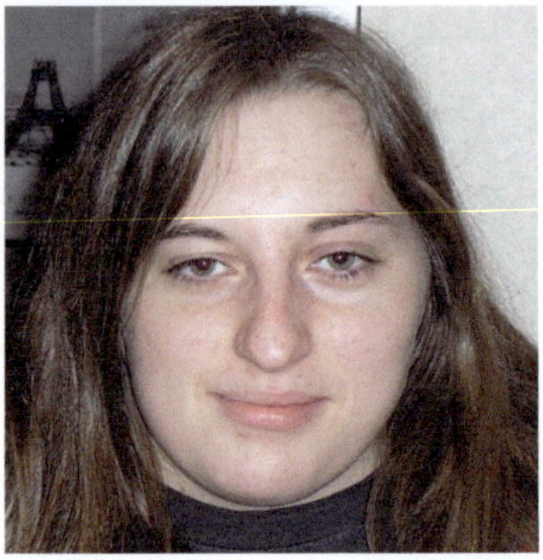

Fig. 14.1 Facial asymmetry. (Published with permission from Debby Feinberg, OD & Mark Rosner, MD). This patient has hemifacial microsomia leading to marked vertical orbital and eye asymmetry

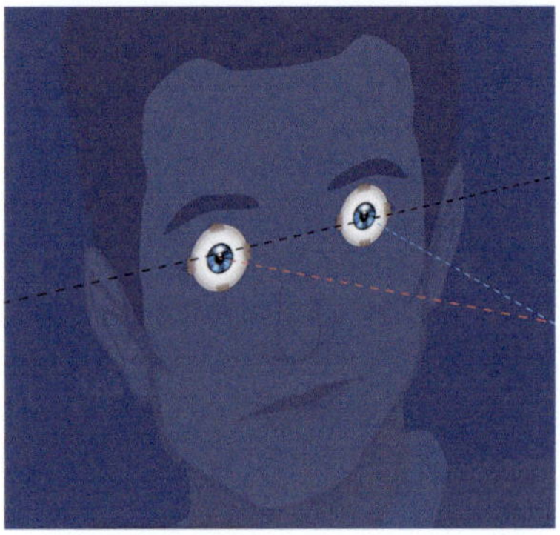

Fig. 14.2 Vertical convergence. (Published with permission from Debby Feinberg, OD & Mark Rosner, MD). Normal vertical convergence. The right eye is lower than the left eye. Note that the higher left eye is hypophoric—the exact opposite of those with superior oblique palsy

Because of this natural vertical asymmetry, the lines of sight of a normal person will not be on the same horizontal plane. The typical angle needed to compensate for typical asymmetry is 1–1.5° (Fig. 14.2).

We theorize that binocular VH is caused by a faulty vertical alignment signal from the utricle that directs the eyes to increase the vertical convergence beyond the amount needed to compensate for that natural asymmetry. The overcompensation appears to be detected by the fusional vergence system as impending diplopia, which results in an adjustment to eliminate the overcompensation. However, the original utricular pathology remains, and once again signals for overcompensation (Fig. 14.3).

This causes a high-frequency cycle of small eye movements, which leads to a remarkably wide range of symptoms. In previous studies, 40–75% of patients reported each of the following symptoms: dizziness, nausea, motion sickness, drifting to one side while walking, sinus pain, neckache, headache, fatigue while reading, eye strain, blurred distance vision, head tilt, losing their place while reading, blurred near vision, light sensitivity, difficulty with reading comprehension, problems with glare, anxiety in crowds, poor depth perception, and anxiety in large spaces. Table 14.1 lists all of the symptoms associated with VH.

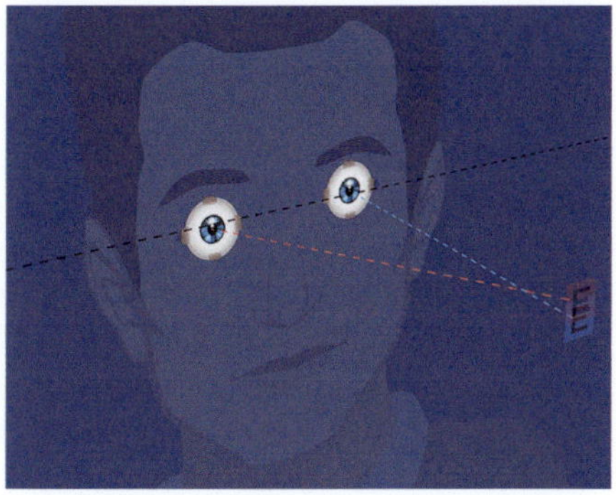

Fig. 14.3 Vertical overconvergence. (Published with permission from Debby Feinberg, OD & Mark Rosner, MD). Note that the line of sight of the lower right eye is hyperphoric, and crosses that of the higher left eye, which is hypophoric, creating impending diplopia

Table 14.1 Symptoms of vertical heterophoria. Published with permission from Debby Feinberg, OD & Mark Rosner, MD

Vestibular symptoms
Dizziness
Drifts to one side while walking
Nausea
Motion sickness
Heterophoria symptoms
Light sensitivity
Problems with reflection or glare
Poor depth perception
Shadowed/overlapping vision
Closing or covering one eye
Double vision
Reading symptoms
Fatigue while reading
Losing your place while reading
Skipping lines while reading
Difficulty with reading comprehension
Pain symptoms
Neck pain
Headache
Head tilt
Sinus pain/pressure
Pain with eye movement
Vision symptoms
Eye strain
Blurred distance vision
Blurred near vision
Anxiety symptoms
Overwhelmed in crowds
Overwhelmed in large spaces

Many patients also report vibrating and shimmering vision, which is also consistent with small, high frequency eye movements.

If this hypothesis is correct, rapid eye motion impairs the ability to fixate. This causes symptoms such as reading difficulty, blurred/shadowed vision or diplopia, and sensitivity to complex visual environments (such as a crowded room, large store, or mall; while watching fast-paced action or 3D in a movie). The extraocular muscles become strained by constant use, causing headache and asthenopia. Vestibular symptoms of dizziness, nausea, impaired gait and balance, and motion sickness are caused by a visual perception of motion that is not matched by the vestibular or proprioceptive systems. Both sensitivity to complex visual environments and dizziness can cause anxiety [13]. Unconscious head tilt, a mechanism to resolve vertical misalignment when the eyes are in a vertically misaligned posture, causes significant neck pain (Fig. 14.4).

The head tilt associated with binocular VH is different from an ocular tilt reaction and from monocular VH (SOP) in its etiology, and effects upon vertical and torsional image displacement (Fig. 14.5).

To correct binocular VH, microprism is introduced base up over the left eye and base down over the right eye, correcting the vertical image disparity, which allows for vertical image fusion and rapid symptom improvement.

Now that the images are realigned, there is no longer impending diplopia, the fusional vergence mechanism is no longer being activated, and the eyes can maintain a stable (though vertically overcompensated) position that is being dictated by the faulty vestibular signal. Our retrospective studies have shown substantial treatment effects [8–10].

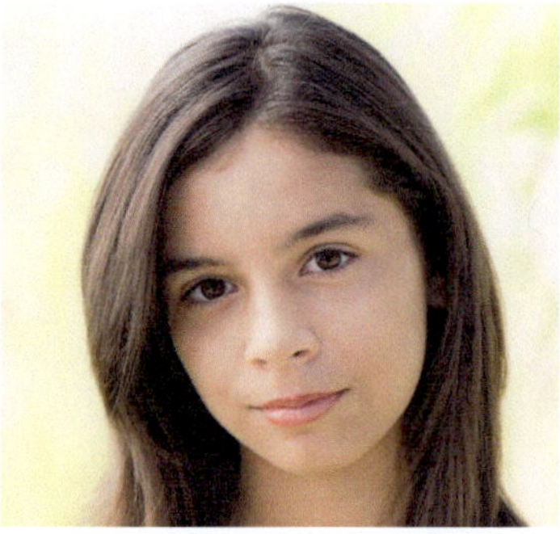

Fig. 14.4 Head tilt to right side. (Photo from Depositphotos, Inc. and was taken by PantherMediaSeller). Note that the hair part is on the high side of the head, which is a "tell" for a chronic head tilt

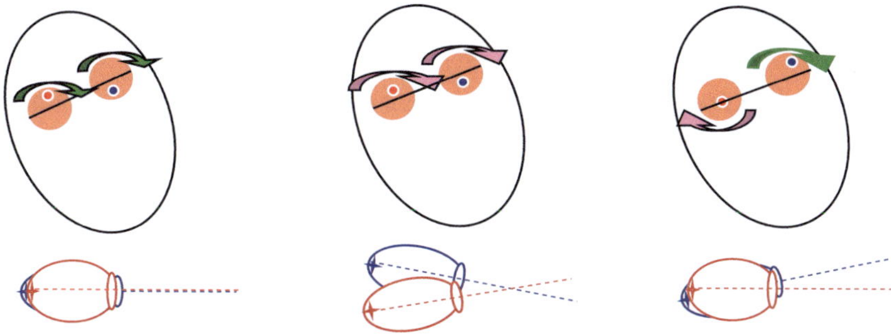

Fig. 14.5 Head tilts: ocular tilt reaction, binocular and monocular VH. (Published with permission from Debby Feinberg, OD & Mark Rosner, MD). The bottom graphic demonstrates eye position and posture at "initial pathology" (sagittal view). The top graphic demonstrates eye position and posture with head tilt

Ocular tilt reaction—Initial "pathology" is a voluntary head tilt, which affects both eyes	**Binocular VH**—Initial pathology (anatomical + vestibular abnormalities) affects both eyes	**Monocular VH**—initial pathology (SOP) affects only 1 eye (high eye = left eye (blue))
Eyes could initially be on the same horizontal plane	Eyes may not initially be on the same horizontal plane	Eyes could initially be on the same horizontal plane
Line of sight/phoric position of high eye is depressed (response to head tilt)—maintains a foveal image—no image misalignment	Line of sight/phoric position of high eye is depressed (initial pathology)—sees a high image	Line of sight/phoric position of high eye is elevated and extorted—see green arrow (initial pathology)—sees a low and extorted image
Line of sight/phoric position of low eye is elevated (response to head tilt)—maintains a foveal image—no image misalignment	Line of sight/phoric position of low eye is elevated (initial pathology)—sees a low image	Line of sight/phoric position of low eye is straight ahead (sees a vertically and torsionally normal image)
Head tilt is the initiating factor, with the eyes changing vertical and torsional position in response. The higher eye depresses, and the lower eye elevates, in order to maintain the image on the foveae and prevent vertical diplopia	Head tilts in an attempt to resolve vertical diplopia causing a compensatory rotary torsion of both eyes (intorsion OD, extorsion OS—see mauve arrows) (secondary pathology)	Head tilts in an attempt to resolve torsional/rotational diplopia, causing an intorsion of the low eye—see mauve arrow (secondary pathology)
Rotary torsion of both eyes in opposite direction as head tilt—see green arrows (response to head tilt)—maintains vertical image alignment	Compensatory rotary torsion keeps image vertical	
	High eye is made even higher with head tilt, placing image closer to fovea	High eye is made even higher with head tilt, worsening vertical image disparity
Patient's perception of diplopia and vertical is not distorted due to phoric and torsional adjustments to head tilt	Prismatic correction of vertical image disparity (base up over left eye; base down over right eye) eliminates head tilt	Prismatic correction of vertical image disparity (base down left eye) does not eliminate extorsion of affected eye—head tilt may still be present

Third Window Syndrome

Serendipitously, one patient reported that upon obtaining an NCD they experienced not only reduction in their sound sensitivity, but also noted marked improvement in their dizziness and gait stability. This led us to investigate our cohort of patients who had persistent dizziness despite microprism correction. At this point we became aware that hyperacusis was present to some degree in this cohort, and that they have a wide array of symptoms (Table 14.2).

We began to administer the Khalfa Sound Sensitivity Questionnaire to these patients and found that a significant number had a high score [14]. Following this evidence, we provided patients with NCDs during their initial examinations and found that they provided significant reduction in symptoms for this group of patients, as well as allowing for a more accurate lens prescription.

This result is consistent with Tullio phenomenon. Additionally, these abnormalities appear to affect the stimulation of the otolith organs (particularly the utricle) in a manner that impacts vertical eye alignment, precipitating a VH. NCDs reduce the amplitude of the sound wave that reaches the ear and the corresponding aberrations to the fluid pressure dynamics that cause Tullio phenomenon.

A study being prepared for publication presents evidence for the effectiveness of NCDs as a method for identifying TWS, as well as a method of treating hyperacusis and dizziness associated with TWS. NCDs attenuate low frequency sound more than ear plugs or muffs, and low-frequency sounds seem to have a disproportionate

Table 14.2 Symptoms of TMW. Published with permission from Debby Feinberg, OD & Mark Rosner, MD

Hyperacusis/sound sensitivity
Sensitive to sound
Sensitivity to the sound of their own heartbeat or voice
Tinnitus
Dizziness/vestibular symptoms
Dizziness or vertigo when producing sound (speaking loudly, singing, coughing)
Dizziness or vertigo caused by physical exertion
Dizziness or vertigo caused by changes in atmospheric pressure
Constant sway in their body
Dizziness or fullness when lying flat
Objects on the horizon appear to move in their field of vision, while walking/running
Physical sensation in ears
Feeling of fluid leaking from ears, without actual fluid leakage
Feeling of fullness in one or both ears
Visual symptoms
Pain while moving eyes
Eye twitching

Table 14.3 Differential diagnoses. Published with permission from Debby Feinberg, OD & Mark Rosner, MD

Atypical Ménière's disease
Migraine-associated vertigo
Vestibular migraine
Labyrinthitis
Vestibular neuronitis
Benign paroxysmal positional vertigo
Chiari malformation
Psychogenic dizziness
Chronic subjective dizziness

effect on the utricle. Some patients report reduction or elimination of hyperacusis and dizziness symptoms when using NCDs (Videos 14.3, 14.4 and 14.5), but others report only limited reduction of symptoms.

In those cases, symptoms can be additionally reduced with medication (carbonic anhydrase inhibitors and/or diuretics) to reduce the fluid pressure in the inner ear. Others have reported additional reduction of Tullio phenomenon symptoms after surgery to repair the dehiscence or the perilymph fistula [15]. There is significant overlap in the presentation and differential diagnoses for TWS and VH, mostly due to the vestibular-type symptoms experienced by those with either condition (Table 14.3).

Feinberg Method for Identifying and Treating Vertical Heterophoria

While there are multiple factors that impede the routine diagnosis of VH by optometrists and ophthalmologists, the most significant is lack of sensitivity of the traditional vertical heterophoria tests. Clinically significant vertical misalignments are too small to be detected reliably by any of the optometric tests for heterophoria. Some of the common tests have never been assessed for test-retest reliability in any published study, but the limited test-retest reliability studies that have been done indicate that the margin of error for the most accurate tests, when performed flawlessly under optimal conditions, is between 2 and 4 D [4, 16–19]. The relationship between test results and actual prescriptions is even more inaccurate: it is common practice to use anywhere from one-third the amount to the full amount of prism indicated by a particular test [20]. We have included multiple tests in our studies, and found that they correctly identify the presence and direction of VH in only 50–60% of patients who respond to treatment with corrective microprism [10].

Because of these limitations of optometric heterophoria tests, other methods are more effective for identifying patients who can be treated with corrective microprism. Patients reporting symptoms that may be related to VH are screened initially with the Binocular Vision Dysfunction Questionnaire (BVDQ), a validated self-reporting instrument that queries VH symptoms including dizziness, anxiety, head and neck pain, reading/comprehension issues, and traditional binocular visual dysfunction at near and far distances [21]. Patients who score at least 15 of a possible

75 points on the BVDQ are candidates for an initial neurovisual examination. The complete exam takes about 80 min and includes the following elements.

1. Trial of NCDs to assess the impact upon gait, balance, and dizziness. If significant, NCDs will be worn throughout the entire exam, as sound will negatively impact the accuracy of the lens prescription, particularly the vertical alignment measurements.
2. Visual acuity examination to identify potential corrections for nearsightedness, farsightedness, and astigmatism.
3. Assessment of discomfort during convergence with a fixation stick (near point of discomfort or NCD testing). The patient brings the fixation stick toward their nose until they experience discomfort, double vision or blur. It is not uncommon for patients to describe discomfort as dizziness, nausea or headache, and for the onset of symptoms to occur prior to diplopic symptoms.
4. Examination for head tilt. Patients with VH often tilt their heads unconsciously to compensate for vertical misalignment by bringing images closer to the foveae (Fig. 14.6).
5. The chronic head tilt leads to overuse of the trapezius muscle and the complaint of neck and upper back pain that is so common in our patients.
6. Gait and balance analysis, used to identify baseline abnormalities. Changes to gait and balance are important indicators of the effectiveness of treatment. The following elements are consistent with different pathologies:

    (a) Unstable rise from seated to standing. Instability with rising indicates a balance problem.

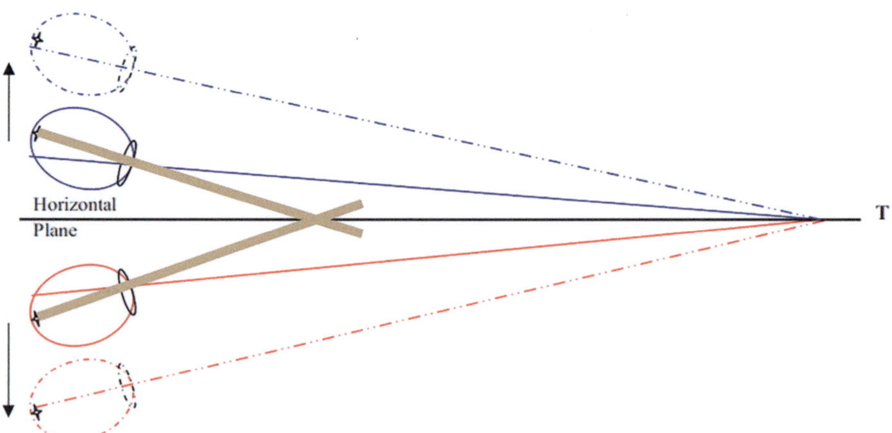

Fig. 14.6 Impact of head tilt on vertical image alignment. (Published with permission from Debby Feinberg, OD & Mark Rosner, MD). Original vertical eye displacement and alignment in solid lines; with head tilt in dotted lines (sagittal view). Beige lines indicate the lines of sight in their vertically crossed position. There is no change in phoric posture/lines of sight when head is tilted. Note that the image strikes the retina a significant distance from the fovea in the original position, but moves much closer to the fovea when the head tilt exaggerates the vertical eye displacement

(b) Drifting to one side with ambulation. A patient who pulls to one side likely has a two-eyed misalignment problem, which is treated somewhat differently than a single-eyed misalignment, as detailed below.
(c) Wobbling side to side ambulation (serpentine gait) which can be indicative of superior oblique palsy.
(d) Unsteady ambulation with head turns ("supermarket walk"). This may indicate a deficiency in visual and vestibular integration.

7. Provocative vestibular tests: bending over and rising quickly, side-to-side head movements.
8. Multiple tests for vertical heterophoria, of which the most consistently useful is the Maddox rod and penlight.

Using the physical findings as a starting point, microprism is added in amounts of 0.25 D until the patient reports a significant reduction in symptoms. The initial exam lasts 80 min.

If a patient's symptoms are caused by VH, treatment with microprism will lead to an immediate and significant reduction in symptoms. If the cause is both TWS and VH, the effect of both is notable (Fig. 14.7).

Rapid resolution of long-term symptoms caused by VH is highly unusual—many patients have reported consistently disabling symptoms for many years. However, from an optometric perspective, there is nothing unusual about treating visual dysfunction with corrective lenses and obtaining rapid results. Better-known symptoms

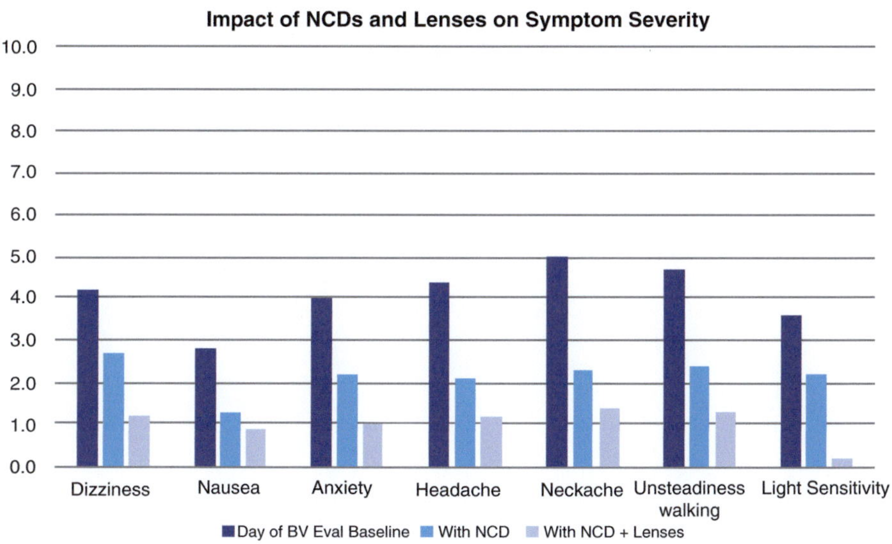

Fig. 14.7 Impact of NCDs and lenses on symptom severity. (Published with permission from Debby Feinberg, OD & Mark Rosner, MD). This patient cohort had both TWS and VH. NCDs were applied first, followed by microprism lenses later in the exam

of heterophoria such as diplopia are readily resolved with corrective lenses, as are severe deficiencies in visual acuity. Correction of heterophoria leads to rapid improvement in functionality.

After the initial exam, patients begin using corrective lenses with the amount of vertical microprism that provides the maximum reduction in symptoms. In most cases, this prescription requires adjustment after 2–4 weeks of use, with a second exam that lasts about 50 min, as the patient's visual system relaxes sufficiently to allow for a more accurate correction. In addition, many patients are prescribed medications that have a significant impact on their muscular and vestibular systems, such as narcotics, benzodiazepines, muscle relaxants or vestibular suppressants. As symptoms improve, the prescribing physicians can reduce or eliminate these medications, which can lead to changes in the vestibular and visual symptoms that require further adjustment to the lens prescription.

Patients who report long-term symptoms as described above are treated for VH with microprism lenses that correct the lines of sight. As demonstrated in the referenced videos, patients respond to treatment quickly and significantly, achieving an average of 80% subjective reduction of symptoms (Videos 14.1, 14.3, 14.4, Fig. 14.8).

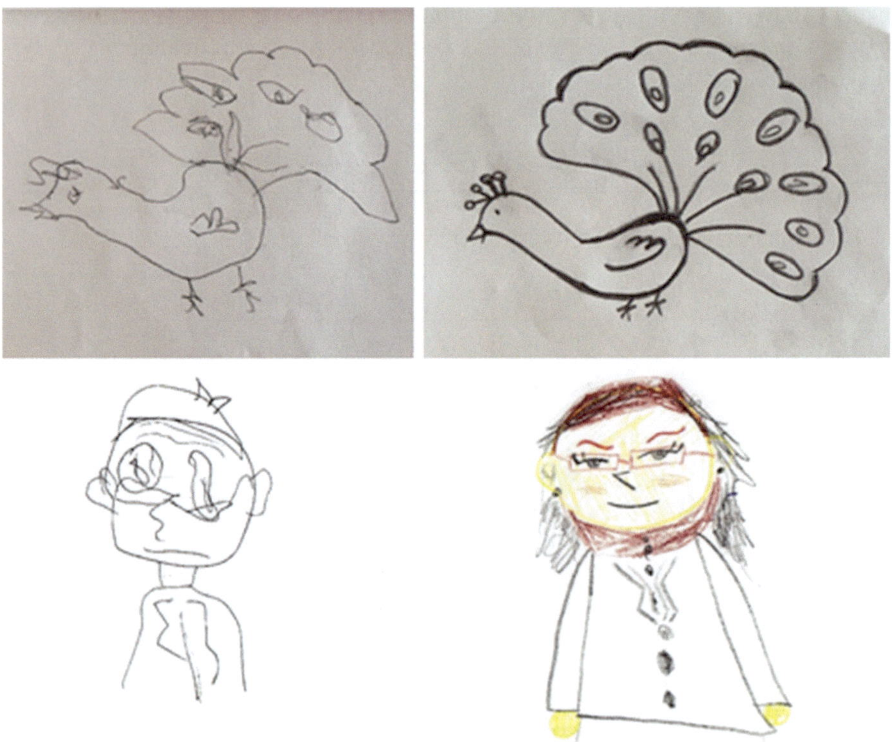

Fig. 14.8 Two examples of fine motor control improvement with microprism lenses in children. (Published with permission from Debby Feinberg, OD & Mark Rosner, MD)

The amount of microprism correction for each of these patients was less than 1 D. In our studies, 68% of patients responded to treatment with a final prescription between 0.5 and 2 D, and 29% had a final prescription of 2.5–4 D. Only 3% had a final prescription greater than 4 D.

Conclusion

TWS and VH share many symptoms, can both be present in the same patient, and are both negatively impacted by sound. This is primarily due to the connectivity of the vestibular and visual systems through the otolith organs and the VOR. NCDs can be utilized to identify those who may have TWS, as a treatment for hyperacusis and its related symptoms, and as an aid to obtain a better microprism lens prescription. Screening patients with TWS for VH using the BVDQ and near point of discomfort testing is straightforward, and helps identify an additional pre- or post-surgical treatment modality for this difficult to treat patient cohort.

Acknowledgment The authors thank Alan Terlep who prepared the text.

References

1. Pullicino R, Grech R. Tullio phenomenon in superior semicircular canal dehiscence (SSCD). BMJ Case Rep. 2015;2015:bcr2015213674. https://doi.org/10.1136/bcr-2015-213674. PMID: 26698215; PMCID: PMC4691913.
2. Fox EJ, Balkany TJ, Arenberg IK. The Tullio phenomenon and perilymph fistula. Otolaryngol Head Neck Surg. 1988;98(1):88–9. https://doi.org/10.1177/019459988809800115. PMID: 3124057.
3. Borish IM. Versions and vergences. In: Clinical refraction. 3rd ed. Chicago, IL: The Professional Press; 1975. p. 189–256.
4. Duke-Elder S, Wybar K. Anomalies of binocular fixation. In: System of opthamology. St. Louis, MO: The C. V. Mosby Company; 1973. p. 513–76.
5. Scheiman M, Wick B. Clinical management of binocular vision: heterophoric, accommodative, and eye movement disorders. 3rd ed. Philadelphia, PA: Wolters Kluwer Health/Lippincott Williams & Wilkins; 2008.
6. Eskridge JB, Amos JF, Bartlett JD. Clinical procedures in optometry. Philadelphia, PA: Lippincott; 1991.
7. Rutstein RP. Anomalies of binocular vision: diagnosis & management. St. Louis, MO: Mosby; 1998.
8. Doble JE, Feinberg DL, Rosner MS, Rosner AJ. Identification of binocular vision dysfunction (vertical Heterophoria) in traumatic brain injury patients and effects of individualized prismatic spectacle lenses in the treatment of postconcussive symptoms: a retrospective analysis. Phys Med Rehabil. 2010;2:244–53.
9. Rosner MS, Feinberg DL, Doble JE, Rosner AJ. Treatment of vertical heterophoria ameliorates persistent post-concussive symptoms: a retrospective analysis utilizing a multi-faceted assessment battery. Brain Inj. 2016;30(3):311–7.

10. Feinberg DL, Rosner MS. Vertical heterophoria treatment ameliorates headache, dizziness and anxiety. Optom Vis Perf. 2020;8(1):24–34.
11. Curthoys IS. The anatomical and physiological basis of clinical tests of otolith function. A tribute to Yoshio Uchino. Front Neurol. 2020;11:566895. https://doi.org/10.3389/fneur.2020.566895.
12. Hohman MH, Kim SW, Heller ES, Frigerio A, Heaton JT, Hadlock TA. Determining the threshold for asymmetry detection in facial expressions. Laryngoscope. 2014;124(4):860–5.
13. Yuan Q, Yu L, Shi D, et al. Anxiety and depression among patients with different types of vestibular peripheral vertigo. Medicine (Baltimore). 2015;94(5):e453.
14. Khalfa S, Dubal S, Veuillet E, Perez-Diaz F, Jouvent R, Collet L. Psychometric normalization of a hyperacusis questionnaire. ORL. 2002;64:436–42. https://doi.org/10.1159/000067570.
15. Suzuki M, Okamoto T, Ushio M, Ota Y. Two cases of Tullio phenomenon in which oval and round window reinforcement surgery was effective. Auris Nasus Larynx. 2019;46(4):636–40. https://doi.org/10.1016/j.anl.2018.10.022. Epub 2018 Dec 17. PMID: 30573214.
16. Gray LS. The prescribing of prisms in clinical practice. Graefes Arch Clin Exp Ophthalmol. 2008;246:627–9.
17. Schroeder TL, Rainey BB, Goss DA, Grosvenor TP. Reliability of and comparisons among methods of measuring dissociated phoria. Optom Vis Sci. 1996;73:389–97.
18. Gall R, Wick B. The symptomatic patient with normal phorias at distance and near: what tests detect a binocular vision problem? Optometry. 2003;74:309–22.
19. Karania R, Evans BJ. The mallett fixation disparity test: influence of test instructions and relationship with symptoms. Opthalmic Physiol Opt. 2006;26:507–22.
20. Wick BB. Prescribing vertical prism: how low can you go? J Optom Vis Dev. 1997;28:77–85.
21. Feinberg DL, Rosner MS, Rosner AJ. Validation of the binocular vision dysfunction questionnaire (BVDQ). Otol Neurotol. 2021;42(1):e66–74. https://doi.org/10.1097/MAO.0000000000002874.

Chapter 15
Surgery, Complication, Revisions

Gerard J. Gianoli

TMWS (third mobile window syndrome) disorders represent a novel era in vestibular diseases. It is not just because of the identification of an anatomic defect on CT scan but they often represent a vestibular problem with a concrete identifiable surgical solution. So much of vestibular medicine is much less tangible, the deficit less readily identifiable, the treatment options less certain, and the results less satisfying.

Surgical Candidacy

When discussing treatment of a TMWS, the first phase is assessing the severity of disease and disability (Table 15.1). There is no definitive formula for this appraisal. While there have been attempts to establish criteria for diagnosis [1], there are no studies published on criteria for who is a surgical candidate. The incidental finding of a dehiscence on a CT scan alone does not fulfill requirements for surgical candidacy. At a minimum, criteria for diagnosis should be met using the triad of (1) historical symptoms consistent with TMWS and symptoms amenable to surgical correction, (2) physiologic testing consistent with a TMWS disorder, and (3) a high-resolution CT scan consistent with a TMWS disorder. A final criterion should include exclusion of other more appropriate diagnoses. Note that in criterion (1) we mention "symptoms amenable to surgical correction." It should be noted that some symptoms are more responsive to surgical intervention than others, and a tailored approach to each patient would be appropriate.

Once a diagnosis has been appropriately made, an assessment of severity of disease burden should be performed. This would include inquiries regarding frequency

G. J. Gianoli (✉)
Ear and Balance Institute, Covington, LA, USA

G. J. Gianoli, P. Thomson (eds.), *Third Mobile Window Syndrome of the Inner Ear*, https://doi.org/10.1007/978-3-031-16586-3_15

Table 15.1 Criteria for surgical intervention in TMWD

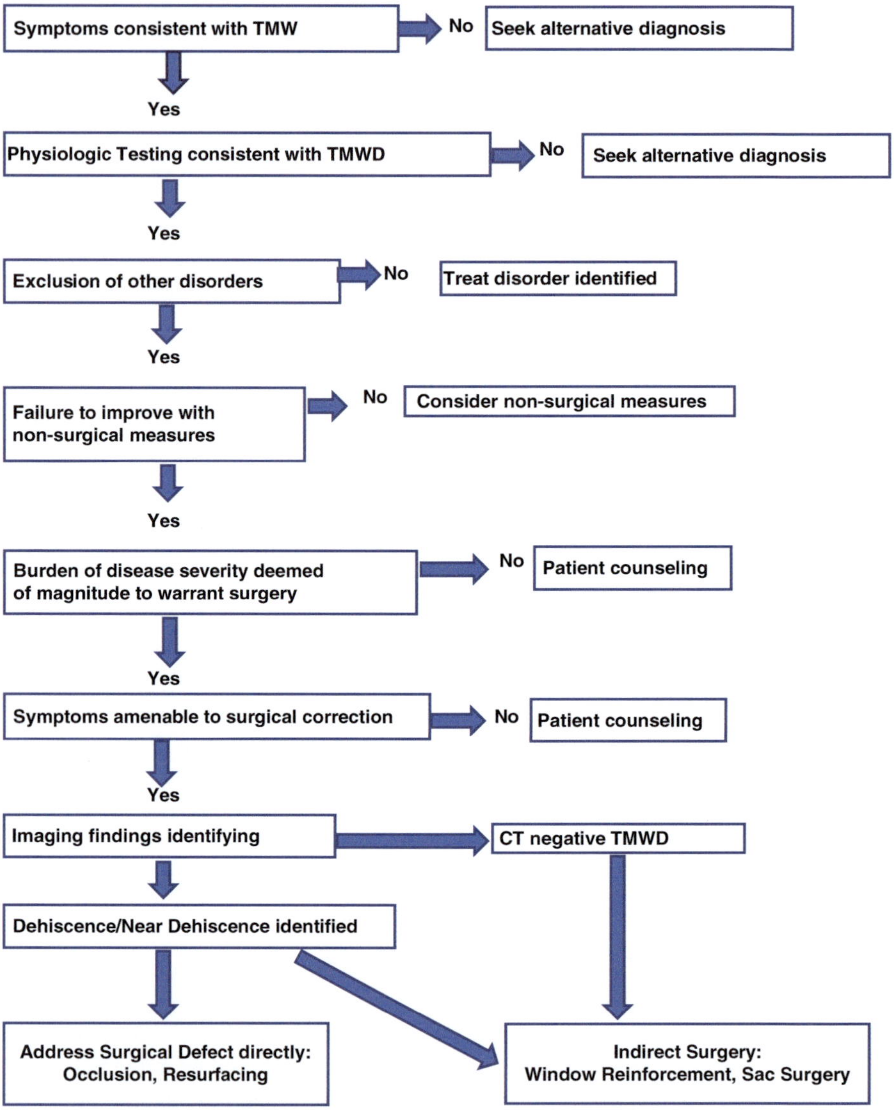

and severity of symptoms, as well as how these symptoms interfere with a major life activity. The same severity and frequency of disease can affect individuals very differently. For example, an episode of vertigo occurring once every three months and lasting a minute per spell with quiescence in between episodes is not considered a major limiting disease for someone who does clerical work. However, the same degree of vertigo can be of disabling severity in an airline pilot. Another example: heartbeat autophony heard only when the surroundings are quiet is not overly concerning. However, heartbeat autophony so loud that it disrupts sleep can destroy one's quality of life.

After severity of disease burden has been evaluated, the next step would be to determine if appropriate non-surgical measures have been considered. These include both non-medical and medical measures. See the chapters on medical therapy, visual manifestations and treatment, and endovascular for an in-depth discussion of non-surgical options. Only once the patient has been diagnosed, assessed for severity of disease, and has been either unsuccessful from appropriate medical therapy or not a candidate for medical therapy, should surgery be considered. Most patients with TMWS will not be candidates for surgical therapy, either because of limited disease burden or effective mitigation of symptoms with medical management.

Preop Counseling

A thorough preoperative audiologic and vestibular evaluation should be performed on any patient undergoing surgery for TMWS. At a minimum, this should include MRI, CT, audiometry, tympanometry, videonystagmography, electrocochleography, and vestibular evoked myogenic potentials (cervical and ocular). Additional studies that are helpful include computerized dynamic posturography (CDP), platform pressure test (PPT), rotational chair, vHIT, and active head rotation testing.

MRI is used to exclude intracranial pathologies that could potentially contribute to or mimic TMWS, such as a meningioma eroding into the semicircular canal [2]. We also like to assess the MRI scan for any soft signs of increased intracranial pressure—cerebellar ectopia/Chiari [3], empty sella, dilated optic nerve sheath diameter, slit-like lateral ventricles, compressed lateral sinuses, etc. [4].

The CT scan, of course, would have been done prior to surgical consideration, but in a case of TMWS it should be scrutinized for areas of dehiscence in addition to the defined lesion. Although most patients with a labyrinthine dehiscence seem to have only one area of dehiscence, there are those with more than one dehiscence [5]. This is more than an academic point. In a patient with superior semicircular canal dehiscence (SCD) and concomitant posterior semicircular canal dehiscence (PCD), failure to repair both will likely result in less than an optimal outcome. Tegmen dehiscences in SCD are found in the vast majority of cases, and preoperative assessment for concomitant encephaloceles is prudent [6]. In TMWS cases where no identifiable dehiscence is noted, a second attempt to identify an otic capsule dehiscence should be performed. In some cases, there may be a near dehiscence identified as the pathologic lesion [7].

Most studies of TMWS have emphasized the importance of audiologic and vestibular testing as a means for diagnosis of the disorder. In addition, preoperative testing should be done to identify vestibular deficits and associated pathologies, such as BPPV, as well as establish a baseline for future comparison should the patient have additional problems in the future. Some unique situations that will be identified with preoperative evaluation include TMWS in the only hearing ear, TMWS in the only vestibular ear, bilateral vestibular hypofunction, concomitant otosclerosis, and bilateral TMWS. Each of these situations require an individualized approach and are addressed in other chapters of this text.

We utilize CDP and PPT on all preoperative TMWS patients. Although CDP can help identify a vestibular cause for balance problems, it is very insensitive in this utility. More importantly, it can help identify non-vestibular causes of balance disorders. In many TMWS cases, the onset of symptoms is coincident with head trauma and frequently followed by litigation. Malingering for monetary gain in such a situation cannot be dismissed out of hand. CDP helps to identify these tendencies in advance [8]. We find PPT (if the patient can maintain good balance on sensory organization test (SOT) #5), an insensitive but very specific test for TMWS and, if needed, can be used postoperatively to assess surgical success. Note that SOT #5 is a condition in computerized dynamic posturography testing with vision denied and the platform surface allowed to sway with center of gravity, thus making it the most challenging for patients with significant vestibular deficits.

Types of Surgery

The principle of surgery for a TMWS disorder is to eliminate abnormal pressure influences on vestibular and auditory sensors. To accomplish this, surgeons have had several different approaches: (1) occlusion of the bony canal to stop pressure transmission, (2) repair of the defect to prevent pressure transmission, (3) a combination of occlusion and repair, and (4) oval and/or round window reinforcement (Table 15.2). Many have used the terms occlusion and plugging synonymously to mean complete blockage of the semicircular canal to prevent stimulation of the canal. Regarding repair, other terms used have been capping and resurfacing.

Table 15.2 Surgical approach for TMWS

Direct surgical approach or window reinforcement	Window reinforcement ± endolymphatic sac decompression
Superior semicircular canal dehiscence Posterior semicircular canal dehiscence Horizontal semicircular canal dehiscence	Cochlear-facial dehiscence Cochlear-internal carotid dehiscence Modiolar defect Hypermobile stapes Vestibule-middle ear dehiscence Large vestibular aqueduct Perilymph fistula (CT negative TMWS) Horizontal canal-facial nerve dehiscence

Dehiscences of the semicircular canals generally lend themselves to direct surgical repair. Other TMWS disorders can be treated with window reinforcement and, in some cases, endolymphatic sac decompression surgery. Note—TMWS with a vascular dehiscence may be candidates for endovascular procedures (Chap. 17)

Generally, capping is meant to include repairs with a solid substance such as bone, cartilage or other synthetic solid substances. Resurfacing is typically used to describe the reformation of bone over the defect by use of hydroxyapatite (HA) cement or bone dust/bone chips. Resurfacing alone has been shown to result in lower success rates, and most surgeons have advocated use of resurfacing only in combination with plugging or capping, but not as a sole repair technique.

Occlusion

The first two reported attempts at surgical occlusion were included in the original report of SCD by Minor et al. [9]. In this approach, a standard middle fossa craniotomy approach was performed, exposing the SCD. The concept of occlusion of the SSC stems from our collective experience with posterior semicircular canal occlusion for intractable BPPV. Occlusion for SSCD is performed similarly. The goal is to occlude the SSC in order to prevent motion of the SSC ampulla. This has led to effective improvement in autophony and vestibular symptoms. By definition, the function of the SSC is removed. This is not significant for most patients, but in some situations the loss of canal function can have significant untoward consequences. In particular, surgical occlusion of bilateral SSCD will result in bilateral loss of SSC function and can be problematic for some [10]. Older patients, patients at risk for poor central compensation and patients who have already lost significant vestibular function should be approached cautiously with plugging. Lastly, in very large defects, occlusion runs the risk of plugging the crus communes which would effectively result in the loss of both superior and posterior semicircular canal function.

Several materials have been used successfully for occlusion techniques. Commonly used materials include bone wax, bone dust, fibrin glue, and fascia. No one material appears to have shown superiority over the others. However, the number of patients in the studies limit the ability for comparison. It should be noted that CT scan would not be useful in determination of adequate plugging postoperatively. MRI has shown utility in demonstration of a plugged superior canal. This is shown in the case discussed under revision surgery.

Repair/Capping

In general, repair involves placing some material over the SSCD to prevent transmission of pressure from the intracranial cavity to the inner ear [8]. Repair and resurfacing techniques also vary quite significantly from surgeon to surgeon. Among the materials used are bone, bone chips, HA bone cement, silastic sheeting, cartilage, and glass ceramic implants [8, 11–13] (Fig. 15.1). There are limited data comparing these techniques but capping (i.e., repair with solid material) has been suggested to be superior to resurfacing (placement of HA cement or bone pate

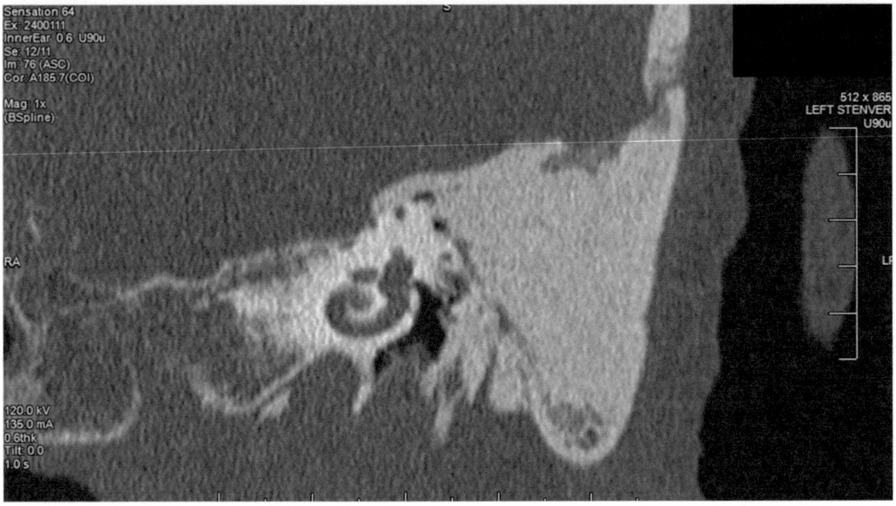

Fig. 15.1 Postoperative CT scan after combined transmastoid/middle fossa craniotomy resurfacing with calvarial bone and obliteration with HA cement

only). Others have combined the use of capping and resurfacing. Similar to occlusion, surgical outcomes for repair/capping are highly successful for controlling vestibular symptoms and autophony. The goal of repair/capping is to completely cover the dehiscent area which is relatively easy with smaller dehiscences, but more challenging with larger dehiscences that extend to the edge of the petrous ridge and into the posterior fossa. The biggest problem with repair/capping is inadequate coverage of the defect which can be due to slippage of the material, incorrect placement, or inadequate curing of the HA cement. However, when successfully performed, this technique gives excellent results while preserving superior semicircular canal patency and function. Some surgeons combine occlusion with repair/capping techniques.

Transmastoid vs. Middle Fossa vs. Combined Approach

Approach for repair or occlusion of an SSCD can be accomplished via a middle fossa craniotomy, a transmastoid approach or a combined middle fossa/transmastoid approach. The advantage of the middle fossa approach [14] is visibility of the defect. The middle fossa approach gives the best exposure of the SSCD defect, but the nature of SSCD anatomy is such that there are usually multiple middle fossa defects. In some cases, the tegmen defects can camouflage the SSCD. Because of this issue, some surgeons have advocated the use of navigational systems to ensure the correct defect is addressed. This point cannot be stressed enough since we have had the occasion to do revision surgery on patients who had the wrong defect plugged or repaired, with obvious consequences. The other disadvantage of the middle fossa craniotomy is the need for a larger craniotomy defect and more extensive brain retraction than the other approaches.

The transmastoid approach [15] has the advantage of very minimal brain retraction which converts the surgery into an outpatient procedure. This "lesser" craniotomy approach, at least theoretically reduces the chance for major intracranial complications such as epidural hematoma, cerebral contusion, and infarction. The major disadvantage of the transmastoid approach is poor visibility of the defect. Although an experienced surgeon should have no trouble identifying the SSC in the mastoid, actual visualization of the SSCD is often difficult or impossible. Therefore, the occlusion or repair is often done without actually seeing the defect. Fortunately, most of the time this is not necessary, but depending on the individual anatomy, it could be problematic. Another disadvantage of the transmastoid approach relates to the "normal" anatomy of most SSCD patients. Most SSCD patients have a very low tegmen and, consequently, there is not much room for dissection superior to the level of the horizontal semicircular canal compared to non-SSCD patients, making dissection somewhat challenging in the area of question.

The combined transmastoid/middle fossa craniotomy approach has the advantage of both approaches, and consequently, this is the one we advocate and utilize in the vast majority of surgery for SSCD. For this approach a standard mastoidectomy is performed with exposure of the superior semicircular canal. The tegmen lateral to the SSC is removed, exposing temporal lobe dura. This tegmen removal is extended laterally to varying degrees, depending on the individual anatomy, angle of tegmen slope and location of SSCD. This may extend onto the lateral skull up to 1–2 cm superior to the tegmen line or be contained within the mastoid itself. The combined approach allows for minimal brain retraction while allowing for excellent visibility of the defect, and localization of the defect obviating the need for a navigational system. The minimal brain retraction also allows this to be an outpatient procedure. The main disadvantage is the need to repair the craniotomy defects afterwards. This can be repaired with silastic sheeting, or the mastoid can be obliterated with fat, HA cement or other material. We utilize either cortical bone taken from the mastoid and/or silastic sheeting for the craniotomy repair (Fig. 15.2).

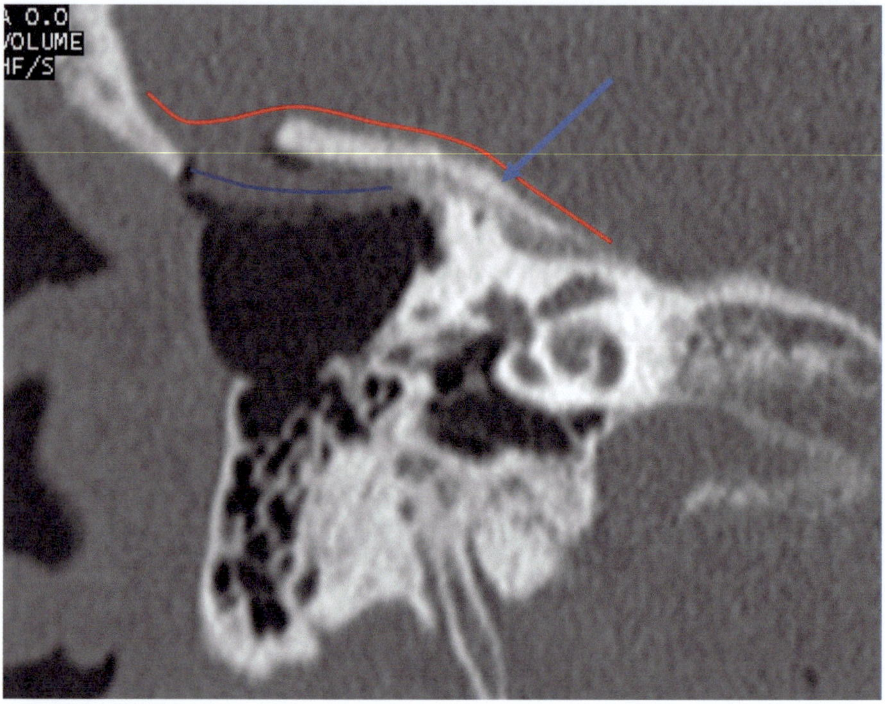

Fig. 15.2 Postoperative CT scan after resurfacing with silastic sheeting (red) and calvarial bone (arrow). The blue line denotes bone wax

Window Reinforcement

One of the more minimally invasive approaches is window reinforcement surgery [16]. In addition to being a minimal approach for SSCD surgery, window reinforcement has become the default surgical procedure for TMWS lesions that do not have a direct surgical correction. Lesions such as cochlear-facial dehiscence, cochlear-internal carotid dehiscence, modiolar defects, hypermobile stapes, large vestibular aqueduct, horizontal semicircular-facial nerve dehiscence, and perilymph fistula (CT negative TMWS) [17].

The technique varies with different surgeons but is basically perilymphatic fistula repair surgery of the round window. We advocate reinforcement of both the round and the oval window if this option is chosen. The outcomes for this procedure are initially quite good but we have witnessed a fairly high recurrence rate within one year after surgery. In general, the larger the dehiscence, the less likely this procedure seems to be adequate for long-term control of symptoms. This procedure, like the others, is most successful in controlling vestibular symptoms. It also seems to be relatively unsuccessful for control of autophony. Its main advantage is its minimally invasive nature and low risk for any serious complications, while its main disadvantage is the low rate of long-term success. While we still offer this minimal approach to patients, we are careful to counsel about the lower success rate. However, we also typically will include window reinforcement concomitantly with resurfacing or occlusion of the SSCD. We find that adjuvant medical therapy postoperatively greatly improves the long-term outlook for these patients.

We have used a variation on window reinforcement in a variety of TMWS patients (SSCD, CFD, and PLF) who have profound hearing loss. Instead of a soft tissue repair of the oval and/or round window, we remove the incus and use HA cement to produce a solid repair of the windows. In this unpublished series of 15 cases, we have had complete resolution of vestibular symptoms in all but one patient. This is a very attractive approach for SCD patients who have profound hearing loss.

Posterior Canal Dehiscence

Less commonly reported is posterior semicircular canal dehiscence (PSCD) [18]. While there are limited reports in the literature regarding surgical intervention for PSCD, theoretically it can be treated in the same manner as SSCD [19]. Occlusion procedures would be most effectively managed through a transmastoid approach, such as transmastoid SSCD occlusion procedures. We have done resurfacing procedures through the transmastoid-posterior fossa approach. Using a wide decompression of posterior fossa plate, inclusive of sigmoid sinus, such as seen with a wide endolymphatic sac decompression procedure, access to the posterior aspect of the petrous bone can be achieved for placement of calvarial bone, cartilage, etc. for PSCD that are dehiscent towards the posterior fossa dura (Fig. 15.3). However, some PSCD do not lend themselves to resurfacing procedures. PSCD that are dehiscent into the vestibular aqueduct can be unapproachable for resurfacing and are

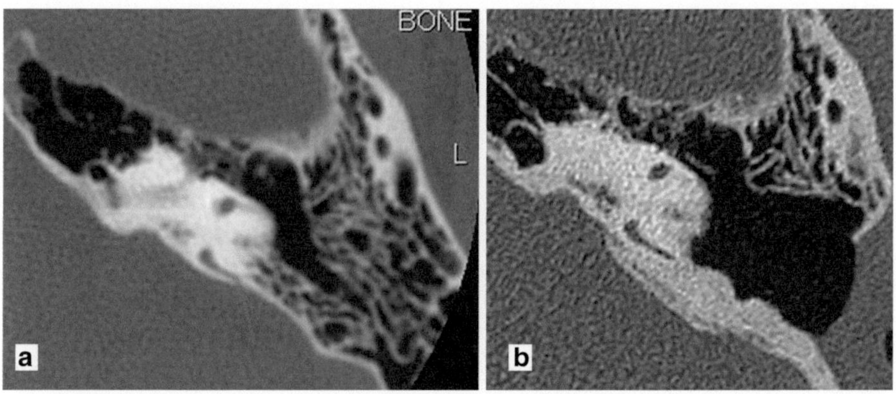

Fig. 15.3 Preop (**a**) and postop (**b**) CT scan of PSCD repair using calvarial bone and HA cement. Arrow points to PSCD, dehiscent toward posterior fossa dura

better managed by other means. PSCD are sometimes dehiscent adjacent to a high jugular bulb. These can sometimes be resurfaced, but other times, if the dehiscence is located on the medial side of the PSC, it may not be accessible. Alternatives to PSCD repair or occlusion in the case of a high jugular bulb can include decompression of the jugular bulb and endovascular procedures (see Chap. 16).

Ancillary Procedures

Endolymphatic Sac Surgery: Although no data currently exist on the use of endolymphatic sac surgery (ESS) for TMWS, ESS has been used as a treatment for endolymphatic hydrops in the past with success [20]. Given that endolymphatic hydrops has been identified in SSCD cases, traditional treatment for endolymphatic hydrops should be explored for TMWS patients [21]. We sometimes utilize ESS in combination with window reinforcement for TMWS involving lesions that are not amenable to a direct surgical repair, such as cochlear-facial dehiscence, IAC-cochlear dehiscence, cochlear-carotid dehiscences, etc. We have also seen patients who were diagnosed as Ménière's/Hydrops and underwent endolymphatic sac decompression with long-term remission of symptoms (13–25 years) only to be later diagnosed with SCD. This leads one to consider whether endolymphatic decompression may have some positive impact on SCD, in particular, and in TMWD, in general.

PE tube placement: [22] PE tube placement was initially recommended as a minimal approach to reduce TMWS symptoms in SCD patients. While this gained some early enthusiasm, it proved to not be universally helpful in SCD. However, we have found PE tube placement a helpful adjuvant in treatment for a select group of TMWS patients. Situations where the patient may be subject to otic barotrauma and patients with intermittent (or chronic) eustachian tube dysfunction (ETD) appear to note benefit from tube placement. We don't think of this as resolving the underlying problem but mitigating one of the factors than can exacerbate TMWS. Obviously, if there are factors other than ETD exacerbating symptoms of TMWS, then PE tube placement will have limited value.

Lumbar puncture (LP): Some patients will have elevated ICP [23], either incidentally or as a contributing factor to TMWS. LP can be performed as both a diagnostic and therapeutic procedure. Control of ICP will help control TMWS symptoms (see Chap. 13 on medical therapy), and in the preoperative setting, to reduce pressure on the oval window/round window repair sites in the immediate postoperative period. We routinely perform LP immediately preoperatively in nearly all TMWS patients for two purposes: (1) to exclude concomitant elevated intracranial pressure as a cause for TMWS and (2) to drain CSF to lower intralabyrinthine pressure temporarily in the early postoperative period which may improve graft success. Like the rationale for using lumbar puncture, many surgeons also employ other techniques to lower intracranial pressure regardless of the approach chosen. This includes hyperventilation to lower CO_2 (26–30 mmHg) and administration of mannitol. This will also allow for easier brain retraction for exposure.

Outcomes

It can be challenging to report outcomes for TMWS due to the varying symptom presentation, difficulties in quantifying the symptoms and the range of approaches [24]. Still much work lies ahead to standardize outcome measures for comparative research in surgical outcomes for TMWS. That said, the most disabling symptoms are typically vestibular in nature, and fortunately, this is the symptom that most reliably can be improved. Unfortunately, this is a symptom not easily measured and does not have a universally agreed upon scale or tool for measurement.

Two large systematic reviews comparing the differing surgical treatments for SSCD have been recently published [25, 26]. The authors note no significant differences in outcomes for the varying approaches to treat SSCD, except for window reinforcement surgery, due to limited numbers presented in the literature. For that matter, the individual surgical techniques vary quite considerably from one surgeon to another, the number of reported surgeries is low, and the reports vary quite a lot in the type of data for outcomes as well as objective measures for outcomes, thus making the reviewers' job of comparison quite difficult. The conclusions are that surgical outcomes provide excellent improvement rates in vestibular symptoms and autophony. There is resolution or significant improvement in vestibular symptoms for over 95% of patients. Autophony is improved in more than 90% of patients. Hearing improvement is seldom seen, so we do not advocate surgery if hearing loss is the sole symptom. Similarly, we do not advocate surgery for the sole symptom of tinnitus. Tinnitus can improve, worsen, or remain unchanged postoperatively. However, one observation we have made is that tinnitus may continue to improve long after the 1-year postop period. One exception for tinnitus: pulsatile tinnitus is frequently improved/resolved with surgery.

One interesting finding, recently reported, demonstrated regrowth of bone over the dehiscent site when treated with a cartilage cap technique [27]. This phenomenon would be expected when bone is used as the cap. This development deserves further study and may shed some light on the pathogenesis of SSCD.

Complications

Complications are typical of what is seen from the approach employed: middle fossa craniotomy, mastoidectomy, and tympanotomy approaches. In general, there are less complications from window reinforcement procedures since this is a less invasive approach. Among the complications specific to the direct approaches for SSCD surgery are early failure, late failure, hearing loss, vestibular loss (concomitant loss of PSC and SSC function), postoperative BPPV, tinnitus, infection, facial paralysis, and other complications seen with major ear surgery [25, 28, 29]. Severe hearing loss is seen in approximately 3% of patients with either of the surgical techniques directly addressing the SSCD, whereas severe hearing loss in window reinforcement does not seem to be a problem. There have been anecdotal reports of higher risk of hearing loss in revision surgery and among patients who had undergone prior stapes surgery. A technique of underwater endoscopic approach has been investigated to reduce the chance of hearing loss [30, 31]. The technique involves a transmastoid approach with drilling and opening of the SSC performed endoscopically underwater, using basic salt solution to fill the mastoid. The concern is that loss of perilymph during surgery may be the etiology for hearing loss postoperatively. Unfortunately, although outcomes for vestibular symptoms seem similarly resolved, preliminary results do not seem to demonstrate any significant difference in hearing outcomes from the limited patients where this has been employed.

Early failure of repair/occlusion is fairly uncommon. Late failures are seen but how common this is will take some time to see. In our experience with over 500 SSCD surgeries since 1998, delayed failure for repair/capping is quite low and is probably <1%. Delayed failures seem to be somewhat higher with occlusion techniques. Some patients who have initially excellent results with occlusion procedures will have recurrence of SSCD symptoms, albeit milder than initially. These patients do quite well with revision surgery. We have postulated that this may be secondary to retraction of the soft tissue plug, allowing movement in the SSCD, aka "loose plug syndrome." This has led some surgeons who had advocated occlusion procedures to adopt an approach of occlusion and resurfacing concomitantly. Other complications typically seen with major ear surgery are, of course, expected but do not seem to be any more common than otologic procedures of similar complexity.

Revision Surgery

Although SSCD surgery has a high success rate, there are failures that may be responsive to revision surgery. The decision to proceed with revision surgery should include an analysis as to why the original surgery was unsuccessful, what symptoms persist, and whether revision surgery can alleviate these symptoms. It should also include a repeat high-resolution CT scan to look for any additional dehiscences that the primary surgery may not have addressed. Figure 15.4 demonstrates a case of a missed second dehiscence. The patient had undergone three prior SSCD procedures—round window reinforcement, transmastoid SSCD occlusion, and then middle fossa SSCD occlusion. The patient had persistent Tullio, autophony, and strain-induced vertigo despite these measures. A follow-up CT demonstrated a concomitant PSCD that had not been addressed. Surgical repair of the PSCD with calvarial bone resolved the patient's symptoms.

Preoperative physiologic testing as mentioned earlier in this chapter should be extensive, since the primary surgery and time will have likely altered vestibular function which may be contributing to the postoperative symptoms. Unless there is an obvious reason for revision surgery, we do not recommend any assessment for this prior to three months postoperative from the primary surgery and this assessment is probably better delayed until at least six months postoperative.

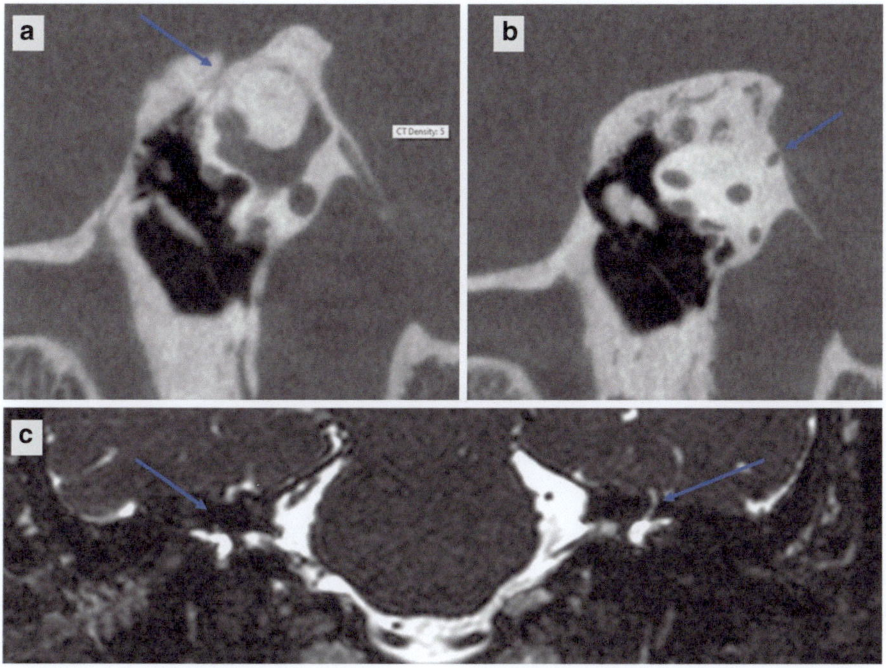

Fig. 15.4 Three prior surgeries—round window reinforcement, transmastoid SSCD occlusion and Middle Fossa SSCD occlusion with persistent symptoms. (**a**) Well occluded and resurfaced SSCD (arrow) with ossification of SSC lumen. (**b**) PSCD (arrow) not yet repaired. (**c**) MRI demonstrating absence of the SSC signal and confirming occlusion. Right arrow points to absent SSC signal and left arrow points to normal SSC signal. Surgical repair of the PSCD with calvarial bone resolved the patient's symptoms

Physiologic testing that reveals the need for revision surgery is not clearly defined. Comparison to testing before the primary surgery should be done. Often the VEMP and ECOG testing may be improved but may still be abnormal and, in some cases, they may have no result postoperatively, leaving the clinician wondering if the surgery was successful or whether otolithic function has been damaged. We find the most helpful determinants as to whether to proceed with revision surgery are (1) the patient's history of strain-induced vertigo or Tullio phenomenon in the suspect ear, (2) ECOG, VEMP testing that has not improved with surgery, and (3) abnormal pressure testing (fistula test, valsalva test, platform pressure test) or abnormal Tullio testing.

Figure 15.5 provides an example of this. It demonstrates a preoperative CT scan of a patient who underwent resurfacing with HA cement but had persistent symptoms. The CT demonstrates a well repaired SSCD. VEMP and ECOG testing were unremarkable and suggested successful surgical repair. However, fistula testing demonstrated vertical/torsional phase-locked eye movements in the plane of superior canal, strongly implicating a persistent SSCD despite the CT scan. Valsalva testing

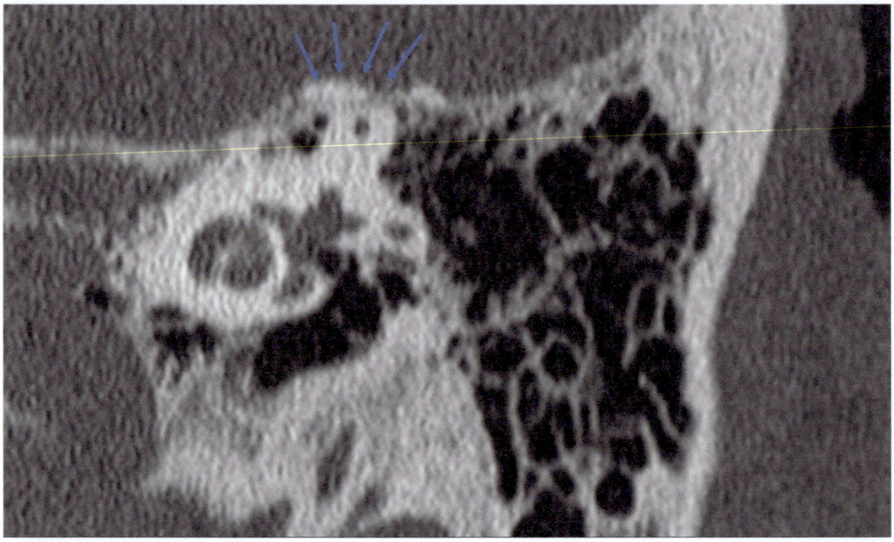

Fig. 15.5 Preoperative CT scan of a patient who underwent resurfacing with HA cement but had persistent symptoms. The CT demonstrates what appears to be a well repaired SSCD. VEMP and ECOG testing were unremarkable and suggested successful surgical repair. However, fistula testing demonstrated vertical/torsional phase-locked eye movements in the plane of superior canal, strongly implicating a persistent SSCD despite the CT scan. Valsalva testing was also abnormal. Surgical exploration revealed HA cement that had failed to cure and was non-rigid, thus allowing continued pressure transmission. Revision surgical repair with calvarial bone resolved his symptoms. Arrows point to the "uncured" HA cement

was also abnormal. Surgical exploration revealed HA cement that had failed to cure and was non-rigid, thus allowing continued pressure transmission. Revision surgical repair with calvarial bone resolved his symptoms. We had a similar case of uncured HA cement early in our surgical experience with SSCD circa 1999 that required revision. At that time, the OR staff mixed the HA cement, and it was suspected that it was inappropriately mixed. Newer HA cement reduces the chance of this happening. However, it is prudent to ensure the HA cement is hardened before closing.

Although revision surgery can provide symptomatic improvement, the success rate is comparatively lower than primary surgery and it has been associated with increased risk of complications such as CSF leak [32, 33]. This reduction may be due to factors such as unrecognized second dehiscences, perilymph fistula, hypermobile stapes, unrecognized IIH or other concomitant processes.

Conclusions

Choosing among the various treatment options for SSCD, and individualizing the care for each patient, can significantly improve the quality of these patients' lives. The range of treatment options include medical and non-surgical strategies, which may be the best option for those averse to surgery or for whom surgery/anesthesia represents great risk. Minimally invasive approaches with window reinforcement procedures can be effective for patients whose main symptoms are vestibular in nature, albeit at a lower success rate and higher recurrence rate than more invasive surgical procedures. For those patients with the most severe vestibular symptoms and incapacitating autophony, more direct surgical alternatives are preferred—occlusion or repair of the SSCD, either through a transmastoid, middle fossa or a combined approach. The recently described endovascular approach for TMWS lesions abutting vascular structures is discussed in a separate chapter.

References

1. Ward BK, van de Berg R, van Rompaey V, Bisdorff A, Hullar TE, Welgampola MS, Carey JP. Superior semicircular canal dehiscence syndrome: diagnostic criteria consensus document of the committee for the classification of vestibular disorders of the Bárány Society. J Vestib Res. 2021;31(3):131–41. https://doi.org/10.3233/VES-200004. PMID: 33522990.
2. Crane BT, Carey JP, McMenomey S, Minor LB. Meningioma causing superior canal dehiscence syndrome. Otol Neurotol. 2010;31(6):1009–10. https://doi.org/10.1097/MAO.0b013e3181a32d85. PMID: 19395985.
3. Kuhn JJ, Clenney T. The association between semicircular canal dehiscence and Chiari type I malformation. Arch Otolaryngol Head Neck Surg. 2010;136(10):1009–14. https://doi.org/10.1001/archoto.2010.169. PMID: 20956749.
4. Barkatullah AF, Leishangthem L, Moss HE. MRI findings as markers of idiopathic intracranial hypertension. Curr Opin Neurol. 2021;34(1):75–83. https://doi.org/10.1097/WCO.0000000000000885. PMID: 33230036; PMCID: PMC7856277.
5. Manzari L. Multiple dehiscences of bony labyrinthine capsule. A rare case report and review of the literature. Acta Otorhinolaryngol Ital. 2010;30(6):317–20. PMID: 21808455; PMCID: PMC3146321.
6. Smullen JL, Andrist EC, Gianoli GJ. Superior semicircular canal dehiscence: a new cause of vertigo. J La State Med Soc. 1999;151(8):397–400. PMID: 10554474.
7. Ward BK, Wenzel A, Ritzl EK, Gutierrez-Hernandez S, Della Santina CC, Minor LB, Carey JP. Near-dehiscence: clinical findings in patients with thin bone over the superior semicircular canal. Otol Neurotol. 2013;34(8):1421–8. https://doi.org/10.1097/MAO.0b013e318287efe6. PMID: 23644303; PMCID: PMC3740012.
8. Gianoli G, McWilliams S, Soileau J, Belafsky P. Posturographic performance in patients with the potential for secondary gain. Otolaryngol Head Neck Surg. 2000;122(1):11–8. https://doi.org/10.1016/S0194-5998(00)70137-9. PMID: 10629476.
9. Minor LB, Solomon D, Zinreich JS, Zee DS. Sound- and/or pressure-induced vertigo due to bone dehiscence of the superior semicircular canal. Arch Otolaryngol Head Neck Surg. 1998;124(3):249–58. https://doi.org/10.1001/archotol.124.3.249. PMID: 9525507.
10. Agrawal Y, Minor LB, Schubert MC, Janky KL, Davalos-Bichara M, Carey JP. Second-side surgery in superior canal dehiscence syndrome. Otol Neurotol. 2012;33(1):72–7. https://doi.org/10.1097/MAO.0b013e31823c9182. PMID: 22158019; PMCID: PMC4082242.
11. Bogle JM, Lundy LB, Zapala DA, Copenhaver A. Dizziness handicap after cartilage cap occlusion for superior semicircular canal dehiscence. Otol Neurotol. 2013;34(1):135–40. https://doi.org/10.1097/MAO.0b013e31827850d4. PMID: 23160454.
12. Kwok P, Gleich O, Spruss T, Strutz J. Different materials for plugging a dehiscent superior semicircular canal: a comparative histologic study using a gerbil model. Otol Neurotol. 2019;40(5):e532–41. https://doi.org/10.1097/MAO.0000000000002205. PMID: 31083091.

13. Mueller SA, Vibert D, Haeusler R, Raabe A, Caversaccio M. Surgical capping of superior semicircular canal dehiscence. Eur Arch Otorhinolaryngol. 2014;271(6):1369–74. https://doi.org/10.1007/s00405-013-2533-x. Epub 2013 May 3. PMID: 23640386.
14. Schwartz SR, Almosnino G, Noonan KY, Banakis Hartl RM, Zeitler DM, Saunders JE, Cass SP. Comparison of transmastoid and middle fossa approaches for superior canal dehiscence repair: a multi-institutional study. Otolaryngol Head Neck Surg. 2019;161(1):130–6. https://doi.org/10.1177/0194599819835173. Epub 2019 Mar 5. PMID: 30832543.
15. Agrawal SK, Parnes LS. Transmastoid superior semicircular canal occlusion. Otol Neurotol. 2008;29(3):363–7. https://doi.org/10.1097/mao.0b013e3181616c9d. PMID: 18180691.
16. Silverstein H, Kartush JM, Parnes LS, Poe DS, Babu SC, Levenson MJ, Wazen J, Ridley RW. Round window reinforcement for superior semicircular canal dehiscence: a retrospective multi-center case series. Am J Otolaryngol. 2014;35(3):286–93. https://doi.org/10.1016/j.amjoto.2014.02.016. Epub 2014 Mar 5. PMID: 24667055.
17. Wackym PA, Wood SJ, Siker DA, Carter DM. Otic capsule dehiscence syndrome: superior semicircular canal dehiscence syndrome with no radiographically visible dehiscence. Ear Nose Throat J. 2015;94(8):E8–E24. https://doi.org/10.1177/014556131509400802. PMID: 26322461.
18. Nomiya S, Cureoglu S, Kariya S, Morita N, Nomiya R, Schachern PA, Nishizaki K, Paparella MM. Posterior semicircular canal dehiscence: a histopathologic human temporal bone study. Otol Neurotol. 2010;31(7):1122–7. https://doi.org/10.1097/MAO.0b013e3181eb3309. PMID: 20657329.
19. Lee JA, Liu YF, Nguyen SA, McRackan TR, Meyer TA, Rizk HG. Posterior semicircular canal dehiscence: case series and systematic review. Otol Neurotol. 2020;41(4):511–21. https://doi.org/10.1097/MAO.0000000000002576. PMID: 32176140.
20. Sood AJ, Lambert PR, Nguyen SA, Meyer TA. Endolymphatic sac surgery for Ménière's disease: a systematic review and meta-analysis. Otol Neurotol. 2014;35(6):1033–45. https://doi.org/10.1097/MAO.0000000000000324. PMID: 24751747.
21. Ray A, Hautefort C, Guichard JP, Horion J, Herman P, Kania R, Houdart E, Verillaud B, Vitaux H, Attyé A, Eliezer M. MRI contribution for the detection of endolymphatic hydrops in patients with superior canal dehiscence syndrome. Eur Arch Otorhinolaryngol. 2021;278(7):2229–38. https://doi.org/10.1007/s00405-020-06282-3. Epub 2020 Aug 14. PMID: 32797276.
22. Limb CJ, Carey JP, Srireddy S, Minor LB. Auditory function in patients with surgically treated superior semicircular canal dehiscence. Otol Neurotol. 2006;27(7):969–80. https://doi.org/10.1097/01.mao.0000235376.70492.8e. PMID: 17006348.
23. Berkiten G, Gürbüz D, Akan O, Tutar B, Tunç MK, Karaketir S, Bircan HS, Berkiten E, Sarı H, Atar Y, Uyar Y. Dehiscence or thinning of bone overlying the superior semicircular canal in idiopathic intracranial hypertension. Eur Arch Otorhinolaryngol. 2021;279:2899. https://doi.org/10.1007/s00405-021-07020-z. PMID: 34424380.
24. Ossen ME, Stokroos R, Kingma H, van Tongeren J, Van Rompaey V, Temel Y, van de Berg R. Heterogeneity in reported outcome measures after surgery in superior canal dehiscence syndrome-a systematic literature review. Front Neurol. 2017;8:347. https://doi.org/10.3389/fneur.2017.00347. PMID: 28790965; PMCID: PMC5523725.
25. Gioacchini FM, Alicandri-Ciufelli M, Kaleci S, Scarpa A, Cassandro E, Re M. Outcomes and complications in superior semicircular canal dehiscence surgery: a systematic review. Laryngoscope. 2016;126(5):1218–24. https://doi.org/10.1002/lary.25662. Epub 2015 Sep 15. PMID: 26371952.
26. Ziylan F, Kinaci A, Beynon AJ, Kunst HP. A comparison of surgical treatments for superior semicircular canal dehiscence: a systematic review. Otol Neurotol. 2017;38(1):1–10. https://doi.org/10.1097/MAO.0000000000001277. PMID: 27861193.
27. Bhatt AA, Vibhute P, Gupta V, Zapala DA, Pooley RA, Lundy LB. New bone formation over dehiscent semicircular canal with cartilage cap. Neuroradiol J. 2022:19714009221096820. https://doi.org/10.1177/19714009221096820. Epub ahead of print. PMID: 35506568.

28. Vlastarakos PV, Proikas K, Tavoulari E, Kikidis D, Maragoudakis P, Nikolopoulos TP. Efficacy assessment and complications of surgical management for superior semicircular canal dehiscence: a meta-analysis of published interventional studies. Eur Arch Otorhinolaryngol. 2009;266(2):177–86. https://doi.org/10.1007/s00405-008-0840-4. Epub 2008 Oct 25. PMID: 18953551.
29. Xie Y, Sharon JD, Pross SE, Abt NB, Varma S, Della Santina CC, Minor LB, Carey JP. Surgical complications from superior canal dehiscence syndrome repair: two decades of experience. Otolaryngol Head Neck Surg. 2017;157(2):273–80. https://doi.org/10.1177/0194599817706491. Epub 2017 Jun 27. PMID: 28653553.
30. Creighton FX Jr, Zhang L, Ward B, Carey JP. Hearing outcomes for an underwater endoscopic technique for transmastoid repair of superior semicircular canal dehiscence. Otol Neurotol. 2021;42(10):e1691–7. https://doi.org/10.1097/MAO.0000000000003238. PMID: 34172657.
31. Kawamura Y, Yamauchi D, Kobayashi T, Ikeda R, Kawase T, Katori Y. Hearing outcomes of transmastoid plugging for superior canal dehiscence syndrome by underwater endoscopic surgery: with special reference to transient bone conduction increase in early postoperative period. Otol Neurotol. 2022;43(3):368–75. https://doi.org/10.1097/MAO.0000000000003461. PMID: 34999616.
32. Mozaffari K, Ghodrati F, Pradhan A, Ng E, Ding K, Rana S, Duong C, Anderson RN, Enomoto A, Sheppard JP, Sun MZ, Phillips HW, Yang I, Gopen Q. Superior semicircular canal dehiscence revision surgery outcomes: a single institution's experience. World Neurosurg. 2021;156:e408–14. https://doi.org/10.1016/j.wneu.2021.09.083. Epub 2021 Sep 25. PMID: 34583007.
33. Sharon JD, Pross SE, Ward BK, Carey JP. Revision surgery for superior canal dehiscence syndrome. Otol Neurotol. 2016;37(8):1096–103. https://doi.org/10.1097/MAO.0000000000001113. PMID: 27348392.

Chapter 16
Endovascular Therapy for Third Mobile Window Syndrome

Pierre Reynard, Eugen Ionescu, Martin Hitier, Charlotte Barbier, and Francis Turjman

P. Reynard · E. Ionescu (✉)
Department of Audiology and Neurotology, Centre Hospitalo-Universitaire Lyon, Lyon, France

Paris Hearing Institute, Research Center of Pasteur Institute, Team Clinical and Translational Exploration of Sensorineural Hearing Loss, Inserm U1120, Paris, France
e-mail: pierre.reynard@chu-lyon.fr; ionescu@chu-lyon.fr

M. Hitier
Department of Otolaryngology Head and Neck Surgery, Centre Hospitalo-Universitaire de Caen, Caen, France

Department of Anatomy, UNICAEN, Caen, France

Inserm, U 1075 COMETE, Caen, France

Normandie University, Caen, France
e-mail: hitier-m@chu-caen.fr

C. Barbier
Department of Radiology, Centre Hospitalo-Universitaire de Caen, Caen, France

F. Turjman
Department of Neuroradiology, Centre Hospitalo-Universitaire Lyon, Groupement Hospitalier Est, Bron, France

Université Claude Bernard Lyon, Villeurbanne, France

UMR5515, INSERM U1206 Centre de Recherche en Acquisition et Traitement d'Images pour la Santé (CREATIS), Villeurbanne, France
e-mail: francis.turjman@chu-lyon.fr

G. J. Gianoli, P. Thomson (eds.), *Third Mobile Window Syndrome of the Inner Ear*, https://doi.org/10.1007/978-3-031-16586-3_16

Introduction

The concept of the third mobile labyrinthine window (TMW) was for the first time used by Cawthorne to describe the principle of semicircular canal (SC) fenestration in patients with advanced otosclerosis [1]. Minor et al. [2] and Smullen et al. [3] described the first clinical observations of superior semicircular canal dehiscence (SSCD) as a distinctive clinical form of spontaneous (or primary) third window abnormality. Merchant et al. further issued the hypothesis regarding the mechanism of this type of conductive hearing loss of the inner ear [4]. Since the 2000s, we have witnessed the progressive appearance of TMW variants with similar clinical and audiological features [5]. The broader concept of otic capsule dehiscence syndrome proposed by Wackym et al. refers to all pathologies of the TMW spectrum whose symptoms, clinical signs, and audiometric aspects correspond to bony defects of the otic capsule confirmed by tomodensitometry [6]. On an anatomical-radiological basis, a classification of TMW subtypes based on anatomical and radiological aspects has recently been proposed [7]. It also includes some intralabyrinthine pathologies that mimic the clinical presentation of a "classical" TMW.

In the classification mentioned above, type II otic capsule dehiscence corresponds to an abnormal contact between the membranous labyrinth and a vascular structure (venous or, less frequently, arterial structure) facilitated by the lack of bony otic capsule. In these TMW variants, the pathomechanism is not yet fully understood. Nonetheless, it can be assumed that non-physiological audio-vestibular stimulation is mainly produced by the pulsating energy of the vascular wall transmitted through the TMW interface to the membranous labyrinth. Obviously, this stimulation would be greater in the case of moderate or intense physical effort as the acceleration of the heart rate and increased cardiac output promotes the appearance of vertigo and tinnitus. This also explains the recurrent presence of pulsatile tinnitus in these variants [8]. When in contact with the perilymphatic space, the vibrations generated by the vascular wall can generate symptoms of different intensities, which depend on the location, surface, and the importance of any mass effect exerted by the vessel on the labyrinthine structure [9]. Other symptoms, including hearing loss, are due to the acoustic energy shunt carried by the vibrating perilymphatic fluid to the zone of minimal resistance generated by the dehiscence, as seen in the classic description of the TMW mechanism.

Three subvariants of labyrinthine-vascular dehiscence will be considered here, as they are accessible for endovascular management.

- The most common symptomatic labyrinthine-vascular TMW subvariant found in our practice involves the vestibular aqueduct (VA) and a high-riding jugular bulb (HRJB). HRJB is an irregular outpouching or protrusion of the vessel that may project into the middle ear cavity, mastoid cavity, or medially toward the petrous apex. The jugular bulb is localized in the upper part of the internal jugular vein and is in close relation with anatomic structures such as the inner ear, carotid artery, and the cranial nerves that pass through the jugular foramen. Jugular bulb abnormalities (JBAs) affect up to 15% of the general population [10] but only very few of these patients are symptomatic. JBAs include high-riding jugular bulb (HRJB), located higher than the basal turn of the cochlea or more than 2 mm from the floor of the internal auditory canal [11], and jugular bulb diverticulum defined as an irregular outpouching issued from the bulb [12]. Venous hypertension and/or turbulent venous flow in the Internal Jugular Vein (IJV) has been suggested as a possible etiologic factor for venous diverticulum with erosion of the overlying bone causing dehiscence through the otic capsule and adjacent structures [13]. Based on various anatomic observations, Couloigner et al. postulated that high jugular bulbs could induce Ménière's disease by a direct or indirect effect on the endolymphatic duct and/or sac, producing a decrease in endolymph resorption [14].

- The second most frequent symptomatic labyrinthine-vascular dehiscence variant involves a HRJB and the posterior semicircular canal (PSC). It should be noted that symptomatic JBAs could be underdiagnosed, and no consensual management has been established. When the symptoms are well tolerated, a "wait-and-see" policy can be adopted [10]. Otherwise, some invasive surgical techniques have been used, such as ligation [15], embolization of the IJV, or surgical lowering of the HRJB [14]. This carries out a high risk of facial palsy, sensorineural hearing loss, jugular hemorrhage, or thrombosis [16]. Alternatively, an endovascular stent-assisted coil implantation has recently been described [17]. The endovascular stent-assisted coil placement technique has been recognized as a safe and effective technique for many years in the treatment of unruptured wide-neck intracranial aneurysms [18]. A similar endovascular technique has been used in the jugular bulb to treat pulsatile tinnitus [19, 20].
- The less frequent labyrinthine-vascular dehiscence (or type II TMW) involves the SSC and the superior petrous sinus (SPS). SSCD by the SPS accounts for 4% to 9% of ears in symptomatic SSCD [21]. Until recently, a surgical procedure like the one proposed in SSCD described by Minor was considered as the only effective method for disabling SPS [22, 23]. Middle cranial fossa or transmastoid approaches are used [24, 25] to reach the dehiscence, and techniques such as plugging, capping or both methods combined can be used to treat this variant. Resurfacing and/or plugging via a middle fossa craniotomy in patients with SSCD by SPS implies mobilizing the SPS which may cause bleeding, thrombosis or complications related to the surgical approach [22, 25, 26]. Recently, an innovative endovascular treatment was proposed [27]. Its principle is to reinforce the vascular wall in contact with the membranous SSC by placing a stent at that level. This procedure aims at reducing the minimal resistance at the dehiscence level, the hypothesis being that the stent rigidifies the SPS walls, minimizing the venous pulsation transmission to the inner ear end organs.

Preliminary Otoneurological and Radiological Investigations

Otoneurological assessment of SSCD classically includes pure tone audiometry showing low-frequency negative bone conduction thresholds on the dehiscent side, and enhanced vestibular-evoked myogenic potentials (VEMPs) responses in air

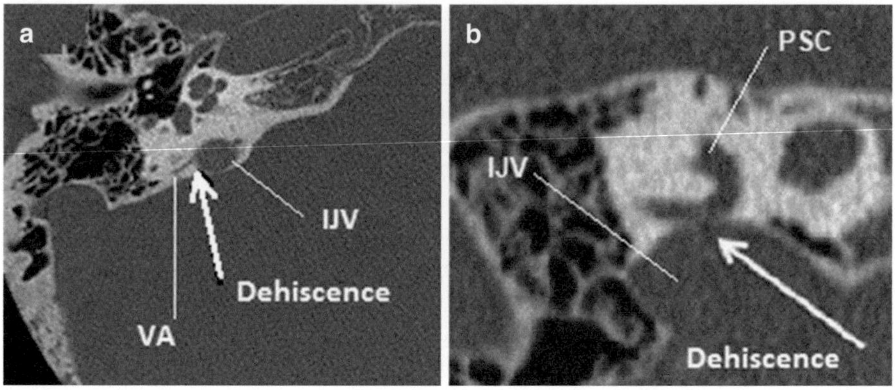

Fig. 16.1 High-riding jugular bulb (HRJB) in contact with a dehiscence of the otic capsule. (**a**) Dehiscence between right IJV and the homonym VA. (**b**) Dehiscence between right IJV and the PSC. *IJV* internal jugular vein, *VA* vestibular aqueduct, *PSC* posterior semicircular canal

conduction [28]. For other TMWs such as dehiscence related to an IJV interface and labyrinthine structures, there are no recommendations although a similar assessment seems well advised.

Commonly, a CT scan of the temporal bone in infra millimetric sections is the gold standard to detect the bony defect [29, 30]. In case of dehiscence involving the jugular bulb, axial slice images are performed, centered on the IJV often associated with a HRJB position (Fig. 16.1a, b). This variant is often observed on the right side, for hemodynamic reasons [31].

In case of dehiscence involving the SPS, a "classic" SSCD image is detected in the plane of this canal (Pöschl plane). However, this image is often more medially located than in a SSCD of the labyrinthine-meningeal interface and has the shape of a "cookie bite" [21] (Fig. 16.2a). We observe the SPS opacification after injection, in the venous phase. MRI of the petrosal bone and inner ear structures has the advantage of being able to improve the diagnosis, and to identify the vascular structure causing the dehiscence [9]. Particularly, 3D T1 weighted sequences can show SPS opacification, and high-resolution labyrinthine sequence 3D T2 could help show the membranous labyrinth morphology and patency [9].

Fusion imaging between HRCT Pöschl plane or 3D T2 and 3D T1 weighted enhanced sequence could help in visualizing the TW's interface (dimensions of the SPS, interface surface, or contact surfaces between vestibular membrane (s) and the walls of the SPS, and an eventual compression effect on the membranous SSC) [9] (Fig. 16.2b, c).

The importance of combining the standard HRCT with 3T MRI to allow a better visualization of the membranous SSC, and an eventual mass-effect by the adjacent SPS at the dehiscence level, has already been described [9].

Before any endovascular procedure, it is essential to check the neuro-vascular anatomy as well as the risk of bleeding. If an endovascular management is chosen

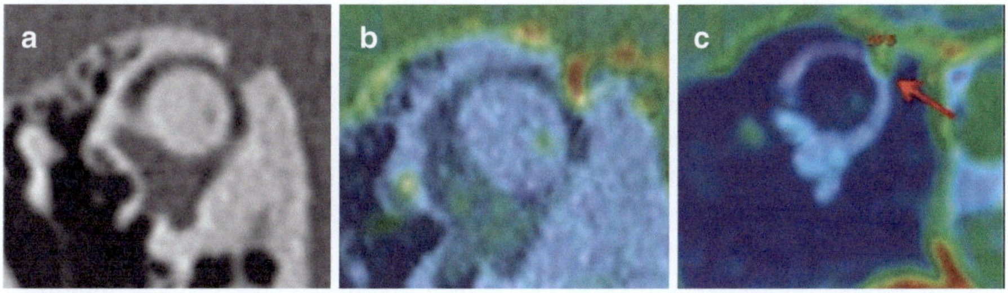

Fig. 16.2 (**a**) high-resolution computed tomography (HRCT) Pöschl plane. "Cookie bite" aspect, SSCD by SPS (length measured at 1.7 mm). (**b**) Fusion between HRCT and 3D T1 weighted enhanced sequence. (**c**) Fusion between 3D T1 weighted enhanced and T2 HR sequences. Compression effect on the SSC (arrow). *SSCD* superior semicircular canal dehiscence, *SPS* superior petrosal sinus

to treat a dehiscence between an HRBJ and the VA or between the HRBJ and a PSC, an evaluation of the IJV in the venous phase of an arteriography carried out by selective catheterization of the ipsilateral internal carotid artery is systematically performed, generally one week before the treatment.

In the case of an SSCD by SPS, the shape and size of the cavernous sinus and the inferior petrosal sinus are assessed to assure retrograde access to the SPS. To avoid possible negative hemodynamic consequences in the venous cerebral circulation in case of SPS thrombosis, alternative accessible retrograde drainage of the SPV through the IJV should be checked beforehand. In addition, if significant anatomic variations of the petrosal venous system (inferior or superior petrosal sinus narrowing or hypoplasia) are found during the preliminary evaluation, stenting of the SPS is not recommended.

Obviously, as for any invasive procedure, the patient must take the decision after being informed of the risks and benefits of the procedure.

Standardized quality of life questionnaires should be used to assess the daily discomfort. The Dizziness Handicap Inventory (DHI) scale in three functional stages proposed by Jacobson and Newman [32] and the Tinnitus Handicap Inventory (THI) scale, classifying tinnitus according to the impact on daily life, [33] seem useful in SSCD [9, 34].

Surgical Treatment

Invasive surgical techniques have been properly described previously. These techniques include ligation, embolization of the jugular vein, or surgical lowering of the HRBJ [18]. The later latter technique requires a deep mastoidectomy with drilling close to the facial nerve, inner ear, and jugular bulb to lower the vein and reconstruct the bony labyrinth with bone dust or cartilage [14, 16].

Endovascular Management

The aim of endovascular management consists in limiting the transmission of vibrations from the vascular wall to the labyrinthine end organs. The TW variants mentioned above can benefit nowadays from alternative endovascular options. These appear to be more conservative than classical surgery, which in some cases may involve sacrificing the venous structures at the origin of possible disturbances of the normal venous return to the base of the skull. In addition, endovascular treatment techniques appear to have an advantage over "classical" surgical techniques because these techniques do not involve manipulating the membranous labyrinth during endovascular procedures. Thus, the risk of hearing or vestibular impairment is estimated to be lower. In fact, the very principle of the endovascular procedure, which aims only to strengthen the vascular resistance at the interface of the dehiscence of the otic capsule, guarantees the preservation of the vestibular function. Thus, in principle, the endovascular procedure is completely opposite to the plugging surgical treatment techniques that propose the anatomical exclusion of SSC involved in non-physiological vestibular stimulation.

Vestibular Aqueduct: Jugular Bulb Dehiscence

The decision to perform endovascular treatment is mutually agreed upon by head and neck surgeons and the neuro-interventional team and is suggested to the patient as an alternative to surgery. Clinicians need to look for signs of Ménière's-like syndrome due to VA compression by JBA [35] as Ménière's syndrome may require a specific treatment, including surgical endolymphatic sac surgery [36].

In case of symptoms due to TW, stent-assisted coil implantation of the JBAs is minimally invasive, preserves venous cerebral blood flow, and gives immediate positive results for pulsatile tinnitus and vertigo [17].

The treatment itself takes place under general anesthesia in a neuro-angiographic suite, after a bolus of heparin. A venous access is performed uni or bilaterally, after femoral venous puncture or direct jugular approach for microcatheter insertion. The guiding catheter is slipped in the jugular vein and two microcatheters are used, one guided in the transverse sinus upstream to the dehiscence to introduce the stent and the other in the outpouching to block it with coils ("jailing technique").

Technically the dehiscence is managed as an aneurysm supplanting the vein, whose treatment is obstruction by placing coils within it, under the protection of a stent forcing the coils to remain in place. The venous sinus thus remains permeable. A stent is deployed to cover the outpouching from top to bottom (Fig. 16.3a, b). If stent deployment is incomplete, it is expanded by stent angioplasty with the use of the same guidewire and a monorail dilation balloon. It is important to perform these stent angioplasties over the jugular foramen to avoid possible compression of the cranial nerves contained in the pars nervosa. Finally, the outpouching is packed with

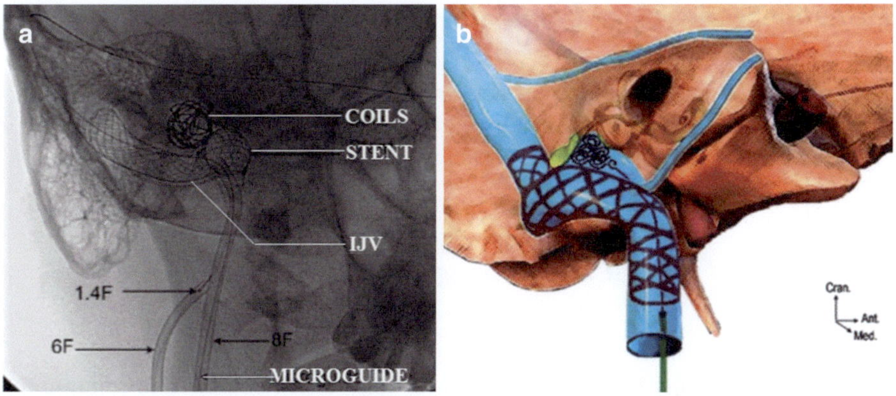

Fig. 16.3 Endovascular procedure for dehiscence of the jugular gulf with the VA. (**a**) Radiography. Coils and stents in place in the right IJV. (**b**) Schematic representation of the jailing technique. *IJV* internal jugular vein. Endolymphatic sac and duct (vestibular aqueduct - *VA*) are displayed in green and brown respectively

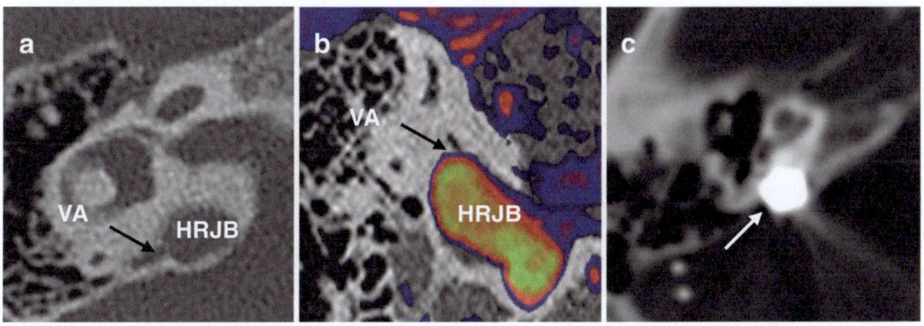

Fig. 16.4 (**a**) right axial petrosal bone high-resolution computed tomography (HRCT). VA in contact with HRJB (black arrow). (**b**) Fusion between HRCT and 3D T1 weighted enhanced sequence of the right petrosal bone—coronal. (**c**) CT—control post treatment: metallic artifact image due to the coils in contact with the right bony labyrinthine structure

detachable bare coils or hydrocoils through the microcatheter (Fig. 16.3a, b). The number of coils depends on the size and filling of the JBA.

At the end of the procedure, the microcatheter is gently removed from the outpouching without disturbing the stent position.

The management of antiplatelet therapy varies; frequently, one antiplatelet drug (clopidogrel) is given for one week before the implantation and is maintained for several months (usually for six months). Some prefer to prescribe two antiplatelet drugs, such as clopidogrel and aspirin.

An immediate postprocedural angiogram can show the placement of the material, with neither coil migration nor interruption of normal venous flow. When performed, postoperative CT scan allows the opportunity to see the coils (metallic artifact) in contact with the dehiscence (see Fig. 16.4 for pre-(a, b) and post-endovascular procedure aspects (c)).

Posterior Semicircular Canal: Jugular Bulb Dehiscence

Although the authors have not yet had any case of this type of dehiscence under clinical observation for which such a treatment could be chosen, we estimate that a similar technique as described above can be successfully applied in this variant.

Dehiscence of the SSCD Involving the Superior Petrous Sinus (SPS)

The first endovascular treatment reported for this variant consisted in stenting the SPS [27]. A standard femoral vein puncture was made under general anesthesia and 500 mg of IV aspirin was injected per procedure. A six French guiding catheter with guide wire was moved forward into the right inferior petrosal sinus, guided by digital subtraction imaging. After accessing the right cavernous sinus, a venogram with retrograde opacification confirmed the presence of a complete petrosal venous system (Fig. 16.5a) Alternatively, the access to the SPS could be made homolaterally to the pathology by catheterization of the SPS abutment in the transverse sinus if the obtuse angle between the two venous structures is sufficiently accessible for navigation. Therefore, the angle formed by SPS with the transverse sinus should be evaluated before choosing the access via the inferior petrosal sinus and cavernous sinus. A single catheter in the SPS will allow the introduction of a stent which has a metal cover and sufficient rigidity to isolate the third window; the stent is placed distally to the cavernous sinus avoiding the obstruction of the superior petrosal vein (SPV) junction to the SPS (Fig. 16.5b). Its size must be chosen with caution, in order to avoid migration or, on the contrary, to avoid labyrinth compression. At the end of the procedure, a venogram showed the patency of both SPS and SPV (Fig. 16.5c). Then, the guidewire and microcatheter are gently withdrawn.

Another case of endovascularly treated SSCD by SPS has been reported in the literature, using a technique inspired by the one described above. The authors

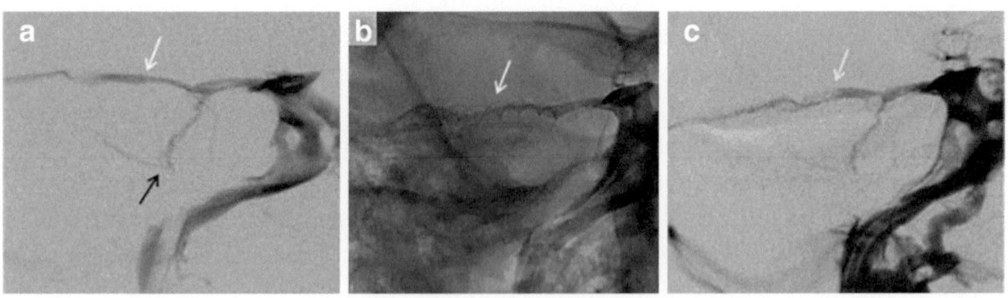

Fig. 16.5 Venogram–frontal views. (**a**) Normal configuration of SPS (white arrow) and SPV (black arrow) before stenting. (**b**) Stents fitted in the SPS (white arrow). (**c**) Venogram at 5 months showing the patency of the SPS (white arrow). *SPS* superior petrosal sinus. *SPV* superior petrosal vein

preferred a coiled SPS thrombosis, a method justified by the presence of a large arachnoid granulation, visualized by angio-MRI. This endovascular procedure was facilitated by the configuration of the deep petrosal venous system. The preoperative anatomic workup had estimated that sacrificing the SPS would leave sufficient alternative venous routes to drain the cavernous sinus and jugular bulb [37].

Post-Treatment Findings

Postoperative clinical assessment often reveals immediate relief of the pulsatile tinnitus. Despite the good results we have obtained and although we have no complications in our small series, these techniques still present a theoretical risk of coil migration and stent thrombosis. The risk of stent thrombosis extrapolated from larger series of venous stents in the transverse sinus seems to be limited. Ahmed et al. reported 52 cases of bilateral transverse sinus stent placement for idiopathic intracranial hypertension without any stent thrombosis or thromboembolic complications [38]. Apart from this, it is known that the peripetrosal sinuses are created by the reflections of the meningeal and periosteal layers of the dura mater, being relatively tense, lined with endothelial cells, which would theoretically limit the risk of thrombosis [39].

A short hospitalization of two days is preferable for anticoagulant treatment surveillance. As the technique uses coils, the same antiplatelet management as described above is recommended after embolization. The rationale for double anti-aggregation in the case of venous stents is not always justified in the absence of a personal history of venous thrombosis. Follow-up angiography at one year may be performed to evaluate the permeability of the stent with stable exclusion of the JBA.

Conclusion

In selected patients, first-line endovascular treatment for vestibular-vascular dehiscence emerges as a new, elegant, and apparently safe alternative to existing surgical techniques. Its principle relies on strengthening the endovascular of the third mobile interface to avoid the transfer of acoustic and/or vibratory energy from the vascular structure to the sensory organs of the inner ear. In addition to classical audiological, vestibular and radiological examinations to diagnose a TMW, additional angio-MRI should be performed in these variants to verify the integrity of the peripetrosal venous circulation.

Obviously our series is still small, our experience being limited to not more than 20 endovascularly treated patients. Therefore, before concluding on the effectiveness and especially the safety of this method, more patients with disabling symptoms should first benefit from it and be followed up enough to assess the real benefit/risk ratio.

Acknowledgment The authors thank Ruxandra C. Ionescu for checking the accuracy of translation in English for this chapter.

References

1. Cawthorne T. Otosclerosis. J Laryngol Otol. 1955;69:437–56. https://doi.org/10.1017/S0022215100050933.
2. Minor LB, Solomon D, Zinreich JS, Zee DS. Sound- and/or pressure-induced vertigo due to bone dehiscence of the superior semicircular canal. Arch Otolaryngol Head Neck Surg. 1998;124(3):249–58. https://doi.org/10.1001/archotol.124.3.249.
3. Smullen JL, Andrist EC, Gianoli GJ. Superior semicircular canal dehiscence: a new cause of vertigo. J Louisiana State Med Soc. 1999;151:397–400.
4. Merchant SN, Rosowski JJ, McKenna MJ. Superior semicircular canal dehiscence mimicking otosclerotic hearing loss. Adv Otorhinolaryngol. 2007;65:137–45. https://doi.org/10.1159/000098790.
5. Ho ML, Moonis G, Halpin CF, Curtin HD. Spectrum of third window abnormalities: semicircular canal dehiscence and beyond. AJNR Am J Neuroradiol. 2017;38(1):2–9. https://doi.org/10.3174/ajnr.A4922.
6. Wackym PA, Wood SJ, Siker DA, Carter DM. Otic capsule dehiscence syndrome: superior semicircular canal dehiscence syndrome with no radiographically visible dehiscence. Ear Nose Throat J. 2015;94:E8–24. https://doi.org/10.1177/014556131509400802.
7. Reynard P, Idriss S, Ltaief-Boudrigua A, Bertholon P, Pirvan A, Truy E, Thai-Van H, Ionescu EC. Proposal for a unitary anatomo-clinical and radiological classification of third mobile window abnormalities. Front Neurol. 2022;12:792545. https://doi.org/10.3389/fneur.2021.792545.
8. Liu Z, Bi W, Li J, Li Q, Dong C, Zhao P, et al. Superior semicircular canal dehiscence in relation to the superior petrosal sinus: a potential cause of pulsatile tinnitus. Clin Radiol. 2015;70:943–7. https://doi.org/10.1016/j.crad.2015.04.017.
9. Ionescu E, Reynard P, Coudert A, Roiban L, Boudrigua AL, Thai-Van H. Superior semicircular canal dehiscence by superior petrosal sinus: proposal for classification. J Int Adv Otol. 2021;17:35–41. https://doi.org/10.5152/iao.2020.9384.
10. Friedmann DR, Eubig J, Winata LS, Pramanik BK, Merchant SN, Lalwani AK. A clinical and histopathologic study of jugular bulb abnormalities. Arch Otolaryngol Head Neck Surg. 2012a;138(1):66–71. https://doi.org/10.1001/archoto.2011.231.
11. Friedmann DR, Le BT, Pramanik BK, Lalwani AK. Clinical spectrum of patients with erosion of the inner ear by jugular bulb abnormalities. Laryngoscope. 2010;120(2):365–72. https://doi.org/10.1002/lary.20699.
12. Friedmann DR, Eubig J, Winata LS, Pramanik BK, Merchant SN, Lalwani AK. Prevalence of jugular bulb abnormalities and resultant inner ear dehiscence: a histopathologic and radiologic study. Otolaryngol Head Neck Surg. 2012b;147(4):750–6. https://doi.org/10.1177/0194599812448615.
13. Otto KJ, Hudgins PA, Abdelkafy W, Mattox DE. Sigmoid sinus diverticulum: a new surgical approach to the correction of pulsatile tinnitus. Otol Neurotol. 2006;28:48–53.
14. Couloigner V, Grayeli AB, Bouccara D, Julien N, Sterkers O. Surgical treatment of the high jugular bulb in patients with Meniere's disease and pulsatile tinnitus. Eur Arch Otorhinolaryngol. 1999;256(5):224–9. https://doi.org/10.1007/s004050050146.
15. Berguer R, Nowak P. Treatment of venous pulsatile tinnitus in younger women. Ann Vasc Surg. 2015;29(4):650–3.
16. El-Begermy MA, Rabie AN. A novel surgical technique for management of tinnitus due to high dehiscent jugular bulb. Otolaryngol Head Neck Surg. 2010;142(4):576–81. https://doi.org/10.1016/j.otohns.2009.12.007.

17. Hitier M, Barbier C, Marie-Aude T, Moreau S, Courtheoux P, Patron V. New treatment of vertigo caused by jugular bulb abnormalities. Surg Innov. 2014a;21(4):365–71. https://doi.org/10.1177/1553350613505918.
18. Thénint MA, Barbier C, Hitier M, Patron V, Saleme S, Courthéoux P. Endovascular treatment of symptomatic vestibular aqueduct dehiscence as a result of jugular bulb abnormalities. J Vasc Interv Radiol. 2014;25:1816–20. https://doi.org/10.1016/j.jvir.2014.07.013.
19. Gard AP, Klopper HB, Thorell WE. Successful endovascular treatment of pulsatile tinnitus caused by a sigmoid sinus aneurysm. A case report and review of the literature. Interv Neuroradiol. 2009;15(4):425–8. https://doi.org/10.1177/159101990901500409.
20. Signorelli F, Mahla K, Turjman F. Endovascular treatment of two concomitant causes of pulsatile tinnitus: sigmoid sinus stenosis and ipsilateral jugular bulb diverticulum. Case report and literature review. Acta Neurochir. 2012;154(1):89–92. https://doi.org/10.1007/s00701-011-1202-3.
21. Schneiders SMD, Rainsbury JW, Hensen EF, Irving RM. Superior petrosal sinus causing superior canal dehiscence syndrome. J Laryngol Otol. 2017;131:593–647. https://doi.org/10.1017/S0022215117001013.
22. Koo JW, Hong SK, Kim DK, Kim JS. Superior semicircular canal dehiscence syndrome by the superior petrosal sinus. J Neurol Neurosurg Psychiatry. 2010;81:465–7. https://doi.org/10.1136/jnnp.2008.155564.
23. Lookabaugh S, Kelly HR, Carter MS, Niesten ME, McKenna MJ, Curtin H, Lee DJ. Radiologic classification of superior canal dehiscence: implications for surgical repair. Otol Neurotol. 2015;36(1):118–25. https://doi.org/10.1097/MAO.0000000000000523.
24. Ziylan F, Kinaci A, Beynon AJ, Kunst HP. A comparison of surgical treatments for superior semicircular canal dehiscence: a systematic review. Otol Neurotol. 2017;38:1–10. https://doi.org/10.1097/MAO.0000000000001277.
25. Ward BK, Agrawal Y, Nguyen E, Della Santina CC, Limb CJ, Francis HW, et al. Hearing outcomes after surgical plugging of the superior semicircular canal by a middle cranial fossa approach. Otol Neurotol. 2012;33:1386–91. https://doi.org/10.1097/MAO.0b013e318268d20d.
26. McCall AA, McKenna MJ, Merchant SN, Curtin HD, Lee DJ. Superior canal dehiscence syndrome associated with the superior petrosal sinus in pediatric and adult patients. Otol Neurotol. 2011;32:1312–9. https://doi.org/10.1097/MAO.0b013e31822e5b0a.
27. Ionescu EC, Coudert A, Reynard P, Truy E, Thai-Van H, Ltaief-Boudrigua A, Turjman F. Stenting the superior petrosal sinus in a patient with symptomatic superior semicircular canal dehiscence. Front Neurol. 2018;9:689. https://doi.org/10.3389/fneur.2018.00689.
28. Ward BK, van de Berg R, van Rompaey V, Bisdorff A, Hullar TE, Welgampola MS, Carey JP. Superior semicircular canal dehiscence syndrome: Diagnostic criteria consensus document of the committee for the classification of vestibular disorders of the Bárány Society. J Vestib Res. 2021;31(3):131–41. https://doi.org/10.3233/VES-200004.
29. Belden CJ, Weg N, Minor LB, Zinreich SJ. CT evaluation of bone dehiscence of the superior semicircular canal as a cause of sound and/or pressure-induced vertigo. Radiology. 2003;226:337–43. https://doi.org/10.1148/radiol.2262010897.
30. Ward BK, Carey JP, Minor LB. Superior Canal dehiscence syndrome: lessons from the first 20 years. Front Neurol. 2017;8:177. https://doi.org/10.3389/fneur.2017.00177.
31. Friedmann DR, Eubig J, McGill M, Babb JS, Pramanik BK, Lalwani AK. Development of the jugular bulb: a radiologic study. Otol Neurotol. 2011;32(8):1389–95. https://doi.org/10.1097/MAO.0b013e31822e5b8d.
32. Jacobson GP, Newman CW. The development of the dizziness handicap inventory. Arch Otolaryngol Head Neck Surg. 1990;116:424–7. https://doi.org/10.1001/archotol.1990.01870040046011.
33. Newman CW, Jacobson GP, Spitzer JB. Development of the Tinnitus Handicap Inventory. Arch Otolaryngol Head Neck Surg. 1996;122(2):143–8. https://doi.org/10.1001/archotol.1996.01890140029007.

34. Crane BT, Minor LB, Carey JP. Superior canal dehiscence plugging reduces dizziness handicap. Laryngoscope. 2008;118(10):1809–13. https://doi.org/10.1097/MLG.0b013e31817f18fa.
35. Hitier M, Roger V, Moreau S, Patron V. High jugular bulb in a cohort of patients with definite Ménière's disease. J Laryngol Otol. 2014b;128(12):1125.
36. Gendre A, Bourget-Aguilar K, Calais C, Espitalier F, Bordure P, Michel G. Evaluation of vestibular function following endolymphatic sac surgery. Eur Arch Otorhinolaryngol. 2022;279(3):1193–201. https://doi.org/10.1007/s00405-021-06743-3.
37. Aw GE, Parker GD, Halmagyi GM, Saxby AJ. Pulsatile tinnitus in superior semicircular canal dehiscence cured by endovascular coil occlusion of the superior petrosal sinus. Otol Neurotol. 2021;42(5):e629–30. https://doi.org/10.1097/MAO.0000000000003012.
38. Ahmed RM, Wilkinson M, Parker GD, Thurtell MJ, Macdonald J, McCluskey PJ, Allan R, Dunne V, Hanlon M, Owler BK, Halmagyi GM. Transverse sinus stenting for idiopathic intracranial hypertension: a review of 52 patients and of model predictions. AJNR Am J Neuroradiol. 2011;32(8):1408–14. https://doi.org/10.3174/ajnr.A2575.
39. Miyawaki EK. Encyclopedia of the neurological sciences. 2nd ed. Cambridge, MA: Academic Press; 2014.

Part IV
Special Situations

Gerard J. Gianoli

Introduction

Unique situations deserve special consideration regarding the diagnosis, treatment, and prognosis of TMWD. So often in medicine we think of individual diseases in a vacuum. Unfortunately, just because a patient has diabetes does not preclude them from also having rheumatoid arthritis. Obviously, the diabetes will influence how the rheumatoid arthritis is treated. Certain immunosuppressants, such as corticosteroids, would want to be avoided due to their untoward effects on diabetic control. Other concomitant disorders can affect or influence the course and prognosis of each other. Such is the case of diabetes and hypertension since both will cause advancement of atherosclerosis.

In the same way, TMWD does not present itself in a vacuum either. There are a number of concomitant disorders/problems that will affect the progression, diagnosis, and treatment of TMWD. Among the most common is bilateral disease. Bilateral disease deserves more attention to diagnosis and counseling of patients than unilateral disease. Concomitant otosclerosis, elevated intracranial pressure, migraine, encephalocele, CSF leak and endolymphatic hydrops present unique problems in diagnosis as well as postoperative management. The special population of the Pediatric, Geriatric, and only hearing ear patient are also unique and may send the clinician down a different treatment based on these factors alone. Lastly, the presentation of TMWS in the postoperative setting is an uncommon presentation but one that we should all be aware of, as well as the diagnostic difficulties in this group.

Chapter 17
Bilateral Superior Semicircular Canal Dehiscence Syndrome

Ariana Chow, Natalie Mahgerefteh, Courtney Duong, Khashayar Mozaffari, Quinton Gopen, and Isaac Yang

Clinical Presentation

Nearly one-third of all SCDS cases present with bilateral pathology [1], however, emerging reports with larger cohorts estimate this number may be closer to 50% [2–4]. The clinical manifestation of bilateral SCDS, similar to its unilateral counterpart, is towards the sixth decade of life and has a modest predilection for females (Table 17.1) [2–4]. Similarly, the diagnostic triad consists of a combination of comprehensive clinical evaluation, including audiogram and vestibular evoked myogenic potential (VEMP) testing, and confirmed with high resolution computed tomography (HRCT) imaging [5–7] (Fig. 17.1). While the characteristic profile of SCDS is similar between unilateral and bilateral disease, specific symptoms such as

Table 17.1 Comparative characteristics of bilateral and unilateral SCDS populations

	Bilateral	Unilateral
Age [2, 3]	Sixth decade	Sixth decade
Sex (female:male) [2, 3]	1.8:1	1.2:1
Head trauma (%) [3]	18.4%	17.4%
Repair side (left:right) [3]	1.3:1	1.2:1

A. Chow · N. Mahgerefteh · C. Duong · K. Mozaffari · I. Yang (✉)
Department of Neurosurgery, University of California, Los Angeles (UCLA), Los Angeles, CA, USA
e-mail: Arianaxchow@ucla.edu; nataliemahg@g.ucla.edu; IYang@mednet.ucla.edu

Q. Gopen
Department of Head and Neck Surgery, University of California, Los Angeles (UCLA), Los Angeles, CA, USA
e-mail: QGopen@mednet.ucla.edu

G. J. Gianoli, P. Thomson (eds.), *Third Mobile Window Syndrome of the Inner Ear*, https://doi.org/10.1007/978-3-031-16586-3_17

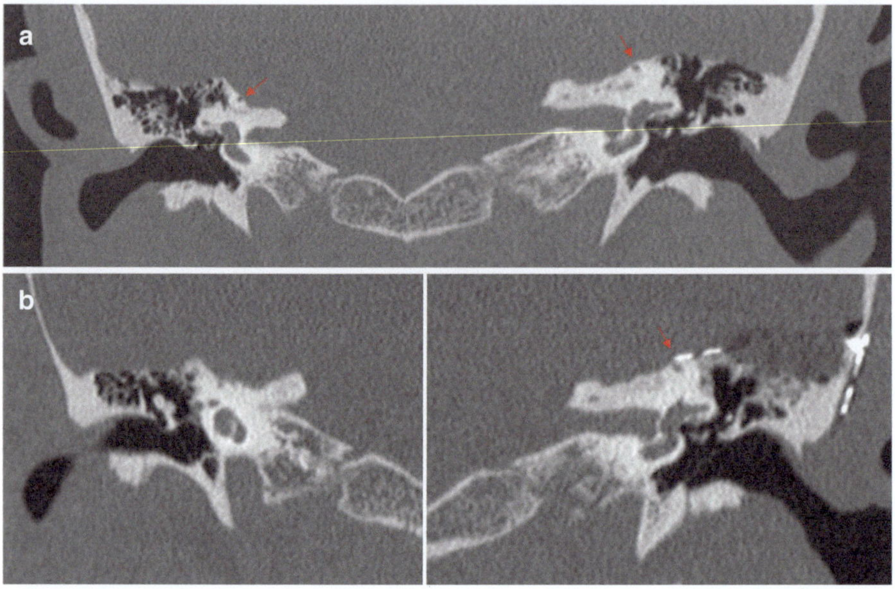

Fig. 17.1 High resolution computed tomography (HRCT) of a 43-year-old male with bilateral SCDS who elected for repair of the left-sided dehiscence. (**a**) Preoperative HRCT of the temporal shows both left and right sided dehiscence (arrows), with symptom presentation of amplification of internal sounds, aural fullness, rapid hearing loss, and tinnitus. (**b**) Postoperative HRCT of the left-sided dehiscence (arrow) with the sealing technique. At the 15-month follow-up, the patient had alleviation of aural fullness and amplification of internal sounds

vertical oscillopsia, impaired visual acuity upon movement, unsteady gait, and vertical and torsional jerk nystagmus have been reported in cases of distinct bilateral presentation [2, 8, 9]. One study found a potential correlation between bilateral disease and history of head trauma [2], and it has also been suggested that dizziness, internal sound amplification, and hearing loss, and disequilibrium may be more common in patients presenting with bilateral pathology as well (Table 17.2) [2–4].

Table 17.2 Comparison of symptom presentation between bilateral and unilateral SCDS populations

	Bilateral	Unilateral
Auditory		
Autophony		✓
Tinnitus		✓
Aural fullness		✓
Hearing loss		✓
Internal amplification		✓
Hyperacusis		✓
Vestibular		
Dizziness		✓
Disequilibrium		✓
Vertigo		✓
Oscillopsia	✓	
Headache		✓

✓ indicates higher prevalence of presentation within the cohort [2, 4]

Management

Asymptomatic patients or those with mild symptoms may choose to pursue more conservative measures such as trigger avoidance and vestibular sedation [2, 5]. However, patients with debilitating and persistent clinical manifestations may require surgical intervention for symptom alleviation. Typically, bilateral SCDS is managed one side at a time, with initial surgical side contingent on the patients' and surgeons' discretion. Generally, the perceiving more symptomatic side receives the first operation, which can at times provide enough symptom alleviation to evade surgical intervention on the contralateral side. This is not always the case as persisting symptoms may still warrant a second surgery. Following the surgical repair of the more severe side, enduring manifestations from the unrepaired ear may become uncovered. Subsequently, patients will require a second surgery if symptoms are intractable [2]. Additional counseling for patients with bilateral SCDS should be spent discussing these potential outcomes so there is a clear understanding of why surgery may be required on both sides [2].

Dehiscence repair is usually accomplished by either plugging, resurfacing, or capping the bony defect in order to re-establish the superior canal roof, and restore the normal transmission of pressure through the inner ear [2–4, 10, 11]. Plugging involves filling the canal with fascia and bone dust to obstruct the canal [12]. Resurfacing entails covering the dehiscence with fascia and a bone graft or bone paste to seal the third window without occlusion of the canal, and capping refers to a procedure in which cartilage or a bone graft is used alone [4, 12–14]. Some evidence suggests that plugging is associated with lower rates of symptom relapse and higher long-term control compared to resurfacing [4, 15]. This may be due to the total occlusion of the canal, which would lead to complete loss of the fluid signal and any subsequent vestibular deficits. This can be an especially key factor in surgical planning, as loss of function in bilateral superior canals can yield a new set of consequences for patients. In a series of 20 surgical repairs, Minor et al. noted complete resolution of vestibular symptoms in 88.9% of patients who received a plugging procedure, compared to 63.6% of patients who underwent resurfacing [15]. When considerable symptomatic impairment is present with bilateral SCDS, the more symptomatic side may be identified and targeted for repair via surgical intervention, and a subsequent repair should generally be pursued only if contralateral symptoms develop, persist, or worsen [2, 5, 6]. In cases where one side is not notably more symptomatic, evaluation of pressure- and sound-induced nystagmus can help select a side for repair [6].

There are various approaches and techniques for surgical management of SCDS [6, 7, 12, 16–18]. A recent review of the literature identified the following four approaches with varying degrees of clinical utility: middle fossa, transmastoid, endoscopic, and transcanal or endaural [7]. However, the two most commonly used approaches are the middle fossa and the transmastoid approach [5]. Many have suggested that the middle fossa approach is the optimal method because it enables a clearer view of the dehiscence [3, 4] and alleviates vestibular symptoms rather effectively [1, 10, 11, 19–21]. However, the transmastoid approach offers its inherent advantages as well. This technique is a more familiar procedure to most otologists, and may present a lower risk of cerebrospinal fluid (CSF) leak, facial nerve injury, and other intracranial complications [1, 12]. Amoodi et al. reported four cases of SCDS that experienced complete resolution following a transmastoid resurfacing procedure [12]. Furthermore, middle cranial fossa resurfacing may confer the attendant risk of seizure due to retraction of the temporal lobe [1, 12, 13, 22, 23]. Although there are always risks associated with surgery, most patients report major improvement in their symptoms [10–14, 16–18, 24–31].

Outcomes

Bilateral SCDS may exhibit a different recovery course compared to unilateral disease. It has been suggested that bilateral SCDS may involve a prolonged recovery time due to the onset of latent contralateral or postoperative symptoms, which may be targeted with subsequent repair [5, 32, 33]. Niesten et al. noted that 54.5% of patients with bilateral SCDS experienced a recovery period of over months, compared to the common duration of a few weeks, and hypothesized that the initial repair may have unmasked symptoms from the contralateral defect and contributed to persisting vestibular symptoms [32]. Furthermore, Wung et al. found that patients with bilateral SCDS had a significantly greater likelihood of experiencing postoperative disequilibrium and autophony than those with unilateral dehiscence [4]. Plugging of the second side has been associated with oscillopsia as well, although the primary, and often more debilitating, symptoms are relieved [2, 5, 33]. Agrawal et al. reported onset of varying degrees of oscillopsia in four patients with bilateral SCDS after a second repair [33]. However, they all still reported general satisfaction with the subsequent repair, which led the authors to suggest that resolution of the initial preoperative bilateral SCDS symptoms may be more significant than the development of temporary to semi-persistent oscillopsia [33].

Bilateral pathology tends to correlate with poorer symptomatic resolution, although overall clinical improvement is reported widely [2, 3, 5, 32]. One study of 41 cases of bilateral SCDS found that patients with bilateral disease experience both greater initial rates and poorer resolution of dizziness [2]. In a large series of 229 surgical repairs, Mozaffari et al. also found that patients with unilateral SCDS saw significantly greater improvement of autophony, aural fullness, tinnitus, hearing loss, dizziness and headache, compared to their bilateral SCDS counterparts [3]. However, patients with bilateral SCDS still benefited from great relief in many of their initial symptoms as dramatic symptomatic resolution was noted in oscillopsia (86.7%), vertigo (75.9%) and hyperacusis (73.0%) [3]. Such results highlight the effectiveness of surgical repair for SCDS patients with bilateral disease, albeit less favorable than their unilateral counterparts.

In addition, it has been suggested that the severity of the bilateral disease itself may also affect outcomes for patients diagnosed with bilateral SCDS. In a series of 179 SCDS patients, researchers noted that patients with bilateral SCDS who underwent unilateral repair experienced significantly greater improvement of hyperacusis, hearing loss, dizziness and disequilibrium, compared to those who required bilateral surgical repair [3]. These findings suggest that there may be salient differences in the clinical courses of patients with unilateral and bilateral SCDS, as well as differences within bilateral patients who have undergone unilateral repair versus those who have undergone bilateral repair.

The underlying reason responsible for some bilateral patients requiring bilateral surgeries, versus others who experience symptomatic improvement following unilateral surgery, is unclear and should be investigated in future studies. Foremost, a large part in surgical management of SCDS relies on the patients' perception of symptom severity and the discussions they have with their surgeons. A study by Mozaffari et al. analyzed outcome differences in bilateral patients who had either unilateral or bilateral repairs [3]. They hypothesize that "unmasking" of contralateral symptoms in unilateral repairs may account for the extended delay of patients seeking repair of the remaining side [3]. Audiologic and cVEMP testing may reliably tell researchers and physicians objective data but if unilateral alleviation provides enough relief, the stress and potential risks of an additional operation can be avoided. Radiographic features of the dehiscence may also contribute, as greater dehiscence volume has been associated with greater impairment on physiologic testing [34, 35] and more severe symptoms [36]. However, such results have mostly been published with unilateral SCDS patients [34–36], and it is important to note that unilateral SCDS may not have an identical clinical presentation to that of bilateral SCDS, thus, such findings may not be applicable to the bilateral SCDS patient population.

More research studies are needed to elucidate the effects of bilaterality on the clinical presentation and outcomes of SCDS. Recognizing the more complex clinical course of bilateral disease compared to unilateral SCDS, and the lower likelihood of achieving symptomatic resolution in such patients, can provide practical information to both neuro-otologists and patients when discussing the repair of this anomaly, especially when considering contralateral repair after the initial surgery.

References

1. Yew A, Zarinkhou G, Spasic M, Trang A, Gopen Q, Yang I. Characteristics and management of superior semicircular canal dehiscence. J Neurol Surg B Skull Base. 2012;73(6):365–70. https://doi.org/10.1055/s-0032-1324397.
2. Jacky Chen CH, Nguyen T, Udawatta M, et al. Clinical assessment of patients with bilateral superior semicircular canal dehiscence. World Neurosurg. 2019;126:e1549–52. https://doi.org/10.1016/j.wneu.2019.03.205.
3. Mozaffari K, Willis SL, Unterberger A, et al. Superior semicircular canal dehiscence outcomes in a consecutive series of 229 surgical repairs with middle cranial fossa craniotomy. World Neurosurg. 2021;156:e229–34. https://doi.org/10.1016/j.wneu.2021.09.038.
4. Wung V, Romiyo P, Ng E, et al. Sealing of superior semicircular canal dehiscence is associated with improved balance outcomes postoperatively versus plugging of the canal in middle fossa craniotomy repairs: a case series. J Neurosurg. 2020;133(2):462–6. https://doi.org/10.3171/2019.4.JNS19264.
5. Bi WL, Brewster R, Poe D, et al. Superior semicircular canal dehiscence syndrome. J Neurosurg. 2017;127(6):1268–76. https://doi.org/10.3171/2016.9.JNS16503.
6. Mikulec AA, Poe DS, McKenna MJ. Operative management of superior semicircular canal dehiscence. Laryngoscope. 2005;115(3):501–7. https://doi.org/10.1097/01.mlg.0000157844.48036.e7.
7. Mau C, Kamal N, Badeti S, et al. Superior semicircular canal dehiscence: diagnosis and management. J Clin Neurosci. 2018;48:58–65. https://doi.org/10.1016/j.jocn.2017.11.019.
8. Deutschländer A, Strupp M, Jahn K, Jäger L, Quiring F, Brandt T. Vertical oscillopsia in bilateral superior canal dehiscence syndrome. Neurology. 2004;62(5):784–7. https://doi.org/10.1212/01.wnl.0000117978.13194.ed.
9. Tilikete C, Krolak-Salmon P, Truy E, Vighetto A. Pulse-synchronous eye oscillations revealing bone superior canal dehiscence. Ann Neurol. 2004;56(4):556–60. https://doi.org/10.1002/ana.20231.
10. Minor LB, Solomon D, Zinreich JS, Zee DS. Sound- and/or pressure-induced vertigo due to bone dehiscence of the superior semicircular canal. Arch Otolaryngol Head Neck Surg. 1998;124(3):249–58. https://doi.org/10.1001/archotol.124.3.249.
11. Minor LB. Superior canal dehiscence syndrome. Am J Otol. 2000;21(1):9–19.
12. Amoodi HA, Makki FM, McNeil M, Bance M. Transmastoid resurfacing of superior semicircular canal dehiscence. Laryngoscope. 2011;121(5):1117–23. https://doi.org/10.1002/lary.21398.
13. Banakis Hartl RM, Cass SP. Effectiveness of transmastoid plugging for semicircular canal dehiscence syndrome. Otolaryngol Head Neck Surg. 2018;158(3):534–40. https://doi.org/10.1177/0194599817751092.
14. Agrawal SK, Parnes LS. Transmastoid superior semicircular canal occlusion. Otol Neurotol. 2008;29(3):363–7. https://doi.org/10.1097/mao.0b013e3181616c9d.
15. Minor LB. Clinical manifestations of superior semicircular canal dehiscence. Laryngoscope. 2005;115(10):1717–27. https://doi.org/10.1097/01.mlg.0000178324.55729.b7.

16. Beyea JA, Agrawal SK, Parnes LS. Transmastoid semicircular canal occlusion: a safe and highly effective treatment for benign paroxysmal positional vertigo and superior canal dehiscence. Laryngoscope. 2012;122(8):1862–6. https://doi.org/10.1002/lary.23390.
17. Limb CJ, Carey JP, Srireddy S, Minor LB. Auditory function in patients with surgically treated superior semicircular canal dehiscence. Otol Neurotol. 2006;27(7):969–80. https://doi.org/10.1097/01.mao.0000235376.70492.8e.
18. Zhao YC, Somers T, van Dinther J, Vanspauwen R, Husseman J, Briggs R. Transmastoid repair of superior semicircular canal dehiscence. J Neurol Surg B Skull Base. 2012;73(4):225–9. https://doi.org/10.1055/s-0032-1312713.
19. Chien WW, Carey JP, Minor LB. Canal dehiscence. Curr Opin Neurol. 2011;24(1):25–31. https://doi.org/10.1097/WCO.0b013e328341ef88.
20. Brantberg K, Bergenius J, Tribukait A. Vestibular-evoked myogenic potentials in patients with dehiscence of the superior semicircular canal. Acta Otolaryngol. 1999;119(6):633–40. https://doi.org/10.1080/00016489950180559.
21. Brantberg K, Bergenius J, Mendel L, Witt H, Tribukait A, Ygge J. Symptoms, findings and treatment in patients with dehiscence of the superior semicircular canal. Acta Otolaryngol. 2001;121(1):68–75. https://doi.org/10.1080/000164801300006308.
22. Mcelveen JT, House JW, Hitselberger WE, Brackmann DE. Retrolabyrinthine vestibular nerve section: a viable alternative to the middle fossa approach. Otolaryngol Head Neck Surg. 1984;92(2):136–40. https://doi.org/10.1177/019459988409200203.
23. Glasscock ME, Davis WE, Hughes GB, Jackson CG. Labyrinthectomy versus middle fossa vestibular nerve section in Menière's disease; a critical evaluation of relief of vertigo. Ann Otol Rhinol Laryngol. 1980;89(4):318–24. https://doi.org/10.1177/000348948008900405.
24. Teixido MT, Artz GJ, Kung BC. Clinical experience with symptomatic superior canal dehiscence in a single neurotologic practice. Otolaryngol Head Neck Surg. 2008;139(3):405–13. https://doi.org/10.1016/j.otohns.2008.06.023.
25. Powell HRF, Khalil SS, Saeed SR. Outcomes of transmastoid surgery for superior semicircular canal dehiscence syndrome. Otol Neurotol. 2016;37(7):e228–33. https://doi.org/10.1097/MAO.0000000000001103.
26. Thomeer H, Bonnard D, Castetbon V, Franco-Vidal V, Darrouzet P, Darrouzet V. Long-term results of middle fossa plugging of superior semicircular canal dehiscences: clinically and instrumentally demonstrated efficiency in a retrospective series of 16 ears. Eur Arch Otorhinolaryngol. 2016;273(7):1689–96. https://doi.org/10.1007/s00405-015-3715-5.
27. Crane BT, Lin FR, Minor LB, Carey JP. Improvement in autophony symptoms after superior canal dehiscence repair. Otol Neurotol. 2010;31(1):140–6. https://doi.org/10.1097/mao.0b013e3181bc39ab.
28. Fiorino F, Barbieri F, Pizzini FB, Beltramello A. A dehiscent superior semicircular canal may be plugged and resurfaced via the transmastoid route. Otol Neurotol. 2010;31(1):136–9. https://doi.org/10.1097/MAO.0b013e3181b76b9e.
29. Deschenes GR, Hsu DP, Megerian CA. Outpatient repair of superior semicircular canal dehiscence via the transmastoid approach. Laryngoscope. 2009;119(9):1765–9. https://doi.org/10.1002/lary.20543.
30. Kirtane MV, Sharma A, Satwalekar D. Transmastoid repair of superior semicircular canal dehiscence. J Laryngol Otol. 2009;123(3):356–8. https://doi.org/10.1017/S0022215108002375.
31. Yuen HW, Eikelboom RH, Atlas MD. Auditory manifestations of superior semicircular canal dehiscence. Otol Neurotol. 2009;30(3):280–5. https://doi.org/10.1097/mao.0b013e31819d895e.
32. Niesten MEF, McKenna MJ, Grolman W, Lee DJ. Clinical factors associated with prolonged recovery after superior canal dehiscence surgery. Otol Neurotol. 2012;33(5):824–31. https://doi.org/10.1097/MAO.0b013e3182544c9e.
33. Agrawal Y, Minor LB, Schubert MC, Janky KL, Davalos-Bichara M, Carey JP. Second-side surgery in superior canal dehiscence syndrome. Otol Neurotol. 2012;33(1):72–7. https://doi.org/10.1097/MAO.0b013e31823c9182.

34. Castellucci A, Piras G, Del Vecchio V, et al. The effect of superior canal dehiscence size and location on audiometric measurements, vestibular-evoked myogenic potentials and video-head impulse testing. Eur Arch Otorhinolaryngol. 2021;278(4):997–1015. https://doi.org/10.1007/s00405-020-06169-3.
35. Rajan GP, Leaper MR, Goggin L, Atlas MD, Boeddinghaus R, Eikelboom RK. The effects of superior semicircular canal dehiscence on the labyrinth: does size matter? Otol Neurotol. 2008;29(7):972–5. https://doi.org/10.1097/MAO.0b013e31817f7382.
36. Lagman C, Beckett JS, Chung LK, et al. Novel method of measuring canal dehiscence and evaluation of its potential as a predictor of symptom outcomes after middle fossa craniotomy. Neurosurgery. 2018;83(3):459–64. https://doi.org/10.1093/neuros/nyx430.

Chapter 18
Otosclerosis

Jonathan Choi and Seilish C. Babu

Introduction

Conductive hearing loss (CHL), defined as an air-bone gap measured by standard audiometry, is most commonly due to middle ear diseases such as otosclerosis [1]. In otosclerosis, abnormal bony metabolism of otic capsule endochondral bone results in progressive hearing loss [2, 3]. Classically, hearing loss is conductive, though sensorineural or mixed hearing loss can occur if the disease extends into the cochlear endosteum. Surgical treatment, by means of stapedectomy or stapedotomy, is extremely effective in correcting the CHL in otosclerosis [4].

CHL can, however, occur in patients without middle ear pathology. Third window syndromes such as enlarged vestibular aqueduct (EVA), X-linked recessive conductive deafness, and superior semicircular canal dehiscence (SCD) have a wide spectrum of clinical manifestations including one that closely mimics the CHL in otosclerosis [5]. It is hypothesized that the CHL from a third window is from the shunting of a portion of the air-conducted acoustic energy entering the vestibule through motion of the stapes away from the cochlea [5, 6]. The hearing loss by air conduction primarily occurs at low frequencies. Concurrently, the third window may improve bone-conducted sound thresholds, resulting in a net CHL audiometric effect [6].

Differentiation of CHL due to third window syndromes from otosclerosis can be challenging because of their overlapping clinical symptoms and presentation. As a matter of fact, there are several reports in the scientific literature of third window syndromes masquerading as otosclerosis that were only discovered after further investigation of post-stapedotomy failure [7–9]. However, there are key distinctions

J. Choi (✉) · S. C. Babu
Michigan Ear Institute, Farmington Hills, MI, USA

G. J. Gianoli, P. Thomson (eds.), *Third Mobile Window Syndrome of the Inner Ear*, https://doi.org/10.1007/978-3-031-16586-3_18

(which will be discussed later in this chapter) to help determine the correct cause of the CHL that will ultimately help make the correct diagnosis and provide the best treatment options for patients.

The greater challenge is correctly identifying patients with concurrent otosclerosis and SCD or any third window syndrome, and determining the appropriate treatment. The incidence of concurrent SCD and otosclerosis is low and purely coincidental given the unique pathogenesis of each. In a 2009 retrospective study, Picavet et al. reported 5.3% of 114 patients with clinical presentations most consistent with otosclerosis demonstrated radiographic evidence of SCD [10]. However, this concurrence rate is likely an overestimate given that middle ear exploration was not offered to this cohort confirming stapes fixation.

Given the rarity of these cases and subsequently our lack of data of stapes surgery outcomes in this group of patients, a better understanding is needed to inform clinical decision making and patient counseling. In this chapter, we will review the presentation, diagnosis, surgical options, and outcomes in treatment of concurrent otosclerosis and third mobile window syndromes, focusing mostly on SCD. We will also discuss potential pitfalls that may be encountered during clinical workup and treatment, with the hope to help others formulate their treatment paradigms.

Otosclerosis

Otosclerosis is a process of progressive pathologic bony remodeling of the otic capsule of the temporal bone [2, 3]. The prevalence of otosclerosis is significantly higher in Caucasians than African Americans and Asians [11]. The ethnic differences in prevalence rates of otosclerosis are largely a reflection of genetic factors, as a positive family history of otosclerosis has been reported in up to 60% of cases. The data in the scientific literature also suggest a higher prevalence in females than males (2:1) [11].

History is one of the most critical aspects of evaluation. The most common clinical presentation is progressive unilateral or bilateral CHL that becomes apparent in individuals between their third and fifth decade of life [11]. Tinnitus and vertigo may also be present. The relationship between otosclerosis and vertigo is less clear, though prior studies mentioned concomitant Ménière's disease and/or otosclerotic foci involving the vestibular labyrinth as potential culprits. This, however, was prior to SCD being a well-established otologic entity and thus should likely warrant reinvestigation to determine the true cause of vertigo in these patients [12, 13]. As mentioned before, there is usually a positive family history of hearing loss and possibly even a history of surgical correction of their hearing loss. Third window symptoms including imbalance, hyperacusis, oscillopsia, autophony, and sound- or pressure-induced vertigo are usually absent.

Otoscopic examination is usually unremarkable. However, some patients will have a red blush over the promontory, which is known as the Schwartze sign. Audiometric evaluation will reveal an air-bone gap, with Carhart's notch and normal bone thresholds [14]. Acoustic reflexes, which are a sensitive measure of the movement of the stapes, will usually be absent in otosclerosis but present in third window syndromes [15].

Often, the diagnosis of otosclerosis can be made with careful history, audiometric evaluation, and acoustic reflexes. However, if there is any doubt with the diagnosis, imaging studies should be obtained with high-resolution computed tomography (HRCT) of the temporal bone being the radiologic method of choice [16]. On CT, otosclerotic lesions appear as hypodense or radiolucent foci in the otic capsule. Careful attention should be paid to the region anterior to the oval window, specifically the fissula ante fenestram, as 70–95% of otosclerotic lesions are seen here [16]. It is important to note, though, that CT is not reliable in detecting otosclerosis when lesions are sclerotic. Air-conduction vestibular evoked myogenic potentials (VEMPs) may also help and will be absent in otosclerosis.

Third Window Syndromes

Enlarged Vestibular Aqueduct

Enlarged vestibular aqueduct (EVA) syndrome was first described by Valvassori and Clemis in 1978 and is a congenital malformation of the temporal bone resulting in an abnormal dilation of the vestibular aqueduct [17]. No universally agreed-upon size criteria exist for when a vestibular aqueduct is considered enlarged—in general, however, vestibular aqueduct diameter larger than 1.5 mm at the midpoint or a vestibular aqueduct wider than the width of the posterior semicircular canal is considered enlarged [18].

Despite being a congenital condition, the age of diagnosis of hearing loss is quite variable, ranging from infancy to adulthood. Moreover, there appears to be significant heterogeneity with the type of hearing loss among individuals with EVA. Most will demonstrate a post-lingual onset of progressive sensorineural hearing loss (SNHL) [19]. The prevalence of EVA in patients with SNHL is estimated to range between 1 and 12% and has increased since the 1990s likely due to implementation of universal newborn hearing screening and HRCT [19].

However, as mentioned before, the clinical presentation is quite variable. Some patients with EVA may have a low-frequency conductive or mixed hearing loss mimicking otosclerosis secondary to a portion of the acoustic energy being shunted away from the cochlea to the third window [7, 20]. Without CT of the temporal bone, it can be extremely difficult to distinguish hearing loss to EVA from otosclerosis. Thus, in the absence of unequivocal evidence in support of otosclerosis such as patients presenting with an unusual clinical history (i.e., hearing loss starting in childhood or hearing loss in patients less susceptible to otosclerosis), a HRCT should be obtained in all these patients as the index of suspicion for EVA will be higher. Furthermore, an otologist should consider EVA in patients with failed stapedectomy or stapedotomy.

Regarding management of patients with concurrent otosclerosis and EVA, the jury is still out on the benefits and risks of stapes surgery due to the rarity of cases. There are reports of profound SNHL following stapedectomy in an ear with EVA due to perilymphatic gusher [7]. Rarely, a patient will have an isolated EVA. Most patients with EVA will have an associated congenital temporal bone anomaly that increases their risk for perilymphatic gusher such as an enlarged cochlear aqueduct or subtle defects in the modiolus and fundus of the internal auditory canal [21, 22]. Irrespective of the mechanism of the perilymphatic gusher, patients should be well informed of this possible risk and our recommendation would be to consider conventional hearing aids or bone-anchored hearing aids.

Superior Semicircular Canal Dehiscence

Since its initial description by Lloyd Minor in 1998, superior semicircular canal dehiscence (SCD) syndrome has been increasingly recognized as a cause of vestibular and/or auditory symptoms in patients [23]. Normally, two functional windows connect the middle and inner ear: the oval window and the round window. In SCD, a pathologic third mobile window into the inner ear is formed from the absence of bone overlying the superior semicircular canal causing a wide variety of symptoms including vertigo/disequilibrium induced by louds sounds (Tullio's phenomenon) or by stimuli that alter middle ear or intracranial pressure (Hennebert's sign), autophony, conductive hyperacusis, CHL, aural fullness, and pulsatile tinnitus [24]. Patients can present with audiovestibular symptoms, vestibular symptoms alone, or auditory symptoms alone.

Diagnosis is confirmed by audiometry, vestibular evoked myogenic potentials (VEMPs), and HRCT with reformatting of the images in planes parallel (Stenvers view) and perpendicular (Pöschl view) to the superior semicircular canal [25]. Surgical repair via resurfacing or plugging of the bony dehiscence is indicated for persistent debilitating symptoms despite conservative management [26].

Identification/Diagnosis of Otosclerosis, SCD, and Concomitant Otosclerosis and SCD

Considering the low-frequency hearing loss and normal otoscopy in both otosclerosis and SCD, it is possible to misdiagnose otosclerosis for SCD and vice versa. There are key distinctions, however, to help differentiate the two. As mentioned before, otosclerosis commonly clinically manifests as progressive CHL with Carhart's notch, normal bone thresholds, and absent acoustic reflexes. Patients with SCD often have CHL with suprathreshold bone lines, present acoustic reflexes, and third window symptoms including conductive hyperacusis (i.e., autophony, somatosounds including hearing eyes move, footsteps, or internal body sounds such as pulsatile tinnitus and mastication/bowel sounds), oscillopsia, autophony, and sound- or pressure-related vertigo [24].

Unfortunately, notwithstanding these distinctions, diagnostic ambiguity occurs in patients with both otosclerosis and SCD. These patients can present with symptoms consistent with otosclerosis—i.e., progressive CHL without sound- or pressure-induced vertigo and air-conduction VEMPs to suggest a third window is present. It is posited that the third window effect becomes obfuscated by closure of one of the three windows via stapes fixation from otosclerosis, resulting in a "normal" two window system [23, 24]. But more commonly, they will continue to have conductive hyperacusis symptoms. This distinction is key to accurate diagnosis and thus performing routine screening for conductive hyperacusis signs is paramount to differentiating patients with otosclerosis alone, SCD alone, or concurrent SCD and otosclerosis [27].

Others have also suggested acoustic reflexes as a diagnostic screening tool [28]. Acoustic reflexes are usually absent and present in otosclerosis and SCD respectively. In patients with both otosclerosis and SCD, acoustic reflexes are also typically absent. However, this is not an infallible approach because we know acoustic reflexes change as otosclerosis progresses. Initially, the acoustic reflexes may be normal but as the stapes fixation advances, thresholds increase, and reflex amplitudes decrease, until eventually reflexes are undetectable [29]. Furthermore, patients with a third window disorder alone can have absent acoustic reflexes.

If there is any suspicion for SCD, further investigation with HRCT and VEMP testing should be prompted, which are not routinely obtained for otosclerosis alone for various reasons including the added cost and radiation incurred with imaging. Table 18.1 compares the findings in otosclerosis alone, SCD alone, and concurrent SCD and otosclerosis. Air-conduction VEMPs are absent in concurrent otosclerosis and SCD and otosclerosis alone. However, bone-conduction VEMPs are present with high amplitudes in patients with both otosclerosis and SCD, and absent in patients with otosclerosis alone [27]. In patients with both otosclerosis and SCD, one should look for fenestral and retrofenestral otosclerosis and a dehiscent superior semicircular canal on HRCT (Fig. 18.1). It is important to note that, with the current fine-cut CT scans, the true prevalence of SCD tends to be overestimated [30]. Thus, a diagnosis of SCD should be made using all the available information including patient symptomatology, VEMP results, audiogram, and radiographic findings.

Table 18.1 Symptoms and diagnostic results in patients with otosclerosis, SCD, and concomitant otosclerosis and SCD

	Otosclerosis	SCD	Otosclerosis and SCD
Sound-induced vertigo	–	+	–
Pressure-induced vertigo	–	+	–
Conductive hyperacusis	–	+	+
Audiogram	CHL with Carhart's notch	CHL Supranormal bone-conduction thresholds	CHL with Carhart's notch Supranormal bone-conduction thresholds
Stapedial reflex	–	+	–
CT	Fenestral ± retrofenestral otosclerosis	Dehiscent superior semicircular canal	Fenestral ± retrofenestral otosclerosis Dehiscent superior semicircular canal
VEMPs	Absent air-conduction VEMPs Present bone-conduction VEMPs	High amplitude, low threshold air- and bone-conduction VEMPs	Absent air-conduction VEMPs High amplitude bone-conduction VEMPs

SCD indicates superior semicircular canal dehiscence, *CHL* conductive hearing loss *CT* computed tomography, *VEMPs* vestibular evoked myogenic potentials

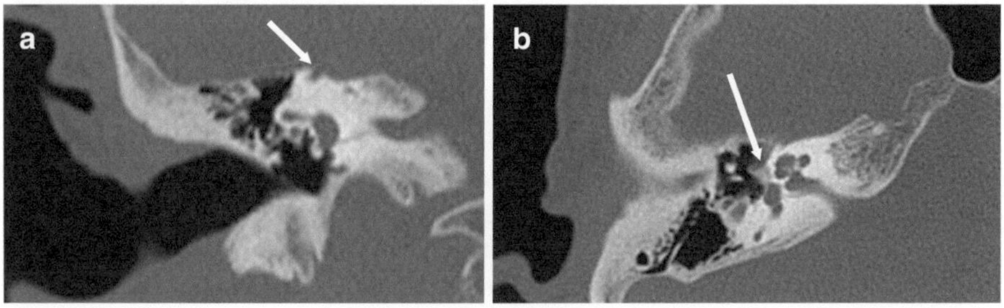

Fig. 18.1 Coronal CT demonstrating SSCD (**a**). Axial CT displaying hypodensity of fissula ante fenestram (**b**). CT indicates computed tomography. (Image courtesy of Eric Sargent, MD, FACS)

Management/Treatment of Concomitant Otosclerosis and SCD

Conflicting opinions exist in literature regarding the role of stapedotomy in individuals with otosclerosis and coexisting SCD. When one considers stapedotomy in these patients, there are four critical issues to address. The first is if significant improvement in hearing can be achieved. Given the rarity of concurrent otosclerosis and true SCD, literature reporting audiological outcomes following stapedotomy is limited to small case series. Most report improved hearing in most patients with partial or complete closure of the air-bone gap [8, 9, 31, 32]. Similar results were seen in the largest primary series to date conducted by Sioshansi et al.; air-bone gap (ABG) improved to 10 dB in 12/20 patients (60%), and 20 dB in 18/20 patients (90%) [27]. One limitation to note in this study, however, is that it is unclear if the patients in this series had true SCD syndrome or merely radiographic evidence of SCD. Regardless, it appears that radiographic evidence of SCD may not be an absolute contraindication for stapedotomy for otosclerosis [33].

Second, is there an increased risk for SNHL following stapedotomy given coexistence of a third window? To date, there are no reports of SNHL following stapes surgery attributed to SCD. However, it is integral to counsel patients of the risk for SNHL in any stapes procedure, regardless of the presence or absence of SCD.

Next, will third window symptoms become unmasked in individuals with true SCD syndrome?

By resolving the fixed stapes in otosclerosis with a mobile stapes prosthesis in the oval window, third window symptoms such as autophony, sound- or pressure-induced vertigo, and hyperacusis can subsequently emerge. Dewyer et al. reported a case series of eight patients, of which seven underwent stapes surgery. Four patients had unmasking of SCD symptoms [8]. More recently, however, Maxwell et al. reported a small case series of four patients with concurrent otosclerosis and true SCD and though one patient reported exacerbation of preoperative pulsatile tinnitus and autophony, none developed new postoperative third window symptoms [9].

Finally, if both are present and a patient wants a surgical intervention, should the otosclerosis or SCD be addressed first? As mentioned before, pressure- or sound-related vertigo symptoms secondary to a third mobile window are often masked. Thus, patients will mostly be bothered by their hearing loss and/or their conductive hyperacusis. If hearing loss is their biggest complaint, then stapes surgery should be considered first. If conductive hyperacusis is their biggest complaint, then the SCD should be addressed first. Staging should also be considered. If stapes surgery is performed, and the patient's third window symptoms are unmasked or more likely if they have persistent conductive hyperacusis, then resurfacing or plugging of the superior semicircular canal bony dehiscence should be offered.

Conclusion

Third window symptoms are often masked in patients with concomitant otosclerosis and true SCD. This is thought to be due to the fixed stapes eliminating the oval window as a functional part of the "three-window" system required to produce third window symptoms. Thus, there can be significant parallels in the clinical presentation between individuals with both true SCD and otosclerosis, and individuals with otosclerosis alone, which presents a diagnostic challenge. The only way to correctly identify patients preoperatively with coexisting otosclerosis and true SCD is via conductive hyperacusis screening and additional testing with fine-cut CT scans and VEMP testing.

Review of the literature shows that most patients achieve partial or complete closure of the ABG with stapedotomy. However, stapedotomy in this cohort of patients carries the risk of unmasking the characteristic audiovestibular SCD symptoms. Thus, surgery should only be pursued on a case-by-case basis after extensive preoperative counseling of patients of not only the aforementioned risk, but also the risk of incomplete closure of ABG.

References

1. Al Muhaimeed H, El Sayed Y, Rabah A, Al-Essa A. Conductive hearing loss: investigation of possible inner ear origin in three cases studies. J Laryngol Otol. 2002;116:942–5. https://doi.org/10.1258/00222150260369507.
2. Makarem AO, Hoang TA, Lo WW, et al. Cavitating otosclerosis: clinical, radiologic, and histopathologic correlations. Otol Neurotol. 2010;31:381–4. https://doi.org/10.1097/MAO.0b013e3181d275e8.
3. Guild SR. Histologic otosclerosis. Ann Otolaryngol. 1944;53:246–67.
4. Spandow O, Söderberg O, Bohlin L. Long-term results in otosclerotic patients operated by stapedectomy or stapedotomy. Scand Audiol. 2000;29:186–90. https://doi.org/10.1080/010503900750042752.
5. Merchant SN, Rosowski JJ. Conductive hearing loss caused by third-window lesions of the inner ear. Otol Neurotol. 2008;29:282–9. https://doi.org/10.1097/MAO.0b013e318161ab24.
6. Rosowski JJ, Songer JE, Nakajima HH, Brinsko KM, Merchant SN. Clinical, experimental, and theoretical investigations of the effect of superior semicircular canal dehiscence on hearing mechanisms. Otol Neurotol. 2004;25(3):323–32. https://doi.org/10.1097/00129492-200405000-00021.
7. Távora-Vieira D, Miller S. Misdiagnosis of otosclerosis in a patient with enlarged vestibular aqueduct syndrome: a case report. J Med Case Reports. 2012;6:178. https://doi.org/10.1186/1752-1947-6-178.
8. Dewyer NA, Quesnel AM, Santos F. A case series of patients with concurrent otosclerosis and superior semicircular canal dehiscence. Otol Neurotol. 2020;41:e172–81. https://doi.org/10.1097/MAO.0000000000002487.
9. Maxwell AK, Slattery WH 3rd, Gopen QS, Miller ME. Failure to close the gap: concomitant superior canal dehiscence in otosclerosis patients. Laryngoscope. 2020;130(4):1023–7. https://doi.org/10.1002/lary.28167.
10. Picavet V, Govaere E, Forton G. Superior semicircular canal dehiscence: prevalence in a population with clinical suspected otosclerosis-type hearing loss. B-ENT. 2009;5:83–8.
11. Gordon MA. The genetics of otosclerosis: a review. Am J Otol. 1989;10:426–38. https://doi.org/10.1097/00129492-198911000-00003.
12. Seligman E, Shambaugh GE Jr. Otosclerosis of the osseous horizontal semicircular canal. Ann Otol Rhinol Laryngol. 1951;60(2):375–81. https://doi.org/10.1177/000348945106000210.
13. Liston SL, Paparella MM, Mancini F, Anderson JH. Otosclerosis and endolymphatic hydrops. Laryngoscope. 1984;94(8):1003–7.
14. Yasan H. Predictive role of Carhart's notch in pre-operative assessment for middle-ear surgery. J Laryngol Otol. 2007;121(3):219–21. https://doi.org/10.1017/S0022215106003343.

15. Foster MF, Backous DD. Clinical evaluation of the patient with otosclerosis. Otolaryngol Clin North Am. 2018;51(2):319–26. https://doi.org/10.1016/j.otc.2017.11.004.
16. Redfors YD, Gröndahl HG, Hellgren J, Lindfors N, Nilsson I, Möller C. Otosclerosis: anatomy and pathology in the temporal bone assessed by multi-slice and cone-beam CT. Otol Neurotol. 2012;33(6):922–7. https://doi.org/10.1097/MAO.0b013e318259b38c.
17. Valvassori GE, Clemis JD. The large vestibular aqueduct syndrome. Laryngoscope. 1978;88(5):723–8. https://doi.org/10.1002/lary.1978.88.5.723.
18. Ascha MS, Manzoor N, Gupta A, Semaan M, Megerian C, Otteson TD. Vestibular aqueduct midpoint width and hearing loss in patients with an enlarged vestibular aqueduct. JAMA Otolaryngol Head Neck Surg. 2017;143(6):601–8. https://doi.org/10.1001/jamaoto.2016.4522.
19. Madden C, Halsted M, Benton C, Greinwald J, Choo D. Enlarged vestibular aqueduct syndrome in the pediatric population. Otol Neurotol. 2003;24(4):625–32. https://doi.org/10.1097/00129492-200307000-00016.
20. Wieczorek SS, Anderson ME Jr, Harris DA, Mikulec AA. Enlarged vestibular aqueduct syndrome mimicking otosclerosis in adults. Am J Otolaryngol. 2013;34(6):619–25. https://doi.org/10.1016/j.amjoto.2013.07.015.
21. Lemmerling MM, Mancuso AA, Antonelli PJ, Kubilis PS. Normal modiolus: CT appearance in patients with a large vestibular aqueduct. Radiology. 1997;204(1):213–9. https://doi.org/10.1148/radiology.204.1.9205250.
22. Hongjian L, Guangke W, Song M, Xiaoli D, Daoxing Z. The prediction of CSF gusher in cochlear implants with inner ear abnormality. Acta Otolaryngol. 2012;132(12):1271–4. https://doi.org/10.3109/00016489.2012.701328.
23. Minor LB, Solomon D, Zinreich JS, Zee DS. Sound- and/or pressure-induced vertigo due to bone dehiscence of the superior semicircular canal. Arch Otolaryngol Head Neck Surg. 1998;124(3):249–58. https://doi.org/10.1001/archotol.124.3.249.
24. Minor LB. Superior canal dehiscence syndrome. Am J Otol. 2000;21:9–19.
25. Ceylan N, Bayraktaroglu S, Alper H, Savaş R, Bilgen C, Kirazli T, Güzelmansur I, Ertürk SM. CT imaging of superior semicircular canal dehiscence: added value of reformatted images. Acta Otolaryngol. 2010;130(9):996–1001. https://doi.org/10.3109/00016481003602108.
26. Minor LB. Clinical manifestations of superior semicircular canal dehiscence. Laryngoscope. 2005;115(10):1717–27. https://doi.org/10.1097/01.mlg.0000178324.55729.b7.
27. Yong M, Zaia E, Westerberg B, Lea J. Diagnosis of superior semicircular canal dehiscence in the presence of concomitant otosclerosis. Otol Neurotol. 2017;38:1071. https://doi.org/10.1097/MAO.0000000000001490.
28. Hong RS, Metz CM, Bojrab DI, Babu SC, Zappia J, Sargent EW, LaRouere MJ. Acoustic reflex screening of conductive hearing loss for third window disorders. Otolaryngol Head Neck Surg. 2015;154(2):343–8. https://doi.org/10.1177/0194599815620162.
29. Hannley MT. Audiologic characteristics of the patient with otosclerosis. Otolaryngol Clin North Am. 1993;26:373–87.
30. Sequeira SM, Whiting BR, Shimony JS, Vo KD, Hullar TE. Accuracy of computed tomography detection of superior canal dehiscence. Otol Neurotol. 2011;32:1500–5. https://doi.org/10.1097/MAO.0b013e318238280c.
31. Hope A, Fagan P. Latent SCD syndrome unmasked by stapedotomy for otosclerosis. J Laryngol Otol. 2010;124:428–30. https://doi.org/10.1017/S0022215109991654.
32. Pritchett CV, Spector ME, Kileny PR, Heidenreich KD, El-Kashlan HK. Surgical treatment of hearing loss when otosclerosis coexists with superior semicircular canal dehiscence syndrome. Otol Neurotol. 2014;35:1163–7. https://doi.org/10.1097/MAO.0000000000000470.
33. Sioshansi PC, Drury EE, Tu NC, Babu SC, Schut CA. Outcomes of stapedotomy in patients with concomitant otosclerosis and superior semicircular canal dehiscence: should a radiographic third window be a contraindication to stapes surgery? Otol Neurotol. 2022;43(2):165–9. https://doi.org/10.1097/MAO.0000000000003429.

Chapter 19
Increased Intracranial Pressure

Karl W. Doerfer, Christopher A. Schutt, Sarah Dwyer, and Karl Kado

Introduction

Superior semicircular canal dehiscence (SSCD) is an example of a "third mobile window" (TMW) condition resulting from dehiscence of middle fossa bone over the superior semicircular canal [1]. While not as well characterized as SSCD, other foci of otic capsule dehiscence have also been described, including the posterior semicircular canal, vestibular aqueduct, internal auditory canal, carotid canal, and fallopian canal [2–7]. TMWs allow aberrant sound and energy transfer through the inner ear, leading to classic findings of mixed hearing loss, autophony and vestibular dysfunction. Less specific symptoms, including pulsatile tinnitus, headache, hyperacusis and visual disturbance, may also be present, resulting in difficulty distinguishing TMW conditions from other entities, including migraine variants and idiopathic intracranial hypertension (IIH) [8].

IIH is of particular interest because, in addition to being an alternative diagnosis for a TMW condition, it may also contribute to the development of a TMW where the otic capsule interfaces with a CSF-containing compartment. The overlapping features of TMW and IIH thus present a challenge when managing patients who present with symptoms suggestive of either or both conditions. Accordingly, this chapter will provide brief overviews of SSCD and IIH and their potential interplay,

K. W. Doerfer (✉)
Department of Otolaryngology & Communication Sciences, Medical College of Wisconsin, Milwaukee, WI, USA

C. A. Schutt · S. Dwyer
Michigan Ear Institute, Farmington Hills, MI, USA

K. Kado
Department of Radiology, College of Human Medicine, Ascension Providence Hospital, Michigan State University, Southfield, MI, USA

G. J. Gianoli, P. Thomson (eds.), *Third Mobile Window Syndrome of the Inner Ear*, https://doi.org/10.1007/978-3-031-16586-3_19

followed by a discussion of evaluation and management of patients presenting with TMW, IIH, or both conditions. Because most existing literature on TMW disorders concerns SSCD, the following discussion will focus primarily on this entity. However, it should be noted that TMWs remain an evolving area of investigation, and future efforts to better characterize non-SSCD variants may provide additional insight regarding etiology, diagnosis, and treatment options for this complex condition.

Etiology of SSCD

Theories for SSCD etiology can be generally grouped into developmental and acquired types. Developmental theories include arrested bone formation and dural-labyrinthine adhesion [9]. Several large radiographic and temporal bone studies support the theory of arrested bone formation. In these series, adult temporal bones with SSCD had overall lateral skull base (LSB) thickness comparable to still-developing neonatal specimens, suggesting that dehiscence arises from impaired LSB development during early childhood [10–12]. Relatedly, the dural adhesion theory, based on the close proximity of the temporal lobe dura and membranous labyrinth during embryonic development, posits that dural adhesions over the superior canal prevent bone deposition, leading to dehiscence [9].

Despite radiographic and histopathologic evidence supporting a developmental etiology, the natural history of SSCD and numerous studies support an acquired basis for the condition. First, despite thin average LSB thickness in young children, symptomatic SSCD is rare in the pediatric population, with most patients presenting in mid-adulthood [13]. Additionally, numerous series show progressive thinning of the LSB with various factors, including age, obesity, obstructive sleep apnea (OSA) and increased intracranial pressure (ICP) [14–19]. In one imaging study, there was a 93% increase in radiographic SSCD in progressive age groupings, suggesting age-related bone remodeling as potential causes of thinning [20]. In other studies, elevated ICP has been shown to be associated with radiographic LSB thinning as well as development of spontaneous encephalocele and cerebrospinal fluid leak, suggesting that high ICP causes erosion and dehiscence through increased force of dural pulsations [15, 16].

An additional consideration for acquired SSCD is the so-called two-hit hypothesis, which posits that dehiscence may occur suddenly due to transient forces along the LSB that fracture or degrade already thin bone over the superior canal. This theory is supported by studies showing that up to 48% of patients with SSCD report symptom onset with a specific event or exposure, including trauma and transient pressure changes [17]. While debate continues regarding the etiology of SSCD, both congenital and acquired theories may hold validity, with developmental arrest occurring in some individuals who go on to have persistently thin LSBs, and a subset of this population developing true dehiscence due to progressive thinning and/or transient microtrauma.

Idiopathic Intracranial Hypertension

Because of its association with other LSB defects, idiopathic intracranial hypertension (IIH) has been proposed as a risk factor for SSCD [18, 19]. Further, IIH and SSCD may present with similar symptoms. Consequently, a more detailed discussion of IIH is warranted.

Early epidemiologic studies performed before 1990 demonstrated IIH incidence to be 0.6–0.9/100,000, although more recent series have shown a significantly higher incidence, with one study reporting rates as high as 7.8/100,000 [21–24]. In general, most series show a dramatically higher incidence among females and patients with obesity. Approximately 90% of patients with IIH are obese women of childbearing age, and rates of IIH in this population are approximately 20 times higher than in the general population [25, 26].

The mechanism for cerebrospinal fluid (CSF) pressure regulation may explain the high rate of IIH in obese patients. Normally, CSF is resorbed into the cerebral venous system via arachnoid granulations that line the dural sinuses. Evidence supports the theory that cerebral venous hypertension causes dysfunction of these one-way valves, impairing CSF resorption and leading to IIH [27–30]. A wide range of experimental and cohort studies show a close relationship between truncal adiposity and cerebral venous pressure, mediated by changes in central venous pressure (CVP) [25, 31–39]. Such CVP increases may be compounded by apneic events in patients with OSA, a condition strongly associated with elevated Body Mass Index (BMI).

Beyond increased intra-abdominal pressure, several other factors may play a role in IIH. Increased levels of pro-thrombotic mediators such as fibrinogen, D-Dimer, and Factors VIII, IX, and XI have been found in obese patients, suggesting that distal venous circulation may be compromised by occult micro-thrombosis in addition to increased intra-abdominal pressure [40]. Further, obesity-related dysregulation of hormonal and neuroendocrine pathways may contribute, as IIH is associated with elevated levels of leptin and steroid regulating enzymes, such as 11β-hydroxysteroid dehydrogenase, which increase CSF production via stimulation of NA+/K+ ATPase transporters in the epithelium of the choroid plexus [41, 42]. Additional research suggests that stenosis and/or increased collapsibility of the dural sinuses may also play a role in the development of IIH. However, other studies suggest that these vascular findings may be a result of IIH and not its cause [27, 43–46].

The classic triad of IIH includes headache, vision changes, and papilledema, although primary otologic symptoms may be present in a subset of patients. Headache, the most common presenting symptom, is often holocranial, pulsatile, and present on waking, although no clear pattern exists [47]. Visual symptoms range from transient obscuration in mild IIH to visual field loss and blindness in advanced disease, which affects 10–20% of patients [23, 25, 48, 49]. Additionally, IIH may cause abducens nerve palsy, which can present as subjective diplopia or clinically apparent disconjugate gaze. This uncommon finding is the only focal neurologic sign permitted in IIH diagnosis and is thought to result from stretch injury along the cisternal course of cranial nerve VI [25, 50]. Papilledema results from increased pressure in the subarachnoid compartment of the optic nerve and is typically present when ICP exceeds 30–35 cmH_2O [35]. When present, fundoscopic findings of papilledema resolve with successful intervention, thus allowing for noninvasive treatment monitoring [32, 34, 51–57]. Pulsatile tinnitus is the most common primary otologic symptom in IIH and is thought to result from turbulent blood flow through stenotic dural sinuses. Although rarely used today, it can be detected with a Toynbee tube [51, 58, 59]. Other otologic symptoms may include hearing loss, aural fullness and vertigo [60].

Role of IIH in Skull Base Defects and SSCD

Numerous studies show a strong correlation between IIH and skull base defects [52, 61–76]. Epidemiologic data also underscore the impact of obesity on this association. In the past two decades, rates of IIH diagnosis and surgical repair of spontaneous CSF leaks rose concomitantly with increasing obesity rates [25, 37, 62]. The prevailing theory for defect formation in IIH involves bony attenuation from repeated pulsations of over-pressurized dura and venous sinuses against the skull base. Erosion may also occur at the site of ectopic arachnoid granulations [28–30, 77, 78]. In the LSB, spontaneous CSF leak and encephaloceles commonly occur along the tegmen tympani and tegmen mastoideum. The anterior skull base is also subject to defect formation, especially at the cribriform plate and lateral recess of the sphenoid sinus [79].

In addition to the association between LSB defects and IIH, studies also demonstrate an association between LSB thinning or defects and SSCD. In one large histopathologic study of 1000 temporal bones by Carey and colleagues, approximately 50% of patients with SSCD had bilateral LSB abnormalities (i.e., bilateral thinning, bilateral SSCD, or unilateral SSCD) [11]. Several other series show a strong association with SSCD and tegmen defects. In a large radiographic series of 604 ears, Crovetto and colleagues demonstrated a higher rate of tegmen dehiscence in 36% of patients with SSCD compared to 10% of those without SSCD [10]. In another large study, which included surgically confirmed pathology, Oh and colleagues demonstrated that 27% of patients with mastoid encephalocele or CSF leak also had concurrent SSCD [80].

Despite the associations between LSB defects and both IIH and SSCD, the role of IIH in the development of SSCD specifically is less well defined. In a retrospective imaging study by Handzel and colleagues, patients with IIH confirmed by lumbar puncture (LP) showed progressive tegmen thinning over a 26-year period. Further, the degree of thinning positively correlated with initial LP opening pressure. However, the authors noted that thinning above the superior semicircular canal did not reach statistical significance [16]. In a similar study by Berkiten and colleagues, patients with IIH showed significantly thinner middle cranial fossa bone thickness compared to controls. However, there was no correlation between bone thickness and CSF pressure. Other investigations examining SSC, obesity and OSA—well-defined risk factors for IIH—have found conflicting evidence that elevated BMI is associated with SSCD [18, 19, 77, 80, 81].

TMW Diagnosis and Management

Several factors complicate SSCD diagnosis. First, the rate of SSCD is overestimated by imaging studies, which show radiographic dehiscence rates between 3.9 and 9% depending on image formatting and level of resolution [10]. However, large temporal bone studies show rates of SSCD to be only 0.5–0.6% [10, 11] This discrepancy is due to limitations of computed tomography (CT) imaging, which may not distinguish very thin bone from true dehiscence even with appropriately formatted, high-resolution scans. Second, as already noted, TMW symptoms can be variable and nonspecific, leading to preliminary diagnosis in patients who ultimately lack objective evidence of dehiscence or, conversely, missed diagnosis in patients with true dehiscence [8]. Further complicating matters, a subset of patients with objective evidence of dehiscence may, for unclear reasons, lack noticeable or bothersome TMW symptoms [82, 83].

Given these challenges, correct diagnosis of SSCD and other TMW conditions requires careful, detailed clinical evaluation. In addition to evaluating for TMW, history taking should include questions directed at alternative or coexisting diagnoses, including migraine, IIH, vascular anomalies, endolymphatic hydrops, canalithiasis, middle ear disease, and nonvestibular balance impairments. Frenzel goggle exam with sound or pressure stimuli to the ear in question may show characteristic vertical-torsional nystagmus [84]. Other vestibular maneuvers, auscultation, position testing, and clinical balance assessment may help identify alternative or contributing conditions.

Diagnostic evaluation requires both audiovestibular testing and imaging. Audiovestibular testing involves audiogram as well as cervical and/or ocular vestibular evoked myogenic potentials (cVEMP, oVEMP). The use of electrocochleography (ECOG) has also been described. Audiogram may show a mixed low-to-mid frequency hearing loss with supranormal bone thresholds, while cVEMP may show decreased thresholds, and oVEMP may show increased amplitude. ECOG may show an increased SP/AP ratio. Recently, oVEMP has been shown to be the most sensitive and specific test to confirm SSCD syndrome suspected from history, physical exam, audiogram and HRCT [85–87]. Radiographic testing requires high-resolution computed tomography (HRCT) with $\leq$0.5 mm cuts performed perpendicular and parallel to the plane of the superior semicircular canal (Stenver and Poschl views). Some reports also suggest that the addition of high-resolution 3D MRI may be helpful to characterize anatomical structures involved at the site of dehiscence [7].

Surgical management of debilitating SSCD involves resurfacing the area of bony dehiscence or occlusion of the superior canal. Middle fossa and transmastoid approaches have been described, with good outcomes reported for both [88]. Similar approaches have been described for posterior canal dehiscence [89]. Round window plugging and reinforcement has also been described for SSCD patients opting for a less involved procedure, and for patients with other TMW variants. While this procedure has a significantly lower risk profile, reports of subjective and objective results are mixed [90].

IIH Diagnosis and Management

Despite the unclear role of IIH in the development of SSCD, otolaryngologists play an important role in the management of this condition, even in the absence of skull base defects. Given the potential risk to vision, patients presenting with symptoms suggesting elevated ICP should receive ophthalmology referral for fundoscopic examination and visual field testing. Additionally, other causes of elevated ICP should be explored before settling on a diagnosis of IIH. Insufficient evaluation may fail to identify conditions or exposures that may raise ICP, including neoplasm, vascular anomalies, endocrine disorders, sleep apnea, renal failure and certain medications (e.g., tetracycline, sulfa, retinoids, lithium, etc.).

Several diagnostic criteria exist for establishing a diagnosis of IIH based on exam findings, imaging and LP results. These include the Modified Dandy Criteria (1937), criteria from the Second Edition of the International Classification of Headache Disorders (2004), and criteria proposed by Friedman and colleagues (2002, 2013) [50, 91, 92]. The most recent revision of the Friedman criteria includes five items required for a diagnosis of Definite IIH, including papilledema, normal brain imaging (except findings consistent with IIH), normal neurologic exam (except cranial nerve abnormalities associated with IIH), LP showing normal CSF composition, and elevated LP opening pressure (i.e., $\geq$250 mmH_2O in adults and $\geq$280 mmH_2O in children) (Table 19.1, Fig. 19.1). Given the potential for fluctuations in CSF pressure, probable IIH may be diagnosed if all conditions are met except elevated opening pressure. Based on evidence that IIH may present without papilledema, these revised criteria also permit diagnosis of IIH without papilledema provided that patients have either (a) bilateral or unilateral abducens nerve palsy or (b) neuroimaging with at least three of the following features: empty sella, flattened posterior globe, perioptic subarachnoid space distention, or transverse venous sinus stenosis. Notably, a diagnosis of IIH without papilledema requires elevated LP opening pressure. However, the threshold of $\geq$250 mmH_2O is the subject of ongoing debate in the neurology literature, given the potential to miss patients with borderline IIH who lack papilledema. A cutoff of $\geq$200 mmH_2O has been suggested to improve sensitivity. However, a recent large population showed that up to 15.8% of normal individuals had an opening pressure above this level [93, 94].

Table 19.1 Diagnostic Criteria for Pseudotumor Cerebri Syndrome (aka Idiopathic Intracranial Hypertension)

1 Required for diagnosis of pseudotumor cerebri syndrome[a]
A. Papilledema
B. Normal neurologic examination except for cranial nerve abnormalities
C. Neuroimaging: Normal brain parenchyma without evidence of hydrocephalus, mass, or structural lesion and no abnormal meningeal enhancement on MRI, with and without gadolinium, for typical patients (female and obese), and MRI, with and without gadolinium, and magnetic resonance venography for others; if MRI is unavailable or contraindicated, contrast-enhanced CT may be used
D. Normal CSF composition
E. Elevated lumbar puncture opening pressure (≥250 mm CSF in adults and ≥280 mm CSF in children [250 mm CSF if the child is not sedated and not obese]) in a properly performed lumbar puncture
2 Required for diagnosis of pseudotumor cerebri syndrome without papilledema
A. In the absence of papilledema, a diagnosis of pseudotumor cerebri syndrome can be made if B–E from above are satisfied, and in addition the patient has a unilateral or bilateral CN-VI palsy
B. In the absence of papilledema or CN-VI palsy, a diagnosis of pseudotumor cerebri syndrome can be suggested but not made if B–E from above are satisfied, and in addition at least three of the following neuroimaging criteria are satisfied: • Empty sella • Flattening of the posterior aspect of the globe • Distention of the perioptic subarachnoid space with or without a tortuous optic nerve • Transverse venous sinus stenosis

Adapted from *Friedman DI, Liu GT, Digre KB. Revised diagnostic criteria for the pseudotumor cerebri syndrome in adults and children. Neurology. 2013;81(*13*):1159–1165*

[a]A diagnosis is **definite** if the patient fulfills criteria A–E. The diagnosis is considered **probable** if criteria A–D are met but the measured CSF pressure is lower than specified for a definite diagnosis

At a minimum, those diagnosed with IIH require multidisciplinary management by a neurologist and ophthalmologist. Other specialty care may also be required depending on specific patient factors. These include neurosurgery, bariatric surgery, sleep medicine, otolaryngology (neurotology, rhinology, sleep surgery) and nutrition. In general, nonsurgical management of IIH involves lifestyle modifications with weight loss, which is often highly effective even at moderate levels, and medical management with carbonic anhydrase inhibitors (e.g., acetazolamide, topiramate) to lower CSF production [34, 54, 95]. Treatment of sleep apnea also plays an important role given its association with obesity and its dramatic, direct effect on ICP levels during apneic events [19, 62, 96]. Several studies have shown that successful management of OSA with either nonsurgical or surgical interventions leads to resolution in elevated ICP [23, 55, 97, 98].

Surgical management of patients with IIH is typically reserved for those with refractory or advanced disease, which affects 10–20% of patients, or those with complications resulting from IIH, including vision loss, encephalocele, and CSF leak [48, 53]. In general, surgical repair of encephalocele and CSF leak is indicated to prevent long-term risk of meningitis [99, 100]. CSF diversion procedures,

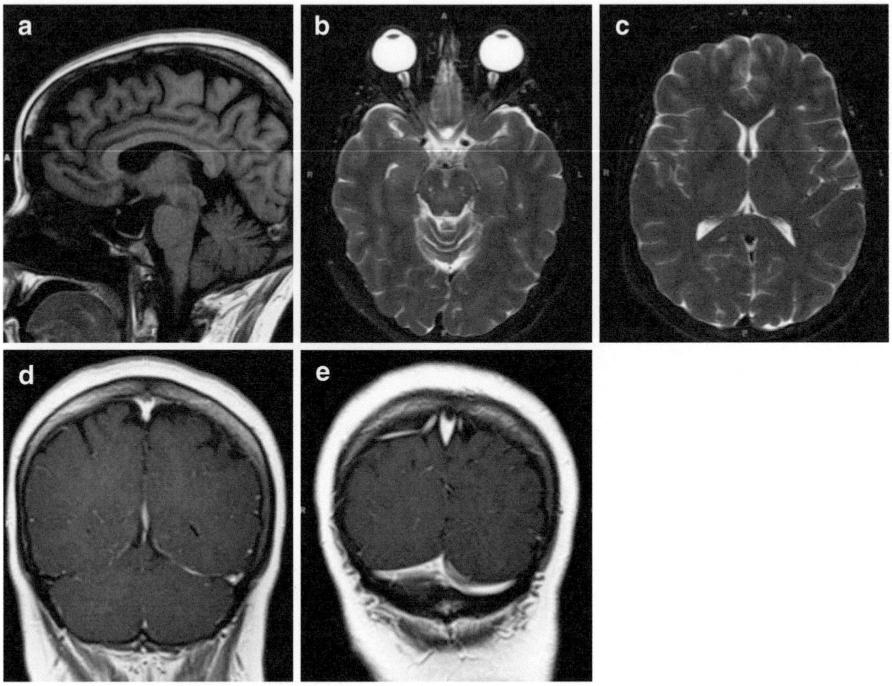

Fig. 19.1 (**a**) Sagittal T1-weighted image in a patient with IIH demonstrates expanded, partially empty sella. (**b**) Axial T2-weighted image in the same patient demonstrates expanded optic nerve sheath CSF and flattening of the posterior optic globes. (**c**) Axial T2-weighted image demonstrates narrowed, slit-like appearance of the lateral ventricles. (**d**, **e**) Coronal post-contrast T1-weighted images demonstrate stenosis of the distal right transverse sinus (**d**) in comparison to the proximal sinus (**e**)

including lumboperitoneal and ventriculoperitoneal shunting, are highly successful at reducing ICP levels to prevent vision loss and reduce headache. However, both are subject to relatively high infection rates and frequently require revision for obstruction [57, 101, 102]. Endovascular stenting for venous outflow obstruction and optic nerve fenestration has also been described, although reported outcomes are limited [44, 57, 103–105]. Otolaryngologists from several subdisciplines also play an important role in surgical management of IIH. As noted previously, IIH can improve or resolve with management of OSA by otolaryngologists specializing in sleep surgery. For patients with encephalocele or CSF leak, rhinologists and neurotologists can offer surgery to correct anterior or lateral skull base defects.

While the role of IIH in the development of SSCD is unclear, the strong association between LSB defects and both IIH and SSCD requires careful neurotologic evaluation and counseling of patients with any concurrent conditions. IIH patients with LSB encephaloceles and/or CSF leaks requiring surgical repair should be carefully evaluated for concurrent SSCD, as surgery may allow correction of both conditions. Similarly, patients with encephaloceles and/or CSF leaks, radiographic

SSCD, but no clinical or audiometric evidence of SSCD, should be counseled regarding the risk of unmasked SSCD or sensorineural hearing loss from otic capsule violation that may occur at the time of surgery. For patients with concurrent IIH and verified SSCD who lack encephalocele and CSF leak, initial management of IIH may provide adequate symptomatic relief and obviate the need for surgical intervention to correct SSCD.

Conclusion

SSCD is a type of TMW condition caused by bony dehiscence over the superior semicircular canal. While etiology is unclear, evidence exists for congenital, acquired, or combined etiologies. The role of IIH in TMW is unclear, although studies show a strong correlation between IIH and lateral skull base attenuation, suggesting an association with SSCD. Symptomatic overlap requires careful consideration of both conditions during patient evaluation and workup. Management of IIH and its complications requires a multidisciplinary approach, with several otolaryngology subdisciplines playing a vital role. Management of patients with both IIH and SSCD depends on the presence of IIH-related complications or, in their absence, the specificity and severity of TMW-related symptoms. Initial conservative management of IIH may provide adequate symptomatic relief obviating the need for intervention to treat TMW syndrome.

References

1. Minor LB, Solomon D, Zinreich JS, Zee DS. Sound- and/or pressure-induced vertigo due to bone dehiscence of the superior semicircular canal. Arch Otolaryngol Neck Surg. 1998;124(3):249. https://doi.org/10.1001/archotol.124.3.249.
2. Merchant SN, Nakajima HH, Halpin C, et al. Clinical investigation and mechanism of air-bone gaps in large vestibular aqueduct syndrome. Ann Otol Rhinol Laryngol. 2007;116(7):532–41. https://doi.org/10.1177/000348940711600709.
3. Blake DM, Tomovic S, Vazquez A, Lee HJ, Jyung RW. Cochlear-facial dehiscence—a newly described entity. Laryngoscope. 2014;124(1):283–9. https://doi.org/10.1002/lary.24223.
4. Karlberg M, Annertz M, Magnusson M. Mondini-like malformation mimicking otosclerosis and superior semicircular canal dehiscence. J Laryngol Otol. 2006;120(5):419–22. https://doi.org/10.1017/S0022215106000934.
5. Kim HHS, Wilson DF. A third mobile window at the cochlear apex. Otolaryngol Head Neck Surg. 2006;135(6):965–6. https://doi.org/10.1016/j.otohns.2005.04.006.
6. Lund AD, Palacios SD. Carotid artery-cochlear dehiscence: a review. Laryngoscope. 2011;121(12):2658–60. https://doi.org/10.1002/lary.22391.
7. Reynard P, Idriss S, Ltaief-Boudrigua A, et al. Proposal for a unitary anatomo-clinical and radiological classification of third mobile window abnormalities. Front Neurol. 2022;12:792545. https://doi.org/10.3389/fneur.2021.792545.

8. Naert L, Berg R, Heyning P, et al. Aggregating the symptoms of superior semicircular canal dehiscence syndrome. Laryngoscope. 2018;128(8):1932–8. https://doi.org/10.1002/lary.27062.
9. Takahashi N, Tsunoda A, Shirakura S, Kitamura K. Anatomical feature of the middle cranial fossa in fetal periods: possible etiology of superior canal dehiscence syndrome. Acta Otolaryngol (Stockh). 2012;132(4):385–90. https://doi.org/10.3109/00016489.2011.637234.
10. Crovetto M, Whyte J, Rodriguez OM, Lecumberri I, Martinez C, Eléxpuru J. Anatomo-radiological study of the superior semicircular canal dehiscence. Eur J Radiol. 2010;76(2):167–72. https://doi.org/10.1016/j.ejrad.2009.05.038.
11. Carey JP, Minor LB, Nager GT. Dehiscence or thinning of bone overlying the superior semicircular canal in a temporal bone survey. Arch Otolaryngol Neck Surg. 2000;126(2):137. https://doi.org/10.1001/archotol.126.2.137.
12. Tóth M, Helling K, Baksa G, Mann W. Localization of congenital Tegmen Tympani defects. Otol Neurotol. 2007;28(8):1120–3. https://doi.org/10.1097/MAO.0b013e31815aee0c.
13. Zhou G, Gopen Q, Poe DS. Clinical and diagnostic characterization of canal dehiscence syndrome: a great otologic mimicker. Otol Neurotol. 2007;28(7):920–6. https://doi.org/10.1097/MAO.0b013e31814b25f2.
14. Davey S, Kelly-Morland C, Phillips JS, Nunney I, Pawaroo D. Assessment of superior semicircular canal thickness with advancing age: SSC thickness and age. Laryngoscope. 2015;125(8):1940–5. https://doi.org/10.1002/lary.25243.
15. Berkiten G, Gürbüz D, Akan O, et al. Dehiscence or thinning of bone overlying the superior semicircular canal in idiopathic intracranial hypertension. Eur Arch Otorhinolaryngol. 2022;279:2899. https://doi.org/10.1007/s00405-021-07020-z.
16. Handzel O, Brenner-Ullman A, Niry D, et al. Tegmen attenuation in patients with idiopathic intracranial hypertension is progressive. Laryngoscope. 2020;130(12):E904. https://doi.org/10.1002/lary.28490.
17. Watters KF, Rosowski JJ, Sauter T, Lee DJ. Superior semicircular canal dehiscence presenting as postpartum vertigo. Otol Neurotol. 2006;27(6):756–68. https://doi.org/10.1097/01.mao.0000227894.27291.9f.
18. Kuo P, Bagwell KA, Mongelluzzo G, et al. Semicircular canal dehiscence among idiopathic intracranial hypertension patients: SSCD among IIH patients. Laryngoscope. 2018;128(5):1196–9. https://doi.org/10.1002/lary.26795.
19. Schutt CA, Neubauer P, Samy RN, et al. The correlation between obesity, obstructive sleep apnea, and superior semicircular canal dehiscence: a new explanation for an increasingly common problem. Otol Neurotol. 2015;36(3):551.
20. Nadgir RN, Ozonoff A, Devaiah AK, Halderman AA, Sakai O. Superior semicircular canal dehiscence: congenital or acquired condition? Am J Neuroradiol. 2011;32(5):947–9. https://doi.org/10.3174/ajnr.A2437.
21. McCluskey G, Mulholland DA, McCarron P, McCarron MO. Idiopathic intracranial hypertension in the northwest of northern Ireland: epidemiology and clinical management. Neuroepidemiology. 2015;45(1):34–9. https://doi.org/10.1159/000435919.
22. Miah L, Strafford H, Fonferko-Shadrach B, et al. Incidence, prevalence, and health care outcomes in idiopathic intracranial hypertension: a population study. Neurology. 2021;96(8):e1251–61. https://doi.org/10.1212/WNL.0000000000011463.
23. Radhakrishnan K, Ahlskog JE, Cross SA, Kurland LT, O'Fallon WM. Idiopathic intracranial hypertension (Pseudotumor cerebri). Descriptive epidemiology in Rochester, Minn, 1976 to 1990. Arch Neurol. 1993;50(1):78–80. https://doi.org/10.1001/archneur.1993.00540010072020.
24. Durcan FJ, Corbett JJ, Wall M. The incidence of pseudotumor cerebri. Population studies in Iowa and Louisiana. Arch Neurol. 1988;45(8):875–7. https://doi.org/10.1001/archneur.1988.00520320065016.
25. Wall M. Idiopathic intracranial hypertension (pseudotumor cerebri). Curr Neurol Neurosci Rep. 2008;8(2):87–93.

26. Jindal M, Hiam L, Raman A, Rejali D. Idiopathic intracranial hypertension in otolaryngology. Eur Arch Otorhinolaryngol. 2009;266(6):803–6. https://doi.org/10.1007/s00405-009-0973-0.
27. De Simone R, Ranieri A, Bonavita V. Advancement in idiopathic intracranial hypertension pathogenesis: focus on sinus venous stenosis. Neurol Sci. 2010;31(Suppl 1):S33–9. https://doi.org/10.1007/s10072-010-0271-z.
28. Kim SW, Choi JH. Cerebrospinal fluid otorrhea caused by arachnoid granulation. Korean J Audiol. 2012;16(3):152–5. https://doi.org/10.7874/kja.2012.16.3.152.
29. Gacek RR. Arachnoid granulation cerebrospinal fluid otorrhea. Ann Otol Rhinol Laryngol. 1990;99(11):854–62. https://doi.org/10.1177/000348949009901102.
30. Yew M, Dubbs B, Tong O, et al. Arachnoid granulations of the temporal bone: a histologic study of dural and osseous penetration. Otol Neurotol. 2011;32(4):602–9. https://doi.org/10.1097/MAO.0b013e3182129026.
31. Bruce BB, Kedar S, Van Stavern GP, et al. Idiopathic intracranial hypertension in men. Neurology. 2009;72(4):304–9. https://doi.org/10.1212/01.wnl.0000333254.84120.f5.
32. Sugerman HJ, Felton WL, Salvant JB, Sismanis A, Kellum JM. Effects of surgically induced weight loss on idiopathic intracranial hypertension in morbid obesity. Neurology. 1995;45(9):1655–9. https://doi.org/10.1212/wnl.45.9.1655.
33. Hannerz J, Greitz D, Ericson K. Is there a relationship between obesity and intracranial hypertension? Int J Obes Relat Metab Disord. 1995;19(4):240–4.
34. Kupersmith MJ, Gamell L, Turbin R, Peck V, Spiegel P, Wall M. Effects of weight loss on the course of idiopathic intracranial hypertension in women. Neurology. 1998;50(4):1094–8. https://doi.org/10.1212/wnl.50.4.1094.
35. Hannerz J, Ericson K. The relationship between idiopathic intracranial hypertension and obesity. Headache. 2009;49(2):178–84. https://doi.org/10.1111/j.1526-4610.2008.01240.x.
36. Nedelmann M, Kaps M, Mueller-Forell W. Venous obstruction and jugular valve insufficiency in idiopathic intracranial hypertension. J Neurol. 2009;256(6):964–9. https://doi.org/10.1007/s00415-009-5056-z.
37. Friedman DI. The pseudotumor cerebri syndrome. Neurol Clin. 2014;32(2):363–96. https://doi.org/10.1016/j.ncl.2014.01.001.
38. Bloomfield GL, Ridings PC, Blocher CR, Marmarou A, Sugerman HJ. A proposed relationship between increased intra-abdominal, intrathoracic, and intracranial pressure. Crit Care Med. 1997;25(3):496–503. https://doi.org/10.1097/00003246-199703000-00020.
39. Michaelides EM, Sismanis A, Sugerman HJ, Felton WL. Pulsatile tinnitus in patients with morbid obesity: the effectiveness of weight reduction surgery. Am J Otol. 2000;21(5):682–5.
40. Kesler A, Kliper E, Assayag EB, et al. Thrombophilic factors in idiopathic intracranial hypertension: a report of 51 patients and a meta-analysis. Blood Coagul Fibrinolysis Int J Haemost Thromb. 2010;21(4):328–33. https://doi.org/10.1097/MBC.0b013e328338ce12.
41. Markey KA, Uldall M, Botfield H, et al. Idiopathic intracranial hypertension, hormones, and 11β-hydroxysteroid dehydrogenases. J Pain Res. 2016;9:223–32. https://doi.org/10.2147/JPR.S80824.
42. Botfield HF, Uldall MS, Westgate CSJ, et al. A glucagon-like peptide-1 receptor agonist reduces intracranial pressure in a rat model of hydrocephalus. Sci Transl Med. 2017;9(404):eaan0972. https://doi.org/10.1126/scitranslmed.aan0972.
43. Higgins JNP, Pickard JD. Lateral sinus stenoses in idiopathic intracranial hypertension resolving after CSF diversion. Neurology. 2004;62(10):1907–8. https://doi.org/10.1212/01.wnl.0000125285.44539.d7.
44. Ahmed RM, Wilkinson M, Parker GD, et al. Transverse sinus stenting for idiopathic intracranial hypertension: a review of 52 patients and of model predictions. AJNR Am J Neuroradiol. 2011;32(8):1408–14. https://doi.org/10.3174/ajnr.A2575.
45. Eisenman DJ. Sinus wall reconstruction for sigmoid sinus diverticulum and dehiscence: a standardized surgical procedure for a range of radiographic findings. Otol Neurotol. 2011;32(7):1116–9. https://doi.org/10.1097/MAO.0b013e31822a1c7d.

46. Goodwin CR, Elder BD, Ward A, et al. Risk factors for failed transverse sinus stenting in Pseudotumor cerebri patients. Clin Neurol Neurosurg. 2014;127:75–8. https://doi.org/10.1016/j.clineuro.2014.09.015.
47. Thurtell MJ, Wall M. Idiopathic intracranial hypertension (pseudotumor cerebri): recognition, treatment, and ongoing management. Curr Treat Options Neurol. 2013;15(1):1–12. https://doi.org/10.1007/s11940-012-0207-4.
48. Acheson JF. Idiopathic intracranial hypertension and visual function. Br Med Bull. 2006;79-80:233–44. https://doi.org/10.1093/bmb/ldl019.
49. Radhakrishnan K, Thacker AK, Bohlaga NH, Maloo JC, Gerryo SE. Epidemiology of idiopathic intracranial hypertension: a prospective and case-control study. J Neurol Sci. 1993;116(1):18–28. https://doi.org/10.1016/0022-510x(93)90084-c.
50. Olesen J. The international classification of headache disorders. 2nd edition (ICHD-II). Rev Neurol (Paris). 2005;161(6-7):689–91. https://doi.org/10.1016/s0035-3787(05)85119-7.
51. Kosmorsky GS. Idiopathic intracranial hypertension: pseudotumor cerebri. Headache. 2014;54(2):389–93. https://doi.org/10.1111/head.12284.
52. Aaron G, Doyle J, Vaphiades MS, Riley KO, Woodworth BA. Increased intracranial pressure in spontaneous CSF leak patients is not associated with papilledema. Otolaryngol Head Neck Surg. 2014;151(6):1061–6. https://doi.org/10.1177/0194599814551122.
53. Bidot S, Clough L, Saindane AM, Newman NJ, Biousse V, Bruce BB. The optic canal size is associated with the severity of papilledema and poor visual function in idiopathic intracranial hypertension. J Neuroophthalmol. 2016;36(2):120–5. https://doi.org/10.1097/WNO.0000000000000318.
54. Johnson LN, Krohel GB, Madsen RW, March GA. The role of weight loss and acetazolamide in the treatment of idiopathic intracranial hypertension (Pseudotumor cerebri). Ophthalmology. 1998;105(12):2313–7. https://doi.org/10.1016/S0161-6420(98)91234-9.
55. Lee AG, Golnik K, Kardon R, Wall M, Eggenberger E, Yedavally S. Sleep apnea and intracranial hypertension in men. Ophthalmology. 2002;109(3):482–5. https://doi.org/10.1016/s0161-6420(01)00987-3.
56. Fridley J, Foroozan R, Sherman V, Brandt ML, Yoshor D. Bariatric surgery for the treatment of idiopathic intracranial hypertension. J Neurosurg. 2011;114(1):34–9. https://doi.org/10.3171/2009.12.JNS09953.
57. Satti SR, Leishangthem L, Chaudry MI. Meta-analysis of CSF diversion procedures and dural venous sinus stenting in the setting of medically refractory idiopathic intracranial hypertension. AJNR Am J Neuroradiol. 2015;36(10):1899–904. https://doi.org/10.3174/ajnr.A4377.
58. Sismanis A, Butts FM, Hughes GB. Objective tinnitus in benign intracranial hypertension: an update. Laryngoscope. 1990;100(1):33–6. https://doi.org/10.1288/00005537-199001000-00008.
59. Murphy TP. Otologic manifestations of pseudotumor cerebri. J Otolaryngol. 1991;20(4):258–61.
60. Shim T, Chillakuru Y, Moncada P, et al. Sensorineural hearing loss and tinnitus characteristics in patients with idiopathic intracranial hypertension. Otol Neurotol. 2021;42(9):1323–8. https://doi.org/10.1097/MAO.0000000000003213.
61. Vivas EX, Mccall A, Raz Y, Fernandez-Miranda JC, Gardner P, Hirsch BE. ICP, BMI, surgical repair, and CSF diversion in patients presenting with spontaneous CSF otorrhea. Otol Neurotol. 2014;35(2):344–7. https://doi.org/10.1097/MAO.0b013e3182a473cf.
62. Nelson RF, Gantz BJ, Hansen MR. The rising incidence of spontaneous cerebrospinal fluid leaks in the United States and the association with obesity and obstructive sleep apnea. Otol Neurotol. 2015;36(3):476–80. https://doi.org/10.1097/MAO.0000000000000535.
63. Stevens SM, Lambert PR, Rizk H, McIlwain WR, Nguyen SA, Meyer TA. Novel radiographic measurement algorithm demonstrating a link between obesity and lateral skull base attenuation. Otolaryngol Head Neck Surg. 2015;152(1):172–9. https://doi.org/10.1177/0194599814557470.

64. Prichard CN, Isaacson B, Oghalai JS, Coker NJ, Vrabec JT. Adult spontaneous CSF otorrhea: correlation with radiographic empty sella. Otolaryngol Head Neck Surg. 2006;134(5):767–71. https://doi.org/10.1016/j.otohns.2006.01.002.
65. Goddard JC, Meyer T, Nguyen S, Lambert PR. New considerations in the cause of spontaneous cerebrospinal fluid otorrhea. Otol Neurotol. 2010;31(6):940–5. https://doi.org/10.1097/mao.0b013e3181e8f36c.
66. Rosenfeld E, Dotan G, Kimchi TJ, Kesler A. Spontaneous cerebrospinal fluid otorrhea and rhinorrhea in idiopathic intracranial hypertension patients. J Neuroophthalmol. 2013;33(2):113–6. https://doi.org/10.1097/WNO.0b013e18274b870.
67. Kenning TJ, Willcox TO, Artz GJ, Schiffmacher P, Farrell CJ, Evans JJ. Surgical management of temporal meningoencephaloceles, cerebrospinal fluid leaks, and intracranial hypertension: treatment paradigm and outcomes. Neurosurg Focus. 2012;32(6):E6. https://doi.org/10.3171/2012.4.FOCUS1265.
68. Stucken EZ, Selesnick SH, Brown KD. The role of obesity in spontaneous temporal bone encephaloceles and CSF leak. Otol Neurotol. 2012;33(8):1412–7. https://doi.org/10.1097/MAO.0b013e318268d350.
69. Schlosser RJ, Bolger WE. Significance of empty sella in cerebrospinal fluid leaks. Otolaryngol Head Neck Surg. 2003;128(1):32–8. https://doi.org/10.1067/mhn.2003.43.
70. O'Connell BP, Stevens SM, Xiao CC, Meyer TA, Schlosser RJ. Lateral skull base attenuation in patients with anterior cranial fossa spontaneous cerebrospinal fluid leaks. Otolaryngol Head Neck Surg. 2016;154(6):1138–44. https://doi.org/10.1177/0194599816630738.
71. Psaltis AJ, Overton LJ, Thomas WW, Fox NF, Banks CA, Schlosser RJ. Differences in skull base thickness in patients with spontaneous cerebrospinal fluid leaks. Am J Rhinol Allergy. 2014;28(1):e73–9. https://doi.org/10.2500/ajra.2014.28.4002.
72. Stevens SM, Rizk HG, McIlwain WR, Lambert PR, Meyer TA. Association between lateral skull base thickness and surgical outcomes in spontaneous CSF Otorrhea. Otolaryngol Head Neck Surg. 2016;154(4):707–14. https://doi.org/10.1177/0194599816628528.
73. Liu Z, Dong C, Wang X, et al. Association between idiopathic intracranial hypertension and sigmoid sinus dehiscence/diverticulum with pulsatile tinnitus: a retrospective imaging study. Neuroradiology. 2015;57(7):747–53. https://doi.org/10.1007/s00234-015-1517-5.
74. Harvey RS, Hertzano R, Kelman SE, Eisenman DJ. Pulse-synchronous tinnitus and sigmoid sinus wall anomalies: descriptive epidemiology and the idiopathic intracranial hypertension patient population. Otol Neurotol. 2014;35(1):7–15. https://doi.org/10.1097/MAO.0b013e3182a4756c.
75. Schlosser RJ, Wilensky EM, Grady MS, Bolger WE. Elevated intracranial pressures in spontaneous cerebrospinal fluid leaks. Am J Rhinol. 2003;17(4):191–5.
76. Wang EW, Vandergrift WA, Schlosser RJ. Spontaneous CSF leaks. Otolaryngol Clin North Am. 2011;44(4):845–56, vii. https://doi.org/10.1016/j.otc.2011.06.018.
77. Rizk HG, Hatch JL, Stevens SM, Lambert PR, Meyer TA. Lateral skull base attenuation in superior semicircular canal dehiscence and spontaneous cerebrospinal fluid otorrhea. Otolaryngol Head Neck Surg. 2016;155(4):641–8. https://doi.org/10.1177/0194599816651261.
78. El Hadi T, Sorrentino T, Calmels MN, Fraysse B, Deguine O, Marx M. Spontaneous tegmen defect and semicircular canal dehiscence: same etiopathogenic entity? Otol Neurotol. 2012;33(4):591–5. https://doi.org/10.1097/MAO.0b013e31824bae10.
79. Georgalas C, Oostra A, Ahmed S, et al. International consensus statement: spontaneous cerebrospinal fluid rhinorrhea. Int Forum Allergy Rhinol. 2021;11(4):794–803. https://doi.org/10.1002/alr.22704.
80. Oh MS, Vivas EX, Hudgins PA, Mattox DE. The prevalence of superior semicircular canal dehiscence in patients with mastoid encephalocele or cerebrospinal fluid otorrhea. Otol Neurotol. 2019;40(4):485–90. https://doi.org/10.1097/MAO.0000000000002155.
81. Jan TA, Cheng YS, Landegger LD, et al. Relationship between surgically treated superior canal dehiscence syndrome and body mass index. Otolaryngol Head Neck Surg. 2017;156(4):722–7. https://doi.org/10.1177/0194599816686563.

82. Erdogan N, Songu M, Akay E, et al. Posterior semicircular canal dehiscence in asymptomatic ears. Acta Otolaryngol (Stockh). 2011;131(1):4–8. https://doi.org/10.3109/00016489.2010.502184.
83. Verrecchia L, Edholm K, Pekkari M. Asymptomatic superior semicircular canal dehiscence. J Laryngol Otol. 2022;136(1):87–90. https://doi.org/10.1017/S0022215121003273.
84. Minor LB, Cremer PD, Carey JP, Della Santina CC, Streubel SO, Weg N. Symptoms and signs in superior canal dehiscence syndrome. Ann N Y Acad Sci. 2001;942:259–73. https://doi.org/10.1111/j.1749-6632.2001.tb03751.x.
85. Zhang L, Creighton FX, Carey JP. A cohort study comparing importance of clinical factors in determining diagnosis and treatment for superior semicircular canal dehiscence syndrome. Otol Neurotol. 2021;42(9):1429–33. https://doi.org/10.1097/MAO.0000000000003274.
86. Zuniga MG, Janky KL, Nguyen KD, Welgampola MS, Carey JP. Ocular versus cervical VEMPs in the diagnosis of superior semicircular canal dehiscence syndrome. Otol Neurotol. 2013;34(1):121–6. https://doi.org/10.1097/MAO.0b013e31827136b0.
87. Janky KL, Nguyen KD, Welgampola M, Zuniga MG, Carey JP. Air-conducted oVEMPs provide the best separation between intact and superior canal dehiscent labyrinths. Otol Neurotol. 2013;34(1):127–34. https://doi.org/10.1097/MAO.0b013e318271c32a.
88. Gioacchini FM, Alicandri-Ciufelli M, Kaleci S, Scarpa A, Cassandro E, Re M. Outcomes and complications in superior semicircular canal dehiscence surgery: a systematic review. Laryngoscope. 2016;126(5):1218–24. https://doi.org/10.1002/lary.25662.
89. Lee JA, Liu YF, Nguyen SA, McRackan TR, Meyer TA, Rizk HG. Posterior semicircular canal dehiscence: case series and systematic review. Otol Neurotol. 2020;41(4):511–21. https://doi.org/10.1097/MAO.0000000000002576.
90. Succar EF, Manickam PV, Wing S, Walter J, Greene JS, Azeredo WJ. Round window plugging in the treatment of superior semicircular canal dehiscence. Laryngoscope. 2018;128(6):1445–52. https://doi.org/10.1002/lary.26899.
91. Friedman DI, Jacobson DM. Diagnostic criteria for idiopathic intracranial hypertension. Neurology. 2002;59(10):1492–5. https://doi.org/10.1212/01.wnl.0000029570.69134.1b.
92. Friedman DI, Liu GT, Digre KB. Revised diagnostic criteria for the pseudotumor cerebri syndrome in adults and children. Neurology. 2013;81(13):1159–65. https://doi.org/10.1212/WNL.0b013e3182a55f17.
93. De Simone R, Ranieri A, Montella S, et al. Intracranial pressure in unresponsive chronic migraine. J Neurol. 2014;261(7):1365–73. https://doi.org/10.1007/s00415-014-7355-2.
94. Wang F, Lesser ER, Cutsforth-Gregory JK, et al. Population-based evaluation of lumbar puncture opening pressures. Front Neurol. 2019;10:899. https://doi.org/10.3389/fneur.2019.00899.
95. Celebisoy N, Gökçay F, Sirin H, Akyürekli O. Treatment of idiopathic intracranial hypertension: topiramate vs acetazolamide, an open-label study. Acta Neurol Scand. 2007;116(5):322–7. https://doi.org/10.1111/j.1600-0404.2007.00905.x.
96. Sugita Y, Iijima S, Teshima Y, et al. Marked episodic elevation of cerebrospinal fluid pressure during nocturnal sleep in patients with sleep apnea hypersomnia syndrome. Electroencephalogr Clin Neurophysiol. 1985;60(3):214–9. https://doi.org/10.1016/0013-4694(85)90033-1.
97. Jennum P, Børgesen SE. Intracranial pressure and obstructive sleep apnea. Chest. 1989;95(2):279–83. https://doi.org/10.1378/chest.95.2.279.
98. Purvin VA, Kawasaki A, Yee RD. Papilledema and obstructive sleep apnea syndrome. Arch Ophthalmol. 2000;118(12):1626–30. https://doi.org/10.1001/archopht.118.12.1626.
99. Poletti-Muringaseril SC, Rufibach K, Ruef C, Holzmann D, Soyka MB. Low meningitis-incidence in primary spontaneous compared to secondary cerebrospinal fluid rhinorrhoea. Rhinology. 2012;50(1):73–9. https://doi.org/10.4193/Rhino11.124.
100. Eljamel MS, Foy PM. Acute traumatic CSF fistulae: the risk of intracranial infection. Br J Neurosurg. 1990;4(5):381–5. https://doi.org/10.3109/02688699008992759.
101. McGirt MJ, Woodworth G, Thomas G, Miller N, Williams M, Rigamonti D. Cerebrospinal fluid shunt placement for pseudotumor cerebri-associated intractable headache: predictors of

treatment response and an analysis of long-term outcomes. J Neurosurg. 2004;101(4):627–32. https://doi.org/10.3171/jns.2004.101.4.0627.
102. Abubaker K, Ali Z, Raza K, Bolger C, Rawluk D, O'Brien D. Idiopathic intracranial hypertension: lumboperitoneal shunts versus ventriculoperitoneal shunts—case series and literature review. Br J Neurosurg. 2011;25(1):94–9. https://doi.org/10.3109/02688697.2010.544781.
103. Kanagalingam S, Subramanian PS. Cerebral venous sinus stenting for pseudotumor cerebri: a review. Saudi J Ophthalmol. 2015;29(1):3–8. https://doi.org/10.1016/j.sjopt.2014.09.007.
104. Carter SR, Seiff SR. Macular changes in pseudotumor cerebri before and after optic nerve sheath fenestration. Ophthalmology. 1995;102(6):937–41. https://doi.org/10.1016/s0161-6420(95)30931-1.
105. Chandrasekaran S, McCluskey P, Minassian D, Assaad N. Visual outcomes for optic nerve sheath fenestration in pseudotumour cerebri and related conditions. Clin Experiment Ophthalmol. 2006;34(7):661–5. https://doi.org/10.1111/j.1442-9071.2006.01301.x.

Chapter 20
Endolymphatic Hydrops

Benjamin R. Johnson, Maroun Semaan, Sarah Mowry, and Alejandro Rivas-Campo

Abbreviations

EH	Endolymphatic hydrops
EVA	Enlarged vestibular aqueduct
GD	Gadolinium
MD	Ménière's disease
MRI	Magnetic resonance imaging
SNHL	Sensorineural hearing loss
SSCD	Superior semicircular canal dehiscence
TWS	Third window syndrome
VEMPs	Vestibular evoked myogenic potentials

Introduction

The aim of this chapter will be to focus on the patient with third mobile window syndrome who also appears to have concomitant hydrops or has hydropic features after successful surgery repair. Research on MRI findings of hydrops in superior canal dehiscence patients will be discussed, and the treatment options available to patients.

B. R. Johnson (✉) · M. Semaan · S. Mowry · A. Rivas-Campo
Department of Otolaryngology-Head & Neck Surgery, University Hospitals Cleveland Medical Center, Cleveland, Ohio, USA

Case Western Reserve University School of Medicine, Cleveland, Ohio, USA
e-mail: Benjamin.Johnson3@uhhospitals.org; Maroun.Semaan@uhhospitals.org; Sarah.Mowry@uhhospitals.org; Alejandro.Rivas@uhhospitals.org

G. J. Gianoli, P. Thomson (eds.), *Third Mobile Window Syndrome of the Inner Ear*, https://doi.org/10.1007/978-3-031-16586-3_20

Endolymphatic hydrops is an excessive build-up of endolymph within the scala media, saccule, utricle, or semicircular canals and is the pathologic correlate of Ménière's disease (MD) [1]. Historically, EH could only be confirmed based on post-mortem temporal bone histology. The changes seen in histology are quite striking, as patients with MD can have up to a 300% increase in the average volume of the endolymphatic space compared to those without MD [2]. While MD has a strong correlation with the presence of EH on temporal bone histology, the reverse is not necessarily true; patients with EH on temporal bone histology may be completely asymptomatic [3]. This suggests that EH is a pathologic hallmark of MD but does not explain the entire disease process which takes place at the subcellular level. In this way EH is similar to amyloid plaques seen in Alzheimer's dementia; they are both a histologic marker of disease but do not offer a complete explanation for symptoms.

Recent advances in magnetic resonance imaging techniques have allowed for contemporaneous confirmation of EH in patients diagnosed with MD. 3T MRI using a combination of intravenous and intratympanic gadolinium contrast administration showed EH in 93% of ears with symptoms attributable to MD and 65% in contralateral asymptomatic ears [4]. This development has given clinicians a less invasive technique for further understanding the relationship between EH and MD.

Multiple theories attempt to explain the relationship between EH and the audio-vestibular symptoms seen in MD [5]. In the "endolymphatic hypertension theory," an abnormally elevated pressure in the endolymphatic system, when compared to the perilymphatic system, is thought to cause a distention of the membranous labyrinth. This distention, in turn, is then thought to cause aberrations in both cochlear and vestibular function. Another hypothesis is the "membrane rupture theory" whereby the acute rupture of the membranous labyrinth and fistula formation between the endolymph and perilymph is thought to cause an acute vertiginous attack. After rupture of the membranous labyrinth, it is thought that either physical distortion or a chemical paralysis of the sense organs causes symptoms. The chemical paralysis is thought to be due to leakage of potassium-rich endolymph into the perilymph which disrupts the vestibulocochlear nerve and delicate hair cell structures. This latter mechanism is called the "K+ intoxication theory" [5]. It is unlikely that any of these theories completely explains the pathophysiology of MD as additional genetic, environmental, and immunologic causes have also been proposed [6–8].

Regardless of the underlying mechanism, there is consensus that MD is an unpredictable and potentially debilitating disease. The prevalence of MD is estimated to be 34–190 per 100,000 [9]. One possible reason for the large variation in prevalence data is because MD is a clinical diagnosis. It can be easily confused with a number of diseases which can cause both vertigo and hearing loss, such as TWS. Consequently, the true prevalence may be lower than previously reported. Female sex, age, and white ethnicity are all associated with increased odds of developing MD. This is also true for several medical comorbidities including severe obesity, arthritis, psoriasis, irritable bowel syndrome, migraines, and gastroesophageal reflux disease.

Table 20.1 Diagnostic Criteria for MD jointly formulated by the Classification Committee of the Bárány Society, The Japan Society for Equilibrium Research, the European Academy of Otology and Neurotology (EAONO), the Equilibrium Committee of the American Academy of Otolaryngology-Head and Neck Surgery (AAO-HNS), and the Korean Balance Society (adapted from Lopez-Escamez et al. [9])

Definite Ménière's disease	Probable Ménière's disease
• Two or more spontaneous attacks of vertigo, each lasting 20 min to 12 h • Audiometrically documented fluctuating low- to mid-frequency sensorineural hearing loss (SNHL) in the affected ear on at least 1 occasion before, during, or after 1 of the episodes of vertigo • Fluctuating aural symptoms (hearing loss, tinnitus, or fullness) in the affected ear	• At least 2 episodes of vertigo or dizziness lasting 20 min to 24 h • Fluctuating aural symptoms (hearing loss, tinnitus, or fullness) in the affected ear • Other causes excluded by other tests

Symptoms of MD include aural fullness, episodic vertigo, fluctuating sensorineural hearing loss and tinnitus. MD can be a diagnostic challenge and is classified into Definite and Probable MD based on joint consensus between the Classification Committee of the Bárány Society, The Japan Society for Equilibrium Research, the European Academy of Otology and Neurotology (EAONO), the Equilibrium Committee of the American Academy of Otolaryngology-Head and Neck Surgery (AAO-HNS), and the Korean Balance Society (Table 20.1) [9].

Third window syndrome (TWS) is a constellation of audiovestibular symptoms due to the presence of a pathologic third window in the bony labyrinth of the inner ear [10].

Normally only two windows are present in the bony labyrinth and mechanical vibration of the stapes footplate generates a fluid pressure wave which travels from the oval to the round window. This results in a pressure gradient across the cochlear partition which activates cochlear hair cells and causes the perception of sound. The presence of a third window allows for an alternative low impedance pathway and alters how a sound pressure wave travels through the membranous labyrinth. The symptoms of TWS are diverse and include autophony, pulsatile tinnitus, aural fullness, low-frequency conductive hearing loss, sound- or pressure-induced vertigo, bone conduction hyperacusis, oscillopsia, nausea, headaches, and chronic disequilibrium (Table 20.3).

Superior semicircular canal dehiscence is the most well-known cause of TWS which was first described by Minor et al. in 1998 [11]. Since then, numerous additional causes of TWS have been discovered as listed in Table 20.2 [12].

Table 20.2 Known causes of third window syndrome

Superior semicircular canal dehiscence
Cochlea-facial nerve dehiscence
Cochlea-internal carotid artery dehiscence
Cochlea-internal auditory canal dehiscence
Lateral semicircular canal-superior semicircular canal ampulla dehiscence
Posterior semicircular canal dehiscence
Posterior semicircular canal-jugular bulb dehiscence
Superior semicircular canal-subarcuate artery dehiscence
Superior semicircular canal-superior petrosal vein dehiscence
Vestibule-middle ear dehiscence
Lateral semicircular canal–facial nerve dehiscence
Enlarged vestibular aqueduct
Post-traumatic hypermobile stapes footplate
CT negative third window syndrome

Concomitant EH and TWS

While TWS and EH appear to be two clinically distinct entities there is emerging evidence that they may frequently occur together. It can be difficult to distinguish between the two on clinical grounds alone given a significant overlap in symptomatology (Table 20.3). Current data regarding concomitant TWS and EH are limited to case series and small retrospective cohort studies. SSCD is the most common TWS and current literature focuses on SSCD and concomitant EH. Studies show a prevalence of EH in patients with SSCD ranging from 23% to 80% [13–15]. This prevalence data should be interpreted with caution given the limited number of patients in each of these studies. All these studies use Gd enhanced 3D-MRI to diagnose EH which is discussed in detail later in this chapter.

The largest study to date found that 9 of 33 (27%) ears with SSCD were also found to have some degree of EH on Gd-enhanced 3D-MRI [13]. Interestingly enough, there was no correlation between clinical symptoms of Ménière's disease and the presence of EH on MRI.

A recent small case series found that 3 out of 16 (23%) patients with SSCD were also found to have concomitant EH [15]. All three cases of concomitant EH were identified only after surgical repair of SSCD failed to resolve the patients' audiovestibular symptoms. Only one of the three patients with SSCD and concomitant EH had VEMP testing reported and it was found to be inconclusive. ECOG testing was not reported for any of these patients.

One retrospective study reported a much higher prevalence of concomitant EH and SSCD with 4 out of 5 ears (80%) with known SSCD showing severe EH of the cochlea on MRI. Additionally 2 out of 5 (40%) ears with SSCD were noted to have mild EH of the vestibule. In contrast to the other two studies mentioned, these authors also explored the relationship between enlarged vestibular aqueduct (EVA),

Table 20.3 Comparison of the symptoms seen in TWS and MD

Third window symptoms	Ménière's disease symptoms
• Autophony • Tinnitus (often pulsatile) • Aural fullness • Low-frequency conductive hearing loss • Sound- or pressure-induced vertigo • Bone conduction hyperacusis • Oscillopsia • Nausea • Headaches • Chronic disequilibrium • Hyperacusis	• Aural fullness • Tinnitus (low-pitch, ocean sound) • Episodic vertigo • Sensorineural hearing loss • Drop attacks • Nausea

as it can be considered a mobile third window, and concomitant EH. They found that 12 ears with an EVA were noted to have mild to severe EH in both the cochlea and vestibule. They hypothesized that the changes in perilymphatic pressure induced by a third window may induce a relative EH [14].

The idea that isolated otologic conditions may actually be related on a fundamental level is not new. It has been hypothesized before that EH and EVA may be related to a similar underlying genetic disease process [16]. The relationship between otosclerosis and EH has also been explored in depth with Shea et al. hypothesizing whether EH may be a result of the otosclerotic process [17–19]. Biomechanical analysis of SSCD has shown that the differential pressure across the scala media and vestibuli is affected by the presence of a third window such as SSCD and that pressure differential increases with increasing size of the dehiscence [20]. To date, the exact relationship between TWS and EH remains unclear; increasing our collective knowledge of this topic is paramount. The remainder of this chapter attempts to explore the relationships between TWS and EH, specifically highlighting important considerations for diagnostic testing and treatment strategies.

Diagnostic Testing

Audiometry

Isolated SSCD is associated with a low-frequency conductive hearing loss below 2 kHz and supranormal bone conduction thresholds [21]. This stands in contrast to EH which is associated with sensorineural hearing loss below 2 kHz. The degree of low-frequency sensorineural hearing loss, however, appears to outweigh the gain in supranormal bone conduction thresholds in SSCD and concomitant EH. Patients with concomitant SSCD and EH have shown an approximately 20 dB increase in air and bone conduction pure tone averages (PTA) when compared to isolated SSCD (Table 20.4). This subtle degree of sensorineural hearing loss can serve as a differentiating factor and aid in the diagnosis of concomitant EH.

Table 20.4 Data adapted from Ray et al. [13] showing an approximately 20 dB increase in air and bone conduction PTA for SSCD and concomitant EH when compared to SSCD alone

	AC PTA	BC PTA
SSCD and EH	47.9 ± 27.7 dB	43.9 ± 29.5 dB
Isolated SSCD	26 ± 18.1 dB	22 ± 14.9 dB

cVEMP/oVEMP

Vestibular evoked myogenic potentials (VEMPs) are frequently used to aid in the diagnosis of complex otologic conditions such as TWS. The cervical VEMP (cVEMP) measures the relaxation of the sternocleidomastoid muscle in response to an ipsilateral auditory stimulus and is thought to reflect saccular function [22]. The ocular VEMP (oVEMP) measures activation of the inferior oblique muscle in response to a contralateral auditory stimulus and is thought to reflect utricular function [23].

VEMP testing is not routinely obtained for a suspected diagnosis of MD as clinical practice guidelines from AAO-HNS recommended against the routine use of vestibular testing in these patients [24]. If obtained, however, cVEMPs can show characteristic changes indicative of MD. cVEMPs were found to be absent in up to 54% of patients with MD [25]. This is consistent with other authors who found that cVEMP responses were significantly reduced or absent in 51% of patients with MD [26]. Tone burst cVEMP thresholds have also been found to be increased in MD and some affected ears showed alterations in frequency tuning. Frequency tuning in unaffected ears means that the 500 Hz threshold is lower than the 1000 Hz but this can be reversed in MD [27]. oVEMPs do not appear to be as sensitive for the diagnosis of MD and are typically only absent in late stage MD [28]. From a physiological standpoint this makes sense as the saccule is more commonly affected than the utricle in MD, and is second only to the cochlea [29].

In contrast to MD, VEMP testing is routinely performed for a suspected diagnosis of TWS. cVEMP testing in patients with SSCD has abnormally low response thresholds and increased peak amplitudes. The thought is that the area of dehiscence reduces impedance and increases the transit of sound/pressure through the vestibular system. Similarly oVEMP testing in patients with SSCD shows abnormally low response thresholds and increased peak amplitudes to an even greater extent. cVEMP sensitivity and specificity for diagnosis of SSCD ranges from 80 to 100% whereas oVEMP sensitivity and specificity ranges from 90 to 100% respectively [23]. One additional note, however, is that VEMP response rates decrease with increasing age and that threshold testing may not be appropriate testing for individuals aged 60 years or older [30]. In a small case series of SSCD and concomitant EH, VEMP testing was reported for only one of the three patients and was found to be inconclusive [15]. A larger retrospective review of SSCD and concomitant EH found that abnormalities in VEMP testing did not correspond with the presence of EH. These authors argue that VEMP testing is confounded in patients with SSCD and concomitant EH, making MRI especially important [12]. Further research is warranted to understand how simultaneous TWS and EH affect the peripheral vestibular system.

ECOG

Electrocochleography (ECOG) is similar to a traditional auditory brainstem response (ABR) in that it measures the electrical response of the auditory system in response to acoustic stimulation. It specifically measures electrical potentials generated by the cochlea and auditory nerve. In contrast to traditional ABR testing, where the recording electrode is placed on the scalp, the recording electrode for ECOG is placed as close to the cochlea as possible. The recording electrode can be placed via a transcanal approach and rests on the tympanic membrane (noninvasive technique) or by inserting it through the tympanic membrane adjacent to the promontory (invasive technique). The responses seen in ECOG consist of the following: the cochlear microphonic (CM), summating potential (SP), and action potential (AP). The CM is an alternating current potential generated by the outer hair cells in response to stimulus. The SP is generated by a combination of both the inner and outer hair cells in response to a stimulus and the AP is equivalent to wave I of the ABR [22]. It is also important to note that tone burst or click stimuli can be both used for ECOG testing and there are some data to suggest that ECOG using tone burst stimuli has a greater sensitivity for detecting EH [31]. The SP/AP ratio is the main diagnostic parameter used to interpret an ECOG, and elevation greater than 0.4 is considered abnormal in most labs. This can be seen in both Ménière's disease and TWS such as SSCD.

Approximately 2/3 of classic Ménière's disease patients have an elevated SP/AP ratio which is thought to reflect the presence of endolymphatic hydrops caused by a distended basilar membrane. The sensitivity and specificity of ECOG ranges from 66.7 to 85.7% and 80% to 100% respectively [32]. Recent clinical practice guidelines from AAO-HNS, however, recommended against the routine use of ECOG for the diagnosis of Ménière's disease because of false negatives for early MD, testing variability, and a lack of protocol standardization [24].

It is interesting to note that elevated SP/AP ratios are also common in SSCD. 93.3% of patients in a small case series with SSCD were noted to have elevated SP/AP ratios. It is important to note that the SP/AP ratio appears to normalize after surgical repair of the dehiscence [33]. For patients with known SSCD or TWS who undergo surgical repair of the dehiscence, a persistently elevated SP/AP ratio should raise suspicion for the presence of concomitant EH or an insufficient repair/occlusion of the SSCD.

Imaging

New MRI modalities have allowed for in vivo evaluation of the presence of EH, something which previously could only be confirmed on post-mortem histology. Initial MRI techniques for evaluation of EH used a three-dimensional (3D) fluid attenuated inversion recovery (FLAIR) sequence after the administration of intratympanic gadolinium (Gd) [34]. The downsides of the intratympanic approach became readily apparent as it was invasive, required an off-label use of Gd, and a 24-h waiting period was needed before the imaging could be obtained. Further research led to the development of a novel MRI technique called the Hybrid of Reversed Image of Positive Endolymph Signal and Native Image of Positive Perilymph Signal (HYDROPS) protocol which uses intravenous Gd administered 4 h before imaging at a standard dose [35]. The HYDROPS protocol subtracts a heavily weighted T2 3D-Flair sequence (Positive Perilymph Image) from a T2-weighted 3D inversion recovery sequence (Positive Endolymph Image). This allows the endolymph to appear black and the surrounding Gd-filled perilymph to appear white (Fig. 20.1). This technique also can differentiate between cochlear and vestibular EH and additionally can classify the EH as mild or severe [36]. The HYDROPS protocol has allowed for the evaluation of concomitant EH in patients

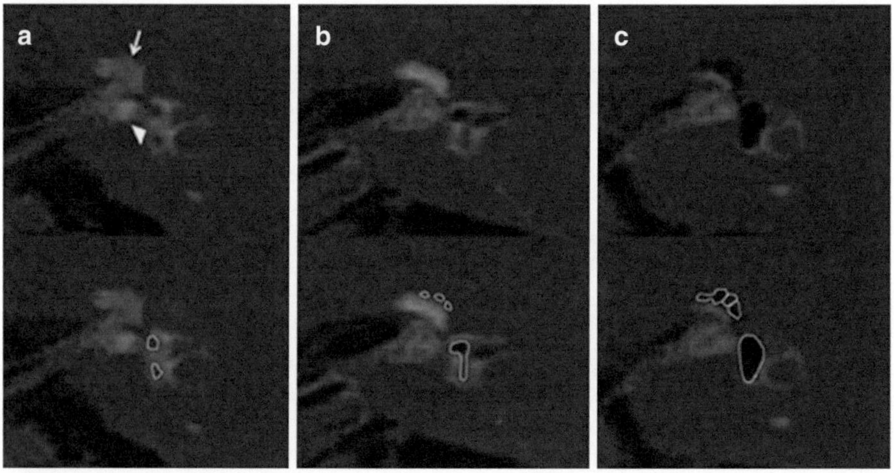

Fig. 20.1 Example images of endolymphatic hydrops (EH) from none (**a**), mild (**b**), and significant (**c**) grades in both the cochlea (arrow) and vestibule (arrowhead). HYDROPS (hybrid of reversed image of positive endolymph signal and native image of positive perilymph signal) was used to detect EH. Original images from the three grades are shown in the upper part, and endolymphatic spaces in the cochlea and the vestibule are traced in the lower part (areas encircled by white lines). (**a**) Gadodiamide hydrate fills the perilymphatic space (white areas), and the endolymphatic space cannot be detected in the cochlea. Mild and severely enlarged endolymphatic spaces can be observed in both the cochlea and the vestibule in **b**, **c**, respectively. (Republished with permission of John Wiley & Sons, from *Laryngoscope*, Vol 126 (1996), Sone et al.; permission conveyed through Copyright Clearance Center, Inc)

with known otosclerosis [18]. More recently it has been used in the setting of TWS and concomitant EH [14]. Other studies simply report the use of 3D-Flair MRI with intravenous Gd contrast to diagnose EH in the setting of SSCD without the HYDROPS protocol [12].

High-resolution temporal bone CT is the first-line imaging modality for the diagnosis of TWS [37]. Stenvers and Poschl views which are orthogonal and parallel to the superior semicircular canal, respectively, can allow for better visualization of SSCD. It is interesting to note that MRI can also be used, showing excellent specificity and sensitivity for SSCD specifically, but it is not as common as CT imaging likely given its increased cost, poor bone visualization, and thicker image slices [38]. Furthermore, since TWS is due to erosion of the otic capsule at multiple possible locations, MRI alone is not able to evaluate for all causes of TWS. For a more detailed discussion of this topic please refer to Chap. 12. There have been reports of CT Negative TWS, however, which by definition would have normal CT imaging but VEMP testing and clinical symptoms similar to CT positive TWS [12].

Treatment

Surgical

Surgery is currently the only reported treatment for TWS and SSCD. Success rates for surgical repair of SSCD via a transmastoid or middle cranial fossa approach (MCF) show high success and low complication rates regardless of the method of repair chosen. These repair techniques include resurfacing, plugging, capping, or a combination of these techniques [39]. Treatments of other forms of TWS such as Cochlear-Facial Dehiscence have successfully been treated with round window reinforcement (RWR) [40]. Advantages of RWR include short operative time, ease of recovery, and lack of significant morbidity apart from a potential slight conductive hearing loss. A minority of patients, however, have persistent symptoms despite surgical repair for TWS. The natural question that arises is what is the cause of treatment failure in these patients, especially when the anatomic third window appears to be adequately addressed. One possibility is that they have concomitant, undiagnosed EH which could lead to refractory audiovestibular symptoms. In a recent case series by Johanis et al., all patients with SSCD and concomitant EH were diagnosed with EH only after failure of surgery to adequately control symptoms [15]. Therefore, patients with persistent symptoms despite surgical repair for TWS should undergo MRI to rule out the presence of EH. Furthermore, an additional argument for obtaining a postoperative MRI in patients with TWS who have failed surgery is to evaluate for the possibility of a small residual dehiscence which may not be evident on CT imaging [41].

It is also important to note that the surgical creation of a third window may in some cases be intentional and therapeutic as in patients with MD who undergo endolymphatic sac decompression. There has been noted to be a positive correlation between the degree of vertigo control and the development of a postoperative low-frequency air bone gap (LFABG) after endolymphatic sac surgery. The development of a LFABG is thought to reflect adequate endolymphatic sac decompression and subsequent formation of a third window [42].

Medical

There are currently no reported studies on medical therapies for SSC [43]. There have, however, been some reports on medical therapies for other TWS (see Chap. 13 for a discussion of medical therapy and TWS). This stands in contrast to MD and EH where medical therapy is well studied and the preferred initial treatment strategy and surgery is reserved for refractory vestibular symptoms. Treatment for MD includes lifestyle modifications such as salt and caffeine restriction. For patients that remain symptomatic, oral pharmacotherapy with diuretics or betahistine (currently not FDA approved in the USA) can be initiated. Specific examples include thiazide diuretics such as hydrochlorothiazide, with or without a potassium sparing diuretic such as triamterene. Acetazolamide, a carbonic anhydrase inhibitor, can also be used. Oral steroids like prednisone are frequently used for acute vertigo or sudden changes in hearing. Benzodiazepines may also be used for symptom control. Intratympanic steroids are also frequently used. Intratympanic gentamicin can also be used but is considered to be ablative and its use varies by institution [44, 45].

Specifically for patients with SSCD who underwent surgical repair and were subsequently found to have concomitant EH, medical therapies including hydrochlorothiazide, acetazolamide, prednisone, or mycophenolate mofetil have been used with anecdotal success [15]. It is important to note that acetazolamide specifically has been noted to improve EH on post-treatment MRI [46], whereas betahistine and furosemide have not [47, 48].

Conclusion

Isolated SSCD is associated with a low-frequency conductive hearing loss and supranormal bone conduction thresholds, while patients with SSCD and concomitant EH are noted to have mild to moderate sensorineural hearing loss. Both TWS and EH are known to cause an increased SP/AP ratio on ECOG. VEMP testing may be unreliable in the setting of TWS and concomitant EH, as EH reduces VEMP response rates. A 3D Flair MRI with intravenous Gd contrast should be obtained for all patients with TWS such as SSCD, who fail surgical management, to rule out concomitant EH. Medical therapy for concomitant EH should be initiated if the patient is symptomatic, with standard therapies used for MD.

References

1. Gürkov R, Pyykö I, Zou J, Kentala E. What is Menière's disease? A contemporary re-evaluation of endolymphatic hydrops. J Neurol. 2016;263(Suppl 1):S71–81. Epub 2016 Apr 15. PMID: 27083887; PMCID: PMC4833790. https://doi.org/10.1007/s00415-015-7930-1.
2. Morita N, Kariya S, Farajzadeh Deroee A, Cureoglu S, Nomiya S, Nomiya R, Harada T, Paparella MM. Membranous labyrinth volumes in normal ears and Ménière disease: a three-dimensional reconstruction study. Laryngoscope. 2009;119(11):2216–20. PMID: 19806642; PMCID: PMC2927481. https://doi.org/10.1002/lary.20723.
3. Merchant SN, Adams JC, Nadol JB Jr. Pathophysiology of Meniere's syndrome: are symptoms caused by endolymphatic hydrops? Otol Neurotol. 2005;26(1):74–81. PMID: 15699723. https://doi.org/10.1097/00129492-200501000-00013.
4. Pyykkö I, Nakashima T, Yoshida T, Zou J, Naganawa S. Meniere's disease: a reappraisal supported by a variable latency of symptoms and the MRI visualisation of endolymphatic hydrops. BMJ Open. 2013;3(2):e001555. PMID: 23418296; PMCID: PMC3586172. https://doi.org/10.1136/bmjopen-2012-001555.
5. Takeda T, Takeda S, Kakigi A. A possible mechanism of the formation of endolymphatic hydrops and its associated inner ear disorders. Auris Nasus Larynx. 2020;47(1):25–41. Epub 2019 Oct 15. PMID: 31623941. https://doi.org/10.1016/j.anl.2019.09.005.
6. Gallego-Martinez A, Lopez-Escamez JA. Genetic architecture of Meniere's disease. Hear Res. 2020;397:107872. Epub 2019 Dec 13. PMID: 31874721. https://doi.org/10.1016/j.heares.2019.107872.
7. Simo H, Yang S, Qu W, Preis M, Nazzal M, Baugh R. Meniere's disease: importance of socioeconomic and environmental factors. Am J Otolaryngol. 2015;36(3):393–8. Epub 2015 Feb 3. PMID: 25771842. https://doi.org/10.1016/j.amjoto.2015.01.009.
8. Derebery MJ. Allergic and immunologic features of Ménière's disease. Otolaryngol Clin North Am. 2011;44(3):655–66, ix. Epub 2011 May 4. PMID: 21621052. https://doi.org/10.1016/j.otc.2011.03.004.
9. Lopez-Escamez JA, Carey J, Chung WH, Goebel JA, Magnusson M, Mandalà M, Newman-Toker DE, Strupp M, Suzuki M, Trabalzini F, Bisdorff A, Classification Committee of the Barany Society; Japan Society for Equilibrium Research; European Academy of Otology and Neurotology (EAONO); Equilibrium Committee of the American Academy of Otolaryngology-Head and Neck Surgery (AAO-HNS); Korean Balance Society. Diagnostic criteria for Menière's disease. J Vestib Res. 2015;25(1):1–7. PMID: 25882471. https://doi.org/10.3233/VES-150549.
10. Iversen MM, Rabbitt RD. Biomechanics of third window syndrome. Front Neurol. 2020;11:891. PMID: 32982922; PMCID: PMC7477384. https://doi.org/10.3389/fneur.2020.00891.
11. Minor LB, Solomon D, Zinreich JS, Zee DS. Sound- and/or pressure-induced vertigo due to bone dehiscence of the superior semicircular canal. Arch Otolaryngol Head Neck Surg. 1998;124(3):249–58. PMID: 9525507. https://doi.org/10.1001/archotol.124.3.249.
12. Wackym PA, Agrawal Y, Ikezono T, Balaban CD. Editorial: Third window syndrome. Front Neurol. 2021;12:704095. Published 2021 Jun 18. https://doi.org/10.3389/fneur.2021.704095.
13. Ray A, Hautefort C, Guichard JP, Horion J, Herman P, Kania R, Houdart E, Verillaud B, Vitaux H, Attyé A, Eliezer M. MRI contribution for the detection of endolymphatic hydrops in patients with superior canal dehiscence syndrome. Eur Arch Otorhinolaryngol. 2021;278(7):2229–38. Epub 2020 Aug 14. PMID: 32797276. https://doi.org/10.1007/s00405-020-06282-3.
14. Sone M, Yoshida T, Morimoto K, Teranishi M, Nakashima T, Naganawa S. Endolymphatic hydrops in superior canal dehiscence and large vestibular aqueduct syndromes. Laryngoscope. 2016;126(6):1446–50. Epub 2015 Nov 3. PMID: 26525170. https://doi.org/10.1002/lary.25747.

15. Johanis M, De Jong R, Miao T, Hwang L, Lum M, Kaur T, Willis S, Arsenault JJ, Duong C, Yang I, Gopen Q. Concurrent superior semicircular canal dehiscence and endolymphatic hydrops: a novel case series. Int J Surg Case Rep. 2021;78:382–6. Epub 2020 Dec 26. PMID: 33421957; PMCID: PMC7804363. https://doi.org/10.1016/j.ijscr.2020.12.074.
16. Spiegel JH, Lalwani AK. Large vestibular aqueduct syndrome and endolymphatic hydrops: two presentations of a common primary inner-ear dysfunction? J Laryngol Otol. 2009;123(8):919–21. Epub 2008 Nov 12. PMID: 19000343. https://doi.org/10.1017/S0022215108004088.
17. Wang F, Yoshida T, Sugimoto S, Shimono M, Teranishi M, Naganawa S, Sone M. Clinical features of ears with otosclerosis and endolymphatic hydrops. Otol Neurotol. 2019;40(4):441–5. PMID: 30870351. https://doi.org/10.1097/MAO.0000000000002175.
18. Mukaida T, Sone M, Yoshida T, Kato K, Teranishi M, Naganawa S, Nakashima T. Magnetic resonance imaging evaluation of endolymphatic hydrops in cases with otosclerosis. Otol Neurotol. 2015;36(7):1146–50. PMID: 25522197. https://doi.org/10.1097/MAO.0000000000000685.
19. Shea JJ Jr, Ge X, Orchik DJ. Endolymphatic hydrops associated with otosclerosis. Am J Otol. 1994;15(3):348–57. PMID: 8579139.
20. Pisano DV, Niesten ME, Merchant SN, Nakajima HH. The effect of superior semicircular canal dehiscence on intracochlear sound pressures. Audiol Neurootol. 2012;17(5):338–48. Epub 2012 Jul 18. PMID: 22814034; PMCID: PMC3541532. https://doi.org/10.1159/000339653.
21. Ward BK, Carey JP, Minor LB. Superior canal dehiscence syndrome: lessons from the first 20 years. Front Neurol. 2017;8:177. PMID: 28503164; PMCID: PMC5408023. https://doi.org/10.3389/fneur.2017.00177.
22. Adams ME, Heidenreich KD, Kileny PR. Audiovestibular testing in patients with Meniere's disease. Otolaryngol Clin North Am. 2010;43(5):995–1009. PMID: 20713239. https://doi.org/10.1016/j.otc.2010.05.008.
23. Zuniga MG, Janky KL, Nguyen KD, Welgampola MS, Carey JP. Ocular versus cervical VEMPs in the diagnosis of superior semicircular canal dehiscence syndrome. Otol Neurotol. 2013;34:121–6.
24. Basura GJ, Adams ME, Monfared A, Schwartz SR, Antonelli PJ, Burkard R, Bush ML, Bykowski J, Colandrea M, Derebery J, Kelly EA, Kerber KA, Koopman CF, Kuch AA, Marcolini E, McKinnon BJ, Ruckenstein MJ, Valenzuela CV, Vosooney A, Walsh SA, Nnacheta LC, Dhepyasuwan N, Buchanan EM. Clinical practice guideline: Ménière's disease. Otolaryngol Head Neck Surg. 2020;162(2_suppl):S1–S55. PMID: 32267799. https://doi.org/10.1177/0194599820909438.
25. De Waele C, Huy PT, Diard JP, Freyss G, Vidal PP. Saccular dysfunction in Meniere's disease. Am J Otol. 1999;20(2):223–32. PMID: 10100527.
26. Murofushi T, Shimizu K, Takegoshi H, Cheng PW. Diagnostic value of prolonged latencies in the vestibular evoked myogenic potential. Arch Otolaryngol Head Neck Surg. 2001;127(9):1069–72. PMID: 11556854. https://doi.org/10.1001/archotol.127.9.1069.
27. Rauch SD, Zhou G, Kujawa SG, Guinan JJ, Herrmann BS. Vestibular evoked myogenic potentials show altered tuning in patients with Ménière's disease. Otol Neurotol. 2004;25(3):333–8. PMID: 15129114. https://doi.org/10.1097/00129492-200405000-00022.
28. Kharkheli E, Japaridze S, Kevanishvili Z, Oz I, Ozluoglu LN. Correlation between vestibular evoked myogenic potentials and disease progression in Ménière's disease. ORL J Otorhinolaryngol Relat Spec. 2019;81(4):193–201. Epub 2019 Aug 7. PMID: 31390639. https://doi.org/10.1159/000496088.
29. Schuknecht HF. Endolymphatic hydrops: can it be controlled? Ann Otol Rhinol Laryngol. 1986;95(1 Pt 1):36–9. PMID: 3947002. https://doi.org/10.1177/000348948609500108.
30. Janky KL, Shepard N. Vestibular evoked myogenic potential (VEMP) testing: normative threshold response curves and effects of age. J Am Acad Audiol. 2009;20(8):514–22. PMID: 19764171; PMCID: PMC2749261. https://doi.org/10.3766/jaaa.20.8.6.

31. Iseli C, Gibson W. A comparison of three methods of using transtympanic electrocochleography for the diagnosis of Meniere's disease: click summating potential measurements, tone burst summating potential amplitude measurements, and biasing of the summating potential using a low frequency tone. Acta Otolaryngol. 2010;130(1):95–101. PMID: 19396716. https://doi.org/10.3109/00016480902858899.
32. Ziylan F, Smeeing DP, Stegeman I, Thomeer HG. Click stimulus electrocochleography versus MRI with intratympanic contrast in Ménière's disease: a systematic review. Otol Neurotol. 2016;37(5):421–7.
33. Arts HA, Adams ME, Telian SA, El-Kashlan H, Kileny PR. Reversible electrocochleographic abnormalities in superior canal dehiscence. Otol Neurotol. 2009;30(1):79–86. PMID: 19092559. https://doi.org/10.1097/MAO.0b013e31818d1b51.
34. Nakashima T, Naganawa S, Sugiura M, Teranishi M, Sone M, Hayashi H, Nakata S, Katayama N, Ishida IM. Visualization of endolymphatic hydrops in patients with Meniere's disease. Laryngoscope. 2007;117(3):415–20. PMID: 17279053. https://doi.org/10.1097/MLG.0b013e31802c300c.
35. Naganawa S, Yamazaki M, Kawai H, Bokura K, Sone M, Nakashima T. Imaging of Ménière's disease after intravenous administration of single-dose gadodiamide: utility of subtraction images with different inversion time. Magn Reson Med Sci. 2012;11(3):213–9. PMID: 23037568. https://doi.org/10.2463/mrms.11.213.
36. Naganawa S, Suzuki K, Nakamichi R, Bokura K, Yoshida T, Sone M, Homann G, Nakashima T, Ikeda M. Semi-quantification of endolymphatic size on MR imaging after intravenous injection of single-dose gadodiamide: comparison between two types of processing strategies. Magn Reson Med Sci. 2013;12(4):261–9. Epub 2013 Oct 29. PMID: 24172793. https://doi.org/10.2463/mrms.2013-0019.
37. Ho ML. Third window lesions. Neuroimaging Clin N Am. 2019;29(1):57–92. PMID: 30466645. https://doi.org/10.1016/j.nic.2018.09.005.
38. Browaeys P, Larson TL, Wong ML, Patel U. Can MRI replace CT in evaluating semicircular canal dehiscence? Am J Neuroradiol. 2013;34(7):1421–7.
39. Gioacchini FM, Alicandri-Ciufelli M, Kaleci S, Scarpa A, Cassandro E, Re M. Outcomes and complications in superior semicircular canal dehiscence surgery: a systematic review. Laryngoscope. 2016;126(5):1218–24. Epub 2015 Sep 15. PMID: 26371952. https://doi.org/10.1002/lary.25662.
40. Wackym PA, Balaban CD, Zhang P, Siker DA, Hundal JS. Third window syndrome: surgical management of cochlea-facial nerve dehiscence. Front Neurol. 2019;10:1281. PMID: 31920911; PMCID: PMC6923767. https://doi.org/10.3389/fneur.2019.01281.
41. Chemtob RA, Epprecht L, Reinshagen KL, Huber A, Caye-Thomasen P, Nakajima HH, Lee DJ. Utility of postoperative magnetic resonance imaging in patients who fail superior canal dehiscence surgery. Otol Neurotol. 2019;40(1):130–8. PMID: 30461526. https://doi.org/10.1097/MAO.0000000000002051.
42. Kim SH, Ko SH, Ahn SH, Hong JM, Lee WS. Significance of the development of the inner ear third window effect after endolymphatic sac surgery in Ménière disease patients. Laryngoscope. 2012;122(8):1838–43. Epub 2012 Jul 2. PMID: 22753085. https://doi.org/10.1002/lary.23332.
43. Eberhard KE, Chari DA, Nakajima HH, Klokker M, Cayé-Thomasen P, Lee DJ. Current trends, controversies, and future directions in the evaluation and management of superior canal dehiscence syndrome. Front Neurol. 2021;12:638574. PMID: 33889125; PMCID: PMC8055857. https://doi.org/10.3389/fneur.2021.638574.
44. Crowson MG, Patki A, Tucci DL. A systematic review of diuretics in the medical management of Ménière's disease. Otolaryngol Head Neck Surg. 2016;154(5):824–34. Epub 2016 Mar 1. PMID: 26932948. https://doi.org/10.1177/0194599816630733.
45. Christopher LH, Wilkinson EP. Meniere's disease: medical management, rationale for vestibular preservation and suggested protocol in medical failure. Am J Otolaryngol. 2021;42(1):102817. Epub 2020 Nov 2. PMID: 33202330. https://doi.org/10.1016/j.amjoto.2020.102817.

46. Sepahdari AR, Vorasubin N, Ishiyama G, Ishiyama A. Endolymphatic hydrops reversal following acetazolamide therapy: demonstration with delayed intravenous contrast-enhanced 3D-FLAIR MRI. Am J Neuroradiol. 2016;37(1):151–4. Epub 2015 Sep 17. PMID: 26381561; PMCID: PMC7960214. https://doi.org/10.3174/ajnr.A4462.
47. Gürkov R, Flatz W, Keeser D, Strupp M, Ertl-Wagner B, Krause E. Effect of standard-dose Betahistine on endolymphatic hydrops: an MRI pilot study. Eur Arch Otorhinolaryngol. 2013;270(4):1231–5. Epub 2012 Jul 4. PMID: 22760844. https://doi.org/10.1007/s00405-012-2087-3.
48. Fiorino F, Mattellini B, Vento M, Mazzocchin L, Bianconi L, Pizzini FB. Does the intravenous administration of furosemide reduce endolymphatic hydrops? J Laryngol Otol. 2016;130(3):242–7. Epub 2016 Jan 14. PMID: 26763125. https://doi.org/10.1017/S0022215115003527.

Chapter 21
Superior Canal Dehiscence Syndrome in the Only Hearing Ear

Miriam R. Smetak, Ankita Patro, and David S. Haynes

Introduction

Operations on the only hearing ear have been given special consideration since the advent of modern otologic surgery [1, 2]. While surgical techniques and outcomes have greatly improved over the past several decades, the risk of decreased or even complete loss of hearing after any otologic surgery can be catastrophic, especially in a patient who relies on one ear as their sole source of auditory input. Hearing loss can result in social isolation secondary to difficulty with communication, the loss of employment, and stigma. In the broader context, severe to profound hearing loss has a societal cost that is estimated to be in the hundreds of thousands of dollars over an individual's lifetime [3].

While surgery on the only hearing ear has been a focus of discussion over the ensuing decades, the diagnosis and management of superior canal dehiscence (SCD) and its associated syndrome (SCDS) are relatively recent. Minor et al. are credited with describing the classic symptoms of SCDS in a series of patients with dehiscences over the superior semicircular canal that were demonstrated on computed tomography (CT) scans in 1998 [4]. Since then, the global literature on SCDS and other third mobile window syndromes (TMWS) continues to expand along with our understanding of the disease process and its surgical management. However, there has been little reported to date on TMWS in the only hearing ear.

As such, this chapter discusses several considerations when managing patients with TMWS in the only hearing ear. First, the natural history of hearing loss in patients with TMWS and the overlap of TMWS with other hearing disorders must

M. R. Smetak (✉) · A. Patro · D. S. Haynes
Department of Otolaryngology-Head and Neck Surgery, Vanderbilt University Medical Center, Nashville, TN, USA
e-mail: miriam.r.smetak@vumc.org; ankita.patro@vumc.org; david.haynes@vumc.org

G. J. Gianoli, P. Thomson (eds.), *Third Mobile Window Syndrome of the Inner Ear*, https://doi.org/10.1007/978-3-031-16586-3_21

be understood. Next, additional care must be taken when weighing the benefits of surgical therapy for TMWS compared to continued conservative management in this patient population. Ultimately, a patient-centered care approach should be used when deciding whether to operate, with open discussions of risks and benefits of each treatment option resulting in shared decision-making between the surgeon and patient. Lastly, special considerations for hearing restoration in the only hearing ear with TMWS will be examined.

Hearing Loss and Superior Canal Dehiscence Syndrome

A low-frequency conductive hearing loss has been associated with SCDS and posterior canal dehiscence since the disease process was first described [5–8]. The mechanism of hearing loss is believed to be secondary to the mobile "third window" introducing an alternative low impedance pathway for sound energy to dissipate, overall lowering the cochlear input impedance and decreasing the amount of sound energy that ultimately reaches the cochlea. A lowering of the bone conduction threshold can also be seen as the summative result of multiple stimulus pathways that results in an overall air-bone gap (ABG) that can be as high as 30 to 60 dB [9]. Typically, hearing loss is greatest at frequencies less than 2000 Hz and remains stable over time [7, 10]. However, the severity of the conductive hearing loss that is experienced by patients with SCDS can vary greatly. This variability may be at least partially explained by the size, shape, and/or location of the dehiscence [9, 11–13].

In addition to low-frequency conductive hearing loss, sensorineural hearing loss (SNHL) can also be seen in patients with radiographic evidence of SCD. The underlying cause of the SNHL is largely unknown but is hypothesized to be due to (1) a common underlying developmental anomaly and/or (2) destructive effects on the cochlea. Alternatively, SCD may simply be an incidental finding during workup of an unrelated SNHL [7]. While it is unknown whether this hearing loss is progressive, progression at the short and intermediate follow-up appears to be similar to that of the normal population [10].

Notably, TMWS may overlap with other otologic disorders such as Ménière's disease and otosclerosis. It is important to determine the etiology of hearing loss in patients with concurrent audiovestibular disorders, as appropriate interventions will vary significantly depending on the etiology of the symptoms [14]. Surgical repair of the dehiscence may sometimes result in closure of a large ABG and improvement in air-conducted pure tone average (PTA), although this result is by no means assured. Typically, surgery is reserved for debilitating vestibular symptoms rather than auditory symptoms alone [15–19].

Surgical Approaches to Superior Canal Dehiscence in the Only Hearing Ear

When planning surgical treatment of SCDS, there are three common approaches to consider: middle cranial fossa (MCF), transmastoid, and round window plugging. A more in-depth discussion of surgical approaches is presented in Chap. 15. Here, we will focus on the special consideration given to each approach in the case of the only hearing ear and the risk of worsening or complete loss of hearing after surgical intervention.

In the MCF approach, a craniotomy with retraction of the temporal lobe directly exposes the site of dehiscence in the floor of the middle fossa. The repair is performed via plugging, resurfacing, or capping with a variety of biologic and synthetic materials. Plugging of the canal is generally considered to have a higher success rate, but manipulation of the membranous labyrinth has raised concerns about the potential for an increased risk of hearing loss. Additionally, the MCF approach is accompanied by more serious risks of nerve injury, CSF leak, stroke, and hemorrhage [20].

The transmastoid approach is performed via a complete mastoidectomy with similar plugging of the superior semicircular canal but without direct visualization of the dehiscence. This approach avoids the morbidity of the craniotomy and temporal lobe retraction. However, it does still carry a significant risk of permanent SNHL. Some surgeons feel that outcomes are less consistent with the transmastoid approach than that of the MCF approach, due to the former's indirect method to addressing the dehiscence [20, 21].

Whether the MCF or transmastoid approach is superior for hearing preservation is unclear [22, 23]. Early reports suggested that surgical repair of SCD via MCF approach had a low risk of SNHL except in cases of revision surgery and could result in normalization of the conductive component of the hearing loss [16]. However, subsequent studies have reported rates of up to 25% for persistent SNHL that is associated with plugging of the canal via the MCF approach [17]. The overall risk of hearing loss greater than 20 dB after either the transmastoid or MCF approach is less than 10%, with a 1–2% risk of profound SNHL. Statistically significant high frequency hearing loss at 8000 Hz has been associated with both procedures [20, 23, 24]. In summary, the MCF and transmastoid approaches have a low but significant risk of permanent change in hearing, and revision surgery has an elevated risk of postoperative SNHL compared to primary surgery [16].

The round window approach has emerged more recently as a less invasive method that circumvents the need for direct manipulation of the membranous labyrinth. In theory, reinforcement of the round window closes off one of the three mobile windows, allowing the labyrinth to return to a more physiologic two-window condition. This approach has shown some success in alleviating the vestibular symptoms of SCDS, although outcomes are variable. Nevertheless, this procedure can be associated with a significant worsening in hearing function. In one study,

46% of patients had a worsening of their conductive hearing loss greater than or equal to 10 dB [25]. In an only hearing ear, this may be an unacceptable consequence and patients should be counseled on the risk of additional hearing loss before pursuing this treatment approach [18, 25].

The Decision to Operate

Parallels can be made to other scenarios, such as chronic ear disease and cerebellopontine angle lesions, where the only hearing ear requires surgical intervention [26, 27]. In general, surgical intervention may be warranted under the following conditions: (1) operative intervention carries relatively low risk to residual hearing or can reasonably be expected to improve hearing, and/or (2) symptoms are debilitating and not responsive to more conservative measures.

> "Surgical intervention may be warranted under the following conditions: (1) operative intervention carries relatively low risk to residual hearing or can reasonably be expected to improve hearing, and/or (2) symptoms are debilitating and not responsive to more conservative measures."

Careful thought should be given when weighing the potential benefits of any surgical intervention against the risk of worsening or complete loss of hearing in the only hearing ear (Fig. 21.1). Surgery should be considered in patients who are most

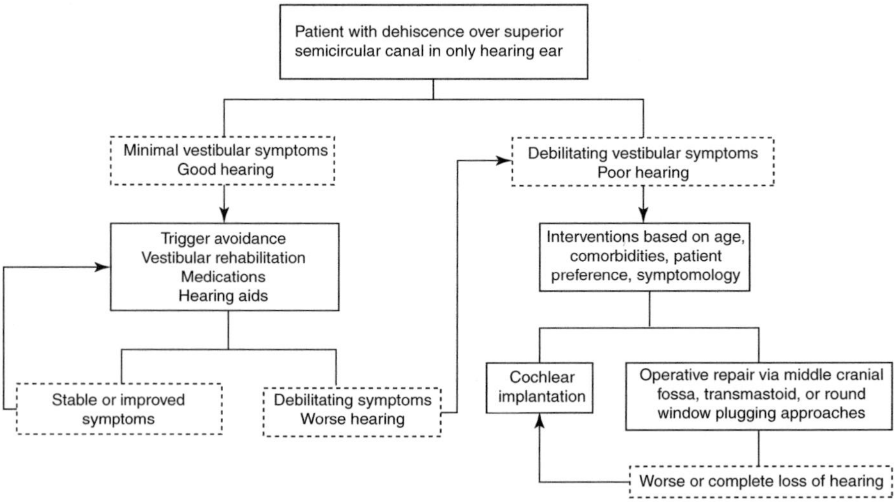

Fig. 21.1 Treatment options for superior canal dehiscence syndrome in the only hearing ear

affected by their symptoms and those who are most likely to benefit from intervention. SCD repair should not be undertaken for repair of conductive hearing loss alone. The transmastoid and MCF approaches to SCD result in no statistically significant changes in ABG compared to preoperative values. Individuals with a large preoperative ABG may experience some improvement in the conductive component of their hearing loss, but this is often not the case. Both approaches carry a small but significant risk of permanent SNHL, especially at high frequencies [24]. The patients most likely to benefit from surgical intervention are those with audiovestibular symptoms related to the third window effect, most notably autophony, pulsatile tinnitus, sensitivity to loud sounds and pressure. Patients with symptoms of imbalance, headache and brain fog are less likely to be responsive to surgical intervention. Although there are no reported medical management options for SCDS, conservative measures with anecdotal benefits including extensive counseling on expectations, medications, trigger avoidance, and vestibular rehabilitation should be trialed first [28–30]. See Chaps. 13, 14, and 16 for discussions of nonsurgical management.

In modern medical care, increasing importance has been placed on patient-centered care, with the practice of shared decision-making as one of its core tenets. The goal of shared decision-making is to maximize patient autonomy. Informed consent entails a complete, honest discussion of the risks of a procedure as well as realistic expectations of the derived benefits. The surgeon's role thus involves providing the patient with complete information that allows him or her to make a decision that aligns with his or her individual goals and values. The result is a treatment plan that is both reasonable and best fits the values of the patient [31]. In the unique case of SCDS in the only hearing ear, the choice to operate must be weighed between not intervening surgically and the low but serious risk of profound hearing loss. Each individual upholds different values that will influence the decision to undergo surgery, and these values must be used as the primary foundation for any treatment plan.

Hearing Rehabilitation in Superior Canal Dehiscence Syndrome

Hearing loss, a major cause of disability globally, has been associated with social isolation, decreased quality of life, and dementia [32–35]. In patients with an only hearing ear, these consequences can be heightened and have even more detrimental impact. Treatment of those with SCDS and an only hearing ear begins with the standard application of hearing aids for amplification in addition to other conservative measures (e.g., trigger avoidance, vestibular rehabilitation, medications) [36]. However, for patients with moderate-to-profound hearing loss who receive limited or no benefit from their hearing aids, cochlear implants (CI) can help restore hearing and lead to improvements in speech perception, quality of life, and cognitive abilities [37–40]. The use of hearing aids may be limited by the individual patient's Tullio response, preventing successful amplification in a significant portion of this patient population.

Specifically, in the SCDS population, few studies have investigated outcomes among CI users. Puram et al. reported a 7% prevalence of SCD among CI patients and significantly worse postoperative speech recognition abilities among SCD patients compared to non-SCD CI recipients [41]. Nevertheless, postoperative speech recognition performance improved significantly compared to preoperative scores for both groups. Subjective rates of dizziness were similar between the SCD and non-SCD groups. The one patient with SCDS in this cohort experienced substantial improvements in both audiologic and vestibular performances after implantation, suggesting the possibility that CI in symptomatic SCD can help ameliorate vestibular symptoms in addition to rehabilitating hearing.

In a more recent study, Matic et al. found comparable speech recognition outcomes between CI recipients with and without SCD [42]. Rates of hearing preservation as well as progress of speech scores in the first 12 months were not significantly affected by whether patients had SCD on imaging. The difference in postoperative scores in Puram et al. can be attributed to their SCD cohort having a significantly longer duration of deafness, a well-known factor that influences CI outcomes, compared to the non-SCD group [43]. On the other hand, duration of deafness was similar between both groups in the Matic et al. study.

When counseling patients with SCD regarding hearing rehabilitation, cochlear implantation thus remains an effective method to improve hearing and even possibly vestibular symptoms. Further studies need to be undertaken with larger cohorts of patients with SCDS as both aforementioned reports primarily report on asymptomatic SCD [41, 42]. In addition, patients with SCDS who forego operative repair appear to have no changes in their autophony, dizziness and hearing over a follow-up period of nearly two years [44]. The natural progression of SCDS needs to be better assessed to help counsel patients on treatment options including CI and operative repair.

Conclusions

Surgical treatment of SCDS can be safe and effective. The risk of profound hearing loss in the operated ear is low but, in patients with contralateral ear deafness, may be devastating. Surgery should be offered to patients with significant audiovestibular symptoms and a diagnosis of SCDS according to the standard of care that would be presented to a patient without contralateral hearing loss. Appropriate counseling should include a focus on realistic expectations of improvement in symptoms and the risk of worsened or complete hearing loss. The discussion should be centered around the patient's individual values and cultivate a shared decision-making process between the patient and the surgeon, upholding the principles of patient-centered care. Ultimately, if the decision is made to operate on the only hearing ear, it is important that special care be taken and that the procedure should be performed by an experienced surgeon, preferably at a high-volume center. Cochlear implantation remains an effective and viable option for hearing restoration in patients with SCDS.

References

1. Althaus SR. Surgery on the only hearing ear. Laryngoscope. 1981;91(5):765–70. https://doi.org/10.1288/00005537-198105000-00009.
2. Chandler JR, Freeman J. Otologic surgery in patients with one hearing ear only. Laryngoscope. 1972;82(5):848–63. https://doi.org/10.1288/00005537-197205000-00012.
3. Mohr PE, Feldman JJ, Dunbar JL, McConkey-Robbins A, Niparko JK, Rittenhouse RK, et al. The societal costs of severe to profound hearing loss in the United States. Int J Technol Assess Health Care. 2000;16(4):1120–35. https://doi.org/10.1017/s0266462300103162.
4. Minor LB, Solomon D, Zinreich JS, Zee DS. Sound- and/or pressure-induced vertigo due to bone dehiscence of the superior semicircular canal. Arch Otolaryngol Head Neck Surg. 1998;124(3):249–58. https://doi.org/10.1001/archotol.124.3.249.
5. Minor LB, Carey JP, Cremer PD, Lustig LR, Streubel SO, Ruckenstein MJ. Dehiscence of bone overlying the superior canal as a cause of apparent conductive hearing loss. Otol Neurotol. 2003;24(2):270–8. https://doi.org/10.1097/00129492-200303000-00023.
6. Merchant SN, Rosowski JJ, McKenna MJ. Superior semicircular canal dehiscence mimicking otosclerotic hearing loss. Adv Otorhinolaryngol. 2007;65:137–45. https://doi.org/10.1159/000098790.
7. McEvoy TP, Mikulec AA, Armbrecht ES, Lowe ME. Quantification of hearing loss associated with superior semi-circular canal dehiscence. Am J Otolaryngol. 2013;34(4):345–9. https://doi.org/10.1016/j.amjoto.2013.01.009.
8. Naert L, Van de Berg R, Van de Heyning P, Bisdorff A, Sharon JD, Ward BK, et al. Aggregating the symptoms of superior semicircular canal dehiscence syndrome. Laryngoscope. 2018;128(8):1932–8. https://doi.org/10.1002/lary.27062.
9. Rosowski JJ, Songer JE, Nakajima HH, Brinsko KM, Merchant SN. Clinical, experimental, and theoretical investigations of the effect of superior semicircular canal dehiscence on hearing mechanisms. Otol Neurotol. 2004;25(3):323–32. https://doi.org/10.1097/00129492-200405000-00021.
10. Patel NS, Hunter JB, O'Connell BP, Bertrand NM, Wanna GB, Carlson ML. Risk of progressive hearing loss in untreated superior semicircular canal dehiscence. Laryngoscope. 2017;127(5):1181–6. https://doi.org/10.1002/lary.26322.
11. Kim N, Steele CR, Puria S. Superior-semicircular-canal dehiscence: effects of location, shape, and size on sound conduction. Hear Res. 2013;301:72–84. https://doi.org/10.1016/j.heares.2013.03.008.
12. Niesten ME, Stieger C, Lee DJ, Merchant JP, Grolman W, Rosowski JJ, et al. Assessment of the effects of superior canal dehiscence location and size on intracochlear sound pressures. Audiol Neurootol. 2015;20(1):62–71. https://doi.org/10.1159/000366512.
13. Castellucci A, Piras G, Del Vecchio V, Crocetta FM, Maiolo V, Ferri GG, et al. The effect of superior canal dehiscence size and location on audiometric measurements, vestibular-evoked myogenic potentials and video-head impulse testing. Eur Arch Otorhinolaryngol. 2021;278(4):997–1015. https://doi.org/10.1007/s00405-020-06169-3.
14. Zhu RT, Van Rompaey V, Ward BK, Van de Berg R, Van de Heyning P, Sharon JD. The interrelations between different causes of dizziness: a conceptual framework for understanding vestibular disorders. Ann Otol Rhinol Laryngol. 2019;128(9):869–78. https://doi.org/10.1177/0003489419845014.
15. Minor LB. Clinical manifestations of superior semicircular canal dehiscence. Laryngoscope. 2005;115(10):1717–27. https://doi.org/10.1097/01.mlg.0000178324.55729.b7.
16. Limb CJ, Carey JP, Srireddy S, Minor LB. Auditory function in patients with surgically treated superior semicircular canal dehiscence. Otol Neurotol. 2006;27(7):969–80. https://doi.org/10.1097/01.mao.0000235376.70492.8e.
17. Ward BK, Agrawal Y, Nguyen E, Della Santina CC, Limb CJ, Francis HW, et al. Hearing outcomes after surgical plugging of the superior semicircular canal by a middle cranial fossa approach. Otol Neurotol. 2012;33(8):1386–91. https://doi.org/10.1097/MAO.0b013e318268d20d.

18. Ziylan F, Kinaci A, Beynon AJ, Kunst HP. A comparison of surgical treatments for superior semicircular canal dehiscence: a systematic review. Otol Neurotol. 2017;38(1):1–10. https://doi.org/10.1097/mao.0000000000001277.
19. Schwartz SR, Almosnino G, Noonan KY, Banakis Hartl RM, Zeitler DM, Saunders JE, et al. Comparison of transmastoid and middle fossa approaches for superior canal dehiscence repair: a multi-institutional study. Otolaryngol Head Neck Surg. 2019;161(1):130–6. https://doi.org/10.1177/0194599819835173.
20. Johanis M, Yang I, Gopen Q. Incidence of intraoperative hearing loss during middle cranial fossa approach for repair of superior semicircular canal dehiscence. J Clin Neurosci. 2018;54:109–12. https://doi.org/10.1016/j.jocn.2018.06.023.
21. Brantberg K, Bergenius J, Mendel L, Witt H, Tribukait A, Ygge J. Symptoms, findings and treatment in patients with dehiscence of the superior semicircular canal. Acta Otolaryngol. 2001;121(1):68–75. https://doi.org/10.1080/000164801300006308.
22. Gioacchini FM, Alicandri-Ciufelli M, Kaleci S, Scarpa A, Cassandro E, Re M. Outcomes and complications in superior semicircular canal dehiscence surgery: a systematic review. Laryngoscope. 2016;126(5):1218–24. https://doi.org/10.1002/lary.25662.
23. Lin KF, Bojrab DI 2nd, Fritz CG, Vandieren A, Babu SC. Hearing outcomes after surgical manipulation of the membranous labyrinth during superior semicircular canal dehiscence plugging or posterior semicircular canal occlusion. Otol Neurotol. 2021;42(6):806–14. https://doi.org/10.1097/mao.0000000000003100.
24. Ellsperman SE, Telian SA, Kileny PR, Welch CM. Auditory outcomes following transmastoid and middle cranial fossa approaches for superior semicircular canal dehiscence repair. Otol Neurotol. 2021;42(10):1544–52. https://doi.org/10.1097/mao.0000000000003323.
25. Succar EF, Manickam PV, Wing S, Walter J, Greene JS, Azeredo WJ. Round window plugging in the treatment of superior semicircular canal dehiscence. Laryngoscope. 2018;128(6):1445–52. https://doi.org/10.1002/lary.26899.
26. Driscoll CL, Jackler RK, Pitts LH, Brackmann DE. Lesions of the internal auditory canal and cerebellopontine angle in an only hearing ear: is surgery ever advisable? Am J Otol. 2000;21(4):573–81. http://ovidsp.ovid.com/ovidweb.cgi?T=JS&PAGE=reference&D=ovftd&NEWS=N&AN=00000455-200007000-00019. Accessed 24 Apr 2022.
27. Sanna M, Shea CM, Gamoletti R, Russo A. Surgery of the 'only hearing ear' with chronic ear disease. J Laryngol Otol. 1992;106(9):793–8. https://doi.org/10.1017/s0022215100120900.
28. Alkhafaji MS, Varma S, Pross SE, Sharon JD, Nellis JC, Santina CCD, et al. Long-term patient-reported outcomes after surgery for superior canal dehiscence syndrome. Otol Neurotol. 2017;38(9):1319–26. https://doi.org/10.1097/mao.0000000000001550.
29. Chung LK, Ung N, Spasic M, Nagasawa DT, Pelargos PE, Thill K, et al. Clinical outcomes of middle fossa craniotomy for superior semicircular canal dehiscence repair. J Neurosurg. 2016;125(5):1187–93. https://doi.org/10.3171/2015.8.jns15391.
30. Jung DH, Lookabaugh SA, Owoc MS, McKenna MJ, Lee DJ. Dizziness is more prevalent than autophony among patients who have undergone repair of superior canal dehiscence. Otol Neurotol. 2015;36(1):126–32. https://doi.org/10.1097/mao.0000000000000531.
31. Beers E, Lee Nilsen M, Johnson JT. The role of patients: shared decision-making. Otolaryngol Clin North Am. 2017;50(4):689–708. https://doi.org/10.1016/j.otc.2017.03.006.
32. Cunningham LL, Tucci DL. Hearing loss in adults. N Engl J Med. 2017;377(25):2465–73. https://doi.org/10.1056/NEJMra1616601.
33. Bainbridge KE, Wallhagen MI. Hearing loss in an aging American population: extent, impact, and management. Annu Rev Public Health. 2014;35:139–52. https://doi.org/10.1146/annurev-publhealth-032013-182510.
34. Dalton DS, Cruickshanks KJ, Klein BE, Klein R, Wiley TL, Nondahl DM. The impact of hearing loss on quality of life in older adults. Gerontologist. 2003;43(5):661–8. https://doi.org/10.1093/geront/43.5.661.

35. Livingston G, Huntley J, Sommerlad A, Ames D, Ballard C, Banerjee S, et al. Dementia prevention, intervention, and care: 2020 report of the lancet commission. Lancet. 2020;396(10248):413–46. https://doi.org/10.1016/S0140-6736(20)30367-6.
36. Cozart AC, Kennedy JT 3rd, Seidman MD. A basis for standardizing superior semicircular canal dehiscence management. Ear Nose Throat J. 2021;100(10):NP444–53. https://doi.org/10.1177/0145561320927941.
37. Wilson BS, Dorman MF. Cochlear implants: a remarkable past and a brilliant future. Hear Res. 2008;242(1–2):3–21. https://doi.org/10.1016/j.heares.2008.06.005.
38. Tang L, Thompson CB, Clark JH, Ceh KM, Yeagle JD, Francis HW. Rehabilitation and psychosocial determinants of Cochlear implant outcomes in older adults. Ear Hear. 2017;38(6):663–71. https://doi.org/10.1097/AUD.0000000000000445.
39. Gaylor JM, Raman G, Chung M, Lee J, Rao M, Lau J, et al. Cochlear implantation in adults: a systematic review and meta-analysis. JAMA Otolaryngol Head Neck Surg. 2013;139(3):265–72. https://doi.org/10.1001/jamaoto.2013.1744.
40. Mosnier I, Bebear JP, Marx M, Fraysse B, Truy E, Lina-Granade G, et al. Improvement of cognitive function after cochlear implantation in elderly patients. JAMA Otolaryngol Head Neck Surg. 2015;141(5):442–50. https://doi.org/10.1001/jamaoto.2015.129.
41. Puram SV, Roberts DS, Niesten ME, Dilger AE, Lee DJ. Cochlear implant outcomes in patients with superior canal dehiscence. Cochlear Implants Int. 2015;16(4):213–21. https://doi.org/10.1179/1754762813Y.0000000044.
42. Matic J, Winklhofer S, Pfiffner F, Roosli C, Veraguth D, Huber A, et al. Influence of semicircular canal dehiscence on Cochlear implant outcome. Audiol Neurootol. 2021;26(3):135–9. https://doi.org/10.1159/000508892.
43. Bernhard N, Gauger U, Romo Ventura E, Uecker FC, Olze H, Knopke S, et al. Duration of deafness impacts auditory performance after cochlear implantation: a meta-analysis. Laryngosc Investig Otolaryngol. 2021;6(2):291–301. https://doi.org/10.1002/lio2.528.
44. Remenschneider AK, Owoc M, Kozin ED, McKenna MJ, Lee DJ, Jung DH. Health utility improves after surgery for superior canal dehiscence syndrome. Otol Neurotol. 2015;36(10):1695–701. https://doi.org/10.1097/MAO.0000000000000886.

Chapter 22
The Pediatric Patient

Gustavo A. Marino and Michael D. Seidman

Semicircular Canal Dehiscence Presenting as a Third Mobile Window Syndrome in the Pediatric Population

A Basis for a Congenital Etiology of Superior Semicircular Canal Dehiscence

The etiology of superior semicircular canal dehiscence (SSCD) in the population is a highly contested subject. Currently, there are two widely accepted theories for the prevalence of SSCD: congenital and acquired. The presence of SSCD in young children supports a congenital cause. Radiographic imaging has shown that superior semicircular canal (sSCC) bone thickness continues to increase between the ages of 2 and 8 years [1]. In a large multicenter review of temporal bone CT images, mean sSCC bone thickness for <2 years was found to be 0.89 ± 0.52 mm, 2 to 8 years was 1.13 ± 0.69 mm, and 3 to 18 years was 1.14 ± 0.82 mm [2]. Similarly, Nadgir's study analyzed 306 CT images and found no significant difference between the sSCC thickness among various age groups, which supports the theory that a plateau in thickness is reached in childhood [3]. This would indicate that the occurrence of a dehiscence is not chronic or gradual, but rather a condition either present from birth, which can remain asymptomatic until adulthood, or acutely acquired later in life.

G. A. Marino
College of Medicine, University of Central Florida (UCF), Orlando, FL, USA

M. D. Seidman (✉)
Otolaryngology Head and Neck Surgery, University of Central Florida, Orlando, FL, USA

Otolaryngology Head and Neck Surgery, University of South Florida, Tampa, FL, USA
e-mail: seidman.md@adventhealth.com

G. J. Gianoli, P. Thomson (eds.), *Third Mobile Window Syndrome of the Inner Ear*, https://doi.org/10.1007/978-3-031-16586-3_22

A large temporal bone study from John Hopkins showed that dehiscence of the sSCC did not have signs of bony remodeling, suggesting that the bone had not changed throughout the individual's life [2]. Furthermore, many studies have shown that the prevalence of superior semicircular canal dehiscence is highest in infants—up to 36.7%—but decreases sharply in early childhood [4]. This provides evidence for a congenital process if the etiology is a failure of bony overgrowth within the first few years of life. In an archival temporal bone study evaluating the incidence and etiology of SSCDs, evidence showed that the thin, inner periosteal layer of bone overlying the superior canal at its protrusion into the middle fossa is not fully covered until as late as ten months of age. Additionally, a similar pattern of dehiscence at the middle fossa was identified in nine adult specimens which may suggest that postnatal failure to develop outer and/or middle layer of bone over the superior canal may be the cause of adult SSCD and third window syndrome. Because the ossification pattern is similar in infants and adults, it indicates that the process that originally brought on the dehiscence likely remained stable for many years [5].

Radiologic studies have also demonstrated that when SCCD is found on one side, the contralateral side is more frequently found to be thin or completely dehiscent, suggesting a developmental etiology. Lagman et al. demonstrated a right-sided predilection (38%) for SSCD (vs. the left 31%, and bilateral SSCD 21%), which is opposite to that more commonly reported in adults, but an association with contralateral thinning or dehiscence was also observed. In larger meta-analyses of SSCD, the incidence of bilaterally identified SSCD ranges between 17 and 37% [6, 7]. One study showed that although no SSCD cases were bilateral, a large proportion displayed "thinning" or "possible dehiscence" on the contralateral side [8]. Due to the prevalence of bilateral thinning, research into etiologies to explain this phenomenon has used computer models to suggest that dystopia of primitive otocysts and migration changes of mesenchymal cells during the formation of the apical cap of the sSCC may contribute to the disease process. A "second hit" such as trauma, infection, inflammation or chronic pressure from the overlying temporal bone or CSF pulsations may then incite or exacerbate the symptoms [9].

Niesten et al. performed a retrospective case report looking at the genetic disposition between patients with SSCD and their first-degree relatives. They noted that first-degree relatives present with similar symptoms; two brothers experienced only conductive hearing loss, whereas two mother-daughter pairs experienced similar hearing deficits, autophony, aural fullness, and pressure- and sound-induced dizziness. CT imaging also showed comparable skull base topography and anatomic abnormalities. Interestingly, all three families developed symptoms in adulthood, and mothers had more severe symptoms than their daughters. Notably, the mother of one family has an established diagnosis of Chiari malformation type-1 (CM-1) [10]. The pathogenesis of CM-1 is believed to come from neuroectodermal developmental abnormalities and overcrowding of the hindbrain which reduces the cerebrospinal fluid space around the cervicomedullary junction and causes amplified fluid pressure waves that can have erosive effects on the surrounding bone. The prevalence of CM-1 is greatly increased in patients with SSCD as opposed to the general population, 23% vs. 0.6% to 1%, respectively. This slow, erosive etiology may affect pre-existing developmental bony abnormalities, thus leading to the development of SSCD concurrently in those with CM-1. Additional genetic and cohort studies are required to confirm the genetic contributions to this pathological process. While the brain does not directly touch the floor of the middle fossa, and intracranial pressures are normally divided evenly throughout the cerebrospinal fluid, structural changes seen in genetic syndromes and outflow obstructions like in CM-1 may better explain the erosive effects of CSF pulsations.

Though very limited research exists on gene mutations that may predispose to SSCD, Hildebrand et al. discuss the potential association between the cochlin (COCH) gene mutation in a patient with SSCD with familial hearing loss. COCH is the most apparent protein in the inner ear and has been associated in playing a role in structural integrity and antimicrobial activity. Individuals with autosomal dominant nonsyndromic hearing loss (ADSNHL), accounting for 15% of congenital hearing loss cases, have been attributed to the COCH gene mutations. Furthermore, they also suggested patients with DFNA9 (a locus within the COCH gene) mutations, which uncharacteristically present with both progressive hearing loss and vestibular deficits, may have underlying SSCD, which would also support a congenital etiology in these cases [11]. Since both the DFNA9-related deafness and SSCD are rare, their occurrence in one patient in their study may suggest a genetic risk factor for developing SSCD. Individuals with these mutations should be recommended for high-resolution temporal bone CT to look for an associated SSCD.

Though SSCD may be present from birth and become an evolving process due to factors like trauma, increased intracranial pressure, and congenital structural or developmental abnormalities, it is important to understand that third mobile window syndrome (TMWS) can only be established following development of clinically relevant symptomology. As aforementioned, studies have shown that bone dehiscence may exist more commonly in the pediatric population, and even may resolve on its own over time. However, the presence of dehiscence alone cannot suffice to diagnose TMWS. There are currently no established guidelines dictating how many relevant symptoms a patient must have to fit the criteria. In this section, SSCD with a TMWS will be referred to as semicircular canal dehiscence syndrome (SCDS)—understood as the presence of a pathological third window on imaging or conduction study with the presence of at least one audiologic or vestibular symptom.

Diagnosing TMWS in a Pediatric Patient with Semicircular Canal Dehiscence

The diagnostic criteria for SCDS include radiologic evidence of dehiscent bone, while third window syndrome requires correlates with clinical symptoms and physiological tests that suggest an abnormality. The most common presenting symptoms necessitating a high-resolution CT image of the temporal bones include otitis media with effusion, hearing loss, temporal bone fracture, cholesteatoma, and other less common symptoms like tinnitus, otalgia, ataxia, a visible mass or a combination of more than one of the aforementioned symptoms [2]. In a systematic review of pediatric SCDS, the most common auditory symptoms included hearing loss, hyperacusis, tinnitus, and autophony. A case series from a children's vestibular center showed that 80% of children with radiologic evidence of SCDS demonstrated mixed or conductive hearing loss, which can be explained by the third window phenomenon [12]. Auditory signs were four times more likely to be the presenting symptom compared to vestibular signs. In adults, the opposite is true, since they most commonly present with vestibular symptoms like noise-induced vertigo or Tullio phenomenon [13]. Vertigo, dizziness, and disequilibrium, and delayed onset of walking and other motor functions were the most reported vestibular symptoms in children [14]. However, dehiscence can also be asymptomatic. Therefore, the actual prevalence and diagnosis of SCDS may not be fully realized. Diagnostic tools to test for mixed or conductive hearing loss include audiometry and tuning fork tests.

Audiological and vestibular symptoms following head injury should also be assessed in the pediatric population. Concussion, or mild traumatic brain injury, related to sports injuries are among the most common type of injury presenting with auditory and vestibular symptoms annually. Many studies have shown that recovery from concussion is both different and prolonged in the pediatric population compared to the adult population. Ommaya et al. suggest that major traumatic brain injury may more commonly result from linear acceleration injuries whereas concussion may result more often from angular head acceleration [15]. Zhou et al. studied patients with a history of concussion and noted that less than 20% had test abnormalities indicative of otolith dysfunction (abnormal VEMP testing and SVV tilt), which are more sensitive to linear acceleration whereas those with a history of major brain injury report much higher incidence [16]. Therefore, it should be considered that concussions in the pediatric population may preferentially affect the semicircular canals sensitive to angular acceleration.

Epidemiological Considerations in SSCD

Lagman et al. reported a 1.65:1 male to female ratio in a systematic review of pediatric SCDS cases. This was in contrast to case reviews in the adult population that show roughly a 1.23:1 female predominance of SCDS. While no exact explanation has been investigated, they proposed that the gender differences are associated with temporal differences in growth and sex hormones. Because skeletal bone development is reliant on thyroid hormones, growth hormone, and insulin-like growth factor 1, it may be significant that growth velocity is slower in males than in females until the age of four. Afterward, the pubertal peak is denoted by a significant increase in IGF-1, which correlates with a spike in the rate of bone growth and height increase, especially in males. In females, estrogen plays a bigger role in bone development. It interacts with GH and IGF-1 to regulate bone catabolism and may add to the reason why female prevalence is more common. Likewise, in older females who suffer from estrogen deficiency or osteopenia/osteoporosis, more bone resorption is seen [14]. Crovetto et al. actually found a decrease in bone thickness overlying the SSC in patients younger than 45 years, compared to those who were older than 45 years of age - 1.14 mm vs. 1.02 mm average thickness, respectively [17].

Neurodevelopmental disorders tend to be the most common similarity across past medical histories in those with reported SSCD, particularly those with autism, cerebral palsy, and Down syndrome. Ear anomalies such as a history of cholesteatoma, recurrent ear infections, and structural abnormalities are also common. A general otologic history is more common than neurodevelopmental history when ear anomalies, ear infections, enlarged vestibular aqueduct, and Ménière's disease are grouped together. Any genetic, neurodevelopmental, or craniofacial abnormality presenting with audiological or vestibular symptoms should be concerning for a third mobile window syndrome [14].

Management

Conservative treatment with the avoidance of provocative stimuli and vestibular rehabilitation is the most encouraged form of symptom management in the pediatric population. In the literature, an overwhelming majority of children with SCDS are not treated surgically, especially since many believe that early onset SSCD is a natural process and symptoms will resolve with more conservative treatment. However, with a lack of case series following pediatric patients with SCDS throughout their life, the success of conservative treatment cannot be adequately assessed. In children who present with hearing loss, the most common form of treatment is the use of a hearing aid. Many children with SCDS fail this therapy due to hyperacusis and Tullio phenomenon. Failure for these reasons may prompt a physician to consider imaging and vestibular testing for a third window syndrome.

For those with predominantly vestibular symptoms, individualized vestibular rehabilitation, including visual stability exercises, has been effective in treating dizziness and imbalance complaints. Operative intervention is often left for children with progressive or intractable vestibular symptoms. Though not commonly implemented according to the literature, surgical options remain the same as in adults—canal plugging and canal roof resurfacing via a middle cranial fossa or transmastoid approach, or round window reinforcement [9, 13, 18]. However, factors such as hearing status, patients' choice, physician comfort and hospital preference can often limit the surgical options available. Lee et al. describe a case of an 11-year-old girl with progressive hearing loss and disequilibrium, pulsatile tinnitus, aural fullness and autophony, later found to have right SSCD with possible left dehiscence on CT. VEMP thresholds were only abnormal on the right. After years of failed attempts at conservative management and using hearing aids, she underwent right SSCD repair via a middle cranial fossa craniotomy. Even as soon as her first preoperative visit, she reported decreased episodes of vertigo and essentially resolved tinnitus and autophony on the right side. Results were confirmed with VEMP conduction studies. Unfortunately, left-sided hearing loss continued to progress [18]. Mignacco et al. reported a new therapy for management of patients with SCDS by using a Vibrant Soundbridge middle ear implant to provide round window reinforcement. The outcomes showed improvement in hearing thresholds and reduction in Tullio phenomenon at the one- and three-month postoperative marks [19]. Sufficient comparative data does not exist between surgical outcomes of pediatric versus adult SSCD repair.

Challenges to Diagnosing SSCD in Children

Children are not able to identify or describe their symptoms in the same way as adults, often precipitating a delay in identification of signs of SCDS. They may also not know that their perceived auditory and vestibular disturbances are pathologic. For example, the hyperacusis they perceive may be seen as a normal process which requires physiological adaptation by avoiding certain triggers and therefore is not reported. Similarly, without any presenting symptoms, the need for a high-resolution CT scan cannot always be justified. When children present with symptoms, they are also typically not the same third window symptoms experienced by adults—such as Tullio phenomenon, Hennebert phenomenon, and conductive dysacusis—that may lead physicians to consider SCDS. Since the identification of SSCD in 1998, the existence of these pathological processes has been questioned. The literature supports these claims, as third window disorders in children may occur without third window syndromic features which are determined by defined symptoms and objective signs normally designed and tested in adult cohorts. A number of factors, like a co-existing cochlear or vestibular dysfunction, may account for these variances. A difference in endolymphatic fluid dynamics in children has also been proposed as a possible explanation [20].

Diagnostic criteria and testing for SCDS have been applied extensively in the adult population, but the application of these same measures to diagnosis in children has rarely been studied. For example, vestibular evoked myogenic potentials (VEMPs) have been found to be 90% sensitive and specific for identifying SSCD by demonstrating a decrease in the impedance of the vestibular system, resulting in lower thresholds and higher amplitudes in the VEMPs [21]. However, the use of VEMPS to assess SSCD in children has not been extensively studied. Kelsch et al. were one of the first to study the feasibility of VEMP testing in children. In a study of 30 children with good hearing established with audiogram, divided into four age groups from 3 to 11 years of age, they were able to successfully record bilateral latencies, amplitudes, compliance, and reflexes to establish a baseline. They demonstrated that VEMP testing is a well-tolerated, reproducible test in children and can be referenced to describe expected latencies and optimal testing parameters in children, and helped to establish the 90-dB normal hearing level baseline used to compare for abnormal responses [22]. With limited research on the topic and a wide range of symptoms that can mimic other diseases, clinical suspicion for SCDS is rare in the diagnosis of pediatric patient with hearing loss. As research into SCDS grows, placement of this disease within the differential diagnosis of clinicians should become more commonplace.

There are also no standard radiologic criteria for identifying dehiscence. Judging as to what is a thinning can be extremely subjective, and there is no agreement or guidelines as to what physical dimensions should be defined as thinning. For example, three different studies, all looking at SSCD, reported different criteria for thinning. Ward established thinning as a thin strip of bone in their study with adults [6]. However, Kaur and Meicklejohn have both shown that actual SCC bone thickness ranges from 0.4 to 2.08 mm with an average of about 1.5 mm. Saxby commented that thinning can be developmental but can lead to a dehiscence in the future [1, 8, 23]. Based on these studies, we suggest that a semicircular canal wall thickness at or below 0.5 mm should be considered as thinning [20].

Because bony capsules in this area in children may be less than 0.1 mm thick, many studies have suggested using the highest resolution CT with cuts smaller than 0.65 mm to better identify instances of SSCD. However, studies continue to report data that use CT slices up to 1 mm in size which can incorrectly rule out SSCD, likely due to old habits, no formal change in protocol broadcasted to providers, and reimbursement remains the same for the radiologist performing the exam, so there has been little effort or motivation to change the standard. Additionally, there is no guideline for establishing a radiologic diagnosis of dehiscence. In 2015, Saxby et al. used a specific classification system where dehiscence was only established if two consecutive images in the perpendicular plane plus at least one image in the corresponding parallel plane (Stenvers and Poschl planes) demonstrated dehiscence. They also identified other pediatric studies, up to that time, and their diagnostic criteria for establishing dehiscence. They found that only five studies used submillimeter imaging, and of those, only two (including their own) used slices in different planes and had at least 100 patients [8]. This lack of standard criteria may account for the large variation in prevalence of SSCD and SCDS in the pediatric population. A standard diagnostic algorithm (Fig. 22.1) should be used as an evaluation scheme to guide the clinician through a potential diagnosis of SCDS [24].

Proposed Standard Diagnostic Criteria

Whether children present with hearing problems or with episodes of dizziness, a detailed history of these events needs to be gathered either from the parents or from the patient themselves. If there are hearing issues, a history of trauma, past infections, or birth defects should be established. If vertigo predominates, considerations like triggering factors, duration of symptoms, and whether the vertigo can be induced should be noted. If answers to these questions cannot be verbalized, it is important to suggest keeping a diary of vertigo for at least two weeks to help the clinician understand the pathological process. Finally, a detailed birth history, family history, and milestone achievement should be documented in order to understand

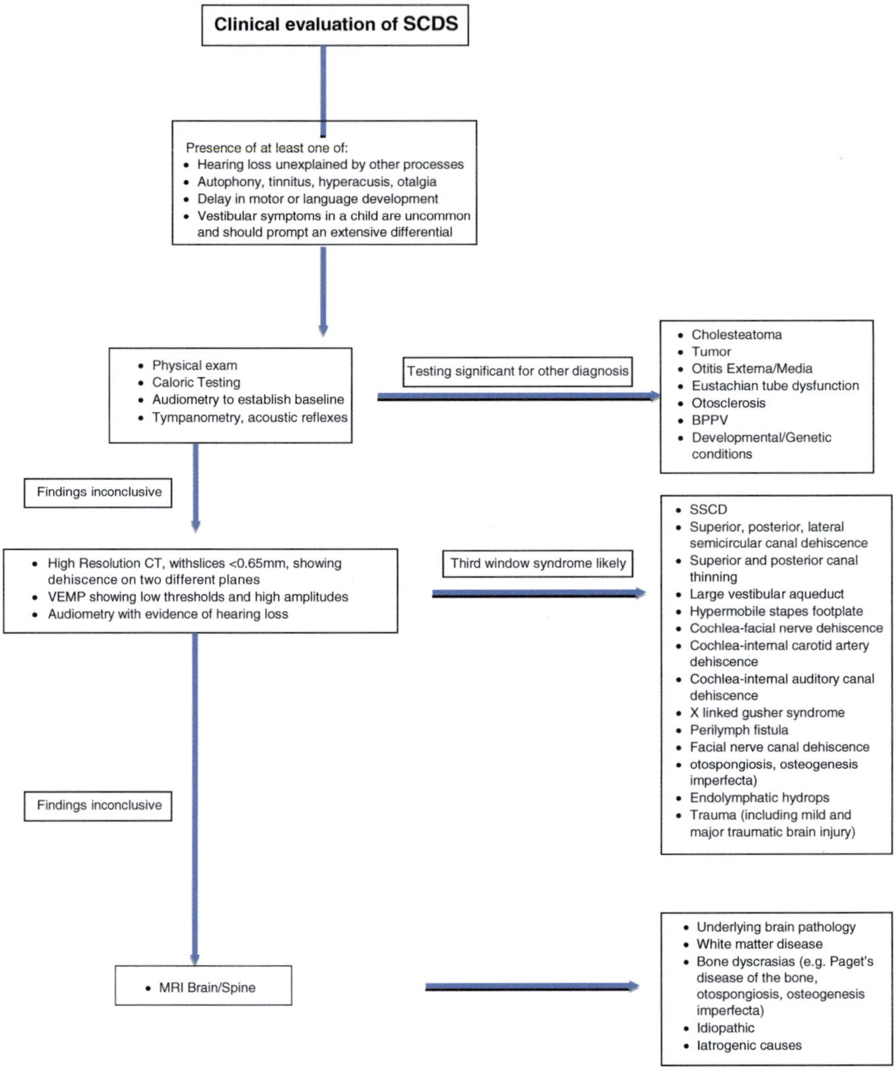

Fig. 22.1 Diagnostic outline for SCDS

motor or language development features that may interact with the current disease process.

An age-appropriate pediatric audiological diagnostic test should be conducted in order to establish a baseline and note any deficits. Weber and Rinne tests have been noted to be successful in children as early as five years of age. While many children do not present with Tullio or Hennebert phenomenon, they should still be tested. Wenzel et al. note a valsalva maneuver in which the examiner motivates the child to cover his/her nose and make a pressure compensation. His/her eyes should remain open as long as possible in order to assess his/her possible eye movements using Frenzel goggles [25].

We propose a standard set of radiological criteria for diagnosing SSCD based on sizing of the images captured and viewing these images in different planes. First, we suggest that the minimum slice be 0.65 mm in size, which has a higher sensitivity for detecting dehiscence as opposed to larger slices. Studies have looked at the CT findings at different collimation widths associated with SSCD and determine the frequency of these findings in a control population. Belden et al. found that in 18 cases where a 1.0 mm collimated CT judged possible or definitive dehiscence, the 0.5 mm collimated CT found overlying bone in all of the same cases. They reported that the positive predictive value of an apparent dehiscence in the diagnosis of SCCD went up from 50% with 1.0 mm slices with transverse and coronal images, to 93% with 0.5 mm slices with reformation in the plane of the SSC [26]. CT scanners, like the Philips MX 16 and Siemens Somatom Sensation 40 or Siemens Somatom Definition AS+, have been used in other studies that can provide images of this size. While CT scanners exist that can provide slices as small as 0.40 mm in size, they may contain unnecessary artifact, or improperly image the semicircular canals without a high enough resolution. Caution should be taken when using slices under 0.65 mm. If any images show an excess of artifact or do not properly image the vestibular organ, these should not be used as evidence for a diagnosis of SSCD. A new, promising technology is the flat panel computed tomography (FPCT). It is routinely used in angiographic studies and has the capability to create higher resolution reconstructions with smaller voxel sizes specifically targeting small organs like the semicircular canals. The voxel is a volume element defining a three-dimensional space, and by targeting a specific organ, slice collimations can be as thin as 0.07 to 0.1 mm. A study looking at the ability of FPCT to identify SCCD in comparison to multi-slice CT (both compared to intraoperative visualization of dehiscence) showed that FPCT was more accurate in detecting SCCD and more precise in predicting the size of the dehiscence than multi-slice CT [27]. Future studies should look to further assess the ability of FPCT to detect SCCD in all age groups, as thinner collimations may be better suited to identify SCCD in the pediatric population. The risks of false positives remain with even the best scans, so the diagnosis of SSCD should never be solely dependent on a CT scan alone.

Various views should be assessed when looking for SSCD. Images should be attained in the coronal and axial planes, and then should be reformatted to include the Poschl and Stenvers planes. Previous case studies have used the "Voxar 3D" or "iSite Philips Picture Archiving and Communication System" software in order to create these reconstructions. We recommend similar technology as the Poschl and Stenvers planes which provide the best views to detect SSCD. Once these four views have been taken, a clear dehiscence in at least more than one plane should be seen in order to provide the diagnosis of SCCD. No other cochlear and/or inner ear malformations, trauma, active infection, ossicular anomalies, and canal atresia should be present. Finally, the images should be read by an experienced neuroradiologist, radiologist, or neurotologist in order to have the highest likelihood of detection. Most published cases use two independent reviewers in order to confirm the diagnosis.

Based on a current review of the literature, these are the best identified tools to achieve an accurate diagnosis of SSCD (Tables 22.1 and 22.2) [8, 28].

Table 22.1 Vestibular exam for third window syndrome

Symptoms of pediatric vestibular disease	Vestibular assessment
1 Reaching out for objects to balance oneself	1 Full neurological examination
2 Delayed motor function and/or development	2 Musculoskeletal exam
3 Clumsiness	3 Oculomotor exam
4 Improper posture or unsteadiness	4 Videonystagmography
5 Abnormal eye movements	5 Video head impulse test
6 Specific triggers to vertigo or imbalance	6 Cervical vestibular evoked myogenic potential test
7 Difficulty walking in the dark	7 Vestibulo-spinal test battery with and without proprioception
8 Difficulty walking unsupported	8 Rotary chair and suppression of visual fixation test
9 Difficulty with running	9 Dix Hallpike, supine roll, and deep hand banging tests
10 Difficult with riding a bike or amusement park rides with complaints of imbalance	
11 Periodic nausea or vomiting	
12 Cyclic nausea or vomiting	
13 Migrainous features	
14 Falls	
15 Abnormal behavior observed by more than one person	
16 Difficulty in challenging movements (sports, dance)	
17 Oscillopsia	
18 Third window symptoms—conductive dysacusis (hearing one's own footsteps), gaze-evoked tinnitus (audible eye movements), autophony (altered perception of one's own voice), Tullio or Hennebert phenomenon, pulsatile tinnitus	
19 Difficulty in challenging visual environments like crowded stores or sports games	
20 Poor hand eye coordination	

Adapted from Dasgupta [20]

Table 22.2 Audiological exam looking for TMWS

Symptoms of pediatric audiological disease	Audiological assessment
1 Autophony 2 Conductive dysacusis 3 Tullio phenomenon 4 Difficulty in crowded environments 5 Hearing or feeling a low frequency tuning fork in an involved ear when applied to a patient's elbow or knee 6 Worsening grades in school 7 Appearance of being inattentive or ignoring a parent/teacher 8 Not responding to name 9 Not responding to commands 10 Not appearing to understand language 11 Motor/language developmental delay 12 Reported hearing loss 13 Tinnitus 14 Aural fullness 15 Sensitivity to loud noises 16 Memory problems	1 Pure tone audiometry with masking 2 Tympanometry 3 Acoustic reflexes 4 Otoscopy 5 Transient otoacoustic emissions 6 Full past medical history, family history 7 History of trauma 8 ECOG

Adapted from Dasgupta [20]

Enlarged Vestibular Aqueduct Syndrome Causing TMWS

Characteristic of Enlarged Vestibular Aqueduct Syndrome

The vestibular aqueduct (VA) is a bony canal in the posterior ridge of the petrous bone, running from the vestibule to the posterior cranial fossa. It holds the endolymphatic duct as it courses to the endolymphatic sac. Large vestibular aqueduct (LVA) syndrome is known to be the most common inner ear abnormality in children with permanent hearing loss. This phenomenon is believed to occur as a result of either impeded embryonic or postnatal development. Clinically, LVA can present with various types of hearing loss including conductive, sensorineural, or mixed. Although auditory symptoms in LVA have been well documented, less research has been done to identify common presenting vestibular symptoms [29]. Berrettini et al. reported vestibular symptoms in less than one-third of patients with MRI-confirmed LVA, though when vestibular function was tested, 13 of 15 patients had vestibular deficits [30]. Symptoms vary within a spectrum of severe episodic vertigo to intermittent unsteadiness in adults, whereas incoordination and imbalance predominate in children [31].

In most cases, LVAS exists as a nonfamilial disease process. However, there have been some cases supporting an autosomal recessive inheritance pattern within families [32–34]. A connection with genetic syndromes, like CHARGE and branchial-oto-renal, also suggest a hereditary component. The association of LVAS and Pendred's syndrome (PS), an autosomal recessive disease characterized by goiter, sensorineural deafness, and defective iodide organification, has garnered extensive research within the literature. PS is the most common form of syndromic SNHL, and the presence of widened endolymphatic duct and sac has been described as a constant feature of the PS inner ear. The pendrin gene (PDS) responsible for PS has been well mapped and is known to work as an iodide-chloride transporter expressed in thyrocytes of the distal nephron. Additionally, this transporter also exists in regions involved in the regulation of the endolymphatic fluid composition and may contribute to subsequent LVA development. There has also been a proposed link between LVAS and distal renal tubular acidosis (dRTA) in which a mutation in the ATP6B1 gene manifests as a dysfunction in a proton pump expressed in the inner ear and could theoretically lead to electrolyte and acid-case imbalance of inner ear fluids. More research on the exact mechanism leading to the development of LVA is ongoing. In a study of 17 patients affected with LVA, 10 had concurrent PS, three had concurrent dRTA, and three were nonsyndromic. Of those with PS, four did not express PDS mutations, but presented clinically indistinguishable to those with the mutations. This suggests that outside elements, like environment or other mutations, may also cause PS.

LVA is characterized on CT imaging studies as having a diameter greater than 1.5 mm at the midpoint of the aqueduct, between the aperture and common crus of the VA in the original paper by Valvasorri using planar tomography [35]. More recent studies have recommended using axial CT scan with criteria for enlarged vestibular aqueduct at 0.9 mm at the midpoint and 1.9 mm at the operculum [36]. However, MRI allows for visualization of the fluid-filled spaces of the inner ear, especially in the membranous labyrinth. 3D reconstructions often assist with visualization of the sac and other inner ear structures, so many authors consider MRI superior in LVA diagnosis.

Recent studies of children with LVAS have been conducted to assess the value of VEMP inner ear anomalies since there have been many previous documented cases of air-bone gaps in these cases, representing a conductive component. Zhou et al. did not find any obvious middle ear pathologies associated with these air-bone gaps. However, they did find abnormally low VEMP thresholds and/or higher VEMP amplitudes, corresponding with augmented VEMP responses, in the majority of LVA cases [37]. These findings correlate with those seen in third mobile window syndrome. LVA can manifest as a third mobile window where air-conducted sounds are deviated from the cochlea to the vestibule, which creates air-bone gaps and can make the semicircular canals and otolith organs more excitable and sensitive.

LVAS presents a challenge for clinicians to treat, and no protocol has been successful in stopping the progression of hearing loss. Typically, conservative measures are tried first, such as counseling patients on avoiding injuries to the head, fluctuations in barometric pressure such as altitude and diving, and immediate treatment with steroids during episodes of acute hearing loss. Previous attempts at endolymphatic sac surgery in patients with progressive sensorineural hearing loss were not efficacious [38]. LVAS treated with cochlear implantation has shown positive outcomes in terms of auditory and speech recognition performance [38, 39]. Other considerations include ensuring proper vaccination of the child against pneumococcal and influenza meningitis, since having an anomalous inner ear structure can predispose to meningitis. Additionally, some centers also prefer vaccination against Haemophilus influenza type b. Additional family screening for those with a family history of hearing loss should also be recommended, including a hearing test for siblings of those with confirmed LVA [30]. As a result of syndromic relationships, thyroid function and perchlorate discharge tests, and molecular evaluation for a PDS gene mutation should be considered.

Other Causes of Third Mobile Window Syndrome in Children

Stapes footplate abnormalities, whether congenital or acquired, can create a third mobile window. Gadre and Matsuda et al. studied 28 patients (33 ears), managed over an 11-year interval, who suffered from unretractable dizziness following head trauma and observed Tullio phenomena or Hennebert sign. Every patient had normal otic capsules confirmed on high-resolution temporal bone CT scans. However, the presence of an abnormal footplate was confirmed with direct visualization. To repair this pathological third window, fat grafting to reinforce the area was performed. None of the patients had worsened hearing immediately after surgery. Ultimately, 24 of the 28 patients (85.7%) demonstrated subjective and objective improvement in hearing and vestibular symptoms following surgery. Based on these findings, it was deduced that congenital or traumatic causes can manifest as a membranous or hypermobile stapes footplate which can cause intractable dizziness typical of third mobile window syndrome [40, 41].

A large retrospective study looking at rare causes of pediatric third window syndrome in a large cohort of 920 children evaluated for audiovestibular function. Of these children, only eight (<1%) had observed pathologic third windows. Three had posterior semicircular canal dehiscence (PSCD), two had posterior semicircular canal thinning (PSCT), two had X-linked gusher, and only one had a combination of dilated internal auditory meatus/irregular cochlear partition/deficient facial nerve canal. They were able to detect mixed/conductive hearing loss in 87.5% of patients, disequilibrium in 75%, and abnormal vestibular function tests in 33%. All had confirmed VEMPs with low thresholds and high amplitudes. Other reported etiologies of third mobile window syndrome have been documented but not well studied (Table 22.3). Despite the small sample size, this study helped to characterize rare variances in anatomy that may result in a third window syndrome.

Pediatric PSCD has hardly been reported in the literature, especially as a single inner ear abnormality. Only one case series has sought to investigate PSCD in children, and it consisted of three children presenting with unilateral PSCD. Dasgupta et al. identified three patients with PSCD who showed a variability in symptoms, whereas the two children with PSCT showed homogeneity in their VEMP results and audiovestibular symptoms. They were the first to document PSCT and a mixed structural abnormality as two new potential causes of a third window syndrome [20].

Table 22.3 Recognized Third Window disorders [30, 42, 43]

1.	Superior, posterior, lateral semicircular canal dehiscence
2.	Superior and posterior canal thinning
3.	Large vestibular aqueduct
4.	Hypermobile stapes footplate
5.	Cochlea-facial nerve dehiscence
6.	Cochlea-internal carotid artery dehiscence
7.	Cochlea-internal auditory canal dehiscence
8.	X-linked gusher syndrome
9.	Perilymph fistula
10.	Facial nerve canal dehiscence
11.	Otosclerosis with internal auditory canal involvement
12.	Bone dyscrasias (e.g., Paget's disease of the bone, otospongiosis, osteogenesis imperfecta)
13.	Endolymphatic hydrops
14.	Trauma (including mild and major traumatic brain injury)

Adapted from Dasgupta [20]

The third window in X-linked gusher is hypothesized to be a result of an anomalous link between the perilymphatic space and the subarachnoid space secondary to incomplete separation of basal turn of cochleas from the fundi of the internal auditory canal [44]. Since 1971, only 89 patients have been reported in the literature. A similar phenotype of progressive mixed hearing loss and a spectrum of vestibular symptoms is common in this population, along with a dilated inner auditory meatus.

Cochlea-facial nerve dehiscence (CFD) presents with the classic symptoms associated with third window syndrome. Wackym et al. conducted surgery for round window reinforcement technique on eight patients, five of which were children, and compared them to outcomes in eight patients with CFD who did not have surgery. All eight had a history of trauma before the onset of their symptoms. DHI, HIT-6, and symptomology were all used to assess for improvement. Surgical management was associated with improved symptoms and outcome measures in all eight patients [42].

Patients experiencing typical signs of TMWS with no otic capsule dehiscence should be treated based on their specific symptoms. If vestibular symptoms predominate, avoiding known triggers, reducing head trauma and bariatric pressure changes, maintaining a detailed account of vestibular symptoms, and undergoing vestibular therapy can often help to alleviate some of the debilitating symptoms of a third mobile window. In the case of auditory symptoms, regular audiograms should be performed to trend the disease progress. Hearing aids are a commonly helpful tool for those with TMWS as they can amplify sounds or reduce noise that may be triggering to some individuals. If hearing loss continues to progress, cochlear implants can be considered. Any episode of acute hearing loss should be treated with a course of corticosteroids as soon as possible and the child evaluated for other underlying causes.

Ongoing Research into Causes of Pediatric TMWS

While researchers are doing a better job at identifying signs and symptoms that may be indicative of a TMWS, more research needs to be done into the different causes and spectrum of presenting symptoms that may be associated with this process. Auditory symptoms seem to be better understood, as a child may present with delayed motor or speech development, ignore a parent when their name is called, or appear inattentive at school, but vestibular symptoms can be harder to verbalize for children. Better tools need to be investigated that may elicit vestibular symptoms on physical exam that may tee a clinician in on a possible TMWS. Studies have shown an excellent response in children when their symptoms are identified early and monitored carefully for disease progression or prepared for surgical treatment. In many who are left untreated, a progression to complete deafness may occur, so swift action is vital to quality of life. Similarly, patients treated with vestibular rehabilitation early have been reported to show better long-term outcomes with their vertigo-related limitations, as opposed to those who receive therapy later in life. A child's ability to adapt to vestibular dysfunction is stronger than that of an adult, but permanent equilibrium effects can result with persistent dysfunction.

There continues to be little guidance on criteria for the diagnosis of SCDS, and even less for other etiologies of TMWS. Extensive progress has been made in the management of SCDS due to the fervor of research surrounding the topic. As more attention is drawn to other etiologies, it is our hope that research will continue to advance on these topics.

It is also important to clarify that acute hearing loss is a medical emergency and should be evaluated in the local emergency department as quickly as possible from the onset of symptoms. Surgical management of SSCD or other forms of TMWS should be reserved for patients who exhibit debilitating clinical signs that have failed to resolve with conservative management. With the knowledge that individuals with the same confirmed disease process, like SCDS, can present with different symptoms, the role of environmental factors in the establishment and progression of the disease should be further investigated.

Conclusion

The prevalence of SSCD has been debated due to bony growth until the age of three, the inability of children to express their symptoms in the same way as adults, and the initial presentation of symptoms that differ from that of the adult population. High-resolution CT images with <0.65 mm slices in at least two planes are considered the gold standard for identification of bony dehiscence. Children more commonly present with auditory symptoms like hearing loss and hyperacusis and tinnitus, and less commonly with vestibular symptoms like vertigo. Management for patients with symptomatic SSCD should begin in a conservative manner, typically with surgery reserved for those with intractable vestibular symptoms. Future investigations should look to follow children with SSCD from a young age through adulthood to see how symptoms progress and which forms of treatment work to minimize symptoms in this population. There also exists a need for standardized diagnostic criteria (clinical, radiological, and using psychological testing) to correctly identify children with SSCD. Research into physiological testing, like that which exists for the adult population, can also help to identify affected children.

The prevalence of other disease processes that may result in a third window syndrome has increased as more research focuses on identifying these, and as technology continues to develop to allow us to see even the smallest defects in bone. Large vestibular aqueduct is the most common inner ear abnormality causing permanent hearing loss. While its diagnosis is better understood, treatment of this process and its correlation with other genetic factors still remains a mystery.

Other third window syndromes have been identified and clinicians should be taught to think about these etiologies when patients present with hearing and vestibular symptoms that do not commonly present in children. Similarities among all third window syndromes exist, including a predominance of audiological or vestibular system, structural abnormalities seen on imaging, and course of management. All acute hearing loss episodes should be evaluated immediately by a physician. Conservative management is emphasized in those who are asymptomatic or express mild, non-debilitating symptoms. Once symptoms significantly affect the patient's day to day life, surgical options exist that seek to reinforce the pathological third window, but these should only be considered in truly severe cases, as the progression of symptoms has not been shown to consistently improve with this treatment.

References

1. Meiklejohn DA, Corrales CE, Boldt BM, et al. Pediatric semicircular canal dehiscence: radiographic and histologic prevalence, with clinical correlation. Otol Neurotol. 2015;36(8):1383–9. https://doi.org/10.1097/MAO.0000000000000811.
2. Sugihara EM, Babu SC, Kitsko DJ, Haupert MS, Thottam PJ. Incidence of pediatric superior semicircular canal dehiscence and inner ear anomalies. Otol Neurotol. 2016;37(9):1370–5. https://doi.org/10.1097/mao.0000000000001194.
3. Nadgir RN, Ozonoff A, Devaiah AK, Halderman AA, Sakai O. Superior semicircular canal dehiscence: congenital or acquired condition? AJNR Am J Neuroradiol. 2011;32(5):947–9. https://doi.org/10.3174/ajnr.A2437.
4. Chen EY, Paladin A, Phillips G, et al. Semicircular canal dehiscence in the pediatric population. Int J Pediatr Otorhinolaryngol. 2009;73(2):321–7. https://doi.org/10.1016/j.ijporl.2008.10.027.
5. Carey JP, Minor LB, Nager GT. Dehiscence or thinning of bone overlying the superior semicircular canal in a temporal bone survey. Arch Otolaryngol Head Neck Surg. 2000;126(2):137–47. https://doi.org/10.1001/archotol.126.2.137.
6. Ward BK, Carey JP, Minor LB. Superior canal dehiscence syndrome: lessons from the first 20 years. Front Neurol. 2017;8:177. https://doi.org/10.3389/fneur.2017.00177.

7. Watters KF, Rosowski JJ, Sauter T, Lee DJ. Superior semicircular canal dehiscence presenting as postpartum vertigo. Otol Neurotol. 2006;27(6):756–68. https://doi.org/10.1097/01.mao.0000227894.27291.9f.
8. Saxby AJ, Gowdy C, Fandiño M, et al. Radiological prevalence of superior and posterior semicircular canal dehiscence in children. Int J Pediatr Otorhinolaryngol. 2015;79(3):411–8. https://doi.org/10.1016/j.ijporl.2015.01.001.
9. Bi WL, Brewster R, Poe D, et al. Superior semicircular canal dehiscence syndrome. J Neurosurg. 2017;127(6):1268–76. https://doi.org/10.3171/2016.9.JNS16503.
10. Niesten MEF, Lookabaugh S, Curtin H, et al. Familial superior canal dehiscence syndrome. JAMA Otolaryngol Head Neck Surg. 2014;140(4):363–8. https://doi.org/10.1001/jamaoto.2013.6718.
11. Hildebrand MS, Tack D, Deluca A, Hur IA, Van Rybroek JM, McMordie SJ, Muilenburg A, Hoskinson DP, Van Camp G, Pensak ML, Storper IS, Huygen PL, Casavant TL, Smith RJ. Mutation in the COCH gene is associated with superior semicircular canal dehiscence. Am J Med Genet A. 2009;149A(2):280–5. https://doi.org/10.1002/ajmg.a.32618.
12. Dasgupta S, Ratnayake SAB. Functional and objective audiovestibular evaluation of children with apparent semicircular canal dehiscence—a case series in a pediatric vestibular center. Front Neurol. 2019;10:306. https://doi.org/10.3389/fneur.2019.00306.
13. Cozart AC, Kennedy JT III, Seidman MD. A basis for standardizing superior semicircular canal dehiscence management. Ear Nose Throat J. 2021;100(10):NP444–53. https://doi.org/10.1177/0145561320927941.
14. Lagman C, Ong V, Chung LK, et al. Pediatric superior semicircular canal dehiscence: illustrative case and systematic review. J Neurosurg Pediatr. 2017;20(2):196–203. https://doi.org/10.3171/2017.3.PEDS1734.
15. Ommaya AK, Gennarelli TA. Cerebral concussion and traumatic unconsciousness: correlation of experimental and clinical observations on blunt head injuries. Brain. 1974;97(4):633–54. https://doi.org/10.1093/brain/97.1.633.
16. Zhou G, Brodsky JR. Objective vestibular testing of children with dizziness and balance complaints following sports-related concussions. Otolaryngol Head Neck Surg. 2015;152(6):1133–9. https://doi.org/10.1177/0194599815576720.
17. Crovetto MA, Whyte J, Sarasola E, Rodriguez JA, García-Barcina MJ. Absence of COCH gene mutations in patients with superior semicircular canal dehiscence. Am J Med Genet A. 2012;158A:251–3. https://doi.org/10.1097/MAO.0b013e3181bc35ce.
18. Lee GS, Zhou G, Poe D, et al. Clinical experience in diagnosis and management of superior semicircular canal dehiscence in children. Laryngoscope. 2011;121(10):2256–61. https://doi.org/10.1002/lary.22134.
19. Mignacco G, Salerni L, Bindi I, Monciatti G, Cerase A, Mandalà M. Case report: local anesthesia round window plugging and simultaneous vibrant soundbridge implant for superior semicircular canal dehiscence. Front Neurol. 2020;11:581783. https://doi.org/10.3389/fneur.2020.581783.
20. Dasgupta S, Ratnayake S, Crunkhorn R, Iqbal J, Strachan L, Avula S. Audiovestibular quantification in rare third window disorders in children. Front Neurol. 2020;11:954. Published 2020 Sep 16. https://doi.org/10.3389/fneur.2020.00954.
21. Mau C, Kamal N, Badeti S, et al. Superior semicircular canal dehiscence: diagnosis and management. J Clin Neurosci. 2018;48:58–65. https://doi.org/10.1016/j.jocn.2017.11.019.
22. Kelsch T, Schaefer L, Esquivel C. Vestibular evoked myogenic potentials in young children: test parameters and normative data. Laryngoscope. 2006;116(6):895–900. https://doi.org/10.1097/01.mlg.0000214664.97049.3e.
23. Kaur T, Johanis M, Miao T, Romiyo P, Duong C, Sun MZ, Ferraro R, Salamon N, McArthur D, Yang I, Gopen Q. CT evaluation of normal bone thickness overlying the superior semicircular canal. J Clin Neurosci. 2019;66:128–32. https://doi.org/10.1016/j.jocn.2019.05.001.
24. Eberhard KE, Chari DA, Nakajima HH, Klokker M, Cayé-Thomasen P, Lee DJ. Current trends, controversies, and future directions in the evaluation and management of superior canal dehiscence syndrome. Front Neurol. 2021;12:638574. https://doi.org/10.3389/fneur.2021.638574.

25. Wenzel A, Stuck BA, Servais JJ, Hörmann K, Hülse M, Hülse R. Superior canal dehiscence syndrome in children—a case report. Int J Pediatr Otorhinolaryngol. 2015;79(9):1573–8. https://doi.org/10.1016/j.ijporl.2015.05.022.
26. Belden CJ, Weg N, Minor LB, Zinreich SJ. CT evaluation of bone dehiscence of the superior semicircular canal as a cause of sound- and/or pressure-induced vertigo. Radiology. 2003;226(2):337–43. https://doi.org/10.1148/radiol.2262010897.
27. Tunkel AE, Carey JP, Pearl M. Flat panel computed tomography in the diagnosis of superior semicircular canal dehiscence syndrome. Otol Neurotol. 2019;40(2):213–7. https://doi.org/10.1097/MAO.0000000000002076.
28. Hagiwara M, Shaikh JA, Fang Y, Fatterpekar G, Roehm PC. Prevalence of radiographic semicircular canal dehiscence in very young children: an evaluation using high-resolution computed tomography of the temporal bones. Pediatr Radiol. 2012;42(12):1456–64. https://doi.org/10.1007/s00247-012-2489-9.
29. Grimmer JF, Hedlund G. Vestibular symptoms in children with enlarged vestibular aqueduct anomaly. Int J Pediatr Otorhinolaryngol. 2007;71:275–82. https://doi.org/10.1016/j.ijporl.2006.10.010.
30. Berrettini S, Forli F, Bogazzi F, et al. Large vestibular aqueduct syndrome: audiological, radiological, clinical, and genetic features. Am J Otolaryngol. 2005;26:363–71. https://doi.org/10.1016/j.amjoto.2005.02.013.
31. Griffith AJ, Arts A, Downs C, et al. Familial large vestibular aqueduct syndrome. Laryngoscope. 1996;106(8):960–5. https://doi.org/10.1097/00005537-199608000-00009.
32. Tong KA, Harnsberger HR, Dahlen RT, Carey JC, Ward K. Large vestibular aqueduct syndrome: a genetic disease? AJR Am J Roentgenol. 1997;168(4):1097–101. https://doi.org/10.2214/ajr.168.4.9124122.
33. Abe S, Usami S, Shinkawa H. Three familial cases of hearing loss associated with enlargement of the vestibular aqueduct. Ann Otol Rhinol Laryngol. 1997;106(12):1063–9. https://doi.org/10.1177/000348949710601210.
34. Satoh H, Nonomura N, Takahashi S. Four cases of familial hearing loss with large vestibular aqueducts. Eur Arch Otorhinolaryngol. 1999;256:83–6. https://doi.org/10.1007/s004050050121.
35. Miyamoto RT, Bichey BG, Wynne MK, Kirk KI. Cochlear implantation with large vestibular aqueduct syndrome. Laryngoscope. 2002;112(7 Pt 1):1178–82. https://doi.org/10.1097/00005537-200,207,000-00006.
36. Valvasori G, Clemis J. The large vestibular aqueduct syndrome. Laryngoscope. 1978;88:723–8.
37. Dewan K, Wippold FJ II, Lieu JE. Enlarged vestibular aqueduct in pediatric sensorineural hearing loss. Otolaryngol Head Neck Surg. 2009;140(4):552–8. https://doi.org/10.1016/j.otohns.2008.12.035.
38. Zhou G, Gopen Q. Characteristics of vestibular evoked myogenic potentials in children with enlarged vestibular aqueduct. Laryngoscope. 2011;121(1):220–5. https://doi.org/10.1002/lary.21184.
39. Au G, Gibson W. Cochlear implantation in children with large vestibular aqueduct syndrome. Am J Otol. 1999;20(2):183–6. PMID: 10100520.
40. Gadre AK, Edwards IR, Baker VM, Roof CR. Membranous or hypermobile stapes footplate: a new anatomic site resulting in third window syndrome. Front Neurol. 2020;11:871. https://doi.org/10.3389/fneur.2020.00871.
41. Matsuda H, Tanzawa Y, Sekine T, Matsumura T, Saito S, Shindo S, Usami S-i, Kase Y, Itoh A, Ikezono T. Congenital membranous stapes footplate producing episodic pressure-induced perilymphatic fistula symptoms. Front Neurol. 2020;11:585747. https://doi.org/10.3389/fneur.2020.585747.
42. Wackym PA, Balaban CD, Zhang P, Siker DA, Hundal JS. Third Window syndrome: surgical management of cochlea-facial nerve dehiscence. Front Neurol. 2019;10:1281. https://doi.org/10.3389/fneur.2019.01281.

43. Scarpa A, Ralli M, Cassandro C, Gioacchini FM, Greco A, Di Stadio A, Cavaliere M, Troisi D, de Vincentiis M, Cassandro E. Inner-ear disorders presenting with air-bone gaps: a review. J Int Adv Otol. 2020;16(1):111–6. https://doi.org/10.5152/iao.2020.7764.
44. El Beltagi AH, Elsherbiny MM, El-Nil H. Congenital X-linked stapes Gusher syndrome. Neuroradiol J. 2012;25(4):486–8. https://doi.org/10.1177/197140091202500412.

Chapter 23
The Geriatric Patient

Michael J. Eliason, Cameron B. Lindemann, and Michael D. Seidman

The World Health Organization (WHO) estimates that between 2015 and 2050, the proportion of the world's population over 60 years will nearly double from 12% to 22% [1]. This aging population provides unique challenges to those responsible for providing medical care. The gradual decrease in mental and physical capacity contributes to multiple comorbidities that affect quality of life and can confound a physician's ability to adequately diagnose and treat this unique cohort of patients. In fact, the United Nations General Assembly asked the WHO to lead the implementation of a "Decade of Healthy Ageing" from 2021 to 2030 [2].

Dizziness and imbalance are widely prevalent symptoms in the elderly population. Population-based studies estimate dizziness as being present in 24–45% of people older than 72 [3–5]. This sensation can lead to falls, bony fractures, extended hospitalizations, and overall decreased quality of life, and often is recognized as a significant public health concern in the context of a growing geriatric and elderly population [6, 7]. In fact, the field of Geriatric Medicine has grown dramatically in recent decades and utilizes a whole-person approach to diagnosing and treating symptomatic dizziness. Figure 23.1 demonstrates the relative morbidity and even mortality that symptomatic disequilibrium has in this unique portion of the population.

M. J. Eliason (✉) · C. B. Lindemann
Department of Otolaryngology-Head and Neck Surgery, Naval Medical Center Portsmouth, Portsmouth, VA, USA

M. D. Seidman
Department of Otolaryngology-Head and Neck Surgery, AdventHealth, Central Florida, Celebration, FL, USA

Oto-HNS, University of Central Florida, Orlando, FL, USA

University of South Florida, Tampa, FL, USA

G. J. Gianoli, P. Thomson (eds.), *Third Mobile Window Syndrome of the Inner Ear*, https://doi.org/10.1007/978-3-031-16586-3_23

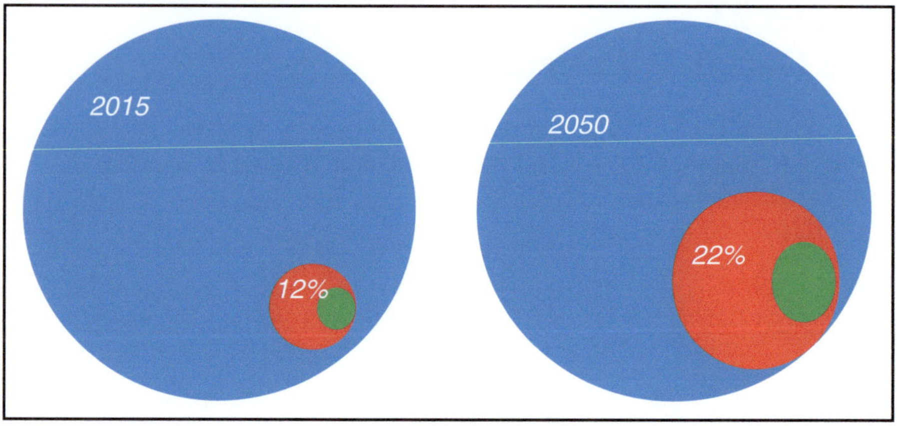

Fig. 23.1 Relative population of elderly patients with symptomatic dizziness. As demonstrated, the amount of the population with age greater than 60 years old will continue to rise relative to the population as a whole as we approach the year 2050. Therefore, the prevalence of symptomatic dizziness in this elderly population will increase significantly and will only cause a larger strain on the healthcare system

The classic teaching is that a person's ability to maintain his or her balance is the summation of inputs from one's vision, peripheral vestibular input, and somatosensory proprioception. Elderly patients often have multiple comorbidities such as hearing and vision loss that can exacerbate underlying peripheral vestibular weakness or dysfunction [8]. Furthermore, polypharmacy, social and emotional vulnerabilities, and declining cognition often cloud the diagnosis of what exactly may be causing the perception of dizziness or imbalance. For these reasons it is paramount that physicians maintain a broad differential diagnosis when a patient or his/her family member claims "dizziness" as the chief complaint.

As demonstrated in Fig. 23.2, Otolaryngologists often play a significant role in the management of geriatric patients with dizziness. Specifically, diagnoses of benign paroxysmal positional vertigo (BPPV), endolymphatic hydrops, labyrinthitis and vestibular migraine are often considered when evaluating these patients. Recently, the role of a third window in the peripheral vestibular system has been recognized as distinct etiology that should be explored in the case of geriatric "dizziness." The objective of this chapter is to review some of the unique characteristics of Third Mobile Window Disorder (TMWD) and specifically superior semicircular canal dehiscence (SSCD) in the geriatric population.

Understanding the role of TMWD, and its relative incidence in the greater scope of peripheral vestibular dysfunction in the geriatric population, requires the consideration of other causes. BPPV is typified by episodic vertigo associated with movement of the head and in inappropriate response of the vestibulo-ocular reflex due to otoliths that have been displaced into at least one of the semicircular canals. This has been estimated as one of the most prevalent causes of peripheral vertigo in up to 42% of all patients with vertigo complaints and is up to seven times higher in the

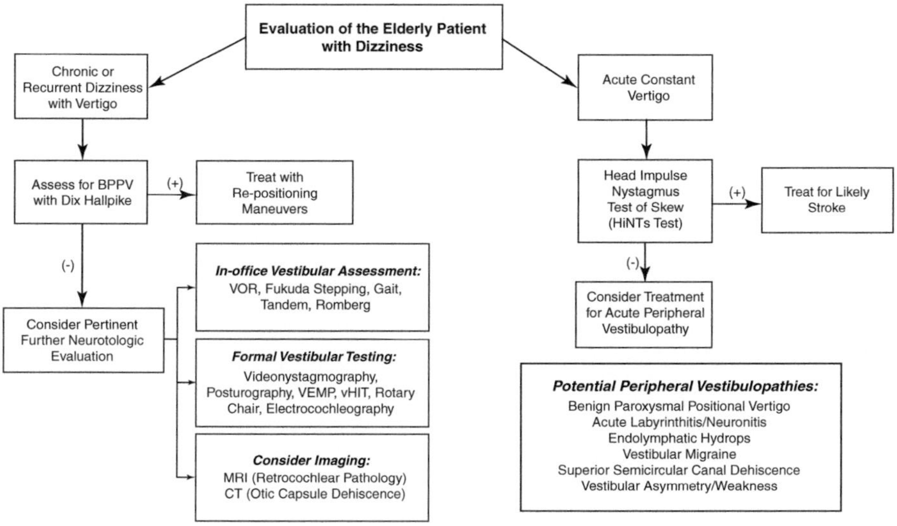

Fig. 23.2 Proposed flowchart for the evaluation of the elderly patient with dizziness. Multiple diagnoses for peripheral vestibulopathies exist in the geriatric population. As delineated in the flowchart, patients with new-onset acute vertigo should be evaluated and treated differently than those with chronic or recurrent dizziness [9]. There exist multiple diagnostic tools for the Otolaryngologist to consider to aid in the diagnosis

population that is greater than 60 years old [10, 11]. A recent review by Balatseuras et al. in 2018 details the likely multifactorial nature as to why BPPV becomes more prevalent and also tends to recur more in the aging population [12].

Endolymphatic hydrops, vestibular migraine, acute labyrinthitis, and weakness secondary to previous labyrinthine inflammation afflict the geriatric population in similar ways as the younger population. Other causes of peripheral vestibular hypofunction unique to the elderly include sensory deficits, such as bilateral vestibular hypofunction, polyneuropathy, impaired visual acuity, polypharmacy, and central disorders such as cerebellar ataxia and normal-pressure hydrocephalus. This population is therefore uniquely at risk for multiple etiologies affecting their imbalance and dizziness. Therefore, an elderly patient who fails to improve with canalith repositioning for BPPV and a trial of vestibular rehabilitation should undergo a more extensive vestibular evaluation. Furthermore, a more holistic approach to the entire patient and all potentially contributing factors should be considered by the treating physician.

SSCD syndrome is the constellation of symptoms that result from the lack of bony coverage of the membranous portion of the superior semicircular canal. Lloyd Minor, MD, and his colleagues first described SSCD in 1998 [13] and since then there has been growth in the understanding of its clinical significance, diagnosis and treatment [14]. Most patients experience symptoms of pressure- or sound-induced vertigo, bone conduction hyperacusis and pulsatile tinnitus. Rosowski and Merchant published a review of multiple cases and concluded that the dehiscence of the inner ear can be from sites of the labyrinth other than the superior canal, and result in symptoms of conductive hearing loss or other symptoms classically associated with SSCD [15, 16]. More recent studies have shown that these patients have a broad range of symptoms that drive patients and surgeons to treat for SSCD [17].

The clinical diagnosis of SSCD in the geriatric patient is similar to that of the general population discussed throughout this text. Symptoms elucidated from the history include the sensation of vertigo when exposed to loud sounds or pressure changes (Tullio and Hennebert phenomena respectively), hearing loss or distortion, pulsatile tinnitus, autophony, aural fullness, and other less specific vestibular complaints. The geriatric population may experience sequelae such as falls or even fractures secondary to the transient vestibular dysfunction caused by SSCD. Therefore, just as General Practitioners are trained to look for other common peripheral vestibulopathies such as BPPV and Ménière's disease, diagnostic criteria for SSCD in the elderly should be readily recognizable and considered at the primary care level as well [18]. Confounding this is the aforementioned multifactorial nature that contributes to this population feeling unsteady on their feet and/or with other imbalance. The combination of musculoskeletal and central nervous system atrophy, polypharmacy, cognitive decline, etc. may preclude a physician from even considering a more rare peripheral vestibular cause like TMWD. Findings such as a conductive hearing loss seen on audiogram and/or supra-threshold bone conduction may be the first and only clues that guide the provider to look closer for possible SSCD or other TMWD.

A mainstay in the diagnostic armamentarium for SSCD is computed tomography (CT). Imaging typically demonstrates dehiscence overlying the superior aspect of the SSC, but it can occur anywhere on the SSC or even other canals. CT will likely prove most useful using oblique planes to the traditional sagittal and coronal planes to get the superior canal either completely in plane or perpendicular to the plane of view. These Stenver (perpendicular to the superior canal) and Poschl (parallel or in plane with the superior canal) views are often useful to adequately characterize the superior canal by allowing measurement of the bony thickness.

A hypothesis unique to the geriatric population is that as people age, their bones are susceptible to becoming less dense and thinner, which predisposes the elderly population to perhaps being more likely to develop symptomatic SSCD. For this reason thickness of bone overlying the superior semicircular canal, as well as the morphology of the temporal bone in general, is of particular interest in studying the etiology of SSCD in the elderly population. However, there is variability in the medical literature regarding whether or not thickness of bone of the middle fossa varies with age [19–21].

Osteopenia and progression to osteoporosis is the manifestation of low bone density that results in fragility of the bony skeleton. The pathophysiology is related to multiple factors, but essentially results from the incongruence between bone formation and resorption. Elderly women are often afflicted due to estrogen deficiency, micronutrient deficiency, and/or other aging effects. Often thought of in terms of the effect on long bones, this has been studied with respect to the bone of the middle cranial fossa.

A retrospective review of 133 high-resolution CT scans demonstrated a mean thickness of bone over the superior canal as 1.25 mm [19]. The team concluded that this thickness of bone was variable, but not dependent on age or gender. Separate studies confirmed that there was no significant difference in superior canal bone thickness nor type of pneumatization based on age [20, 21]. However, others have reported the opposite, stating that age does in fact place elderly patients at increased risk for SSCD. Davey et al. demonstrated a linear relationship–for every unit increase in age the predicted bony thickness reduced by 0.0047 mm [22].

Additional data by Crovetto et al. support the hypothesis that there is slight osteopenia of the roof of the superior canal associated with aging. Furthermore, their data suggest that this effect is more pronounced in the post-menopausal period where bone resorption is known to be most prevalent [23]. Other studies have also shown correlation in symptomatic SSCD in those who are at higher risk of osteoporosis [24].

Additionally, some have described the effects of varying radiographic patterns of the tegmen tympani as it related to SSCD, as opposed to thickness of the bone overlying the superior canal alone, as a function of age. The general tegmen tympani classification system described is as follows: dehiscent, papyraceous, normal, thick and pneumatized [25–27]. In this classification scheme, thickness of bone certainly plays a role; however, appearance of bone is the primary target. There are data suggesting that the morphology of the tegmen tympani demonstrates a 4.1% increased risk of tegmen dehiscence for every year of increasing age in normal and thick patterns. The risk increases even more for dehiscent and papyraceous patterns, with increased risk of SSCD of 12 and 20 times respectively [26, 27]. Other authors report that SSCD risk and tegmen tympani morphology are not related to advancing age [20].

Overall, the data seem to indicate that SSCD is related to the tegmen morphology present in the patient rather than solely thickness of the temporal bone in this region alone. Additionally, the morphology of the temporal bone appears to change with advancing age, placing patients at increased risk for SSCD based on the tegmen pattern, rather than simple decrease in the thickness of bone overlying the superior canal.

A limitation to interpreting the data with regard to bone type and thickness compared to patient age represents some of the conflicting data between studies and publications. Though the data available currently do not provide a perfectly clear picture on the role of age and changes to the character of the temporal bone, anatomic changes with advancing age should be a consideration in diagnosing and treating geriatric patients with SSCD.

In addition to the thinning of bone and differing bone morphologies as a potential contributor to symptomatic SSCD, the concept of varying dural thickness as a factor is considered as well. The thickness of the dura is known to negatively correlate with age with significantly thinner dura in older patients [28]. The thinning of the dura with age is perhaps what converts a previously asymptomatic bony dehiscence over the superior canal to one that is symptomatic due to an easier transmission of intracranial process to the peripheral vestibular system.

Treatment options for symptomatic SSCD in the geriatric population are generally the same as the rest of the population. Surgical approaches are via a transmastoid approach, middle cranial fossa craniotomy approach, or a combination of the two. Most surgeons utilize a microscopic technique, but others have described the use of endoscopic techniques. Dr. Silverstein et al. published a relevant multi-center cases series regarding the use of round window reinforcement as a means to reduce symptoms of SSCD [29]. Given its low risks compared to middle cranial fossa or transmastoid occlusion, round window reinforcement may be appropriate for a geriatric patient who may not tolerate surgery requiring longer anesthesia time or significant surgical risk.

Central compensation of a unilateral peripheral vestibulopathy tends to take longer and may be less complete in the elderly population when compared to younger patients with similar insults. This potential for lack of effective central compensation should be considered when deciding on surgical management of SSCD for someone of advanced age. Specifically, plugging or complete occlusion of a semicircular canal requires a period of central compensation after surgery. Therefore, given the lack of data to guide these surgical decisions in the elderly population, it may be worth considering a less invasive procedure like round window reinforcement.

Frailty of the geriatric patient must be considered when discussing surgical options and approaches. The neurosurgical literature has demonstrated increased postoperative complications following craniotomy in those with higher frailty index scores [30, 31]. Specifically, the risk of 30-day mortality, postoperative complications, and discharge to destinations other than home are increased as an elderly patient is determined to be more frail. These risks must be considered and openly discussed with patients and their families when determining surgical candidacy for what is ultimately an elective procedure. When considering alternatives to middle fossa craniotomy, a transmastoid procedure may be better tolerated. In fact, a 2012 study looking at mastoidectomy in the elderly population for inflammatory disease concluded that there should be no reason to withhold mastoidectomy surgery for older patients on the basis that the procedure is too risky [32].

With the benefit of advanced healthcare capabilities and a better knowledge of healthy lifestyles, the portion of the population exceeding 65 years old will continue to grow over the coming decades. As we have discussed, the elderly population experiences dizziness at rates far greater than younger adults or children. SSCD and other TMWD can often be a more difficult diagnosis to clinch in this population for multiple confounding reasons, but should certainly be considered especially in the setting of hearing distortions. The literature remains unclear on the role of osteopenia and osteoporosis on predisposing this older population to SSCD, but there is some evidence that the morphologic type of bone in the tegmen region may correlate to one's age. Treatment options in the geriatric population are the same, but prudent attention to frailty and its potential associated risks after craniotomy need to be considered.

References

1. WHO. Ageing and health. Geneva: WHO; n.d.. https://www.who.int/news-room/fact-sheets/detail/ageing-and-health. Accessed 6 Mar 2022.
2. Decade of Healthy Ageing. n.d. The platform. https://www.decadeofhealthyageing.org/. Accessed 6 Mar 2022.
3. Tinetti ME, Williams CS, Gill TM. Dizziness among older adults: a possible geriatric syndrome. Ann Intern Med. 2000;132(5):337–44.
4. Albuquerque de Moraes S, Jefferson de Souza Soares W, Rodrigues RAS, Fett WCR, Ferriolli E, Perracini MR. Dizziness in community-dwelling older adults: a population-based study. Braz J Otorhinolaryngol. 2011;77(6):691–9.
5. Jönsson R, Sixt E, Landahl S, Rosenhall U. Prevalence of dizziness and vertigo in an urban elderly population. J Vestib Res. 2004;14(1):47–52.
6. Iwasaki S, Yamasoba T. Dizziness and imbalance in the elderly: age-related decline in the vestibular system. Aging Dis. 2015;6(1):38–47.
7. Stel VS, Pluijm SM, Deeg DJ, Smit JH, Bouter LM, Lips P. A classification tree for predicting recurrent falling in community-dwelling older persons. J Am Geriatr Soc. 2003;51(10):1356–64.
8. Barin K, Dodson EE. Dizziness in the elderly. Otolaryngol Clin N Am. 2011;44(2):437–54.
9. Hartholt K, Lee R, Burns E, et al. Mortality from falls among US adults aged 75 years or older, 2000-2016. JAMA. 2019;321(21):2131–3. https://doi.org/10.1001/jama.2019.4185.
10. Hanley K, O'Dowd T, Considine N. A systematic review of vertigo in primary care. Br J Gen Pract. 2001;51(469):666–71.
11. Neuhauser HK, von Brevern M, Radtke A, Lezius F, Feldmann M, Ziese T, Lempert T. Epidemiology of vestibular vertigo: a neurotologic survey of the general population. Neurology. 2005;65(6):898–904.
12. Balatsouras DG, Koukoutsis G, Fassolis A, Moukos A, Apris A. Benign paroxysmal positional vertigo in the elderly: current insights. Clin Interv Aging. 2018;13:2251–66.
13. Minor LB, Solomon D, Zinreich JS, Zee DS. Sound- and/or pressure-induced vertigo due to bone dehiscence of the superior semicircular canal. Arch Otolaryngol Head Neck Surg. 1998;124:249–58.
14. Ward B, Carey J, Minor L. Superior canal dehiscence syndrome: lessons from the first 20 years. Front Neurol. 2017;8:177.
15. Merchant SN, Rosowski JJ. Conductive hearing loss caused by third-window lesions of the inner ear. Otol Neurotol. 2008;29:282–9.
16. Rosowski JJ, Songer JE, Nakajima HH, Brinsko KM, Merchant SN. Clinical, experimental, and theoretical investigations of the effect of superior semicircular canal dehiscence on hearing mechanisms. Otol Neurotol. 2004;25:323–32.
17. Cozart A, Kennedy J, Seidman M. A basis for standardizing superior semicircular canal dehiscence management. Ear Nose Throat J. 2021;100(10):444–53.
18. Thomson P. Ménière's: why its diagnosis calls for more careful evaluation. Br J Gen Pract. 2017;67(665):569–70.
19. Kaur T, Johanis M, Miao T, et al. CT evaluation of normal bone thickness overlying the superior semicircular canal. J Clin Neurosci. 2019;66:128–32. https://doi.org/10.1016/j.jocn.2019.05.001.
20. Evlice B, Çabuk DS, Duyan H. The evaluation of superior semicircular canal bone thickness and radiological patterns in relation to age and gender. Surg Radiol Anat. 2021;43(11):1839–44. https://doi.org/10.1007/s00276-021-02797-4.
21. Mahulu EN, Fan X, Ding S, et al. The variation of superior semicircular canal bone thickness in relation to age and gender. Acta Otolaryngol. 2019;139(6):473–8. https://doi.org/10.1080/00016489.2019.1595721.

22. Davey S, Kelly-Morland C, Phillips JS, Nunney I, Pawaroo D. Assessment of superior semicircular canal thickness with advancing age. Laryngoscope. 2015;125:1940–5.
23. Crovetto MA, Whyte J, Rodriguez OM, et al. Influence of aging and menopause in the origin of the superior semicircular canal dehiscence. Otol Neurotol. 2012;33(4):681–4. https://doi.org/10.1097/MAO.0b013e31824f9969.
24. Yu A, Teich DL, Moonis G, Wong ET. Superior semicircular canal dehiscence in East Asian women with osteoporosis. BMC Ear Nose Throat Disord. 2012;12:8. https://doi.org/10.1186/1472-6815-12-8.
25. Cisneros AI, Whyte J, Martínez C, et al. Radiological patterns of the bony roof of the superior semicircular canal. Surg Radiol Anat. 2013;35(1):61–5. https://doi.org/10.1007/s00276-012-1019-7.
26. Whyte J, Tejedor MT, Fraile JJ, et al. Association between tegmen tympani status and superior semicircular canal pattern. Otol Neurotol. 2016;37(1):66–9. https://doi.org/10.1097/MAO.0000000000000918.
27. Suryanarayanan R, Lesser TH. 'Honeycomb' tegmen: multiple tegmen defects associated with superior semicircular canal dehiscence. J Laryngol Otol. 2010;124(5):560–3. https://doi.org/10.1017/S0022215109991411.
28. Fam M, Potash A, Potash M, et al. Skull base dural thickness and relationship to demographic features: a postmortem study and literature review. J Neurol Surg B Skull Base. 2018;79:614–20.
29. Silverstein H, Kartush J, Parnes L, et al. Round window reinforcement for superior semicircular canal dehiscence: a retrospective multi-center case series. Am J Otolaryngol. 2014;35(3):286–93.
30. Sastry RA, Pertsch N, Tang O, Shao B, Toms SA, Weil RJ. Frailty and outcomes after craniotomy or craniectomy for atraumatic chronic subdural hematoma. World Neurosurg. 2021;145:e242–51.
31. Mulligan P, Raore B, Liu S, Olson JJ. Neurological and functional outcomes of subdural hematoma evacuation in patients over 70 years of age. J Neurosci Rural Pract. 2013;4:250–6.
32. Ahn JH, An YS, Bae JS, Kim DY. Postoperative results of tympanoplasty with mastoidectomy in elderly patients with chronic otitis media. Ann Otol Rhinol Laryngol. 2012;121(3):168–73.

Chapter 24
Cerebrospinal Fluid Fistulas and Encephaloceles in the Setting of Superior Semicircular Canal Dehiscence

J. Walter Kutz Jr. and Donald Tan

Introduction

The cause of superior canal dehiscence (SCD) is likely a combination of congenitally thin bone and acquired changes from elevated cerebrospinal fluid (CSF) pressure or trauma. Dehiscence of the tegmen (the bone that separates the middle fossa from the mastoid and middle ear) is also a result of the same factors and is often present in patients with superior canal dehiscence. The combination of a dehiscent tegmen and elevated cerebrospinal fluid pressure may result in a spontaneous cerebrospinal fluid fistula or encephalocele. This chapter will discuss the association between superior canal dehiscence and spontaneous cerebrospinal fluid fistula and encephaloceles. Next, appropriate imaging and laboratory investigation will be discussed. Finally, the nuances of treating superior canal dehiscence in the setting of CSF fistulas and encephaloceles will be examined.

J. W. Kutz Jr. (✉)
Otolaryngology and Neurological Surgery, The University of Texas Southwestern Medical Center, Dallas, TX, USA
e-mail: walter.kutz@utsouthwestern.edu

D. Tan
The University of Texas Southwestern, Dallas, TX, USA
e-mail: DONALD.TAN@phhs.org

G. J. Gianoli, P. Thomson (eds.), *Third Mobile Window Syndrome of the Inner Ear*, https://doi.org/10.1007/978-3-031-16586-3_24

Association of CSF Fistula and Encephaloceles with Superior Canal Dehiscence

Superior canal dehiscence is more common in patients with tegmen defects, CSF fistula, and encephaloceles. In the most extensive series to date, Oh et al. demonstrated that among 83 case subjects, superior canal dehiscence was present in 35% of subjects with an encephalocele and 21% in those with CSF fistula [1]. A similar case series by Allen et al. reported a 16.1% incidence of SCD in patients with spontaneous CSF fistula [2]. In comparison, the reported rate of superior canal dehiscence in the general population ranges between 0.5% with histologic evaluation and up to 9% when looking at CT alone [3–6]. Although SCD may be present on imaging and testing, many patients with SCD will be asymptomatic. However, when repairing cerebrospinal fluid fistula and encephaloceles, the dura is often elevated off the superior semicircular canal. The concern by lifting the dura from the dehiscent superior canal is creating a third window of the labyrinth resulting in symptoms of sound- or pressure-induced vertigo, enhanced bone conduction, pulsatile tinnitus, autophony, and aural fullness. The possibility of unmasking symptoms creates a conundrum as to whether to repair the SCD during surgery for the cerebrospinal fluid fistula and encephalocele. How to address incidental superior canal dehiscence during surgical repair of a tegmen defect will be addressed later in this chapter.

Crovetto et al. and el Hadi et al. have examined the relationship in reverse, reporting the rate of tegmen dehiscence in patients with SCD to be 36.4% and 56.5% in their respective series [6, 7]. The bidirectional association has led authors to theorize plausible etiologies, although none have been proven definitively [1, 7, 8]. Because tegmen dehiscence is more common in patients with superior canal dehiscence, addressing the thin or absent tegmen during repair of SCD should be considered and will be discussed later in this chapter.

Presentation and Complications of Spontaneous CSF Fistulas and Encephaloceles

Middle ear effusion and copious otorrhea after placement of a tympanostomy tube are the most common presentation in patients with a CSF fistula. Less commonly, patients will present with meningitis, and the CSF fistula or encephalocele is discovered when looking for the cause of meningitis. In patients undergoing repair of superior canal dehiscence, a CSF fistula may occur during the surgical approach when the dura is elevated from the middle fossa floor. Carefully reviewing the CT scan before surgery may prevent this complication or prepare the surgeon to address an intraoperative CSF fistula or encephalocele.

An active CSF fistula or encephalocele places the patient at risk for meningitis. The incidence in patients with an active CSF fistula or encephalocele is unknown and is likely low, but it does occur and can be life-threatening. The reported rate of preoperative meningitis in patients with spontaneous CSF fistula of the lateral skull base ranges from 6% to 58% [9–11]. A study by Rao et al. reported no cases of meningitis in a series of patients who refused or could not undergo repair of an active CSF fistula, which included patients with active chronic otitis media [12]. However, in patients who can undergo surgical repair, it is advisable to repair the fistula or encephalocele to prevent meningitis. To lower the risk of meningitis, the Centers for Disease Control and Prevention (CDC) recommend pneumococcal vaccines for patients with a CSF fistula [13].

Imaging and Laboratory Evaluation for CSF Fistula and Encephaloceles

Fortunately, imaging for CSF fistula, encephalocele, and superior canal dehiscence is the same. A high-resolution non-contrasted computed tomography of the temporal bone with <1 mm slice thickness is recommended [9, 14]. Please see Chap. 12 for more discussion on imaging. The tegmen is best evaluated in the coronal plane, while the posterior fossa is better assessed with axial images. Magnetic resonance imaging is a valuable adjunct to CT for the evaluation of encephaloceles as well as stigmata of idiopathic intracranial hypertension[14] (Fig. 24.1). See Chap. 19 for more discussion on IIH.

In the setting of an actively draining tympanostomy tube or perforation, the diagnosis can often be made by the history of copious and constant clear otorrhea. A chronic middle ear effusion should raise the suspicion of a CSF fistula. Confirmation can be achieved by sampling middle ear fluid via tympanocentesis and sending the fluid for beta-2 transferrin analysis. Beta-2 transferrin has a reported sensitivity of 99% and a specificity of 97%, although it may have a false-negative result for intermittent leakage and in the setting of meningitis [15, 16].

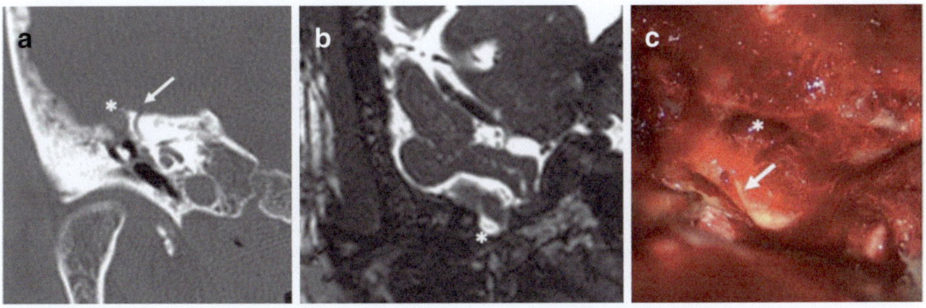

Fig. 24.1 Concurrent encephalocele of the right temporal bone. (**a**) Coronal high-resolution CT of the temporal bone showing a concurrent encephalocele (*) and superior canal dehiscence (arrow). (**b**) Heavily weighted T2 coronal MRI confirming the encephalocele. (**c**) Intraoperative photo showing the superior canal dehiscence (arrow) and the tegmen tympani defect (arrow)

Surgical Repair of CSF Fistula and Encephaloceles

When approaching a CSF fistula or encephalocele of the temporal bone, the surgeon must choose the appropriate repair technique based on the location, size, number of defects, surgeon preference, and patient factors.

The most common surgical approaches include:

- Middle fossa approach
- Transmastoid approach
- Combination of the middle fossa and transmastoid approaches
- Subtotal petrosectomy with eustachian tube obliteration and closure of the external auditory canal

When repairing a tegmen defect, special considerations include awareness of the possibility of exposed ossicles and dehiscence of the geniculate ganglion. When repairing defects of the tegmen tympani, the ossicles can be found superior to the defect (Fig. 24.2). In this situation, elevation of the dura may result in disarticulation of the ossicles and conductive hearing loss. A thorough review of the coronal CT scan will identify this situation. If the ossicles are superior to the defect, the ossicles are identified by carefully elevating the dura. A bone chip from the craniotomy flap can be placed over the ossicles to create a "neoepitympanum." This will allow the ossicles to move freely and also repair the tegmen defect [14]. Another potential pitfall is facial nerve injury in the setting of a dehiscent geniculate ganglion. In the

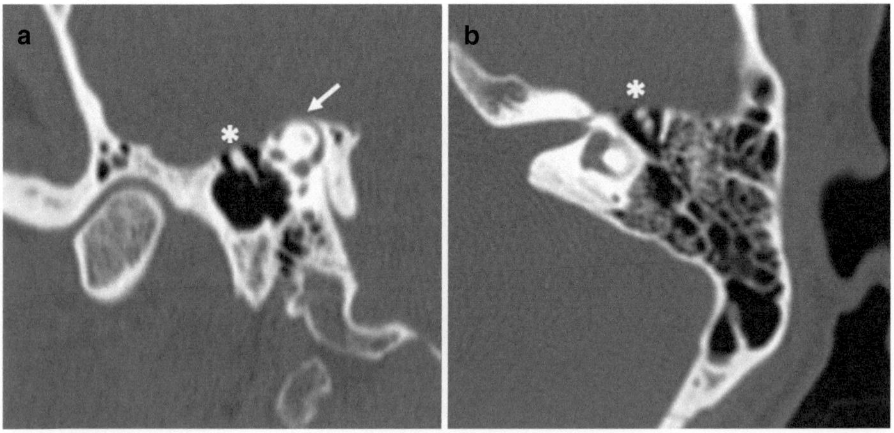

Fig. 24.2 A thin tegmen tympani in a patient with superior canal dehiscence shows the ossicles contacting the dura. (**a**) Coronal high-resolution CT temporal bone in oblique, reformatted plane showing superior canal dehiscence (arrow) and the ossicles (*) contacting the dura. (**b**) Axial high-resolution CT showing the ossicles (*) contacting the dura

normal temporal bone, the geniculate ganglion is dehiscent approximately 15% of the time; however, the geniculate ganglion is dehiscent in about 38% with a CSF fistula or encephalocele, so awareness of a possible dehiscent geniculate ganglion will prevent facial nerve injury during the process of dural elevation [17].

A middle fossa approach is preferred for the tegmen tympani defects since the ossicular chain can be avoided. The middle fossa approach is also preferred when there are multiple defects since the entire middle fossa floor is exposed. In addition, the middle fossa approach allows easy identification and repair of a dehiscent superior semicircular canal. The downside of the middle fossa craniotomy is the need for overnight observation in the intensive care unit and the additional risks of a craniotomy, including hemorrhage, cerebrovascular accident, memory loss, and rarely seizures.

The transmastoid approach can avoid a craniotomy and address tegmen mastoideum and posterior fossa defects. Tegmen tympani defects are more difficult to access unless the body of the incus and head of the malleus are removed. When superior canal dehiscence is also present, the canal can be gently opened on both sides of the defect and judiciously packed with bone pate, fascia, bone wax, or a combination of these materials [18–20]. Another alternative method to repair the superior semicircular canal defect is to elevate the dura over the superior semicircular canal and resurface the canal with cartilage or bone cement. However, a resurfacing technique has a higher recurrent symptoms rate than plugging the canal [21].

Many available materials are used to repair the dural defects, including autologous and other materials, such as bone cement and allograft fascia. Multiple layer closure with soft tissue, such as fascia, fat, or muscle, and more durable materials such as bone flaps, cartilage and bone cement, provides the best chance of long-term repair [14, 22–26].

Treatment of Asymptomatic Superior Canal Dehiscence During Repair of CSF Fistulas and Encephaloceles

There is no clear evidence that asymptomatic superior canal dehiscence found during repair of CSF fistula or encephalocele should be repaired. However, the elevation of the dura near the SCD carries the theoretical risk of inadvertently creating a third window and making a previously asymptomatic patient symptomatic [27]. If the superior canal dehiscence is not repaired and the patient becomes symptomatic after repairing a CSF fistula or encephalocele, revision surgery to repair the superior canal dehiscence has an increased risk of permanent sensorineural hearing loss [28]. Conversely, there is no apparent symptomatic benefit to addressing the SCD of an asymptomatic patient. In a series of patients who underwent surgical repair of a CSF fistula or encephalocele through a middle fossa craniotomy approach, patients with simultaneous repair of asymptomatic SCD had increased requirement for postoperative anti-emetics and increased incidence of postoperative complaints of imbalance at the 1-month postoperative visit [2]. The decision to repair incidentally noted

SCD during repair of a CSF fistula or encephalocele should therefore be made on a case by case basis, taking into account patient characteristics and whether the patient has bilateral superior canal dehiscence. For instance, in the case of bilateral dehiscence, plugging one canal may increase the chance of long-term vestibular problems if the contralateral canal requires repair in the future. In this case, a more conservative management strategy of resurfacing, rather than plugging, the dehiscent canal should be considered.

Postoperative Considerations

Patients with spontaneous CSF fistula and encephaloceles should be evaluated for elevated intracranial CSF pressure. One of the more common causes of chronically elevated intracranial pressure is idiopathic intracranial hypertension (IIH). MRI may show findings of IIH including an empty sella, dilated optic nerve sheath thickening and tortuosity, arachnoid granulations of the cranial sinuses, posterior globe flattening, Meckel's cave enlargement, and sigmoid sinus narrowing [29]. After repairing the CSF fistula, idiopathic intracranial hypertension is evaluated by obtaining opening CSF pressure through a lumbar puncture [9, 30]. It is imperative to assess intracranial pressure at some point after repair of a CSF leak since the leak itself may have lowered ICP. Some of these patients will be found to have IIH and will need ongoing treatment to prevent symptoms and other complications of IIH. Sleep apnea is another common cause of elevated CSF pressure that can lead to spontaneous CSF fistula and encephaloceles, so obtaining a history of possible sleep apnea and obtaining a sleep study should be considered [31, 32].

In summary, there is a significant association between superior canal dehiscence and spontaneous defects of the tegmen. Therefore, preoperative evaluation for SCD repair should include high-resolution CT of the temporal bone to evaluate the status of the tegmen. If spontaneous CSF fistula or encephaloceles are detected or occur during surgery, concurrent repair is indicated to prevent bacterial meningitis. The optimal management of asymptomatic superior canal dehiscence in the setting of a spontaneous CSF fistula or an encephalocele is nuanced. Since there is no clear evidence on whether to repair the incidental superior canal dehiscence, addressing the superior canal dehiscence should be determined on a case-by-case basis.

References

1. Oh MS, Vivas EX, Hudgins PA, Mattox DE. The prevalence of superior semicircular canal dehiscence in patients with mastoid encephalocele or cerebrospinal fluid otorrhea. Otol Neurotol. 2019;40(4):485–90. https://doi.org/10.1097/MAO.0000000000002155.
2. Allen KP, Perez CL, Isaacson B, Roland PS, Duong TT, Kutz JW. Superior semicircular canal dehiscence in patients with spontaneous cerebrospinal fluid otorrhea. Otolaryngol Head Neck Surg. 2012;147(6):1120–4. https://doi.org/10.1177/0194599812457545.

3. Carey JP, Minor LB, Nager GT. Dehiscence or thinning of bone overlying the superior semicircular canal in a temporal bone survey. Arch Otolaryngol Head Neck Surg. 2000;126(2):137–47. https://doi.org/10.1001/archotol.126.2.137.
4. Williamson RA, Vrabec JT, Coker NJ, Sandlin M. Coronal computed tomography prevalence of superior semicircular canal dehiscence. Otolaryngol Head Neck Surg. 2003;129(5):481–9. https://doi.org/10.1016/s0194-5998(03)01391-3.
5. Masaki Y. The prevalence of superior canal dehiscence syndrome as assessed by temporal bone computed tomography imaging. Acta Otolaryngol. 2011;131(3):258–62. https://doi.org/10.3109/00016489.2010.526145.
6. Crovetto M, Whyte J, Rodriguez OM, Lecumberri I, Martinez C, Elexpuru J. Anatomo-radiological study of the Superior Semicircular Canal Dehiscence Radiological considerations of Superior and Posterior Semicircular Canals. Eur J Radiol. 2010;76(2):167–72. https://doi.org/10.1016/j.ejrad.2009.05.038.
7. El Hadi T, Sorrentino T, Calmels MN, Fraysse B, Deguine O, Marx M. Spontaneous tegmen defect and semicircular canal dehiscence: same etiopathogenic entity? Otol Neurotol. 2012;33(4):591–5. https://doi.org/10.1097/MAO.0b013e31824bae10.
8. Hildebrand MS, Tack D, Deluca A, et al. Mutation in the COCH gene is associated with superior semicircular canal dehiscence. Am J Med Genet A. 2009;149A(2):280–5. https://doi.org/10.1002/ajmg.a.32618.
9. Lobo BC, Baumanis MM, Nelson RF. Surgical repair of spontaneous cerebrospinal fluid (CSF) leaks: a systematic review. Laryngosc Investig Otolaryngol. 2017;2(5):215–24. https://doi.org/10.1002/lio2.75.
10. Son HJ, Karkas A, Buchanan P, et al. Spontaneous cerebrospinal fluid effusion of the temporal bone: repair, audiological outcomes, and obesity. Laryngoscope. 2014;124(5):1204–8. https://doi.org/10.1002/lary.24484.
11. Markou K, Goudakos J, Franco-Vidal V, Vergnolles V, Vignes JR, Darrouzet V. Spontaneous osteodural defects of the temporal bone: diagnosis and management of 12 cases. Am J Otolaryngol. 2011;32(2):135–40. https://doi.org/10.1016/j.amjoto.2009.12.003.
12. Rao N, Redleaf M. Spontaneous middle cranial fossa cerebrospinal fluid otorrhea in adults. Laryngoscope. 2016;126(2):464–8. https://doi.org/10.1002/lary.25461.
13. Centers for Disease Control and Prevention. Pneumococcal vaccination: summary of who and when to vaccinate. Atlanta, GA: Centers for Disease Control and Prevention; 2022. Accessed 22 Apr 2022.
14. Kutz JW Jr, Tolisano AM. Diagnosis and management of spontaneous cerebrospinal fluid fistula and encephaloceles. Curr Opin Otolaryngol Head Neck Surg. 2019;27(5):369–75. https://doi.org/10.1097/MOO.0000000000000568.
15. Warnecke A, Averbeck T, Wurster U, Harmening M, Lenarz T, Stover T. Diagnostic relevance of beta2-transferrin for the detection of cerebrospinal fluid fistulas. Arch Otolaryngol Head Neck Surg. 2004;130(10):1178–84. https://doi.org/10.1001/archotol.130.10.1178.
16. Korem M, Ovadia H, Paldor I, et al. False negative beta-2 transferrin in the diagnosis of cerebrospinal fluid leak in the presence of Streptococcus pneumoniae. Laryngoscope. 2015;125(3):556–60. https://doi.org/10.1002/lary.24940.
17. Isaacson B, Vrabec JT. The radiographic prevalence of geniculate ganglion dehiscence in normal and congenitally thin temporal bones. Otol Neurotol. 2007;28(1):107–10. https://doi.org/10.1097/01.mao.0000235968.53474.77.
18. de Wolf MJF, Dawe N, Jervis S, et al. Transmastoid occlusion surgery for superior semicircular canal dehiscence syndrome improves patient-reported quality-of-life measures and corrects cVEMP thresholds and amplitudes. Otol Neurotol. 2021;42(10):1534–43. https://doi.org/10.1097/MAO.0000000000003329.
19. Banakis Hartl RM, Cass SP. Effectiveness of transmastoid plugging for semicircular canal dehiscence syndrome. Otolaryngol Head Neck Surg. 2018;158(3):534–40. https://doi.org/10.1177/0194599817751092.

20. Rodgers B, Lin J, Staecker H. Transmastoid resurfacing versus middle fossa plugging for repair of superior canal dehiscence: comparison of techniques from a retrospective cohort. World J Otorhinolaryngol Head Neck Surg. 2016;2(3):161–7. https://doi.org/10.1016/j.wjorl.2016.11.001.
21. Al Afif A, Farmer R, Bance M. Outcomes of transmastoid resurfacing for superior canal dehiscence using a cartilage overlay technique. Laryngoscope. 2019;129(9):2164–9. https://doi.org/10.1002/lary.27789.
22. Brown NE, Grundfast KM, Jabre A, Megerian CA, O'Malley BW Jr, Rosenberg SI. Diagnosis and management of spontaneous cerebrospinal fluid-middle ear effusion and otorrhea. Laryngoscope. 2004;114(5):800–5. https://doi.org/10.1097/00005537-200405000-00002.
23. Carlson ML, Copeland WR III, Driscoll CL, et al. Temporal bone encephalocele and cerebrospinal fluid fistula repair utilizing the middle cranial fossa or combined mastoid-middle cranial fossa approach. J Neurosurg. 2013;119(5):1314–22. https://doi.org/10.3171/2013.6.JNS13322.
24. Gubbels SP, Selden NR, Delashaw JB Jr, McMenomey SO. Spontaneous middle fossa encephalocele and cerebrospinal fluid leakage: diagnosis and management. Otol Neurotol. 2007;28(8):1131–9. https://doi.org/10.1097/MAO.0b013e318157f7b6.
25. Nelson RF, Roche JP, Gantz BJ, Hansen MR. Middle Cranial Fossa (MCF) approach without the use of lumbar drain for the management of spontaneous cerebral spinal fluid (CSF) leaks. Otol Neurotol. 2016;37(10):1625–9. https://doi.org/10.1097/MAO.0000000000001208.
26. Kveton JF, Goravalingappa R. Elimination of temporal bone cerebrospinal fluid otorrhea using hydroxyapatite cement. Laryngoscope. 2000;110(10 Pt 1):1655–9. https://doi.org/10.1097/00005537-200010000-00016.
27. Mikulec AA, Khan AM, Barker FG, McKenna MJ. Bilateral meningoencephalocele repair complicated by superior semicircular canal dehiscence: case report. Skull Base. 2008;18(6):423–8. https://doi.org/10.1055/s-0028-1087217.
28. Locketz G, Margalit N, Gonen L, Fliss DM, Handzel O. Dilemmas in the treatment of concurrent bilateral meningoencephalocele and superior semicircular canal dehiscence. Otol Neurotol. 2015;36(5):932–5. https://doi.org/10.1097/MAO.0000000000000729.
29. Batur Caglayan HZ, Ucar M, Hasanreisoglu M, Nazliel B, Tokgoz N. Magnetic resonance imaging of idiopathic intracranial hypertension: before and after treatment. J Neuroophthalmol. 2019;39(3):324–9. https://doi.org/10.1097/WNO.0000000000000792.
30. Kutz JW Jr, Johnson AK, Wick CC. Surgical management of spontaneous cerebrospinal fistulas and encephaloceles of the temporal bone. Laryngoscope. 2018;128(9):2170–7. https://doi.org/10.1002/lary.27208.
31. Bakhsheshian J, Hwang MS, Friedman M. Association between obstructive sleep apnea and spontaneous cerebrospinal fluid leaks: a systematic review and meta-analysis. JAMA Otolaryngol Head Neck Surg. 2015;141(8):733–8. https://doi.org/10.1001/jamaoto.2015.1128.
32. Nelson RF, Gantz BJ, Hansen MR. The rising incidence of spontaneous cerebrospinal fluid leaks in the United States and the association with obesity and obstructive sleep apnea. Otol Neurotol. 2015;36(3):476–80. https://doi.org/10.1097/MAO.0000000000000535.

Chapter 25
Migraine, Headache, and Third Mobile Window Syndrome

P. Ashley Wackym, Carey D. Balaban, and Todd M. Mowery

An illustrative summary that highlights the spectrum of the most common complaints from patients with perilymph fistula (PLF) was published over a quarter century ago [1]. No doubt many of these patients had third mobile window syndrome (TMWS) due to bony sites of dehiscence not yet discovered. In this publication the authors reported the percentage of their patients reporting each of the 13 most common complaints. The three most frequent complaints were disequilibrium, headache and dizziness. Other important clinical symptoms included cognitive dysfunction, nausea, visual disturbance, and objective as well as subjective hearing loss. The most common symptoms of superior semicircular canal dehiscence (SSCD), and other sites of TMWS, include pseudoconductive hearing loss (bone conduction hyperacusis), autophony, pulsatile tinnitus, and sound- or pressure-induced vertigo [2–11]. Some of the internal sounds that patients report as being particularly disturbing include hearing their eyes move and/or blink, hearing their heels strike loudly, chewing (often so loud they need to stop chewing to hear what others say), belching or borborygmi. Patients also experience aural fullness typical of endolymphatic hydrops. This spectrum of symptoms observed is summarized in Chap. 1.

P. A. Wackym (✉) · T. M. Mowery
Department of Otolaryngology – Head and Neck Surgery, Rutgers Robert Wood Johnson Medical School, New Brunswick, NJ, USA

Rutgers Brain Health Institute, Piscataway, NJ, USA
e-mail: wackym@neurotology.org

C. D. Balaban
Departments of Otolaryngology, Neurobiology, Communication Sciences & Disorders, and Bioengineering, University of Pittsburgh School of Medicine, Pittsburgh, PA, USA

G. J. Gianoli, P. Thomson (eds.), *Third Mobile Window Syndrome of the Inner Ear*, https://doi.org/10.1007/978-3-031-16586-3_25

Headache and Migraine

Migraine is a symptomatically heterogeneous condition, of which headache is just one manifestation. Migraine is a disorder of altered sensory thresholding, with hypersensitivity among sufferers to sensory input. Advances in functional neuroimaging have highlighted that several brain areas are involved even prior to pain onset. Clinically, patients can experience symptoms hours to days prior to migraine pain, which can warn of impending headache. These symptoms can include mood and cognitive change, fatigue and neck discomfort. Epidemiological studies have suggested that migraine is associated with other systemic conditions such as depression, anxiety, irritable bowel syndrome, fibromyalgia, sleep disorders, and chronic fatigue, as well as cognitive disorders (for review see Karsan and Goadsby [12]). The association between migraine and psychiatric disorders has been well documented through numerous population-based studies. The results of these studies show an increased risk of suffering from depression, bipolar disorders, numerous anxiety disorders, especially posttraumatic stress disorder. Many reasons have been postulated for these associations, including comorbidities, cause and effect, and shared pathophysiological mechanisms [13]. Sarif et al. completed a systematic review of the association of migraine and cognitive dysfunction, including dementia [14]. All the reviewed studies put together showed an association between headache and cognitive dysfunction of any form. They showed that the frequency and duration of headache is a determinant for dementia. However, few studies also focused on how treating headaches with certain drugs can lead to dementia. The reviewed published literature showed that headaches of any sort and their treatment are potentially linked to dementia [14].

As one of the most common chronic daily headache (CDH) disorders, chronic migraine (CM) is featured by frequent headache attacks with at least 15 headache days per month [15, 16]. Chronic migraine sufferers usually have a history of episodic migraine (EM) and their headache frequencies increase with time. It is estimated that approximately 3% EM patients evolve to CM per year [17, 18]. This transformation can be bidirectional with about 26% of CM patients reverting to EM in a cohort followed for two years [19]. Because of this, it is difficult to confirm the true prevalence of CM. With the increasing headache frequency, CM can become less intense, but is associated with worse response to treatment. Both the undertreated headache and associated comorbidities cause greater disease burden for CM compared with EM [20–22]. Although regarded as the same spectrum illness with EM [23], the detailed pathophysiology of CM is not fully understood. The role of vestibular dysfunction due to TMWS in EM and/or CM remains understudied. Studies have recognized several predisposing factors and triggers such as specific olfactory stimuli, sleep deprivation, hunger, bright light, medication overuse, insufficient migraine prophylactic treatment, low socioeconomic status, stressful events and depression [19, 24]. Some epidemiological studies have suggested that migraine is associated in a bidirectional fashion with other disorders, such as mood disorders and chronic fatigue, as well as with other pain conditions such as fibromyalgia [12].

In a series with three different TMWS cohorts, depression, as measured with Beck's Depression Inventory (BDI), was significantly reduced after surgical management [5]. These same cohorts had significant reduction in their Headache Impact Test (HIT-6) scores after surgical management, underscoring the potential contribution of TMWS to depression and migraine. Moreover, recent neurophysiological and imaging studies have indicated that CM may be associated with both structural and functional alterations in some brain regions, especially cortical hyperexcitability and brainstem dysfunction [25–27]. Sensitization of the trigeminal system also plays a vital role, as allodynia is quite common in CM patients [28]. In addition, several molecular mechanisms have been implicated in the pathogenesis of CM, such as calcitonin gene-related peptide (CGRP), serotonin (5-HT), pituitary adenylate cyclase activating polypeptide (PACAP), and others [29–31]. Migraine should be considered a neural disorder of brain function, in which alterations in networks integrating the limbic system with the sensory and homeostatic systems occur early and persist after headache resolution and perhaps interictally. The associations with some of these other disorders may allude to the inherent sensory sensitivity of the migraine brain and shared neurobiology and neurotransmitter systems, rather than true comorbidity [32].

Pathophysiology of Chronic Migraine

Like EM, the pathophysiological basis of CM is not fully understood. However, recent data indicate that migraine is a disorder of brain dysfunction with both the genetic background and environment triggering [33]. The transformation of EM to CM is also related to the brain. Recent evidence has demonstrated both structural and functional alterations in the brain, in particular cortical hyperexcitability and abnormities in the brainstem [27]. More CM patients than EM patients report cutaneous allodynia [34], suggesting that sensitization of trigeminal system is involved in the development of the disease. Seo and Park investigated the clinical significance of allodynia compared with other sensory hypersensitivities in migraine patients [35]. They found that migraine particularly combined with allodynia resulted in poor clinical outcomes. In addition, several molecules, such as CGRP and 5-HT [29, 30], have been reported to be correlated with the transition from occasional migraine to EM to CM. In brief, both recurring headache attacks and the comorbid conditions (medication over use, anxiety, and depression) promote the derangement of top-down pain modulation and also atypical release of nociceptive molecules, which aggravates trigeminal sensitization induced by repeated nociceptive inputs. With this hypersensitive state, the EM finally progresses to CM. The neural plasticity induced by the risk factors of CM may in turn exert an influence.

Since migraine is characterized by altered sensory thresholding with hypersensitivity among sufferers to sensory input, we believe that the gravitational receptor asymmetries seen in TMWS are triggering migraine via this hypersensitivity-associated mechanism.

Measuring the Impact of Headache

When measuring the magnitude of headache and migraine headache in patients with TMWS and, equally importantly, the response to surgical intervention it is essential to incorporate a validated survey instrument into clinical practice. We have found the six-item HIT-6 to be an outstanding tool to accomplish these goals. The short-form HIT-6 is a widely used patient-reported outcome measure that assesses the negative effects of headaches on normal activity. Houts et al. completed a narrative literature review to examine existing qualitative research in patients with migraine and headache, and to provide insight into the relevance and meaningfulness of HIT-6 items to the lives of migraine patients [36]. This review demonstrated qualitative support for the relevance of the items of the HIT-6 in migraine patients, supporting its ongoing use in clinical migraine research and practice. The six-item HIT-6 includes the following questions: Question 1: *When you have headaches, how often is the pain severe?*; Question 2: *How often do headaches limit your ability to do usual daily activities including household work, work, school, or social activities?*; Question 3: *When you have a headache, how often do you wish you could lie down?*; Question 4: *In the past 4 weeks, how often have you felt too tired to do work or daily activities because of your headaches?*; Question 5: *In the past 4 weeks, how often have you felt fed up or irritated because of your headaches?*; Question 6: *In the past 4 weeks, how often did headaches limit your ability to concentrate on work or daily activities?* Each item has five descriptive response options, with each awarded a specific number of points: "Never" (6 points), "Rarely" (8 points), "Sometimes" (10 points), "Very often" (11 points), and "Always" (13 points). The score is the sum of item (points) responses. The index score ranges from 36 to 78, where scores 36–49 indicate little to no impact on life (Class I); 50–55 indicates some impact on life (Class II); 56–59 indicates substantial impact on life (Class III); and 60–78 indicates very severe impact on life (Class IV).

There are alternative validated survey instruments such as the Chronic Headache Quality of Life Questionnaire (CHQLQ) which is a 14-item questionnaire, assessing the functional aspects of headache-related quality of life, producing three domain scores (role prevention, role restriction and emotional function) [37]. Haywood et al. compared the quality and acceptability of a new headache-specific patient-reported measure, the CHQLQ, with the six-item HIT-6, in people meeting an epidemiological definition of chronic headaches [37]. They concluded while both measures are structurally valid, internally consistent, temporally stable, and responsive to change, the CHQLQ has greater relevance to the patient experience of chronic headache. However, for the patient with TMWS, the CHQLQ questions are too similar to the Dizziness Handicap Inventory domains (functional, physical, and impact on disability) and it is likely that the TMWS patients would answer the CHQLQ questions based upon their vestibular dysfunction symptoms/experiences. For this reason, we find the HIT-6 to be more useful in this specific patient population.

Headache and Migraine in Third Mobile Window Syndrome

It is common for patients with TMWS to experience symptom complexes associated with headache and migraine headache. They can also experience the variants of migraine: vestibular migraine (VM), ocular migraine, and hemiplegic migraine. Table 25.1 summarizes the character of the headache, presence of headache, and the prevalence of migraine variants in six cohorts of patients that included: SSCD with plugging, TMWS with no visible site of dehiscence by high-resolution temporal bone CT (CT− TMWS) with round window reinforcement (RWR), both SSCD plugging and CT− TMWS with RWR, cochlea-facial nerve dehiscence (CFD) with RWR, CFD without RWR and surgically managed PLF. Of note there were patients with TMWS and no headache. In these same series the prevalence of no headache was 9.1% in SSCD with plugging, 7.1% in CT− RWR, 12.5% in CFD without RWR, and 12% surgically managed PLF [1, 4–6]. The remaining cohorts all experienced headache preoperatively. Ward et al. [38] reviewed the first 20 years of literature after SSCD, and regarding migraine and SSCD they stated, "*Many patients with [SSCD] also have migraine, but this may represent the high prevalence of migraine in the general population and that [SSCD] is an effective migraine trigger.*" Another way of restating that is that SSCD and other sites creating TMWS induce migraine, in the same way that trigeminal nerve stimulation, olfactory stimulation, and ocular stimulation can induce episodes of migraine. Of course, both possibilities can be true and using a validated survey instrument, the HIT-6, to measure the scores before and after surgical intervention supports this.

Table 25.2 summarizes the HIT-6 scores and classifications before and after surgical intervention, as well as the statistical significance, for four different cohorts of patients with TMWS. Note that for all four comparisons, the improvement in the HIT-6 score was highly statistically significant ($p < 0.001$). However, based upon the postoperative classifications, there were a few patients with HIT-6 Class III or Class IV (next to worst and worst Class) suggesting that they were migraine patients whose TMWS made their migraine worse, but it persisted after surgical intervention. Figure 25.1 shows an example of individual patient data for eight CFD patients preoperatively and after RWR surgery.

As shown in Table 25.1, patients with TMWS can also experience VM (migraine-associated dizziness) which is recognized as a distinct clinical entity that accounts for a high proportion of patients with vestibular symptoms (for review see Furman et al. [39]). It is so common that VM should be considered in any patient presenting with dizziness, vertigo, or disequilibrium. A temporal overlap between vestibular symptoms, such as vertigo and head-movement intolerance, and migraine symptoms, such as headache, photophobia, and phonophobia, is a requisite diagnostic criterion. Physical examination and laboratory testing are usually normal in VM but can be used to rule out other vestibular disorders with overlapping symptoms such as TMWS. The pathophysiology of VM is incompletely understood but plausibly

Table 25.1 Presence and characteristics of chronic headache/migraine and migraine variants in six cohorts of patients with third mobile window syndrome of different etiologies

Etiology of third mobile window syndrome and cohort studied	Chronic headache/ migraine	24/7 while awake	Daily or frequent	Occasional headache	No headache	Vestibular migraine	Ocular migraine	Hemiplegic migraine
SSCD with plugging (Wackym et al. [4, 5])	91% (10/11)	9.1% (1/11)	81.8% (9/11)	9.1% (1/11)	9.1% (1/11)	9.1% (1/11)	9.1% (1/11)	None
CT− with RWR (Wackym et al. [4, 5])	92.9% (13/14)	71.4% (10/14)	21.4% (3/14)	None	7.1% (1/14)	14.3% (2/14)	21.4% (3/14)	7.1% (1/14)
SSCD plugging + CT− with RWR (Wackym et al. [5])	100% (4/4)	None	100% (4/4)	None	None	None	25% (1/4)	None
CFD with RWR (Wackym et al. [6])	75% (6/8)	25% (2/8)	75% (6/8)	None	None	37.5% (3/8)	62.5% (5/8)	None
CFD without RWR (Wackym et al. [6])	87.5% (7/8)	None	75% (6/8)	12.5% (1/8)	12.5% (1/8)	62.5% (5/8)	25% (2/8)	None
PLF (Black et al. [1])	88% (51/58)	NR	NR	NR	12% (7/58)	NR	NR	NR

24/7 indicates migraine headache present constantly, 24 h and 7 days per week while awake; *CFD with RWR*, cochlea-facial nerve dehiscence with round window reinforcement surgery; *CFD without RWR*, cochlea-facial nerve dehiscence without round window reinforcement surgery; *CT− with RWR*, third window syndrome with no bony site of dehiscence seen on high-resolution temporal bone CT with round window reinforcement surgery; *PLF*, perilymphatic fistula; SSCD with plugging, superior semicircular canal dehiscence with plugging and resurfacing; *SSCD with plugging + CT− with RWR*, superior semicircular canal dehiscence with plugging and resurfacing plus third window syndrome with no bony site of dehiscence seen on high-resolution temporal bone CT with round window reinforcement surgery; *RWR*, round window reinforcement surgery. Published with permission, copyright © P.A. Wackym, MD

Table 25.2 Headache Impact Test (HIT-6) score preoperatively and postoperatively, statistical significance, and preoperative and postoperative classification

Etiology of third mobile window syndrome and cohort studied	Mean preoperative HIT-6 score	Mean postoperative HIT-6 score	Statistical significance (paired *t*-test)	Preoperative HIT-6 classifications	Postoperative HIT-6 classifications
SSCD with plugging ($n = 5$) ($n = 4$ with headache) (Wackym et al. [5])	69.8 (range 61–76, SD ± 6.34)	44.5 (range 36–61, SD ± 11.27)	$p < 0.001$	4 Class IV (plus 1 with no headache)	3 Class I, 1 Class IV
CT− with RWR ($n = 8$) ($n = 7$ with headache) (Wackym et al. [5])	74 (range 68–78, SD ± 4)	45.7 (range 42–49, SD ± 3.14)	$p < 0.001$	7 Class IV	7 Class I
SSCD plugging + CT− with RWR ($n = 4$) (Wackym et al. [5])	69.3 (range 57–78, SD ± 9.7)	46.8 (range 36–53, SD ± 8.10)	$p < 0.001$	3 Class IV, 1 Class III	2 Class I, 2 Class II
CFD with RWR ($n = 8$) (Wackym et al. [6])	64.9 (range 52–69, SE ± 1.1)	42.4 (range 36–55, SE ± 2.7)	$p < 0.001$	8 Class IV	7 Class I or Class II, 1 Class III

CFD with RWR, cochlea-facial nerve dehiscence with round window reinforcement surgery; *CT− with RWR*, third window syndrome with no bony site of dehiscence seen on high-resolution temporal bone CT with round window reinforcement surgery; *HIT-6*, Headache Impact Test 6; *SD*, standard deviation, *SE*, standard error; *SSCD with plugging*, superior semicircular canal dehiscence with plugging and resurfacing; *SSCD with plugging + CT− with RWR*, superior semicircular canal dehiscence with plugging and resurfacing plus third window syndrome with no bony site of dehiscence seen on high-resolution temporal bone CT with round window reinforcement surgery; *RWR*, round window reinforcement surgery. HIT-6 classification: Class I (36–49), Class II (50–55), Class III (56–59), Class IV (60–78). Published with permission, copyright © P.A. Wackym, MD

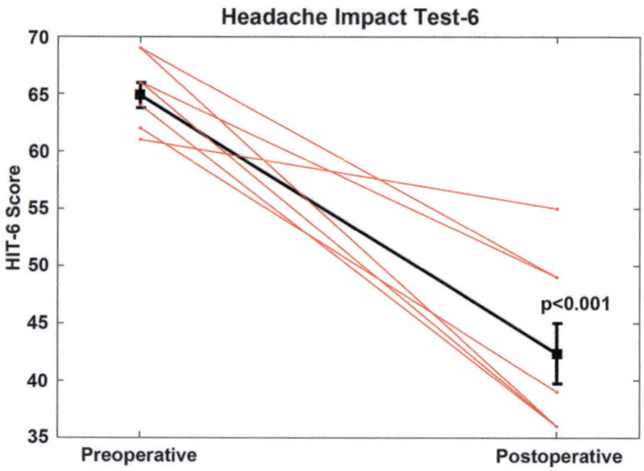

Fig. 25.1 Example of individual patient data for preoperative and postoperative Headache Impact Test (HIT-6) scores. The patients depicted are a cochlea-facial nerve dehiscence cohort who had round window reinforcement procedures performed. The preoperative mean HIT-6 score was 64.9 (SE 1.1, range 52–69). The postoperative mean HIT-6 score was 42.4 (SE 2.7, range 36–55). This improvement was highly statistically significant (paired *t*-test, $p < 0.001$). These data are plotted as a single black line. Individual patients are plotted as separate lines (red). (Used with permission, copyright © P.A. Wackym, MD)

could include neuroanatomical pathways to and from central vestibular structures and neurochemical modulation via the locus coeruleus and raphe nuclei. In the absence of controlled trials, treatment options for patients with VM largely mirror those for migraine headache. These treatment approaches include the prophylactic prevention of migraines with: (1) antiseizure medications such as topiramate (Topamax) or zonisamide (Zonegran); (2) calcium channel blockers such as verapamil (Verelan); (3) tricyclic antidepressants such as nortriptyline (Pamelor); or beta-blockers, for children, such as propranolol (Inderal). Approximately one-third of vestibular migraine patients have endolymphatic hydrops, which is typically bilateral.

VM patients do not have sound-induced dizziness and nausea or autophony; however, when these patients have endolymphatic hydrops, they can have sound sensitivity that borders on a Tullio phenomenon. For this reason, when a high-resolution temporal bone CT shows no evidence of TMWS, all patients suspected of having CT− TMWS are treated as a VM patient since medical management, if successful, avoids unnecessary surgery. Typically, CT− TMWS patients will have some improvement with medical management, and then regression as the dose is increased resulting in switching to another class of medication. Ultimately the patients never come under control and reassessment leads to a decision for surgical intervention.

Vestibular migraine is an example of the integral overlap between vestibular pathways and migraine circuit triggers and central mechanisms for premonitory symptom generation [39]. Information transmitted by peripheral vestibular sensory organs and the vestibular nerve to the medulla and pons is an external trigger within the migraine circuit construct proposed by Ho and coworkers [40, 41]. This model is based upon the distribution of the neuropeptide CGRP, which has a complex distribution within the vestibular periphery [42]. The neurotologist author (PAW) has observed that migraine headache is nearly always present in patients with gravitational receptor dysfunction type of vertigo caused by TMWS, but infrequently with rotational receptor dysfunction type of true rotational vertigo [4–6, 8–10]. This is an important concept as TMWS can induce migraine symptoms consistent with three variants of migraine—ocular migraine, hemiplegic migraine and VM. This is why patients with TMWS, who normally have gravitational receptor dysfunction type of vertigo (disequilibrium) as their dominant vestibular dysfunction, can have episodes of vestibular migraine and infrequent true rotational vertigo attacks. However, as shown in Table 25.1, surgical management of TMWS typically improves the migraine symptoms. However, sometimes there is a marked decrease of the frequency and intensity of the migraines, as migraine has a high incidence overall (Table 25.2 and Fig. 25.1) [4–6, 8–10].

Headache and migraine headache have been reported to be associated with idiopathic intracranial hypertension (IIH), which has also been reported in patients with SSCD and CT− TMWS [43–45]. Visual alterations and headache are the two main symptoms of idiopathic intracranial hypertension, although additional features including cranial nerve palsies, cognitive deficits, olfactory deficits, and tinnitus are not uncommon [43]. The headache associated with idiopathic intracranial hypertension frequently has a migrainous phenotype. The underlying cause of the disorder has not yet been determined, although obesity is thought to be a risk factor. In a series of 12 patients with comorbidities complicating the recovery of their surgical management of TMWS, Wackym and collaborators reported a patient with bilateral SSCD who had recurrent TMWS symptoms and subsequently had multiple bilateral middle ear surgeries to manage her CT− TMWS [44]. She was ultimately found to have IIH and it was only after ventriculoperitoneal shunt placement to control her intracranial pressure that her migraine headaches were controlled and she no longer experienced recurrent CT− TMWS symptoms that required surgical intervention. Berkiten et al. studied 57 patients (114 ears), 20 who were controls and 37 who were IIH [45]. All patients were evaluated with high-resolution temporal bone CT for superior semicircular canal bony roof thickness and SSCD. In the IIH group, while dehiscence was detected in 25 of 74 ears, no dehiscence was detected in 49 ears. In the control group, while dehiscence was detected in five ears, no dehiscence was detected in 35 ears. The difference was statistically significant ($p = 0.015$). In contrast, Kuo et al. reported 121 patients who had both a lumbar puncture performed to determine opening pressure and high-resolution temporal bone CT imaging, of which 24 patients (19.8%) met the criteria for IIH with an opening pressure >25 cm H_2O [46]. The remaining 97 patient cohort (80.2%) did not have elevated opening pressures and served as the controls. None of the 24 patients with IIH had radiographic SSCD, whereas eight of the 97 patients (8.2%) without IIH had radiographic SSCD. The average opening pressure in patients without radiographic SSCD was 20.2 cm H_2O compared to 19.3 cm H_2O in patients with radiographic SSCD ($p = 0.521$). These findings suggest that the relationship between IIH and

SSCD is not clear. Finally, Kutz and Tolisano reported a series of patients with spontaneous CSF leaks and encephaloceles [47]. They noted that there was an increased incidence of obesity in this cohort and that concurrent superior semicircular canal dehiscence was seen in up to 15% of cases.

Summary

Migraine is a symptomatically heterogeneous condition, of which headache is just one manifestation. Migraine is a disorder associated with altered sensory thresholding, with hypersensitivity among sufferers to different sensory inputs. Hence, we suggest that sensitivity to the gravitational receptor asymmetries seen in TMWS is triggering migraine symptoms via this hypersensitivity-associated mechanism. When measuring the magnitude of headache and migraine headache in patients with TMWS and, equally importantly, the response to surgical intervention it is essential to incorporate a validated survey instrument into clinical practice. We have found that the six-item HIT-6 has documented a highly statistically significant improvement postoperatively in symptom reporting.

References

1. Black FO, Pesznecker S, Norton T, et al. Surgical management of perilymphatic fistulas: a Portland experience. Am J Otolaryngol. 1992;13:254–62.
2. Minor LB, Solomon D, Zinreich JS, Zee DS. Sound- and/or pressure-induced vertigo due to bone dehiscence of the superior semicircular canal. Arch Otolaryngol Head Neck Surg. 1998;124(3):249–58. https://doi.org/10.1001/archotol.124.3.249.
3. Minor LB. Clinical manifestations of superior semicircular canal dehiscence. Laryngoscope. 2005;115:1717–27. https://doi.org/10.1097/01.mlg.0000178324.55729.b7.
4. Wackym PA, Wood SJ, Siker DA, Carter DM. Otic capsule dehiscence syndrome: superior canal dehiscence syndrome with no radiographically visible dehiscence. Ear Nose Throat J. 2015;94(7):E8–24. https://doi.org/10.1177/014556131509400802.
5. Wackym PA, Balaban CD, Mackay HT, et al. Longitudinal cognitive and neurobehavioral functional outcomes after repairing otic capsule dehiscence. Otol Neurotol. 2016;37(1):70–82. https://doi.org/10.1097/MAO.0000000000000928.
6. Wackym PA, Balaban CD, Zhang P, Siker DA, Hundal JS. Third window syndrome: surgical management of cochlea-facial dehiscence. Front Neurol. 2019;10:1281. https://doi.org/10.3389/fneur.2019.01281.
7. Wackym PA, Agrawal Y, Ikezono T, Balaban CD. Editorial: Third window syndrome. Front Neurol. 2021;12:704095. https://doi.org/10.3389/fneur.2021.704095.
8. Wackym PA. Right cochlea-facial nerve dehiscence: 16 year old thought to have conversion disorder. 2019. https://doi.org/10.13140/RG.2.2.27418.90564. https://youtu.be/fTjsnnU-ALBw. Accessed 1 Sep 2022. Copyright © P.A. Wackym, MD, used with permission.
9. Wackym PA. Right superior semicircular canal dehiscence repair: symptoms and recovery. 2017. https://doi.org/10.13140/RG.2.2.32032.79361. https://youtu.be/er4k8NZrG2I. Accessed 1 Sep 2022. Copyright © P.A. Wackym, MD, used with permission.

10. Wackym PA. Cochlea-facial nerve dehiscence: traumatic third window syndrome after a snowboarding accident. 2019. https://doi.org/10.13140/RG.2.2.17283.76327. https://youtu.be/NCDMD5FGf-w. Accessed 1 Sep 2022. Copyright © P.A. Wackym, MD, used with permission.
11. Naert L, Van de Berg R, Van de Heyning P, et al. Aggregating the symptoms of superior semicircular canal dehiscence syndrome. Laryngoscope. 2018;128(8):1932–8. https://doi.org/10.1002/lary.27062.
12. Karsan N, Goadsby PJ. Migraine is more than just headache: is the link to chronic fatigue and mood disorders simply due to shared biological systems? Front Hum Neurosci. 2021;15:646692. https://doi.org/10.3389/fnhum.2021.646692.
13. Radat F. What is the link between migraine and psychiatric disorders? From epidemiology to therapeutics. Rev Neurol (Paris). 2021;177(7):821–6. https://doi.org/10.1016/j.neurol.2021.07.007.
14. Sharif S, Saleem A, Koumadoraki E, Jarvis S, Madouros N, Khan S. Headache - a window to dementia: an unexpected twist. Cureus. 2021;13(2):e13398. https://doi.org/10.7759/cureus.13398.
15. IHS. Headache Classification Committee of the International Headache Society (IHS) the international classification of headache disorders, 3rd edition. Cephalalgia. 2018;38(1):1–211. https://doi.org/10.1177/0333102417738202.
16. Su M, Yu S. Chronic migraine: a process of dysmodulation and sensitization. Mol Pain. 2018;14:1744806918767697. https://doi.org/10.1177/1744806918767697.
17. Lipton RB, Fanning KM, Serrano D, Reed ML, Cady R, Buse DC. Ineffective acute treatment of episodic migraine is associated with new-onset chronic migraine. Neurology. 2015;84(7):688–95. https://doi.org/10.1212/WNL.0000000000001256.
18. Scher AI, Buse DC, Fanning KM, et al. Comorbid pain and migraine chronicity: the Chronic Migraine Epidemiology and Outcomes Study. Neurology. 2017;89(5):461–8. https://doi.org/10.1212/WNL.0000000000004177.
19. Manack A, Buse DC, Serrano D, Turkel CC, Lipton RB. Rates, predictors, and consequences of remission from chronic migraine to episodic migraine. Neurology. 2011;76(8):711–8. https://doi.org/10.1212/WNL.0b013e31820d8af2.
20. Adams AM, Serrano D, Buse DC, et al. The impact of chronic migraine: the Chronic Migraine Epidemiology and Outcomes (CaMEO) Study methods and baseline results. Cephalalgia. 2015;35(7):563–78. https://doi.org/10.1177/0333102414552532.
21. Lipton RB, Manack Adams A, Buse DC, Fanning KM, Reed ML. A comparison of the Chronic Migraine Epidemiology and Outcomes (CaMEO) Study and American Migraine Prevalence and Prevention (AMPP) Study: demographics and headache-related disability. Headache. 2016;56(8):1280–9. https://doi.org/10.1111/head.12878.
22. Buse DC, Manack A, Serrano D, Turkel C, Lipton RB. Sociodemographic and comorbidity profiles of chronic migraine and episodic migraine sufferers. J Neurol Neurosurg Psychiatry. 2010;81(4):428–32. https://doi.org/10.1136/jnnp.2009.192492.
23. Aurora SK. Spectrum of illness: understanding biological patterns and relationships in chronic migraine. Neurology. 2009;72(5 Suppl):S8–13. https://doi.org/10.1212/WNL.0b013e31819749fd.
24. Cho SJ, Chu MK. Risk factors of chronic daily headache or chronic migraine. Curr Pain Headache Rep. 2015;19(1):465. https://doi.org/10.1007/s11916-014-0465-9.
25. Aurora SK, Barrodale PM, Tipton RL, Khodavirdi A. Brainstem dysfunction in chronic migraine as evidenced by neurophysiological and positron emission tomography studies. Headache. 2007;47(7):996–1003. https://doi.org/10.1111/j.1526-4610.2007.00853.x; discussion 1004–7.
26. Lai TH, Chou KH, Fuh JL, et al. Gray matter changes related to medication overuse in patients with chronic migraine. Cephalalgia. 2016;36(14):1324–33. https://doi.org/10.1177/0333102416630593.

27. Mathew NT. Pathophysiology of chronic migraine and mode of action of preventive medications. Headache. 2011;51(Suppl 2):84–92. https://doi.org/10.1111/j.1526-4610.2011.01955.x.
28. Schwedt TJ, Larson-Prior L, Coalson RS, et al. Allodynia and descending pain modulation in migraine: a resting state functional connectivity analysis. Pain Med. 2014;15(1):154–65. https://doi.org/10.1111/pme.12267.
29. Cernuda-Morollón E, Larrosa D, Ramón C, Vega J, Martínez-Camblor P, Pascual J. Interictal increase of CGRP levels in peripheral blood as a biomarker for chronic migraine. Neurology. 2013;81(14):1191–6. https://doi.org/10.1212/WNL.0b013e3182a6cb72.
30. Rossi C, Pini LA, Cupini ML, Calabresi P, Sarchielli P. Endocannabinoids in platelets of chronic migraine patients and medication-overuse headache patients: relation with serotonin levels. Eur J Clin Pharmacol. 2008;64(1):1–8. https://doi.org/10.1007/s00228-007-0391-4.
31. Han X, Dong Z, Hou L, et al. Interictal plasma pituitary adenylate cyclase-activating polypeptide levels are decreased in migraineurs but remain unchanged in patients with tension-type headache. Clin Chim Acta. 2015;450:151–4. https://doi.org/10.1016/j.cca.2015.08.017.
32. Balaban CD, Black RD, Silberstein SD. Vestibular neuroscience for the headache specialist. Headache. 2019;59:1109–27. https://doi.org/10.1111/head.13550.
33. Goadsby PJ, Holland PR, Martins-Oliveira M, Hoffmann J, Schankin C, Akerman S. Pathophysiology of migraine: a disorder of sensory processing. Physiol Rev. 2017;97(2):553–622. https://doi.org/10.1152/physrev.00034.2015.
34. Bigal ME, Ashina S, Burstein R, et al. Prevalence and characteristics of allodynia in headache sufferers: a population study. Neurology. 2008;70(17):1525–33. https://doi.org/10.1212/01.wnl.0000310645.31020.b1.
35. Seo JG, Park SP. Clinical significance of sensory hypersensitivities in migraine patients: does allodynia have a priority on it? Neurol Sci. 2019;40(2):393–8. https://doi.org/10.1007/s10072-018-3661-2.
36. Houts CR, Wirth RJ, McGinley JS, et al. Content validity of HIT-6 as a measure of headache impact in people with migraine: a narrative review. Headache. 2020;60(1):28–39. https://doi.org/10.1111/head.13701.
37. Haywood KL, Achana F, Nichols V, et al. Measuring health-related quality of life in chronic headache: a comparative evaluation of the Chronic Headache Quality of Life Questionnaire and Headache Impact Test (HIT-6). Cephalalgia. 2021;41(10):1100–23. https://doi.org/10.1177/03331024211006045.
38. Ward BK, Carey JP, Minor LB. Superior canal dehiscence syndrome: lessons from the first 20 years. Front Neurol. 2017;8:177. https://doi.org/10.3389/fneur.2017.00177.
39. Furman JM, Marcus DA, Balaban CD. Vestibular migraine: clinical aspects and pathophysiology. Lancet Neurol. 2013;12:706–15. https://doi.org/10.1016/S1474-4422(13)70107-8.
40. Ho TW, Edvinsson L, Goadsby PJ. CGRP and its receptors provide new insights into migraine pathophysiology. Nat Rev Neurol. 2010;6:573–82. https://doi.org/10.1038/nrneurol.2010.127.
41. Xu D, Chen D, Zhu LN, et al. Safety and tolerability of calcitonin-gene-related peptide binding monoclonal antibodies for the prevention of episodic migraine - a meta-analysis of randomized controlled trials. Cephalalgia. 2019;39(9):1164–79. https://doi.org/10.1177/0333102419829007.
42. Wackym PA. Ultrastructural organization of calcitonin gene-related peptide immunoreactive efferent axons and terminals in the rat vestibular periphery. Am J Otolaryngol. 1993;14:41–50.
43. Raoof N, Hoffmann J. Diagnosis and treatment of idiopathic intracranial hypertension. Cephalalgia. 2021;41(4):472–8. https://doi.org/10.1177/0333102421997093.
44. Wackym PA, Mackay-Promitas HT, Demirel S, et al. Comorbidities confounding the outcomes of surgery for third window syndrome: outlier analysis. Laryngosc Invest Otolaryngol. 2017;2(5):225–53. https://onlinelibrary.wiley.com/doi/full/10.1002/lio2.89.

45. Berkiten G, Gürbüz D, Akan O, et al. Dehiscence or thinning of bone overlying the superior semicircular canal in idiopathic intracranial hypertension. Eur Arch Otorhinolaryngol. 2022;279(6):2899–904. https://doi.org/10.1007/s00405-021-07020-z.
46. Kuo P, Bagwell KA, Mongelluzzo G, et al. Semicircular canal dehiscence among idiopathic intracranial hypertension patients. Laryngoscope. 2018;128(5):1196–9. https://doi.org/10.1002/lary.26795.
47. Kutz JW Jr, Tolisano AM. Diagnosis and management of spontaneous cerebrospinal fluid fistula and encephaloceles. Curr Opin Otolaryngol Head Neck Surg. 2019;27(5):369–75. https://doi.org/10.1097/MOO.0000000000000568.

Chapter 26
Postoperative Third Mobile Window Syndrome

Alexander L. Luryi and Dennis I. Bojrab

Introduction: Iatrogenic Third Window Phenomena

Prior to the discovery of superior semicircular canal dehiscence and its associated vestibuloacoustic syndrome, non-iatrogenic Tullio phenomenon, pressure-induced vertigo, and other symptoms now associated with TMWD were attributed to perilymph fistulae, congenitally abnormal contact between the stapes and the vestibule, or presumed brainstem or cerebellar lesions [1, 2]. Likewise, these symptoms were frequently reported following surgery of the middle ear, mastoid, or skull base, and the causes of these postoperative findings were unknown or similarly attributed to undiagnosed perilymph fistulae or central nervous system injury [3, 4]. It is now suspected that many of these symptoms were caused by undiagnosed third mobile window phenomena [5]. Any surgical procedure in which dissection includes or affects the bony inner ear may lead to TMWD. This chapter discusses specific procedures which may lead to development of new-onset TMWD, typical presentations of these phenomena, their diagnosis and their management.

Stapes Surgery

Dizziness after stapes surgery is common. Temporary, mild to moderate vertigo is presumed to result from intraoperative physical disruption of the endolymphatic space, while more severe or longer-lasting symptoms can result from TMWD as

A. L. Luryi (✉)
Division of Otolaryngology-Head and Neck Surgery, Department of Surgery, Cooper University Hospital, Camden, NJ, USA

D. I. Bojrab
Department of NeurotologyMichigan Ear InstituteFarmington Hills, MI, USA

G. J. Gianoli, P. Thomson (eds.), *Third Mobile Window Syndrome of the Inner Ear*, https://doi.org/10.1007/978-3-031-16586-3_26

well as benign paroxysmal positional vertigo, pneumolabyrinth, or intralabyrinthine protrusion of the prosthesis [6–8]. Stapes surgery can lead to TMWD through several mechanisms, including the formation of a perilymph fistula, total stapedectomy resulting in a membranous or hypermobile footplate, or unmasking of SCDS in the setting of a pre-existing dehiscence of the superior semicircular canal.

Perilymph fistula is a known complication of stapes surgery and has been reported for decades [9]. A vestibulotomy and perilymph fistula must be created in the otosclerotic oval window to accommodate a prosthesis and restore hearing. Post-stapedectomy perilymph fistulas occur when this vestibulotomy does not adequately close and communication between the inner and middle ears persists. Patients with post-stapedectomy fistula present with dizziness, disequilibrium, and a positive fistula sign, with or without recurrent conductive or sensorineural hearing loss [10]. Revision stapes surgery is more likely to result in perilymph fistula than primary stapes surgery due to scarring of the oval window and loss of normal anatomic landmarks. Likewise, total stapedectomy is more likely to result in perilymph fistula than stapedotomy due to the greater area of exposed vestibule [10, 11]. Patients with suspected perilymph fistula after stapes surgery should undergo exploration of the middle ear and reinforcement of the oval window with fascia or fat [12]. To prevent perilymph fistula formation after stapedotomy, some authors advocate reinforcing the oval window during primary surgery with soft tissue rather than blood patching or other techniques, although this has not been proven to affect outcomes [13].

When total or partial stapedectomy is performed, a part of the stapes footplate is removed and the vestibule is covered with soft tissue (typically fat, fascia or vein tissue) [14]. Eventually, this soft tissue is expected to undergo fibrosis and contract into a rigid structure. However, the replacement of the bony footplate with a soft or fibrous covering may create a mobile third window around the implanted stapes prosthesis. Prior to the discovery of SCDS, transient Tullio phenomenon following stapes surgery was attributed to perilymph fistula or overly long prosthesis impacting the saccule. [15] It is likely that some of these cases could be attributed to postoperative hypermobility of the membranous oval window leading to a third mobile window. Although this phenomenon has not been conclusively demonstrated in extant literature, a hypermobile or membranous footplate has been shown to lead to third window phenomena following middle ear trauma [16]. Patients with persistent and debilitating noise- or pressure-induced vertigo after stapes surgery may be offered exploration of the middle ear and reinforcement of the oval window to address this.

Stapes surgery may also exacerbate or unmask symptoms of previously subclinical TMWD in patients with dehiscence of the superior semicircular canal or other inner ear structures [17]. In these patients, the otosclerotic focus of the oval window is thought to prevent acoustic impulses from disrupting endolymph in the labyrinth. Upon stapedectomy or stapedotomy, a third mobile window is restored in the oval window. These patients develop typical TMWD symptoms including Tullio phenomenon, dizziness and disequilibrium and exhibit characteristic abnormal findings on vestibular evoked myogenic potentials [18]. If imaging had not been obtained prior to stapes surgery, computed tomography of the temporal bone without intravenous contrast should be obtained and may reveal a dehiscence of the superior semicircular canal. Decreased thresholds on vestibular evoked myogenic potential (VEMP) also supports this diagnosis. If necessary, these patients can be surgically managed with superior semicircular canal plugging or resurfacing via standard middle cranial fossa or transmastoid routes with good success [17].

Surgery for Cholesteatoma

Depending on the extent of disease, surgery for cholesteatoma can lead to TMWD in multiple ways. Patterns of origin and spread of cholesteatoma are highly variable, and erosion of the lateral [19], posterior [20], and superior [21] semicircular canals, as well as the cochlea [22] has been reported. Any full- or near-full-thickness erosion of the bony inner ear by cholesteatoma without breach of the membranous inner ear can lead to TMWD. Furthermore, surgery for cholesteatoma in which a mass of debris or matrix is removed from a dehiscent or thin inner ear wall can unmask a third window phenomenon.

Management of symptomatic labyrinthine fistulae in the setting of cholesteatoma is controversial. If cholesteatoma can be confidently cleared, the labyrinthine fistula can be resurfaced with bone pate, hydroxyapatite cement, cartilage, or other hard biocompatible materials. Alternatively, plugging of the affected semicircular canal has been shown to be effective in managing symptoms of TMWD in cholesteatoma, although this will adversely affect the function of the involved canal [23].

However, traditional teaching dictates that in cases of labyrinthine fistula resulting from cholesteatoma, the mastoid cavity should be exteriorized and cholesteatoma matrix should be left covering the fistula itself to reduce the risk of inner ear damage [19]. Management of patients with disabling noise- and pressure-induced vertigo following modified radical mastoidectomy with labyrinthine fistula is a technical and decisional challenge. Some patients may manage these symptoms with tight-fitting ear plugs in the operative ear, although this can worsen aeration of the cavity during wear [24]. Surgical repair of the labyrinthine fistula after exteriorization has been described [25]. This operation involves elevation of all epithelium surrounding the fistula, removal of granulation tissue present, and placement of a graft (bone pate, cartilage, fascia, etc.) to cover the fistula. Care must be taken to ensure that all epithelium has been elevated over the graft to prevent further labyrinthine injury. Favorable outcomes for this technique have been reported, but patients must be counseled of the risk of profound sensorineural hearing loss resulting from direct trauma or suppurative labyrinthitis.

Surgery of the Lateral Skull Base

Depending on initial pathology and surgical approach, lateral skull base surgery which spares the inner ear may create a third mobile window in any segment of the cochlea or labyrinth, leading to iatrogenic TMWD. Violation of inner ear structures has been reported in up to 20% of hearing-preservation approaches to vestibular schwannoma [26]. Resection of vestibular schwannomas via the retrosigmoid or suboccipital approaches can be complicated by dehiscence of the medial portion of the superior or posterior semicircular canals as well as the medial portion of the vestibule [27, 28], particularly when aggressive exposure of the internal auditory canal is undertaken (Fig. 26.1). Surgery via the middle cranial fossa approach can result in, or unmask, superior semicircular canal dehiscence or cochlear dehiscence, depending on the extent of anterior dissection [29].

Iatrogenic TMWD may also result from transmastoid approaches to the lateral skull base. Transtemporal approaches to the petrous apex, including supralabyrinthine, retrofacial, and subarcuate approaches, require thinning of bone over one or more semicircular canals and can result in exposure of the membranous labyrinth and TMWD. Similarly, the retrolabyrinthine approach for hearing-preservation resection of a small vestibular schwannoma at the porus acusticus may lead to dehiscence of the posterior semicircular canal. Excessive superior drilling during endolymphatic sac procedures for recalcitrant Ménière's disease may also result in posterior semicircular canal dehiscence [27, 30] (Fig. 26.2).

Management of iatrogenic TMWD resulting from skull base surgery is complex and depends on initial pathology, surgical approach, and size and location of the defect. Injuries which result in non-serviceable hearing in addition to vestibular symptoms may be managed with ablative therapy such as vestibular nerve section or labyrinthectomy with or without concurrent cochlear implantation [28]. For patients without significant hearing loss, surgical repair of the inner ear fistula is

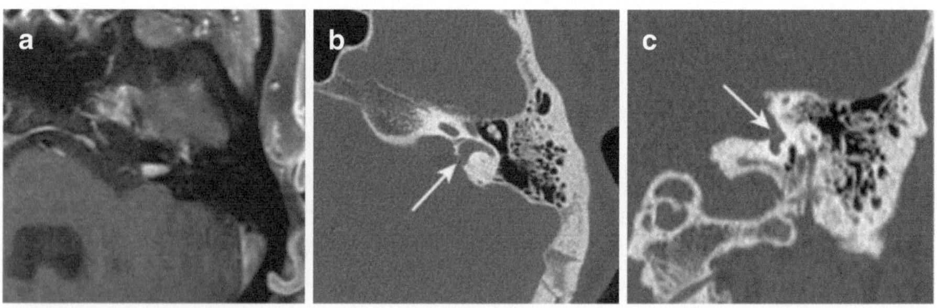

Fig. 26.1 T1-weighted gadolinium-enhanced magnetic resonance image demonstrating a left intracanalicular vestibular schwannoma in axial view, which was subsequently removed via the retrosigmoid approach (**a**). Computed tomographic scan of the left temporal bone demonstrating postoperative dehiscence of the vestibule in axial view (**b**) and superior limb of the posterior semicircular canal in coronal view (**c**), with arrows pointing to site of dehiscence. (Adapted with permission from Bartholomew et al., 2019 [27])

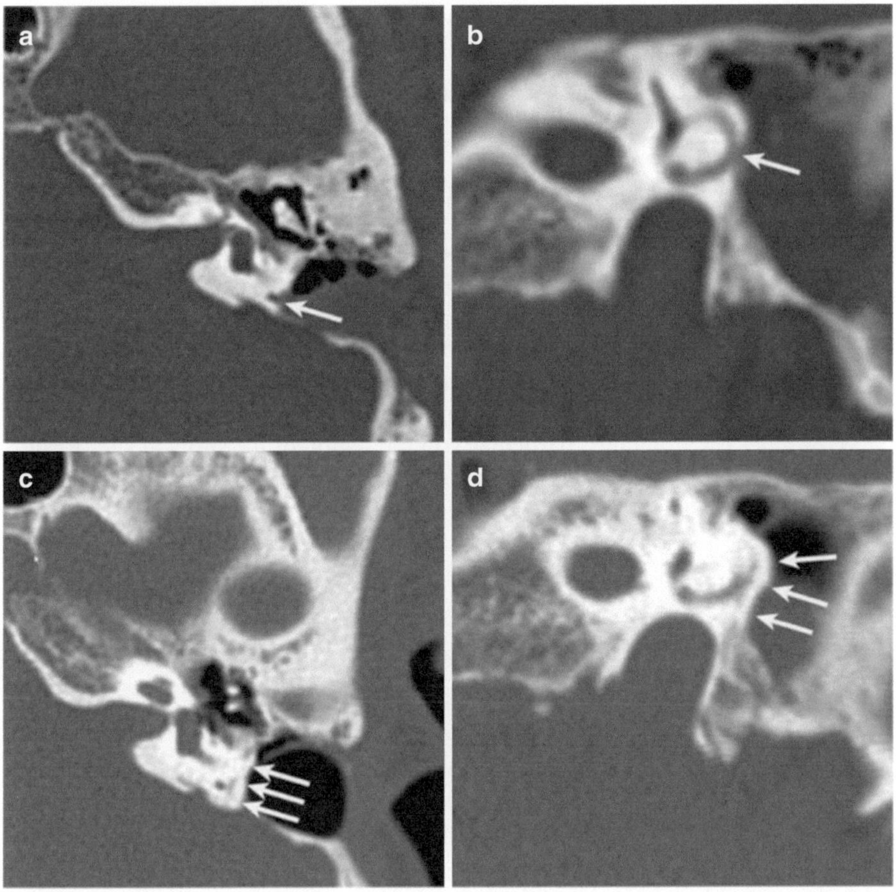

Fig. 26.2 Computed tomographic scan of right temporal bone demonstrating dehiscence of the posterior semicircular canal in axial (**a**) and coronal view (**b**) following endolymphatic sac surgery, with arrows pointing to site of dehiscence. Scans demonstrating subsequent repair with arrows pointing to hydroxyapatite resurfacing in axial (**c**) and coronal view (**d**). (Adapted with permission from Bartholomew et al., 2019 [27])

preferred. Defects in the semicircular canals caused during transmastoid [27] or middle cranial fossa approaches can be readily repaired via the same approach [31]. Repair of cochlear defects or medial labyrinthine or vestibular defects sustained via middle cranial fossa or retrosigmoid approaches to the skull base may not be feasible due to their intracranial location and proximity to surrounding structures. Patients with these defects, serviceable hearing, and debilitating TMWD symptoms can be offered a transcanal round window reinforcement procedure. While less effective than repair of the primary defect, this procedure is minimally invasive and reduces symptoms of TMWD in approximately two-thirds of patients. Successful management of defects of the medial vestibule sustained during retrosigmoid skull base surgery has been reported with this technique [27, 32].

Diagnosis of Postoperative TMWD

Postoperative TMWD presents a diagnostic challenge. Patients undergoing otologic surgery may be left with a conductive hearing loss, which is therefore not specific for TMWD in this population. Likewise, depending on their initial pathology and surgery, they may have altered vestibular function and VEMP testing may be unreliable or impossible due to the degree of conductive hearing loss, which reduces sound pressure impulses reaching the inner ear. Therefore, diagnosis of this condition relies heavily on a thorough patient history and physical examination. Reported symptoms of Tullio phenomenon or Valsalva-associated vertigo and a positive fistula sign are specific, although insensitive, findings for TMWD and should prompt further consideration of this diagnosis. Furthermore, high-resolution non-contrasted computed tomography of the temporal bone should be carefully examined for dehiscence of inner ear structures, particularly in the region of the surgical site. Results of audiologic and vestibular testing should be interpreted with consideration of the effects of the patient's pre-existing otologic pathology.

Case Example

Case Details

A 50-year-old woman presented for evaluation of left-sided hearing loss and non-pulsatile tinnitus. She had undergone a left stapedectomy 25 years prior for presumed otosclerosis which had improved her hearing at the time. She had since had progressive left-sided hearing loss for 10 years. Audiologic examination revealed a moderate mixed hearing loss on the left side with a Carhart notch present and an air-bone gap of approximately 30 dB. She underwent a middle ear exploration, during which the prosthesis was found to have migrated out of the oval window, which had re-obliterated. A new stapedotomy was created and a new piston was placed.

Following surgery, she reported an improvement in her left-sided non-pulsatile tinnitus and hearing loss. However, she reported new symptoms of autophony, pulsatile tinnitus, and hyperacusis on the left. A repeat audiogram revealed persistent but improved primarily low-frequency conductive hearing loss, with an air-bone gap of approximately 15 dB. VEMP testing revealed ocular VEMPs with increased amplitudes and decreased thresholds and symmetrical cervical VEMPs. A computed tomography scan of the temporal bone was performed, and a representative section is shown in Fig. 26.3. The patient subsequently underwent a transmastoid plugging of the left superior semicircular canal which resulted in resolution of her pulsatile tinnitus, autophony, and hyperacusis.

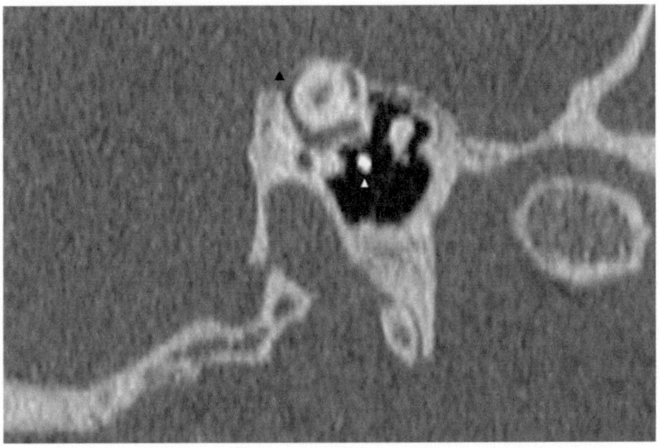

Fig. 26.3 Non-contrasted Stenvers view computed tomography of the left ear, revealing a dehiscent superior semicircular canal (black arrow). The stapes prosthesis was visualized (white arrow) and was in adequate position in the vestibule

Case Discussion

This patient had true left otosclerosis which was initially surgically treated 25 years ago with subsequent prosthesis displacement. Her oval window sealed off again resulting in recurrent conductive hearing loss. Presumably, she developed a dehiscence of the superior semicircular canal in the intervening time. Upon revision stapedotomy, the opening of the oval window unmasked her superior semicircular canal dehiscence syndrome, resulting in characteristic acoustic symptoms of hyperacusis and autophony. As with this patient, patients with unmasked TMWD following stapes surgery can usually be treated with standard transmastoid or middle cranial fossa repair of the superior canal dehiscence with excellent results.

Conclusions

Iatrogenic third window phenomena can occur after a multitude of otologic and neurotologic procedures, including stapes surgery, surgery for cholesteatoma and chronic ear disease, and lateral skull base surgery. The resultant bony dehiscence can be located anywhere in the inner ear, including the labyrinth, vestibule and cochlea. Many postoperative vestibular syndromes which have been known for decades have been attributed to third window phenomena since the discovery of SCDS, leading to significant strides in our ability to treat these conditions. Over the next several decades, further discoveries in the field of TWMD may illuminate additional conditions and treatments for patients with these complex disorders.

References

1. Rottach KG, von Maydell RD, DiScenna AO, et al. Quantitative measurements of eye movements in a patient with Tullio phenomenon. J Vestib Res. 1996;6:255–9.
2. Vogel P, Tackmann W, Schmidt FJ. Observations on the Tullio phenomenon. J Neurol. 1986;233:136–9. https://doi.org/10.1007/bf00314417.
3. Moffat DA, Gray RF, Irving RM. Mastoid obliteration using bone pâté. Clin Otolaryngol Allied Sci. 1994;19:149–57. https://doi.org/10.1111/j.1365-2273.1994.tb01201.x.
4. Seltzer S, McCabe BF. Perilymph fistula: the Iowa experience. Laryngoscope. 1986;96:37–49. https://doi.org/10.1288/00005537-198601000-00007.
5. Hornibrook J. Perilymph fistula: fifty years of controversy. ISRN Otolaryngol. 2012;2012:281248. https://doi.org/10.5402/2012/281248.
6. Atacan E, Sennaroglu L, Genc A, et al. Benign paroxysmal positional vertigo after stapedectomy. Laryngoscope. 2001;111:1257–9. https://doi.org/10.1097/00005537-200107000-00021.
7. Mandalà M, Colletti L, Carner M, et al. Pneumolabyrinth and positional vertigo after stapedectomy. Auris Nasus Larynx. 2011;38:547–50. https://doi.org/10.1016/j.anl.2010.12.010.
8. Toirkens JP, Kelders WPA. Intravestibular stapes prosthesis protrusion causing post stapedectomy vertigo. J Belg Soc Radiol. 2015;99:92–4. https://doi.org/10.5334/jbr-btr.951.
9. Farrior J, Sutherland A. Revision stapes surgery. Laryngoscope. 1991;101:1155–61. https://doi.org/10.1288/00005537-199111000-00003.
10. Vincent R, Rovers M, Zingade N, et al. Revision stapedotomy: operative findings and hearing results. A prospective study of 652 cases from the Otology-Neurotology Database. Otol Neurotol. 2010;31:875–82. https://doi.org/10.1097/MAO.0b013e3181e8f1da.
11. Ozüer MZ, Olgun L, Gültekin G. Revision stapes surgery. Otolaryngol Head Neck Surg. 2012;146:109–13. https://doi.org/10.1177/0194599811423523.
12. Lesinski SG. Causes of conductive hearing loss after stapedectomy or stapedotomy: a prospective study of 279 consecutive surgical revisions. Otol Neurotol. 2002;23:281–8. https://doi.org/10.1097/00129492-200205000-00009.
13. Lin KF, Selesnick S. Stapedotomy with adipose tissue seal: hearing outcomes, incidence of sensorineural hearing loss, and comparison to alternative techniques. Otol Neurotol. 2016;37:851–8. https://doi.org/10.1097/mao.0000000000001117.
14. Wiet RJ, Battista RA, Wiet RM, et al. Hearing outcomes in stapes surgery: a comparison of fat, fascia, and vein tissue seals. Otolaryngol Head Neck Surg. 2013;148:115–20. https://doi.org/10.1177/0194599812463184.
15. Huy PTB. Physiopathology of peripheral non-Menière's vestibular disorders. Acta Otolaryngol Suppl. 1994;513:5–10. https://doi.org/10.3109/00016489409127320.
16. Gadre AK, Edwards IR, Baker VM, et al. Membranous or hypermobile stapes footplate: a new anatomic site resulting in third window syndrome. Front Neurol. 2020;11:871. https://doi.org/10.3389/fneur.2020.00871.
17. Hope A, Fagan P. Latent superior canal dehiscence syndrome unmasked by stapedotomy for otosclerosis. J Laryngol Otol. 2010;124:428–30. https://doi.org/10.1017/s0022215109991654.
18. Pritchett CV, Spector ME, Kileny PR, et al. Surgical treatment of hearing loss when otosclerosis coexists with superior semicircular canal dehiscence syndrome. Otol Neurotol. 2014;35:1163–7. https://doi.org/10.1097/mao.0000000000000470.
19. Sheehy JL, Brackmann DE. Cholesteatoma surgery: management of the labyrinthine fistula--a report of 97 cases. Laryngoscope. 1979;89:78–87. https://doi.org/10.1288/00005537-197901000-00008.
20. Fowler J, Dhaliwal S, Parnes LS. Congenital cholesteatoma of the mastoid causing posterior semicircular canal dehiscence. Otol Neurotol. 2019;40:e56–7. https://doi.org/10.1097/mao.0000000000002053.
21. Moon IS, Kwon MO, Park CY, et al. Surgical management of labyrinthine fistula in chronic otitis media with cholesteatoma. Auris Nasus Larynx. 2012;39:261–4. https://doi.org/10.1016/j.anl.2011.06.002.

22. Chao YH, Yun SH, Shin JO, et al. Cochlear fistula in chronic otitis media with cholesteatoma. Am J Otolaryngol. 1996;17:15–8.
23. Chen Z, Dongzhen, Wu Y, et al. Surgical treatment of labyrinthine fistula caused by cholesteatoma with semicircular canal occlusion. Acta Otolaryngol. 2010;130:75–8. https://doi.org/10.3109/00016480902875083.
24. Blake P, Morrissey G. Canal wall down techniques for managing cholesteatoma. Aust N Z J Surg. 1991;61:914–8. https://doi.org/10.1111/j.1445-2197.1991.tb00009.x.
25. Hakuba N, Hato N, Shinomori Y, et al. Labyrinthine fistula as a late complication of middle ear surgery using the canal wall down technique. Otol Neurotol. 2002;23:832–5. https://doi.org/10.1097/00129492-200211000-00003.
26. Ben-Shlomo N, Rahimi A, Abunimer AM, et al. Incidence of iatrogenic inner ear breaches from vestibular schwannoma surgery: a review of 1,153 hearing preservation approaches. J Neurol Surg B Skull Base. 2020;81(S 01):S1–S272. https://doi.org/10.1055/s-0040-1702361.
27. Bartholomew RA, Poe D, Dunn IF, et al. Iatrogenic inner ear dehiscence after lateral skull base surgery: therapeutic dilemma and treatment options. Otol Neurotol. 2019;40:e399–404. https://doi.org/10.1097/mao.0000000000002162.
28. Deep NL, Kay-Rivest E, Roland JT Jr. Iatrogenic third window after retrosigmoid approach to a vestibular schwannoma managed with cochlear implantation. Otol Neurotol. 2021;42:1355–9. https://doi.org/10.1097/mao.0000000000003267.
29. Kosty JA, Stevens SM, Gozal YM, et al. Middle fossa approach for resection of vestibular schwannomas: a decade of experience. Oper Neurosurg. 2019;16:147–58. https://doi.org/10.1093/ons/opy126.
30. Kiumehr S, Mahboubi H, Djalilian HR. Posterior semicircular canal dehiscence following endolymphatic sac surgery. Laryngoscope. 2012;122:2079–81. https://doi.org/10.1002/lary.23474.
31. Phillips DJ, Souter MA, Vitkovic J, et al. Diagnosis and outcomes of middle cranial fossa repair for patients with superior semicircular canal dehiscence syndrome. J Clin Neurosci. 2010;17:339–41. https://doi.org/10.1016/j.jocn.2009.06.021.
32. Silverstein H, Kartush JM, Parnes LS, et al. Round window reinforcement for superior semicircular canal dehiscence: a retrospective multi-center case series. Am J Otolaryngol. 2014;35:286–93. https://doi.org/10.1016/j.amjoto.2014.02.016.

Part V
From the Patient Perspective

Philippa Thomson

Introduction

It was in 2016 that I published a memoir of my experiences as a sufferer of bilateral SCDS [1]. The book covered the extreme difficulty I had in getting a diagnosis, the complexities encountered when it came to treatment and the very damaging effects of the condition during a substantial part of my life. I sincerely hoped back then that I would be one of the last patients with this disorder who had to endure such a horrendous time, but through maintaining contact with numerous patients of inner ear problems from around the world, it rapidly became clear to me that very little was improving for so many of these people. My bafflement turned to frustration, which then quite often switched to anger when I was told some of the stories. My drive to change the situation eventually led me to contact a commissioning editor at Springer, and here we are.

An isolated email from Kenneth in America came to me out of the blue one day, and its succinct message lodged in my mind: *I had botched surgery on my left superior semicircular canal. The doctor ignored my complaints until she realized I had a brain leak. She did the surgery again but my symptoms were worse than ever. I went to a doctor at another clinic and she completely removed my superior canal. I have imbalance, tinnitus, anxiety and possible SCDS in the right ear. The first doctor ruined my life. She never should have operated, because she had little experience with the condition. I just had to get this off my chest.* Of course we all know that things can go wrong in medicine, but a selection of personal stories gathered together by me in the next chapter present a snapshot of what patients with Third Mobile Window Syndrome are regularly up against. The vast majority experience difficulty obtaining a diagnosis—an accurate one that is—and there are countless cases of substandard care, overlooked symptoms and bureaucratic bungling. And for some there have been tragic consequences.

A nurse once suggested that to really 'get it', an inner ear disorder has to be lived and felt, minute by minute, hour by hour, for weeks to years on end [2]. Unfortunately it isn't possible for medical professionals to simply step into their patients' shoes, nor would we want them to have to, so the next best thing is to listen very carefully to the voices of patients, absorb their messages and then construct an action plan around them. First-person narratives can make a significant contribution to patient-centred care, and they invite an emotional response, engaging our curiosity and imagination. They are helpful for seeing patients as individuals, rather than lumped together as a group. There can often be a transformative power to storytelling, and it can act as an aid to informing service improvement and development. It ties in with the principles of evidence-based practice, by means of a three-pronged approach: personal stories increase the health professionals' understanding of the issues that affect patients; the stories reframe and refocus the priorities of care; and the accounts help to close the gap between human experience and theory.

Third Mobile Window Syndrome is an invisible condition. Unless someone is being physically sick as a result of it, or literally falling over or unable to stand, there are no outward signs of how incredibly unwell it is making a person feel. There is considerable variety and fluctuation in the presentation of symptoms, and the severity of the disorder is on a spectrum, ranging from manageable to completely debilitating. It can also involve hearing loss, which may increase isolation, something the London ear surgeon Jeremy Lavy has acknowledged: 'Hearing is so central to who we are. Of the five senses, I think it's probably the one we underestimate the most. What we have realised with hearing problems is it isolates you incredibly socially' [3].

These facts make the job of dealing with the illness even harder, and the need for understanding from others even greater. Communication and trust between doctor and patient become paramount, and establishing a clear medical history has to be a collaborative process. Lisa Sanders has described it as being like 'two writers collaborating on a manuscript, passing drafts of the story back and forth until both are satisfied. What the patient brings to the process is unique: the particular and private facts of his life and illness. And what the physician brings is the knowledge and understanding that will help him order that story, so that it makes sense both to the doctor and the patient' [4]. The depersonalising language and process of medicine need to be counteracted with kindness, openness and honesty, and when health professionals start to see the world as their patients are seeing it, the experience can inspire empathy.

A breach of trust can cause a patient to feel disempowered and isolated, and then a most important component, hope, starts to fade away too. The combined feelings of loneliness and uselessness ripple outwards as well, affecting family and friends, as the patient may become unable to work and fulfil responsibilities or enjoy their usual activities, and then depression and despair start to take hold. Stories of patients feeling dismissed are all too common with Third Mobile Window Syndrome—they frequently don't feel believed, they may be accused of overreacting, it's often suggested that their story is unlikely, and worst of all, they are told, 'It's all in your head'. In my own case, many doctors could not comprehend what was wrong with me and I was made to feel that was my fault somehow. Sympathy and understanding were sometimes in very short supply, and there was almost always insufficient time allowed at consultations.

Listening to patients' voices, and believing them, is just the start, as the challenge is then to employ the stories to correct and advance practice, and to truly position the patients at the centre of treatment. With any illness, 'the knowledge can be summarised as WHAT we do and HOW we do it. What we do is usually seen as being informed by the scientific evidence base; how we do it is informed by the sort of knowledge that comes from reflection on narrative' [5].

References

1. Thomson P. A hole in my life. Battling chronic dizziness. Createspace. 2016.
2. Haybach P. Inner ear balance and dizziness disorders. Booksurge, LLC. 2005.
3. Sanders L. Every patient tells a story. New York: Broadway Books; 2009.
4. Merriman H. Room 5: 8. Helena. BBC Sounds, Feb 15, 2022.
5. Buckley A, et al. Patient narratives 1: using patient stories to reflect on care. Nurs Times. 2016;112(10):22–5.

Chapter 27
Patient Stories

Philippa Thomson

When Despair Sets In

In October 2017, **Kelvin Edmunds** went missing from his home near Cardiff, in Wales. His body was discovered a few days later about 20 miles away, in Cwmbach woods, near where he used to play as a young boy. He had taken his own life at the age of 61.

As a young man in the 1970s and 1980s Kelvin had been an aspiring guitarist and toured all over the place in a band called *Ohibo Paronti*. Ian Davies, the drummer who had known him since school, described Kelvin as 'such an outgoing guy who could turn his hand to anything.' Stardom in the music world never materialised and Kelvin moved abroad for a while to work, but the band members always kept in touch. 'By the late 90s, he just wasn't the same bloke', said Ian. 'He was having terrible trouble with his hearing, but none of us realised how bad it was. He couldn't function properly at all.' Kelvin had eventually been diagnosed with SCDS and the condition was making him hypersensitive to sound. 'He resorted to putting tissues in his ears to muffle exterior sounds. Everywhere he went he just couldn't escape it. Imagine being able to hear your own eyeballs moving from side to side in your head and your heart beating.' Some of the details recalled by Ian and another close friend, Jon, remain hazy but they agree that a surgery was undertaken in the UK. It didn't relieve the torture, however, and over a number of years Kelvin's mental health deteriorated dramatically. Kelvin made an unsuccessful suicide attempt earlier in 2017 and then voluntarily admitted himself to a psychiatric unit. Sadly, it wasn't enough to save his life.

Any loss of life that can be avoided is lamentable, but Kelvin is far from the only person to have contemplated this means of escape from Third Mobile Window

P. Thomson (✉)
North Berwick, East Lothian, UK

G. J. Gianoli, P. Thomson (eds.), *Third Mobile Window Syndrome of the Inner Ear*, https://doi.org/10.1007/978-3-031-16586-3_27

Syndrome. And the fact is, we have no way of knowing how many other people may have resorted to taking their own lives for this reason. Another UK patient, **David**, shot himself in the head in a fit of depression in 2015, but has fortunately survived to tell the tale. ‘I’m 56 now and I first experienced strange symptoms in 2000, when I was 35. They began after some strenuous bedroom antics followed by an intense migraine-like headache. My GP was concerned it may be a stroke or aneurysm, and so the rollercoaster ride began. It took almost eight years to finally diagnose me. Being his first SCDS op, my surgeon should have done more research and actually read the medical journal article that helped a junior audiologist figure out what my condition was. Secondly, the surgeon should agree a procedure with the patient and then stick to the plan … not change his damn mind en route to theatre when his patient is already out for the count. I was to undergo a mid fossa approach and it was only several months later I was told by a registrar that the doctor had changed his mind and gone in transmastoid. I was left with 90% deafness on the operated side, and raging tinnitus. In 2014, pushing a fully laden wheelbarrow up a plank while working on my kitchen extension, I experienced an intense headache and major dizziness. To circumvent the long-winded referral process, I paid privately for an MRI and to see the same surgeon again. He sat me and my wife down in front of a screen and joyfully pointed out where his original repair had failed, insisting he must re-repair it before he would consider a procedure on my right side dehiscence.’

‘Carnage ensued,’ reports David. ‘It was only after I later began my legal case that I obtained my full medical records, wherein I found a radiologist’s report of March 2015, which stated the MRI showed a right side dehiscence and evidence of a previous left side repair which remained fully intact. It was the arrogance and reckless indifference displayed by my surgeon, resulting in me needing six operations instead of two, that drove me to suicide. Once inside my skull the second time, seeing the repair was intact, he decided (without my consent) to obliterate my left superior canal. Unfortunately he also mostly destroyed the other two canals and saccule, and damaged the utricle. All this caused major depression and PTSD, and ultimately cost me my career, my marriage, my home and my future.’ It was a different surgeon who in 2016 successfully undertook a right side resurfacing for David, ‘following a complete raft of testing, the like of which I’d never had before.’

Despair felt by patients can be caused by a variety of factors, but for **Joanne** in Canada it also resulted from mishandled surgery. ‘I have bilateral SCDS. The vestibular system was completely destroyed during surgery on one side. I lost most of my hearing on that side as well. I have struggled so much with my condition and have resigned myself to the fact that this is my lot in life. I cannot explain to anyone (maybe my husband) how I feel. I will never seek sympathy but I do feel quite alone in this battle. It actually feels good to explain myself—thanks for listening.’ **Suzanne** in New York was diagnosed with bilateral SCDS in 2021, after being misdiagnosed with Ménière’s disease for four years, but ‘the ENT physician did not advise surgery’, she explained. ‘He said to get different hearing aids and try

Klonopin. I have severe hearing loss, horrible tinnitus and hyperacusis, and I hear my heartbeat in my left ear. I feel like my life is falling apart—I can hardly work, my marriage is strained and I find myself isolating because it is really difficult to enjoy anything because of the hearing loss and distortion.'

Fernando in Spain 'has been suffering for many years, and now I'm on a waiting list for surgery in a public hospital. It's been two years so far and I really don't know how I can continue like this. Sometimes I think I may be better off dead than to have to live with this condition.' **Anil's** situation in India is even worse. 'I am 45 now and my symptoms started at the age of 42. I have been diagnosed with SCDS in my left ear but I'm still not able to find a specialist who does these surgeries in India. Life has changed completely for me having this disorder. Patients like us need family support, medical support and financial assistance. In India, people also seem to find it hard to understand what I am going through, and that applies even to my family. I'm no longer able to lead an active professional or social life, and yet going to America for an operation is a very difficult proposition, both financially and logistically.'

For **Rob**, in the UK, 'life has stopped.' He expounds: 'I'm 54, slim, and up until two years ago I ran 20 miles a week. Out running one day I became dizzy and unsteady on my feet. I had a CT scan, two MRI scans and a neck MRI, and I've seen three ENT doctors. I can hear my neck creaking, there's screaming tinnitus and a full feeling of pressure in my left ear. I am at my wit's end, nobody seems able to help. It's gone on for so long, I've now got anxiety stepping in. I can get out of bed sometimes to go for a short walk or make tea, but I have to sit on the barstool. I'm in a bit of a mess. I'm in tears as I write this.' **Rita**, a woman in her sixties living in New York, also wants her life back. The insensitivity of doctors and dismissal of her concerns have worn her down. 'My odyssey began six years ago when I ignored pressure from exercise headaches. I was initially diagnosed with an ear infection, but I did finally visit another ENT who carried out some tests and informed me I had lost significant hearing on my left side. Within a couple of months I was experiencing low level 24/7 dizziness, anxiety, vision problems, nausea, brain fog and a feeling of unwellness. This started my journey to find a diagnosis and I saw eight top specialists in NYC. They either didn't believe me or, when they did, they diagnosed me as having Ménière's disease. A neurologist referred me to a psychiatrist and prescribed Xanax! Because these doctors saw me as functioning, they dismissed the severity of my symptoms. After about 18 months I was referred to another doctor who, without testing, indicated I probably had a perilymph fistula and undertook a procedure. But the dizziness never really went away, in fact it has worsened. The doctor has basically moved on from me and has pretty much told me that since I am still working I should be able to live with the problem. I do continue to go to work every day because if I didn't I would probably just sit on the couch and cry. I know this, because that is what I do most weekends.'

The Psychological Impact

Michael in America doesn't mince his words: 'SCDS is literally an indescribable torture. And that's coming from a fellow who was once told by his physician he'd probably die of appendicitis due to his high threshold of pain. The psychological aspect, in my honest opinion, is the most oppressive part. I only recently started to feel I was free of that, and that was one and half years after my surgery. It was a cross-country flight when I was 54 that was the tipping point. During the trip I told my wife, "I need to go to the ER, but I honestly wouldn't know how to describe what's wrong with me." Over time, as none of the tests showed any specific issues, during one of the ER visits I was held in isolation from my family to be seen by a psychiatrist, who tried to tie it all to PTSD and depression. I knew it wasn't those issues, so I continued to fight to find out what was going on—and keep in mind, the symptoms are partly why it is hard to identify SCDS, as you just can't think straight. It wasn't until making a phone call one day that I noticed the pulse tone during the ringing was causing my field of vision to correspondingly vibrate. That was my epiphany.'

Joanne in Canada developed an issue with her heart beating in her right ear in 2018, but in 2021 was still no further forward in getting relief, despite an ENT doctor having informed her she 'had a hole in her ear.' His advice was 'to visit a psychiatrist and talk about living with this condition, as there is no fix and it will continue until your heart stops beating. He could/should have been kinder', she remarked. 'Sometimes I feel like I'm losing my mind with the noise. And during this period with pulsatile tinnitus, I can't seem to read anything and absorb it.' Her niece has been a vital support in this respect.

The struggle and horribly prolonged length of time to get a diagnosis is a constant refrain among TMWS patients. For **Philippa** in New Zealand, it took 'about 20 years, and during that time I was accused of all sorts of things—panic disorder, Ménière's, imaginitis, viral labyrinthitis, putting it on!! When I look back over my life, I'm pretty sure I've been dealing with symptoms throughout it.' For **Jeff** in America, the journey took 10 years, and it all started with a scuba dive in Hawaii in 2003. 'I had made several hundred dives up to this point and never had any problems. This time I heard a loud pop when clearing my ears and instantly got very dizzy. By the time I saw an ENT I had a number of symptoms—dizziness when hearing loud sounds, hearing my own heartbeat, a deafening noise when eating crunchy foods—but he quickly dismissed them, and I went home disappointed as I knew there was something wrong.' Over subsequent years, four more ENT doctors were visited but his bilateral SCDS diagnosis remained out of reach: 'My perception is that most doctors exit medical school and never learn anything new. Fortunately, I eventually found one exceptional doctor who's not that way.' At one point, Jeff had even seen a cardiologist 'because I was hearing very irregular heartbeats and it scared me into thinking there was something wrong there too. The cardiologist found nothing abnormal and asked what I was hearing. I described the rhythm and skipping of beats so he hooked me up to the EKG, and asked me to raise my finger every time I heard a skipped beat. After a minute of doing that, the doctor rolled his chair over and said quietly, "I want to hear ALL about this SCDS!" Apparently the heartbeat I was hearing was perfectly normal, but no one ever hears that without a stethoscope.'

Alice in America, now 57, 'saw close to 30 doctors and had probably twice as many tests—it was awful. No matter what they told me, I know myself and I knew something was wrong. I knew I wouldn't give up until I figured it out—being blown off, not taken seriously, being misdiagnosed, thinking cancer would be easier, the despair creeping in, and taking time out as I knew if yet another doctor dismissed me I may not be able to get back up. August 2015 was when it all began but with no known trigger.' Alice now knows she has SCDS, perilymph fistula, a Chiari malformation and increased cranial pressure, as she eventually found her way to a physician with extensive SCDS experience.

Paul in the UK is 55, and started having major ear trouble in his teens, so he has 'suffered for nearly 40 years and been diagnosed with just about every ear disorder going. When I've mentioned SCDS to ENT "specialists" I almost get laughed at, and one even intimated that there was no such disease. I remember having a form of tinnitus at a young age and I recall asking my mam why pictures on the wall would move from time to time. I clearly remember the first full dizzy bout at the age of 18, but I couldn't figure out a trigger. I was on a building site, as a plumber by trade, and it was an awful experience.' Paul's symptoms have recently progressed further and on top of the pounding heartbeat, he's experiencing whooshing tinnitus, deafness, disequilibrium and a considerable amount of stress. But he's yet to be given a firm diagnosis. The focus for medical professionals surely needs to be on how individuals such as Paul have fallen through the cracks—either through seeing clinicians who have concluded they are crazy, or by the lack of a referral on to someone who may be able to provide the answer. Far too many are ending up in limbo.

A Diagnostic Maze

Graham's experiences in the UK have been easier, but it still took a long time for him to be diagnosed. He is 48 now and estimates the main symptoms began when he was about 34, although he does recall 'when a teenager, having a problem with my dad in the garden, bending over doing work for a bit and feeling very light-headed on getting up. That happened several times. I have always wondered whether a car accident in 1997 was the significant trigger, when a car ran into me from behind and I hit my head on the rear view mirror and had mild concussion. After that I started to have problems with getting words muddled up, although it was another few years before the autophony developed, and hearing my eyes move.' Graham's profession is as a librarian and in the end it was his own research skills that led to his discovery about SCDS. Before that 'a local ENT decided to insert grommets, and when that didn't work, he wanted me to take anti-depressants. Not for depression, but to numb the nerves in my head to relieve the symptoms. That's when I decided to go off on my own research journey.'

Carolyn in America has reached the age of 83, but it was a fall back in 1980 that kicked off the dizzy spells. 'I went to 12 different doctors and spent $15,000 worth of tests to find out what was wrong. The doctors were still scratching their heads and telling me nothing was wrong with me. But I had so many symptoms, and they would not go away unless I was lying down. I was working full time as a nurse so I would get off work from night shift, lay down, get up to make meals, lay down again until it was time to get up to go back to work. Things became so bad that I ended up in the emergency department for three days and nights, but two weeks later the doctor dismissed me and released me back to work, with just some Valium to take.' Regular visits to a dentist and oral surgeon resulted in treatment for TMJ, but things deteriorated further after another fall in 2008 and then a flight in 2011 caused a very sharp pain in Carolyn's left ear. It wasn't until 2018 that the root of her problems was at long last unmasked. 'I noticed that I was hearing my voice louder in my right ear than before the crown work on my teeth had been started. I was often being told by my husband that I talked too softly whereas I thought I was yelling my way through many years. I visited a new ear doctor and he ordered the CT scan to check for SCDS. Sure enough, it turned out I have that.'

Ian in Canada 'wishes he had found online communities for support sooner, given how confusing and disorienting my condition of SCDS has been. It took 2+ years of being misdiagnosed with BPPV, Ménière's and other things before being referred to a vestibular clinic.' Ian is 48 and his symptoms began when he was about 44. 'I feel that I put a great deal of burden onto my family and friends. They've all been amazingly supportive, but I do feel the burden that I've created.' If a diagnosis is not only delayed but continues to be unattainable, all the negative effects are ramped up for the patient. **Maxine** has seen 'so many doctors with the diagnosis just of anxiety. I can hear internal bodily sounds, my neck, spine and jaw vibrating in my ears very loudly, and the sound of my eyes moving loudly when I'm in a quiet room. Occasionally I have ringing in my ears and hearing my heartbeat, and I constantly feel out of sorts. I'm sometimes very dizzy, and my hearing can be really sensitive to sounds such as when my partner puts his keys in the door. I feel as though I can't go to the doctors any more. That they are getting fed up with me.'

It's a situation not far removed from **Cindy's** in Canada. 'I ended up seeing an ENT who had treated SCDS before. He was horribly patronising and treated me as if I was hoping for this diagnosis, when it was my neurologist who suggested that diagnosis in the first place. No one has really been able to settle on a diagnosis. I am 59 years old and first noticed symptoms after flying with a cold in the fall of 2017. After that flight the symptoms really escalated. For me, something which is quite distressing is that I'm having trouble finding words. I stumble along and finally get it, but I'm a nurse and it's very embarrassing at work when I'm talking to patients.' **Andrea** in America is having an equally difficult time. 'I'm 47, I don't know if I have SCDS. So many tests but with all of those tests, nobody can truly figure it out. It makes me very sad, I feel alone, and I sort of feel like a hypochondriac when I try to explain what I feel. So I don't even tell my husband anymore … he thinks everything I feel is an excuse. Some days, or even weeks, are good, but most aren't. I have those days where everything is just OFF. My mind does not work, I can't see things clearly. I can't find my words or concentrate. I'm dizzy, nauseous; I vomit, or at least dry heave, many mornings. I notice it even more when I leave the house—just walking down the aisles in the grocery store is horrible. I told my neurologist that there are days I feel I can't drive. And he just said, "So don't drive." It's a helpless feeling that no one can even comprehend.'

The Knock-Backs

Some of the responses that patients receive are astonishing. Take **Barb** in America. 'I'm having issues with ringing in the ears, light sensitivity, whooshing sounds at times with different head positions. I've also got sensorineural hearing loss. I feel like I'm floating, unable to tolerate stores and busy places, and at times it feels like things are moving while I'm still. I feel out of sorts, I have noise intolerance, I get sharp pains in my ears, and am unable to have anything at all blowing in my ear. Now when I try doing certain things like bending frequently, I get dizzy. And some days I actually feel even confused. A CT scan was undertaken and showed thinning of the bone consistent with SCDS. The doctors at a major medical institution said I was making up my symptoms and since I could not hear my eyes move, I did not have it. I am at my wit's end. I need help.' **Mel** in Australia has been led to conclude 'the only way to get information is to research it yourself, as the majority of the medical fraternity seem not to look any further than the end of their nose. I'm 49 and I've had a lifetime of migraines with aura, sinusitis, ear infections and most recently vertigo attacks. I have thought I was going a little nutty, in that nothing was ever really clearly a specific diagnosis for all my years of misery. In 2021 the otolaryngologist told me that he can't do anything to help me. I have more than one factor at play and as he doesn't know precisely what is causing the vertigo, I have to learn to live with it.'

In many of the cases it is hardly surprising how low expectations fall when it comes to what ENT physicians will do to provide help. **Frank's** first appointment in America with an ENT doctor 'was pretty much a waste of time, except for the fact that she gave me the option to have an MRI. At a follow up appointment with her after the scan, I discovered she had no idea what SCDS was and really didn't seem very interested. I learned more from the internet than I did from her.' He was diagnosed with bilateral SCDS by a different doctor in 2019, at the age of 62.

Two women in Canada have had the unenviable task of trying to convince medical professionals that something had gone seriously awry, after each of them had fallen and hit their heads. **Cheryl**, a nurse aged 60, hit her head on the right side behind the ear, and from that moment all her symptoms started. 'It is one of the most frustrating things when you have to do your own research and then convince specialists to listen to you. I just didn't trust that my doctor told me it was stress and would go away. I didn't have that stress the day before I hit my head, and I did not have the sounds either. Now I hear my eyes moving, my footsteps, I hear my chewing, my pulse, and I get dizziness after reading for a while.'

Caroline, age 38, started experiencing symptoms when she was 28. She is very keen for her story to be heard. 'I fell on a concrete floor and lost consciousness, hitting my head very badly at the back of it. From that day, I became really sick. Many people said to me that it was traumatic brain injury, concussion, or post-concussion syndrome. I made no progress at the rehabilitation center and then the diagnosis arrived: invalidity for work at 31 years old! No, no, I did not accept that. I was upset, tired, confused. I was not able to improve from this traumatic brain injury and nobody could explain why. I want to open the eyes of many people who thought this was all in my head. Yes, it was in my head, but it was not somatic, psychological or whatever, it was a physical problem. Years later, seven years later, I was given the hypothesis of SCDS. It was a doctor with significant expertise in this field who explained to me that when someone is not able to recover from brain injury, they can expect the possibility of SCDS. That possibility had been removed far too quickly in the earlier stages. I always had good hearing and so others thought it was not possible that I had SCDS. And yet it proved to be bilateral. It was a long hard road for me with many trials and failures, and I'm sad because I'm sure there are patients out there who give up early, because they find few people believe in them.'

Don, aged 63, who is only on Medicaid in America, has almost given up hope of receiving treatment as his insurer will not pay for him to go out of state. 'My frustration has been great as my struggle to get answers finally resulted in a CT scan that found bilateral dehiscence. However, since then I have been told that my symptoms are not from the dehiscence. They include constant noise, bad head days, brain fog, extreme fatigue, standing spins, pressure in my head and the feeling that there is a low voltage shorted wire in my brain. On bad days I feel like my voice is in my head, but the ENT told me that it would not come and go, it would always be like that if it was SCDS. This last year the hissing sound has gotten worse and the other symptoms seem to be mounting. I think it was my move to the mountains. The weather changes often and there's a lot of rain. My work is also very physical and with a few days of heavy lifting, my head feels as though it is about to explode. The only cure I have found is rest.'

Theresa, also in America, considers her symptoms mild in comparison with many others, but she nevertheless 'has hearing loss and a real loss in processing abilities. Sometimes my brain simply can't understand what my ears are hearing. I have brain fog, tinnitus, pulsatile tinnitus and hyperacusis.' Nothing in particular happened to cause an uptick in her symptoms, some of which started at a very young age, but by 2014 'I had lost a job due to my brain fog, and by 2016 I no longer felt comfortable working outside of my home.' She is now 60 and was diagnosed with SCDS in 2019. 'It took many years to finally diagnose the issue and in the meantime I was misdiagnosed and told it was all in my head. That was one of the most difficult things—medical professionals just simply not believing me and chalking it up to anxiety. Anxiety seems to be the catch-all term for doctors when they can't work out the problem. It seems hard for them to admit they don't have the answer and instead they put the blame on an elusive anxiety diagnosis. I can't begin to tell you how many times this has happened to me. Being diagnosed was like a breath of fresh air and I so badly wanted to wave it in the faces of all the physicians that had told me it was just my imagination. It was the dismissive nature of a lot of physicians that was one of my biggest issues.'

Lewis is 43 and resides in the UK. His obstacle relates to the sparsity of expertise in the field. 'I started experiencing pretty minor tinnitus at about 30 years of age, then out of the blue it got much louder about 10 or 11 years later. Since then I have been unable to get on top of it. Slowly but surely I have had tests and scans, and thus far they have interpreted the results as suggesting that the tinnitus is likely due to either the high riding jugular bulb on that side, and/or very thin bone forming the posterior semicircular canal, and/or the very thin bone between the mastoid and the right sigmoid bone. On my last visit, I spoke to a young lady who is very pleasant but rather early on in her training, and not clued up about issues of bone thinning and dehiscence. I hold out hope that there might be a possible surgical intervention, but if it is possible it would almost certainly only be available in the US.'

Affliction at a Young Age

Age isn't the determining factor either, as **Sam** in New Zealand knows only too well. He was just 29 when he was diagnosed with SCDS on the right side. 'I'd had anxiety and some brain fog for about three years but then I took a long haul flight and as soon as I landed my right ear was blocked. Over the next 12 months I had fatigue and headaches along with the continuation of the brain fog. I was a fit gym guy doing lots of weight lifting, so maybe the bone thinned during those five years. I feel so, so unwell with this. My life is on hold. I lost my job and house.' **Ulfur**, who lives in Norway, was a mere 11 years of age when severe dizziness turned his life upside down in 2010. He was hospitalised in Norway to undergo a battery of medical tests and the first diagnosis was a virus affecting his balance nerve. Two weeks later Ulfur was worse, not better as the doctors had predicted, and one evening after a bath he deteriorated significantly and was developing vision problems. More tests in hospital followed, and a hole was even drilled in the young boy's head in an effort to release pressure from a suspected CSF leak. His mother Arna describes the extent of her son's suffering: 'He couldn't even sit up to eat, brush his teeth, take a sip of water or read. Light and sound bothered him greatly and he was disengaged.' A CT scan was eventually undertaken, and SCDS identified. Very fortunately for Ulfur, the Norwegian healthcare system allows for treatment abroad if it cannot be provided appropriately at home, and he was flown all the way to Louisiana for surgery. 'The recovery was miraculous. The day after surgery he sat up, then stood up and walked. It was almost biblical', said Arna.

McKenzee, a determined young woman in Canada, was diagnosed as a teenager 'but it took five years .... five painful years. I feel like my first, regular doctor treated it as a joke and put it all down to puberty and hormones, but the majority of the doctors did try very hard and they truly had no clue what was going on. I feel like it is a lack of education, as I wasn't following the textbook in terms of age and symptoms. Many medications for my brain were tried and also for depression and anxiety. Then I was tested for POTS, and next for seizures manifesting as dizziness. After all those results were negative, I was referred to a cardiologist, and again I was told I was "normal" and told to go home. I was still complaining of dizziness, so the doctors essentially told me I was crazy and sent me to a psychologist, where I was told it was "all in my head". I was at a point where I was taking eight Gravol a day, and sleeping maybe 2 h a night, with multiple anxiety attacks. I begged them to try more things as I could not spend my life like that. It was my mother's insistence that made them finally send me to an ear specialist. He actually said, "I bet my career that you don't have this rare condition called SCDS", and wasn't going to do any testing, except we pleaded with him. That is how I was diagnosed.' It seems important to reflect on McKenzee's summing up of her situation: 'I can't even explain how alone I felt. If it was not for my family, I would not be here. I would be lying if I said I didn't think about taking my life. I was on the low priority list for the doctors because I was a "young healthy girl". I didn't have an obvious tumor and I wasn't dying, so I feel I was overlooked. Another thing that was very difficult is that people did not believe me, so they would always say "well, you don't look sick, you look fine". It was so frustrating that no one believed me.'

Max, also in Canada, had the same feeling that 'doctors and ENT specialists disregarded my statements about the weird plethora of symptoms I was experiencing.' He is now 39 and was eventually diagnosed with bilateral SCDS but 'for a long time the doctors I encountered seemed to belittle, or be misinformed on SCDS, or any health issues related to my symptoms. They seemed totally ok about taking another five years before coming up with a diagnosis. I'm also getting sick of trying to educate "specialists" who don't want to hear my "crazy" talk about hearing my eyes move. I'm a professional musician and singer, which makes me even more aware of sounds. Anyone with autophony can feel like they are losing their mind, so imagine the pain I deal with every day being a musician. But the go-to response from doctors is "well you're a musician, no wonder you have ear problems"—basically saying it's me, the fool musician who turns up his amp too loud. But I was one of the musicians in my circle who took way more care than the average. I wore ear plugs frequently and I was very focused on playing at a safe volume at shows. My voice is loud, I hear my heartbeat during physical activity, I hear my eyes move, and my footsteps when I walk. And then a new symptom was a sudden loss of hearing, weirdly enough while I was at a spa, in a super quiet setting. All the high frequencies and clarity have diminished to a point where I may need a hearing aid.' Blaming noise exposure as the cause of hypersensitive hearing/hyperacusis is completely the opposite of what is actually known about noise-induced hearing loss. Musicians such as Max are *less* sensitive to sound than others, not more sensitive.

Deciding on Surgery

For the patients who obtain a TMWS diagnosis, it is very important that the surgical options are accurately explained to them, along with the pros and cons, depending on their own particular symptoms and their severity. This certainly does not happen as a matter of course, and scare stories abound too. **Cheri** in Canada is 54 and has been living with her varied and fluctuating SCDS symptoms since her late 20s. 'Based on what my ENT told me and reading up on the outcomes possibly not working, and even making a person worse, I wouldn't get the surgery. If I became completely debilitated and did not have any quality of life, my decision may be a different one.' **Jane** was diagnosed relatively quickly with bilateral SCDS, but only offered a craniotomy as her surgical option. 'I'm a nurse, I know that a lot can go wrong in surgery, especially with a craniotomy, but I wasn't told about the trans-mastoid approach. At this time I'm trying to just tolerate my symptoms day to day, but there are periods when I think I really can't handle them any more. I still have a young child; I want at least a near normal life.' **Shannon** in Australia is not 'planning on having surgery anytime soon, because I am too scared. I wouldn't want to risk being in a worse condition than I am now, as my wife and I are trying to start a family. My doctor explained to me that I should only consider surgery if I felt it was absolutely necessary. He explained the risks, as well as the recovery aspect, and possible follow up surgery if something wasn't done right the first time.' Shannon is now 43 and admits her condition 'has really changed me as a person. I've tried to explain SCDS to my employer, staff and friends and I feel like it gets brushed off really easily, as though what I'm going through doesn't sound bad. But in fact it really is bad, when you live with it day by day—it's life changing.'

Sarah in America is another musician for whom bilateral SCDS brought a career, as a violinist, to an end—in her case at the age of 48. Her symptoms crept into her life over time, as she explains: 'I kept finding ways to blame myself for what was happening. Many doctors thought I was just highly-strung and stressed out. After my diagnosis, I realized I had to reinterpret the previous 14 years with this new knowledge. I had accepted depression, pain, anxiety, insecurity and hypersensitivity as par for the course. Ever-increasing anxiety was easily attributable to unresolved psychological issues from my past, and I only learned recently that anxiety is a very common symptom for people with vestibular disorders. Violinists often suffer from tension, especially neck and back pain, so there was no way for me to know that pain from playing was being compounded by pain from my condition. It's now evident that I was combating sensory overload and a collapsed tolerance to everyday noises, as well as the panic response that is hard-wired into the brain to guard against imbalance. By 2016, my condition had progressed to the point that I was crying through concerts and falling over after them, and then throughout the day. I think about how my heart raced and I wanted to forcibly stop certain colleagues from bludgeoning me with sound from their instruments. How I felt as though I either couldn't hear myself when the music was loud, or I was convinced I was bellowing atop the rest of the orchestra when it was soft. There was a feeling of not just losing my confidence, more like losing my mind.' Sarah, who is now 52, is holding off from surgery, largely because she is concerned that her migraines are not well controlled, but she does also worry that her consultant may not totally understand her headaches. 'I don't want to criticise him, because I truly appreciate his caution and fear of making things worse for me with surgery. But he outright admitted during an appointment, "The problem with you is I just don't know what to do." I have not completely ruled it out because there are times when I start to despair, and I believe I must consider surgery before considering ending my pain by ending my life.'

Happier Days Ahead

For **Chris** in Tasmania, just one week after surgery at the age of 63, there was the realisation that 'my operation has been an amazing success. It was by far the scariest decision I've ever had to make in my life but so far I feel it's one of the best decisions I've ever made. My recovery is improving rapidly every day. All the debilitating SCDS symptoms have gone and what's incredible is my demeanour. I'm so positive, happy and talkative already—I haven't felt like this for such a long time. I was hardly speaking before, as it was so uncomfortable and loud inside my head.' Her symptoms had been triggered by a flight and it got to the stage 'where it impacted my quality of life to the point where I didn't feel confident driving, I couldn't cope well in social situations and I was just having too many really bad days. I've doubted myself so much over the last three or more years, wondering if I was imagining or exaggerating my symptoms, especially when I had some good days. It's just so incredibly hard to articulate to friends and family and doctors what I've been going through, and that in turn used to feed the little doubting person inside my head.'

Robert in the UK decided his 82 years make him an unsuitable candidate for surgery which was disappointing, but he has no criticism with regard to the doctors' approach in his case. His symptoms appeared rather rapidly at the age of 78 when he turned his head sharply to the right in the process of driving onto a motorway, and a CT scan revealed a dehiscence to be the cause of his vertigo. He was warned that an operation might increase the vertigo and possibly cause deafness, so he is working on balance exercises to help relieve his dizziness. **Maureen**, aged 72, in the UK 'has always felt that my consultant had my best interest at heart. He was very approachable and easy to talk to, and everything was explained to me. Her surgery in 2020 'was partly successful from my point of view, in that I lost some of the symptoms, but my balance issues have remained. However, this possibility was explained to me, of not losing all the symptoms. I decided to go ahead; I was feeling so awful before the operation, I felt I couldn't live with all those symptoms.'

Jeff, also in the UK, was surprised to be offered surgery as quickly as he was. 'I jumped at the chance even though I was scared at the thought and I knew the potential risks. I'm 60 and I thought about younger people having this ghastly condition.

I may only have another 20 years or so left, but the thought of having the disorder for the rest of my days was daunting. I didn't want my retirement to be so challenging. Following surgery, most symptoms have gone away. To start with, I was a little bit on edge during my walking, and about allowing so much general noise to surround me without throwing both hands up to cover my ears. I'd been programmed to protect my ears from noise getting in, and breaking this habit has been difficult.' Jeff's problems had begun with a traffic accident, when a vehicle crashed into the side of his car and the airbag failed to inflate. Overall, he believes, 'I can't really fault the NHS at all. The only thing that got to me was coping with so many noisy ENT waiting areas. Not all of us are deaf in that department!'

Like Mother, Like Daughter

TMWS has been identified as sometimes occurring in more than one member of a family, and **Bernie** and her daughter **Danell** in America are a case in point. Bernie is now 83 and has decided against surgical intervention to repair the very large dehiscence found in her left ear and a potentially very small one, plus sensorineural hearing loss, on the right side. She says she is 'able to lead a fairly good quality of life. My dizziness is minimal, I have no headaches, mostly fullness inside my head and I hear my voice and many other sounds, especially high-pitched tones which are very painful. I have a strong support group and I take my daily walks with my walking stick, and it keeps me from drifting.' She is happy now that she better understands the nature of the condition she is choosing to live with. Sometimes just having validation that there is a physiological problem can be very satisfying for a patient.

Bernie is 'so aggressive about new information, but that's because I am thinking of my daughter and her family. I am always looking on websites for more knowledge.' Her daughter Danell is 62. 'My first symptom was probably sometime in my mid to late 30s. I began experiencing what felt like water plugging my left ear, and I mentioned this to my doctor during annual physical checks over the years. I also saw at least two ENT physicians. I tried ear candling, acupuncture and a chiropractor. No one found any problem, so no one had any solutions. Shortly after my mother's diagnosis, I decided to see whether I might have the same problem and made an appointment with an audiologist and another ENT doctor. Insignificant hearing loss was found and a nasal hygiene routine was recommended, with the use of Flonase. When no improvements occurred, I mentioned that my mom had been diagnosed with SCDS. The doctor told me the condition was rare and not hereditary, so it would be very unlikely I had the same thing. I asked to be tested anyway, and that was when the dehiscence was discovered—much to the doctor's surprise!'

Like her mother, Danell is not opting for surgery at this point in her life. 'I am feeling quite lucky. I can withstand being in loud situations if I am just listening. If I have to shout above the noise, however, that will irritate or even hurt the ear with dehiscence. I usually just hold the ear shut with my finger if I need to talk in a loud place. I have some balance-related issues that may have gotten a little worse in the last few years, but I have not ever had vertigo. I can drift slightly at times—I notice it when walking with my husband as I occasionally bump into him or into the wall in a hallway, or when going through a door. I will be very grateful if these are the only symptoms I continue to have as I age.'

Conclusion

All the remarkable patients in this chapter have given permission for their names, ages and locations to be published. There is so much to learn from their stories, the ups the downs, the good and the bad, and that is what they all wish for most of all—greatly increased awareness about TMWS and all its complexities, and an educated understanding of what it means for those unfortunate enough to have their lives affected by it. It is also worthy of note that patients receive some degree of relief even if their physicians are unable to make a diagnosis, so long as those physicians make sure to show empathy and don't simply write them off as 'crazy' people.

If doctors elicit a full history from their patients, the chance of a wrong diagnosis being handed out is greatly reduced. In the cases listed, many of the doctors who either missed a diagnosis or attributed the problems to anxiety alone, had overlooked the potential second events—head trauma, otic barotrauma resulting from air travel, and so on—so cause must always be investigated within the person's medical history. Making a diagnosis of anxiety may often be very appropriate within the context of TMWS, but failing to look for an inner ear cause for it is totally inappropriate. As with most vestibular disorders, TMWS requires extensive testing to arrive at the correct diagnosis, and that makes it possible to objectively identify specific disorders that can support the subjective input from the history. To exclude a diagnosis of TMWS in a patient with TMWS symptoms, when they haven't undergone adequate testing is just plain wrong.

This book aims to fill the gap in education about TMWS for medical professionals, but if it still proves impossible to determine what is wrong with a patient, then they need to be sent to someone else. Many places only discuss the treatment that they can provide, or have experience with, whereas it is important to explain what can be offered elsewhere, including medical therapy. Ego can sometimes stand in the way of referrals happening, and embarrassment may prevent some others still. The simple truth, however, is that no physician is right all the time, and every physician will come across cases for which they are unable to find the answer. Keep the patient's best interest in mind at every step of the way, and then everything else falls into place.

Chapter 28
Patient Experiences of Living with Superior Semicircular Canal Dehiscence Syndrome

Krister Tano and Anette Sörlin

In the autumn of 2015, we made an interview study of 12 of our 13 patients with a diagnosed case of SCDS (superior canal dehiscence syndrome) at our clinic. The interviews were semistructured and lasted for about 30–60 min per patient. The interviews were digitally recorded and later transcribed verbatim. In all, the material consisted of about 100 written pages with citations from these 12 patients who expressed their experiences of living with SCDS. Most of the patient citations in this chapter emanate from the interviews of these 12 patients [1]. After the interviews, the patients also completed four different questionnaires that have been used for SCDS patients at different hospitals in Sweden. We will see the results of one of these questionnaires later in this chapter.

According to Mau et al. [2], the most debilitating symptoms were phonophobia and chronic disequilibrium, which also reflects our experience after the patient interviews. Moreover, in the recently published consensus document from the Bárány society [3] one also can find a range of symptoms associated with SCDS disease. Furthermore, also in Naert et al. [4] one can find a rather complete list of the most common SCDS symptoms.

The symptoms of SCDS can be divided into symptoms mainly related to the cochlear part of the inner ear and those mainly related to the vestibular part and if we organize the common symptoms of SCDS in such a way, we can visualize them as in Table 28.1 (from Öhman et al. [1]).

K. Tano (✉)
ENT, Umeå University/Sunderby Hospital, Luleå, Sweden
e-mail: Krister.tano@umu.se

A. Sörlin
ENT/Audiology, Sunderby Hospital, Luleå, Sweden
e-mail: anette.sorlin@norrbotten.se

G. J. Gianoli, P. Thomson (eds.), *Third Mobile Window Syndrome of the Inner Ear*, https://doi.org/10.1007/978-3-031-16586-3_28

Table 28.1 Common symptoms of SCDS. Adapted from Öhman et al. [1]

Symptom		Meaning
Cochlear symptoms	Hearing loss	Especially low frequency sounds
	Pulsatile tinnitus	An ever-present sound in the ear, for example from hearing the heart or the pulse
	Aural fullness	A sensation that the ears feel blocked up or stuffy
	Autophony	To hear one's own voice as changed and too loud
	Cochlear hyperacusis	Sensitiveness to normal sound, causing pain and/or discomfort in the head
	Conductive hyperacusis	To hear sounds that are "conducted" and amplified throughout the body
Vestibular symptoms	Chronic disequilibrium	A general sensation of lack of balance
	Tullio phenomenon	Vertigo, nystagmus, and oscillopsia induced by sound
	Hennebert sign	Vertigo and/or nystagmus induced by pressure changes

Below, we have connected the symptoms described in Table 28.1 with citations from patients with SCDS. In this way, these symptoms become more vivid, when they are coupled with the patient citations.

Experiencing New and Strange Symptoms

Some patients are able to describe a rather rapid onset of the symptoms, for example after an upper respiratory tract infection (URTI). Other patients describe a more gradual onset:

"*When I was in the forest hunting elk, I suddenly noticed an unsteadiness when I walked on uneven surfaces, which I hadn't noticed before*".

Usually these symptoms get worse with time, and new symptoms often appear after a while, as one of the patients put it:

At first I noticed hypersensitivity to sounds, for example when people used their cutlery. After a while, I felt a pressure (or blockage) in the ear, which was constant, but worsened if I performed physical work. Then, I also started to notice a kind of disturbed balance—a feeling of drifting towards one side when I was walking. These symptoms developed during a period of 2–3 years.

This progression of SCDS is also described by Saliba et al. [5]. In the study of Saliba et al., the patients had suffered from symptoms of SCDS for an average of about five years prior to diagnosis. These patients reported progressively increasing symptoms, on average four debilitating cochlear symptoms and two debilitating vestibular symptoms per patient at the time of diagnosis.

Furthermore, many of the initial symptoms of SCDS are able to provoke anxiety and even panic:

"And when she laughed, it would be terrible in my right ear. And I thought, 'what is this?', it felt really strange. And then I started to get inexplicable dizziness; not all the time but from time to time … And then I started to hear my pulse very clearly, mainly in the right ear … And then I felt dizzy when I lifted something heavy, for example, and when I blew my nose, many such strange things would happen. And this dizziness began to appear more and more. And by the end, it started to be difficult when I was out and about—I could suddenly get very wobbly and unstable. And I was actually afraid, because I thought 'what is this?' It was very unpleasant … And I was so unsure. I felt like … many of these symptoms were very strange and so I thought 'I'm going crazy'."

"It's a trauma for many people before you come to know what you have. You may experience it as having a brain tumor, or a brain injury, but you don't know what to blame it on. It has been so unpleasant. If I hadn't known this, then I don't think I could have managed … I would have gone crazy, and jumped off a bridge. Do you understand? It is really a shame that there are people out there who do not know what they have."

Cochlear Symptoms

Regarding ***hearing loss***, it is not typical for SCDS to result in a sensorineural hearing loss, but many patients describe how difficult it is to hear other people, because of the unsettling surrounding sounds and also due to the disturbing noises from their own bodies (pulse, etc.):

"I cannot determine how loud I am speaking when I talk to people … If I am talking with people during a dinner, I have to quit chewing in order to hear what other people are saying to me."

Tinnitus is often described as pulsatile and follows the heart beating. It can be worse if the patient is speaking, or during physical exertion. Tinnitus as a constant tone can sometimes be a side effect of surgery and can be very disturbing.

Aural fullness is often an early symptom, and it is not unusual to find patients have been to primary care because of this and were advised to perform Valsalva's maneuver (trying to blow the nose while pinching the nose at the same time) without any effect on the "blockage" feeling in the ear. One patient formulated it this way: "*It was as if you had suctioned something into the ear and it never disappeared.*" Other patients describe the feeling like having water in the ear.

Autophony is one of the prominent symptoms of SCDS and can be very disturbing, especially for people that have to speak a lot at work: "*I first noticed that I could hear my heart beating and it felt like my heart was inside my ear, and also when I spoke, it was as if my voice was outside my head and I felt as if I was inside a glass bowl.*"

A patient who worked as a teacher complained that due to the autophony, she could not tell how loud she was speaking—the higher she raised her voice, the more difficult it was to speak due to the echo in her head. Another patient said that the SCDS symptoms started with: "*a terrible noise in my head when I was talking, and it just got worse and worse over the subsequent years.*"

Another patient complained: "*It feels like I am inside a metal drum all the time, and everything I say echoes in my head. These resonance sounds worsen if I raise my voice. I also feel constantly tired due to the ever-present sounds.*"

Cochlear hyperacusis is one of the most distressing symptoms of SCDS disease for many patients. Some patients experience a worsening of this sound sensitivity over a period of 5–10 years. The hypersensitivity to sounds from the environment (doing the dishes, children's voices, etc.) is often much more distressing than hearing sounds from the body, like hearing your own pulse, for example. One patient put it this way: "*If I am exposed to loud sounds, I get dizzy. Low frequency sounds more often lead to dizziness, but high frequency sounds are more painful. It is never quiet in my head, which makes me super tired almost all the time. It does not matter if I sleep well, so it is a different kind of tiredness.*" It is our experience that the patients with significant cochlear symptoms are the patients most affected by such fatigue.

Several patients say that they are highly sensitive to sudden, loud sounds, and that they eventually become scared of such sounds: "*It is as if you are standing very close to a loudspeaker, and suddenly the sound comes on abruptly at its highest level—it feels like your head will explode.*"

Another, similar experience: "*I slowly noticed that I had become more and more sensitive to sound. I worked in an environment with a lot of sound, so I had to get stronger and stronger sound protection devices, but eventually that did not help either. The symptoms kept getting worse and worse during the years. The hypersensitivity to sound is the most debilitating symptom. The worst kind of sounds are clattering porcelain, children's voices, and music. Also, when I go to the dentist and they use the drill on my teeth—I just can't stand it, so I prefer to have teeth extracted, rather than mend a cavity with the drill.*"

Another example: "*I am sensitive to loud sounds—it becomes like a piercing sensation and an echo in my head. It is difficult for me to use a hearing aid, because of the amplification of all the surrounding sounds.*"

A 51-year-old man put it like this: "*It feels that all loud sounds go straight into my bone marrow and lead further into my eyes.*" Furthermore, another patient said: "*If a member of my family unloaded the dishes from the dishwashing machine, I had to go to the bedroom and hold my ears. The sound from the porcelain was so piercing that I could not stand it.*"

Philippa Thomson describes in her book *A Hole in My Life* [6] a long journey of more or less successful contacts with the healthcare system due to her SCDS. She also describes the typical ***conductive hyperacusis***, which involves hearing the normal internal body sounds at disturbingly loud volume: "*I have popping and crackling sounds in my ears and jaw, and I can hear my heart pounding up in my ear; so* *if I'm stressed or I've been running and am out of breath, there's a terrible, loud thumping noise. I hear my own voice echoing around my head when I speak—it's awful when I am angry and have to raise my voice to tell my daughter off, as it really hurts my head.*"

Other similar experiences from patients: "*I hear my heart beating all the time.*"

"*After a year or so, I started to feel strange symptoms in my eyes—a kind of eye dizziness. Later on, it got worse, and I also heard when my eyes moved, and I heard my pulse all the time.*"

"*When I walked on the snow, I heard the sound loudly and when I drove on the road with winter tires, I got a vibrating sound in my head.*"

"*When I walked on gravel it was like I had my head inside a bag of potato chips.*"

Vestibular Symptoms

There are some vestibular symptoms that are typical of SCDS, and some of the most common are listed below with actual patient citations. In some patients, the vestibular symptoms are more prominent and disturbing than the cochlear symptoms.

Chronic disequilibrium is a swaying feeling and a drifting towards one side, especially when walking and when doing physical exercise: "*I have balance problems as if I am drifting towards one side when I walk. It is a feeling of swaying. It has not worsened over the years, but it gets worse if I work a lot, especially doing physically demanding work.*"

"*I started to hear my body sounds and develop dizziness. It was very traumatic until I got the diagnosis after several years—I thought that I was going crazy. I was scared to death of the dizziness, because I could not understand what it was.*"

These balance problems also led to difficulties in maintaining a good physique because the training induced vertigo: "*I also get dizzy and unsteady, especially during physical exertion, for example if I am walking up a hill.*"

"*When I exercise, the balance problems get worse—when I stand up, or lift up something heavy, walk up a hill, etc. On the other hand, the dizziness fades away when you stop the exercise.*"

The ***Tullio phenomenon*** was described as follows by a patient working as a pilot:

"*I noticed when I heard the electronic alert voice that we have as pilots, for example 'landing gear, landing gear', my eyes started to jump and my vision became blurred. The same thing happened after a while when I listened to loud music when I drove the car. During the same time period, I also noticed that I could hear my muscles when I moved my eyes. After this, I started to search on the internet and eventually found a description for the Tullio phenomenon, which in turn led me to the ENT clinic and to the diagnosis of SCDS.*"

The ***Hennebert sign*** is characterized by dizziness caused by pressure changes in the ear: "*It started with a bad URTI. I blew my nose with force, and then I became so dizzy that I fell on the floor. It was like being on a carousel. It passed rather quickly, but since then I have noticed that I have a hypersensitivity to loud sounds. When this rotatory dizziness starts, it is like you are inside a rolling sphere which rolls in all directions, and not only horizontally like in a carousel.*"

The progression of symptoms is very varied among the patients with SCDS. Some patients describe a history of the addition of different symptoms over a period of years: "*It started with a piercing pain in my ear after a sudden, loud sound. After a while I noticed intermittent dizziness. Then I started to hear my pulse in the ear and an echo in my head when I spoke. The unsteadiness increased during physical exertion, when I blew my nose, and when I was outside walking.*"

Some patients, however, did not experience such a progression, but adapted to the situation: "*I noticed a feeling like if you have water in the ear. If it is a bit dark or the surface is uneven—then I feel unsteady. I also hear my pulse and when I am walking, I can hear my footsteps clearly, but I cannot say that I suffer much because of this. I do not really suffer from loud sounds either.*"

So there is a large variation between patients in terms of how intense the symptoms of SCDS are, and also how much these symptoms affect their daily life, as we will see below.

In addition to these cochlear and vestibular symptoms, SCDS could affect both cognitive and emotional functions:

"*I could sit and read one page and then when I turned the page and thought about it, I didn't remember what had been on the previous page. I thought, 'what the hell, have I started to become senile or what is going on?' I couldn't remember anything. And, yes, it went on for a while, and I started to get worried, simply because there could be something wrong, something seriously wrong with my brain.*"

"*So, it is something that shows up sometimes, a type of fatigue. And maybe as my family said at the time, I'm more … have less patience sometimes. And I'm a person who has a great deal of patience. So maybe, from here to here [showing levels with hands], it is a small difference anyway. And it's a shame if you have less patience with your children or things like that. You get angry and irritated because you are really tired. And usually I say to them at home 'can you be quiet because my ear hurts'.*"

"*Yes, I felt very alone, because I withdrew. And I was a bit depressed by it from the beginning. I haven't been bothered about it so much any more since as they say, it gets easier over time. It was a new thing for me. I could not understand what it was.*"

A Restricted Life Due to SCDS Disease

Many patients with SCDS are so frightened of being exposed to loud sounds that it affects their social lives: "*Everything I say echoes in my head, and if I raise my voice the echo becomes painful, which means that I avoid situations where I must speak with a loud voice. When my husband and I are watching TV, I have to put in earplugs, because I cannot stand it even when the sound level is very low.*"

One patient who was very sensitive to pressure changes found it hard to travel by car, especially when the car changed altitudes (from the top of a hill to the bottom of a hill). She also didn't want to travel by plane, because she was scared of getting dizzy due to the pressure changes.

The hypersensitivity to loud sounds is a major obstacle for many patients: "Y*ou get very tired of hearing your own voice this loud. I had to stop singing in a choir due to the massive amounts of sound that entered my brain when I was singing.*"

Another patient said: "*I can't go to music events or sing myself, because I hear my own voice that loud. Sometimes I put earplugs in the ear so that I can get at least some rest from sounds outside the body—the sounds coming from inside your body are there all the time.*"

"*I cannot go to the pub—there are too many sounds in a small area. I have learned to live with it, and I have adjusted my life so it is becoming bearable. It was important to get the diagnosis so that you knew what it was and that it was not a tumor or anything dangerous. I have a type of hearing aid, which prevents sounds from coming into the ear, and I use this when I am together with other people.*"

Another similar experience: "*You are always on high alert when you are at a restaurant, if anybody would make a sound from a glass—then I have to hold my ears. These symptoms have worsened over time.*"

"*I was really tired—I would wake up in the morning and after breakfast it felt like it was time to go to bed again. The extreme tiredness was the worst symptom. You just wanted to lie in bed and have quiet around you. You tried to keep all conversations to a minimum—just 'yes, yes', 'no'. It was so hard to endure the sound of your own voice. When I was together with other people, it was like having a party with 25 kids running around all the time—just unbearable and extremely tiring.*"

One patient complained that she could never take an escalator—it felt that she was going to fall down.

Some of the patients reported that they did not participate in birthday parties or other gatherings where there were a lot of people. Furthermore, the balance problems could also lead to a restricted social life and to sick leave: "*This swaying dizziness led to the need to use a walker when I was outdoors. Especially during wintertime when I was walking on ice and snow … I became extremely tired in my head and could not understand why. I cannot go to the movies due to the high sound levels in there. If I am out in the city where there are a lot of people, I get dizzy because of all the motion due to the people around me. I am on sick leave, but it is difficult to explain to other people why I cannot work … They say: 'You look fine!'*"

Having SCDS was described as having an invisible disability—friends and colleges could not understand why it was necessary to be on sick leave when they looked healthy.

Even for patients who didn't exercise very much, balance issues were described as a restriction in their everyday life. Some patients found it troublesome to carry out various household activities that included climbing, such as cleaning the windows, changing curtains and so on.

However, most patients reported that, despite having SCDS, they managed to go to work, even though some of the employers had to make some environmental adjustments at work, such as sitting alone in the office for example.

Coping Strategies

From the examples above, we have seen that the typical SCDS symptoms can be of such a magnitude that they have a significant impact on the patient's social life. Many of these patients have developed different coping strategies in order to "survive." Some of the patients had stopped going to the gym, others wear earplugs when they are in shops or in the city when there is a lot of traffic around them. Some of the patients have even stopped going to the dentist because of the uncomfortable noise from the drill.

People with tinnitus can often be helped with therapy, where they learn to accept the sound and their situation. It is also evident that many of the SCDS patients that have chosen not to undergo surgery have learned to accept their situation. One patient that had been to a psychologist said: "*I am not as afraid of loud sounds as I was before—before I just went around and waited for a sound to come, and I was on high alert all the time due to this. I have been taking exercises in relaxation and yoga, and these things have been helpful … a lot of the coping strategies that I learned and that work are designed to help you endure and accept the situation.*"

Some of the patients have chosen not to talk much about their problems. According to these patients, it is very much about attitude, and a strategy of not letting the disease take too much of their mental energy. They try to make everyday life run as smoothly as possible, even if they have to abstain from some things.

However, the dizziness can also be a challenge for patients and thus demands coping strategies:

"*If I am going somewhere, I have to get ready three hours before so I can rest a while if I get dizzy. The balance problems are the symptoms that affect my daily life the most—I could not work in healthcare any longer, so I eventually took permanent sick leave.*"

Another patient stated that: "*It was a big relief to get the diagnosis, then you could start to learn to accept the condition … But you still live with fear in a way, because you can never really plan something in case you happen to have a bad day. The dizziness is the worst symptom, because it is this rotatory dizziness that prevents you from coping with your situation.*"

The most important coping strategy among the patients was to protect their ears. Earplugs of different kinds were often a big help. Although sounds coming from inside of the body became louder, many patients felt that the use of earplugs was an absolute necessity if they were going to meet people: "*I have headphones on all day with faint music—then I can cope with my symptoms. The worst is if high sounds come, and you are not prepared—then you have to hyperventilate. You are very tense all the time because you always have to be prepared to meet a sudden sound. All this makes you very tired. The tin can sensation and the hypersensitivity to sound is absolutely the worst thing about this disease.*"

Another patient reported that the family had to replace all porcelain dishes at home with paper dishes due to the pain he felt inside his head because of this sound hypersensitivity.

Many patients with SCDS have developed strategies in order to eliminate the impact of possible upcoming loud sounds, for example, by reaching for a closing door before it slams, pulling in the leash before the dog barks, or positioning their head when talking to people so that the affected ear is pointing away from the voices. These kinds of maneuvers tend to take place automatically, without patients even thinking about it.

Why are many SCDS patients so extremely tired? In our experience, this fatigue is more common among the patients with predominantly cochlear symptoms. It is not clear if this fatigue is secondary to the stress produced by the efforts to avoid sound, or if it is due to a direct effect on the brain due to the constant prevalence of sounds from inside the body and from the environment. As one patient put it: "*There is sound all the time, especially from within the body, and eventually you get tired of it.*"

Encounters with Healthcare

Since many of the symptoms of SCDS mimic many other diseases, it is understandable that these patients are often misunderstood by the primary healthcare providers. Pressure in the middle ear or fluid in the middle ear (secretory otitis media) is a common and harmless condition, which often follows an URTI, and these conditions often produce a sensation of "blockage" or fullness in the affected ear.

A poor sense of balance when walking outdoors could be related to aging, especially in combination with impaired vision. Other common explanations from healthcare providers for the disequilibrium experienced by the SCDS patients were either high or low blood pressure levels, anxiety, or problems deriving from the shoulders and neck.

Thus, it would be desirable if the primary healthcare provider could be more aware of the typical combination of symptoms in SCDS disease: sensation of ear fullness, hypersensitivity to loud sounds, hearing the body's sounds and dizziness, especially during physical exercise. Patients contacting the primary care with dizziness, aural fullness, and sound sensitivity should be asked what provokes the dizziness, rather than if it is rotatory or not [7]. If the answer is: "Sound and straining," SCDS should be considered as one of the differential diagnoses.

The most important thing, however, is to be aware of the existence of this syndrome, because if you don't know what to look for, you will not find it.

Some voices from the patients: "*I went to primary care, and they told me that it was a muscular thing from the neck, and they sent me to the physiotherapist, but it did not get any better.*"

"*At the primary care center, they told me that I had fluid in my ear, and that I should do the Valsalva maneuver, but it only led to increased dizziness. You start to doubt yourself in the end: Am I just imagining it? Can it really be that I have these weird symptoms? The primary care team needs to learn more about this disease!*"

A 50-year-old woman was told: "*When you become older, it is normal to get these kinds of problems.*" She felt that she was not taken seriously. Her dizziness escalated, and she decided to change to another healthcare center, which in turn sent her to the ENT clinic, which led to a rapid diagnosis.

Another 70-year-old woman visited the emergency unit twice due to her dizziness and disequilibrium, without getting the correct diagnosis. After a while, she was sent to the ENT clinic, where she was quickly diagnosed. This patient also underlines the importance of a respectful attitude by the healthcare personnel, not to make light of the problem.

Other patient voices: "*I contacted the primary healthcare provider, and I got a nasal cortisone spray against the sense of aural fullness. It did not help at all and after one year I contacted the healthcare provider again and was referred to the ENT clinic, where I was quickly diagnosed.*"

And yet another witness: "*It took two years before I received the diagnosis. I thought that I had a brain tumor because of the unsteadiness and balance problems when I walked.*"

Hence, getting a diagnosis was of great importance. The experience of having these strange and often debilitating symptoms did not become easier when they were told that everything looked fine.

When they received the diagnosis, they felt substantial relief, both in the sense of rehabilitation—"*I told you it was something wrong with my ear*"—and a confirmation that they were not about to go insane or had a brain tumor.

Another patient expressed: "*It is extremely important that you have contact with a doctor that understands you—I cannot emphasize this enough. Otherwise, it would be awful if you didn't have anyone to ask when symptoms come and go, and when questions come up.*"

Why Surgery?

Based on our data, about half of the patients chose to undergo an operation. The surgery is not without risks, which is why the preoperative information is very important. The main symptoms alleviated with surgery are dizziness/vertigo and autophony, according to a study by the Hopkins group [8].

One can use a questionnaire to help the doctor to estimate the burden of the SCDS disease. However, when one just looks at the results of the answers to the questionnaire (Table 28.2), one finds that some of the patients with low scores still undergo surgery, and some patients with a high score have chosen not to undergo surgery.

Table 28.2 Monitored using the modified THI questionnaire

Pat no	Sex and age[a] (years)	Diseased ear (L/R/B)[b]	Disease duration (years)	MTQ score 2015	MTQ score 2021	Surgery (Yes/No) (L/R/B)[b]
1	F (59)	B	15	AS:54	AS:26[c]	Yes/B
2	F (53)	L	15	46	42	No
3	F (63)	B	13	AS:4	AS:24	Yes/L
4	M (44)	B	7	BS:92, AS:0	AS:0	Yes/B
5	M (51)	L	4	52	24	No
6	M (55)	R	2	AS:4	AS:8	Yes[d]/R
7	F (72)	L	4	10	2	No
8	M (43)	R	2	28	AS:0	Yes/R
9	F (54)	B	3	AS:70	AS:78	Yes/R × 2
10	F (65)	R	12	54	34	No
11	M (67)	L	10	AS:24	X	Yes/L
12	F (67)	L	5	46	36	No

Twelve patients with SCDS monitored between 2015 and 2021. X = deceased. MTQ = The THI (Newman et al. 1996) modified by changing the word "tinnitus" to "SCDS." This questionnaire is composed of 25 questions. The score is calculated as follows: "Do you have difficulties concentrating due to SCDS?" "NO" = 0 points, "Sometimes" = 2 points, and "Yes" = 4 points. Thus, if the answer is "yes" on all the 25 questions the total score will be 100 points. BS = Before surgery. AS = After surgery. "Disease duration" was at the time of the first MTQ (2015). The second MTQ was performed 6 years after the first MTQ, which was 2021

[a] Age at the time of the first MTQ (2015)

[b] Left/Right/Both

[c] After the second operation

[d] Reinforcement of the round window

So how did the patients motivate their decisions?

"I felt that I had no choice, especially because I experienced that it became worse with time."

"I can live with the dizziness but not with the sounds."

"I had no choice—the symptoms were so tormenting that I felt that I have to do something."

"I wanted to have the surgery because of the balance problems. I did not have many symptoms, which is why I chose the easier operation when they reinforced the round window, but I have not noticed any improvement since the surgery."

"As a pilot, I was grounded because of my SCDS, but after surgery to address the defect, I was astonished—it was completely quiet. After a little more than six months, I was back as a pilot again. Five years later, the same symptoms popped up again after I fell during a downhill skiing accident. Now it was the other ear that had developed the same disease, so I returned to the USA for another surgery—also with good results."

Of course, there are risks associated with the surgery, and this is something that patients also must be prepared to encounter: "*The first months after the surgery, I had more problems with sensitivity to sounds and also with balance,*" one patient said after an operation with transmastoid plugging of the defect.

"I hear it very clearly, if something touches the affected ear: hair, glasses etc. The surgery was not successful, and after the surgery I was very dizzy. I have been retraining my balance a lot afterwards, and slowly I became better so that I can walk outside without help."

Cozart et al. (2021) reported that aggressive vestibular rehabilitation was needed in more than 50% of the patients after surgery [9].

"*I was operated on about a year after the diagnosis, but I got very tiring tinnitus after the surgery. The echo in my head due to hypersensitivity to sounds disappeared after the surgery, but I developed disturbing tinnitus instead and some balance problems, however I am feeling better.*" The surgery performed involved plugging the superior canal.

Hence, it seems that although some patients experienced side effects such as tinnitus and balance problems, they still appreciated undergoing the surgery, especially if the sound hypersensitivity/autophony disappeared.

The Place of Questionnaires

There are not many studies investigating the impact of SCDS on the quality of life of the patients [10]. Most often, questionnaires are used as a tool for evaluating surgery for SCDS [11]. We have been using a modified version of the THI (tinnitus handicap inventory) questionnaire, developed by Newman et al. [12]. The THI is a self-reporting measure that can be used in clinical practice to quantify the impact of tinnitus on daily living. We used the same questionnaire, but replaced the word "tinnitus" with "SCDS" instead. In this way, we believe that we can appreciate how much the patient is affected by the SCDS disease on a daily basis. Furthermore, it was also possible to follow the progress of the disease over time. In addition, it can be used to evaluate the effects of surgery over time.

In Table 28.2, we have listed 12 patients that have been monitored using the modified THI questionnaire. One can see that it is not easy to predict which patients will benefit from surgery, based on the answers in the questionnaire. This is, of course, because there are so many other factors that are involved in the decision to operate or not.

However, patient number 1 is rather satisfied two years after her second operation. She thinks that her hearing is better, her balance has improved, and she experiences less dizziness. The hypersensitivity to loud sounds has diminished, although she still uses ear plugs in some situations. Now, she can handle occasions where there are a lot of environmental sounds and there is no echo in her head when she speaks. Moreover, she is now working full time and can even manage visiting the dentist.

Patient number 3 has deteriorated over these six years (score from 4 → 24), but as she has SCDS on both sides, it is most likely the other, nonoperated ear that is now producing the most symptoms. Patients number 4 and 8 showed full recovery after surgery.

Patient number 6 only had reinforcement of the round window membrane, which had no improvement on his symptoms, but he can manage his disease without further surgery. The low score underlines that he probably manages well in his daily life.

Patient number 9 had surgery twice on the right ear but is now considering surgery also on the left ear. According to her score (78/100), she is probably highly affected by the disease in her daily life.

Patients number 2, 5, 7, 10, and 12 are examples of patients adapting to their disease by acceptance and coping strategies, and have so far not wanted any surgery.

References

1. Öhman J, Sörlin A, Forssen A, Tano K. Patients' experiences of living with superior canal dehiscence syndrome. Int J Audiol. 2018;57:825–30. https://doi.org/10.1080/14992027.2018.1487086.
2. Mau C, Kamal N, Badeti S, Reddy R, Ying Y-LM, Jyung RW, Liu JK. Superior semicircular canal dehiscence: diagnosis and management. J Clin Neurosci. 2018;48:58–65. https://doi.org/10.1016/j.jocn.2017.11.019.
3. Ward BK, van de Berg R, van Rompaey V, Bisdorff A, Hullar TE, Welgampola MS, Carey JP. Superior semicircular canal dehiscence syndrome: diagnostic criteria consensus document of the committee for the classification of vestibular disorders of the Bárány Society. J Vestib Res. 2021;31:131–41. https://doi.org/10.3233/VES-200004.
4. Naert L, Ocak I, Griet M, Van de Berg R, Stultiens JJA, Van de Heyning P, Bisdorff A, Sharon JD, Ward BK, Van Rompaey V. Prospective analysis of an evidence-based symptom set in supe-

rior canal dehiscence syndrome. Otol Neurotol. 2021;42:e186–92. https://doi.org/10.1002/lary.27062.
5. Saliba I, Maniakas A, Benamira LZ, Nehme J, Benoit M, Montreuil-Jacques V. Superior canal dehiscence syndrome: clinical manifestations and radiologic correlations. Eur Arch Otorhinolaryngol. 2014;271:2905–14. https://doi.org/10.1007/s00405-013-2711-x.
6. Thomson P. A hole in my life. Memoir. 2016. ISBN 978-0-9935989-0-6.
7. Newman-Toker D, Edlow J. TiTrate: a novel approach to diagnosing acute dizziness and vertigo. Neurol Clin. 2015;33(3):577–99. https://doi.org/10.1016/j.ncl.2015.04.011.
8. Ward B, Carey J, Minor L. Superior canal dehiscence syndrome: lessons from the first 20 years. Front Neurol. 2017;8:177. https://doi.org/10.3389/fneur.2017.00177.
9. Cozart AC, Kennedy JT III, Seidman MD. A basis for standardizing superior semicircular canal dehiscence management. Ear Nose Throat J. 2021;100:444–53. https://doi.org/10.1177/0145561320927941.
10. Ocak I, Topsakal V, Van de Heyning P, Van Haesendonck G, Jorissen C, van de Berg R, Vanderveken OM, Van Rompaey V. Impact of superior canal dehiscence syndrome on health utility values: a prospective case-control study. Front Neurol. 2020;11:552495. https://doi.org/10.3389/fneur.2020.552495.
11. Ossen ME, Stokroos R, Kingma H, van Tongeren J, van Rompaey V, Temel Y, van de Berg R. Heterogeneity in reported outcome measures after surgery in superior canal dehiscence syndrome – a systematic literature review. Front Neurol. 2017;8:347. https://doi.org/10.3389/fneur.2017.00347.
12. Newman CW, Jacobson GP, Spitzer JB. Development of the tinnitus handicap inventory. Arch Otolaryngol Head Neck Surg. 1996;122(2):143–8. https://doi.org/10.1001/archotol.1996.01890140029007.

Chapter 29
Doctor-Patient Communication

Gerard J. Gianoli and Philippa Thomson

Effective and collaborative doctor-patient communication is central to building a therapeutic relationship between the two parties, and it enables the patient to make well-informed decisions about their treatment as well as to set expectations that can be met. Positive exchanges of this kind can be a source of motivation and support, helping both sides achieve their agreed-upon goals.

Philippa Thomson, a patient with bilateral SCDS, outlines a series of questions that arise regularly for TMWS patients and they are answered by Dr Gerard Gianoli. The direct questions seek specific information related to the topics that concern most patients who are affected by this disorder.

Symptoms

- **Q. Is there an association between a patient's symptoms and the size of their dehiscence?**
  - **A.** Size does seem to play a part in symptoms associated with Superior Semicircular Canal Dehiscence (SCD). The size of the dehiscence has been correlated with the size of the air-bone gap on audiometry [1]. The longer the dehiscence, the larger the air-bone gap noted on audiometry, in general. Specifically, a 3 mm dehiscence has been demonstrated to be a potential "critical point" at which defects shorter than 3 mm don't tend to have conductive gaps and those greater than 3 mm do, with an increasing gap for sizes greater

G. J. Gianoli
Ear and Balance Institute, Covington, LA, USA

P. Thomson (✉)
North Berwick, East Lothian, UK

G. J. Gianoli, P. Thomson (eds.), *Third Mobile Window Syndrome of the Inner Ear*, https://doi.org/10.1007/978-3-031-16586-3_29

than 3 mm [2, 3]. The expected symptoms associated with this would be more difficulty with hearing loss and greater degree in autophony. However, the perception of symptoms and how they are expressed by individual patients varies greatly.

- While VEMP testing is not a symptom, the size of dehiscence has demonstrated a positive correlation between the length of SSCD and the cVEMP and oVEMP (500 Hz) thresholds and cVEMP amplitude [4]. Similar to an increasing conductive gap, one would expect a lower VEMP threshold and greater VEMP amplitude to generally result in greater sound-induced symptoms, specifically Tullio phenomenon and sound sensitivity. However, vestibular symptoms have not been correlated with the length of dehiscence.
- Concurrent tegmen defects [5] have been shown to correlate with increasing SSCD length. These, of course, do not cause any symptoms, unless there is an associated encephalocele or CSF leak.

- **Q. Patients often find their ears popping, and they feel full, when symptoms start. Why is this the case—are the Eustachian tubes affected by TMWS?**
  - **A.** The literature is silent on any effects of TMWS on eustachian tube function. However, there is an overlap of symptoms in patients who have patulous eustachian tubes and SCD—autophony to voice and breathing. Patients who hear loud popping in their ears are likely hearing some internal noise that is normal (such as eustachian tube opening) but is perceived louder due to their TMWS. As for the fullness sensation, this is a symptom well described to be part of TMWS. Its etiology is debatable. Lastly, eustachian tube dysfunction (ETD) is extremely common. The concurrence of ETD and a TMWD is almost assuredly to occur on a regular basis.
- **Q. When might a ventilation tube in the eardrum be helpful?**
  - **A.** In the early years after SCD was identified and surgical occlusion/repair was shown to be successful, several surgeons anecdotally noted that ventilation tube (VT) placement alleviated their patients' symptoms. However, the initial enthusiasm for VT placement as a means for treatment of SSCD did not bear out, with most patients finding no influence on their symptoms. With that qualifier, in my practice I have found VT placement very helpful in two specific situations. The first is the patient who has otic barotrauma with air travel. Most patients with otic barotrauma will have no more problems than otalgia upon descent of the aircraft. However, the TMWS patient who suffers otic barotrauma will not just have pain, but also have nausea, vertigo/dizziness, and, in some cases, labyrinthine damage. VT placement can allow these patients to fly in comfort and potentially prevent more significant problems. The second group of patients are those who have chronic or recurrent eustachian tube dysfunction. Besides having the usual symptoms due to negative middle ear pressure, the TMWS patients also will suffer from its effect on the TMWD. Furthermore, the inevitable urge to auto-inflate can exacerbate or trigger vestibular events in the TMWS patient. Placement of VT can prevent

this. I suspect many of my colleagues I mentioned above, who noted VT placement benefitting their patients, may have had patients with concomitant eustachian tube dysfunction.

- **Q. Do the majority of patients with TMWS hear their eyes move? Those who do not are sometimes told, wrongly, that they cannot therefore be suffering from that condition.**
  - **A.** My experience is that most patients do not hear their eyes move. The symptoms associated with TMWS are varied. It has been called the great Otologic Mimicker due to its varied presentation and its ability to present like many other otologic conditions. Not all patients with TMWD have autophony or bone conduction hyperacusis and not all patients with autophony or bone conduction hyperacusis have TMWD. As mentioned above, patulous eustachian tube is a condition with the prominent symptom of hearing one's own voice and breathing. Autophony to eye movement is more specific to TMWS. The Barany Society, in an attempt to organize a diagnostic criterion for SSCD listed several symptoms that are needed for diagnosis [6]:
  - *At least one of the following symptoms consistent with the presence of a 'third mobile window' in the inner ear:*

    Bone conduction hyperacusis [1]
    Sound-induced vertigo and/or oscillopsia time-locked to the stimulus [2]
    Pressure-induced vertigo and/or oscillopsia time-locked to the stimulus [3]
    Pulsatile tinnitus

    Bone conduction hyperacusis is defined as: "Symptoms can include hearing one's voice loudly or distorted in the affected ear (auto-phony), abnormal perception of one's own internal body sounds like hearing loudly one's eye movements or blinking, borborygmi, crepitus from jaw or neck movements, and footfalls."
  - According to these criteria, not only is "hearing your eyes move" not necessary to make the diagnosis, bone conduction hyperacusis (of any internal noises) is not necessary to make the diagnosis.

- **Q. Hyperacusis can be debilitating. It is complicated by the diversity of its cause and clinical presentation. Four subtypes have been identified: excessive loudness, annoyance, fear, and pain. Do you agree that a question for future research remains as to how these overlap, or whether they are mechanistically distinct disorders?**
  - **A.** The investigation into hyperacusis has been ongoing prior to its current intersection with TMWS. The advent of TMWS as a progenitor of hyperacusis will likely reveal that much of what was considered a psychological disorder or a central nervous system disorder is originated in the peripheral end organ. I suspect the four types described are simply differing manifestations of the same process. Early in my career (prior to the discovery of SSCD), I felt

frustrated in treating these patients and felt I had little to offer them for treatment. However, now it seems like virtually all of my TMWS patients have hyperacusis to some degree. I am happy to tell them that there are treatment options that can successfully control their symptoms. That said, I think this subject is one that has much to be explored in the future of TMWS research.

- **Q. Patients of TMWS often suffer from neck stiffness or pain, without realizing that symptom is connected to their inner ear disorder. Can you explain why this happens—does the vestibular system partly control the neck muscles?**
  - **A.** While the vestibulo-ocular reflex is the most well known of the vestibular reflexes, there are several others. Abnormal vestibular stimulation will result in symptoms associated with these reflexes when provoked. The vestibulocollic reflex (VCR) is a well-described reflex to the neck muscles whose purpose is to stabilize the head. Labyrinthectomized animals will demonstrate the classic head tilt reaction (head tilted to the labyrinthectomized side) due to abnormal stimulation of the VCR. In humans, the head tilt reaction is muted by comparison to lower animals. The main symptom from abnormal VCR stimulation is neck pain/stiffness. The most common location for this discomfort is the upper part of the neck near the insertion into the occiput.
- **Q. Many also complain of more generalized head pressure—is there anything in particular that might be contributing to that, or are various factors involved?**
  - **A.** Generalized head pressure is a symptom of elevated intracranial pressure (ICP). In my practice, we routinely measure ICP. Some patients with TMWS are found to have Pseudotumor Cerebri and will benefit greatly from efforts to lower ICP. There are other patients with TMWD who do not have Pseudotumor Cerebri but appear to be much more sensitive to mildly elevated ICP. These patients also note significant benefit from lowering ICP and specifically the symptom of head pressure improves.
- **Q. In connection to the previous question, low barometric pressure has adverse consequences for a lot of patients. Is the biggest issue the change in pressure differential at the round and oval windows, with the inner ear reflecting the intracranial pressure and the other side the barometric pressure?**
  - **A.** While it has been observed that low barometric pressure can cause exacerbation of otologic symptoms in TMWD patients, there have been no studies regarding this topic. That said, the only place the inner ear interfaces with atmospheric pressure is through the oval and round windows. Consequently, it would seem logical that the oval and/or round window (OW/RW) would be involved somehow in barometric pressure affecting the inner ear in TMWD. Most likely the change in the pressure across the OW/RW would cause a shift in pressure across the inner ear due to the relatively higher intra-

cranial pressure (compared to higher barometric pressure). We know that increased pressure into the middle ear (via Nasal Valsalva) and at the OW (via Fistula Testing) can provoke vestibular stimulation in TMWS patients. It would seem likely that a similar mechanism occurs with a change to lower barometric pressure.
  - Alternatively, low barometric pressure has been seen as an exacerbant of Migraine, and the co-occurrence of Migraine with TMWS would seem to be assured given the prevalence of Migraine.

- **Q. Have you ever encountered a patient whose dehiscence has closed up on its own, or who has improved dramatically without surgery?**
  - **A.** While I have never encountered a patient whose dehiscence has closed spontaneously, recently Bhatt et al. [7] reported five cases of superior canal bone growth after cartilage capping procedures. These were patients who had preoperative CT scans demonstrating SSCD and postoperative CT scans demonstrating growth of bone covering the prior SSCD. There was one additional patient who had ectopic bone growth adjacent to the dehiscence.
  - Symptom resolution or improvement without surgery is not unusual. It has been observed in the past that symptoms can wax and wane with long periods of remission. It appears that much of the symptom improvement (or worsening) is correlated with patient activity—the more strenuous activity, the more symptoms. Some patients recognize this and avoid triggers thus minimizing vestibular stimulation, while other patients fail to recognize this. We have advocated a number of medical measures to minimize TMWS (see Chap. 13 on Medical Therapy) as an alternative to surgical intervention, while leaving surgery for those who fail to have adequate resolution with such measures.

- **Q. Is it the case that TMWS symptoms quite often trigger migraine symptoms? And can treatment of the migraine sometimes give a patient sufficient relief to avoid surgery?**
  - **A.** Migraine is a very common disorder and concomitant Migraine in TMWS occurs. It has been observed that Migraine patients have a prolonged recovery and somewhat less successful outcome from surgical repair than those without Migraine. Because Migraine and TMWS have overlapping symptoms, it would seem prudent to maximize therapy for Migraine before recommending surgery for TMWS. There is also a subgroup of patients with TMWS and headache that will have resolution of headache after surgery. Whether this represents a Migraine resolved by treatment of TMWS or a different headache disorder entirely is up for debate.

- **Q. With regard to the progression of symptoms, is there a point at which you would advise someone not to drive?**
  - **A.** I always advise extreme caution with driving, climbing, operating heavy machinery, or any other activity where poor balance places the patient or others at risk of injury. I advise the patients to err on the side of caution, and I

remind them that TMWS is not a fatal disease unless it results in trauma due to a fall or motor vehicle accident. However, I find it hard to make a blanket statement for a patient to not drive. Many patients have significant time where they are free of symptoms and the restriction from driving is very limiting in our society. Most patients know when to drive and when not to drive. However, there are some who do not. For those patients, I advise against driving. I also advise professional drivers (such as truck drivers and airline pilots) to discontinue until their disease is under control.

- **Q. Patients who have been diagnosed with TMWS are usually nervous about flying. Should they try to avoid flying, or are there just precautionary measures they can sensibly take to prevent their symptoms worsening?**
  - **A.** For all TMWS patients we advocate avoidance of air travel if they have a URI or sinusitis. However, most patients with TMWS can fly without problems. The ones that have problems are those with borderline eustachian tube function and consequently are prone to otic barotrauma. For those patients, we recommend nasal decongestants prior to travel, Earplanes, and, if necessary, myringotomy and/or VT.
- **Q. For a pregnant woman who has already been diagnosed with TMWS, would you always advise a C-section delivery or are there circumstances in which that can be avoided?**
  - **A.** We generally advocate C-sections for all TMWS patients due to the observation of TMWS worsening/onset with vaginal delivery. At present, I am not aware of a circumstance that would mitigate this.

Diagnosis

- **Q. The diagnostic process for TMWS needs speeding up, most would agree about that. Can you see wider use of the skull vibration-induced nystagmus test helping with that, as it is a noninvasive rapid first-line test which has shown to be well tolerated by adults and children? It reveals any vestibular asymmetry, so should it be used regularly by physicians in primary care?**
  - **A.** Vibration-induced nystagmus (VIN) is a very nonspecific test that demonstrates nystagmus with vestibular function asymmetry regardless of the cause. In SSCD, VIN tends to be a torsional-vertical nystagmus suggestive of superior canal stimulation, but this can be seen with other conditions. We like the VIN test as a confirmation of vestibular asymmetry and helpful in pointing to a vestibular cause of the patient's symptoms but do not see it as particularly useful in the specific diagnosis of TMWD.

- **Q. Could you please put to rest a matter that has often delayed an accurate diagnosis for TMWS patients. If a VEMP test result is normal, can a person still potentially be suffering from the disorder?**
  - **A.** VEMP testing includes both oVEMP (testing principally the utricle) and cVEMP (testing principally the saccule). cVEMP testing is the most widely available and the test most commonly referred to as "VEMP testing." While it is often abnormally present at higher amplitude responses and lower threshold levels in SSCD, it is a test dependent on the patient's volitional contraction of their sternocleidomastoid muscle. Inadequate muscle contraction or inadequate muscle size can result in less responsiveness unrelated to SSCD. So, a patient who does not contract the muscle (or does not adequately contract the muscle) can have an absent cVEMP response, regardless of the status of their saccule or SSCD. Further, any labyrinthine damage can cause damage to the saccule and reduce its responsiveness to sound stimulation. Many TMWS patients have evidence of inner ear damage, and concomitant damage to the saccule cannot be ruled out. oVEMP testing is less commonly employed but appears to be more sensitive and specific to TMWS. oVEMP is less plagued with the problem with volitional muscle contraction since the only instruction for the patients is to keep their line of site elevated. However, the utricle can be damaged by the same processes that cause caloric weakness (horizontal canal dysfunction). While abnormal cVEMP or oVEMP results support the diagnosis of TMWS, normal results do not rule out the diagnosis.
- **Q. Aural fullness is so often a first or early symptom. The person then goes along to their doctor who frequently advises them to perform a Valsalva maneuver and take decongestants. Is there more that such a doctor could be doing at this initial stage that would move the patient closer to a diagnosis of TMWS?**
  - **A.** The recommendation to perform a nasal Valsalva maneuver stems from the presumed diagnosis of eustachian tube dysfunction (ETD), which is certainly much more common than TMWS. So, it is not surprising for this to be the first recommendation given to patients with aural fullness. I suspect the best piece of advice for both patients and physicians is that, if autoinflation or other methods directed towards ETD does not resolve the problem, then further investigation is warranted.
- **Q. The diagnosis of Vestibular Migraine is possibly overused, and some might argue it has become the "trash can" diagnosis when a physician doesn't know what is wrong with a patient. Is there something specific that could be done to prevent this happening?**
  - **A.** I do believe the diagnosis of Migraine is often used as a default diagnosis when a physician is unsure of the diagnosis. That said, a trial of anti-migraine therapy is very reasonable as an initial treatment strategy. However, if a patient does not respond to conventional anti-migraine therapy, the clinician should

be prompted to look for other diagnoses. Unfortunately, in medicine patients often get a label that becomes difficult for doctors to look beyond, despite evidence to the contrary and despite failed therapy directed towards that diagnosis.

- **Q. How do you think hypothyroidism in a patient may contribute towards TMWS symptoms? Do you rule it in or out with all your vestibular patients, and how do you treat it in the positive cases?**
  - **A.** Hypothyroidism has long been associated with Ménière's disease and treatment of Hypothyroidism has been associated with improvement of Ménière's disease [8]. Given that there is a significant overlap in symptoms for Ménière's and TMWS, as well as the recent studies demonstrating a high incidence of endolymphatic hydrops among SSCD patients, it would seem prudent to screen for and treat hypothyroidism. Besides the benefit of relief from symptoms of hypothyroidism, I have witnessed significant improvement in TMWS symptoms among patients I have treated. So, from a pragmatic as well as a possible etiologic standpoint, it seems to make sense to screen for hypothyroidism. My experience has demonstrated that the most common patient that benefits from this is the patient who was already diagnosed with hypothyroidism many years earlier and is currently getting treatment. However, their current treatment has not been assessed in quite some time and, when assessed, is found to be subtherapeutic.
- **Q. When diagnosing a truly bilateral patient, do they always have more symptoms from one ear, and how do you determine which ear that is?**
  - **A.** Most patients with bilateral disease will have one ear that gives them the most symptoms, and this will be evident from the history prior to any testing. In fact, many times the symptoms from the more symptomatic ear will overshadow symptoms from the contralateral ear. Keep in mind that auditory symptoms are usually able to be lateralized (i.e., do you have aural fullness in your right ear?), whereas vestibular symptoms are typically not able to be lateralized (i.e., is your right ear giving you vertigo?). The auditory symptoms are always in comparison of the "bad ear" to the "good ear" with the patient's presumption that the "good ear" is normal, regardless of whether that is the case. It is not unusual for a patient with "unilateral autophony" to have resolution of autophony after surgery but then to notice autophony in the contralateral ear postoperatively since they are now comparing it to an ear without autophony. So, from an auditory standpoint it is relatively easy to determine the more affected ear. From a vestibular standpoint, testing is usually necessary. Among the tests that correlate with vestibular problems and help determine the more affected ear we use cVEMP, oVEMP, Fistula test, Tullio test, ECOG, and the Platform Pressure Test. The more severely affected vestibular ear will tend to be more abnormally stimulated with this battery of tests. These test results are used in combination with the patient's history, the audiometric results, and the patient's wishes to help determine which ear should

first undergo surgery. In general, we try to do surgery on the most affected ear first with the hope that it will give the most benefit and possibly allow the patients to avoid a contralateral surgery. Interestingly, we have found the anatomic findings on CT scan to have little impact on this decision.

- **Q. The progression of TMWS symptoms for a musician can frequently signal the end of their musical career. Are there words of hope that you can offer for such individuals? Is there a chance they might resume playing their instrument?**
  - **A.** Musicians are affected by TMWS like other patients but because of their profession the manifestations can be disproportionate. Two factors loom large for musicians: (1) Tullio Phenomenon and (2) Strain-induced dizziness/vertigo. Many patients can avoid Tullio phenomenon by avoiding the offending noise or using noise-canceling headphones. This is not a viable tactic for many musicians. Strain-induced vertigo/dizziness is a problem more prominent for singers and for musicians who use brass and wind instruments. The Valsalva maneuver required for these activities will exacerbate their symptoms. TMWS can cripple a career in music. The good news is that I have had several musicians return to their profession after surgical repair, and recently, I had an opera singer who returned to singing with medical management of SSCD.

Surgery

- **Q. I think there may be a certain amount of misunderstanding among the patient population about what a plugging surgery does. Plugging a semicircular canal decreases its function, rather than completely destroying it—is that correct? And the function of the canal may even have been diminished before surgery if the overlying dura was compressing it—does that happen often?**
  - **A.** The concept behind plugging of the superior semicircular canal dehiscence is to prevent endolymphatic motion through the superior canal. Theoretically, this would in fact completely remove superior canal function from the plugged canal and prevent otolithic stimulation. In reality, there is still some residual movement and consequently function of the superior canal, albeit quite diminished from preoperatively. In contrast, resurfacing or capping procedures at least theoretically preserve or improve superior canal function. In practical application, however, sometimes these approaches result in partial occlusion and reduction in superior canal function.
  - Regarding superior canal function, our only clinically available means for testing is vHIT. Keep in mind that vHIT only assesses the very high frequency of vestibular response, and we have no means to assess the rest of the vestibular response frequency spectrum such as we have for the horizontal semicir-

cular canal. Regarding reduced vHIT responses in SSCD preoperatively, it has been noted to be a frequent finding but, interestingly, vHIT of the other canals (posterior and horizontal) have also demonstrated reduced response on the side affected by SSCD [9]. There does appear to be a size effect that is associated with reduced function. This has been ascribed to the possibility of herniated dura plugging a portion of the superior canal. Postoperatively for SSCD plugging, vHIT has demonstrated reduced VOR response for the surgically plugged superior canal, but also for the ipsilateral horizontal and posterior canals [10]. This has been attributed to a possible inflammatory response in the postoperative labyrinth.

- **Q. Occlusions/plugging surgeries have been known to fail after being initially successful. Have you ever known a successful resurfacing surgery suddenly fail?**
  - **A.** I have certainly encountered failed capping and resurfacing procedures—both my own and other surgeons'. However, the more common history of failed surgery is either (1) failure to relieve symptoms, noted almost immediately postoperative, or (2) slow return of symptoms. The typical reason for failed resurfacing surgery is failure of the resurfacing material to provide a solid repair. In this scenario, the patient may have a short reprieve from symptoms due to swelling in the area and reduced transmission of pressure from the dura. However, once this has resolved, the symptoms return to become almost identical to preoperative. In surgical exploration, these cases usually demonstrate "soft" or semisolid HA cement, or no residual resurfacing material, suggesting that it had been completely resorbed. The cases of failed capping procedures are usually due to either improper placement or slippage of the capping material. These cases usually have a similar clinical course as the resurfacing failures, with symptoms returning shortly after surgery. By contrast, failure of occlusion surgeries can sometimes be delayed by a year postoperatively. This is likely due to scar contracture of the plugging material, eventually reaching a critical point where the plug is no longer of sufficient size to prevent endolymphatic movement.
- **Q. Is a resurfacing surgery less likely to be successful if a significant amount of the canal is eroded?**
  - **A.** In general, resurfacing techniques have shown to have a somewhat lower success rate than plugging or capping procedures. A very large SSCD would seem to be more easily approached and more successfully approached by a capping or plugging procedure than resurfacing. With resurfacing, the larger the area that needs to be resurfaced, the larger the area at risk for failure.
- **Q. To get the best seal, one that is truly pressure-tight, is it advisable for surgeons to always use a patient's own tissues, i.e., fascia and bone?**
  - **A.** This is a question that has not yet been answered. My general impression is that as long as the repair is extradural in a capping procedure, the edges of

the cap (whether bone, cartilage, or other substance) will seal with scarring at the edges that eventually form an adequate seal. With plugging procedures, most surgeons will perform either a resurfacing or capping on top of the plug. I think the same applies in this situation. However, I think the more important principle to consider is whether the repair is rigid or not. A non-rigid repair will result in persistent symptoms postoperatively.

- **Q. At either end of the spectrum, young or old, are there age limits beyond which you believe it is unwise to operate?**
  - **A.** Yes. In those less than 5 years of age, we need to be mindful that the superior canal ossification may not yet be complete. In some cases, the finding of SSCD may be a transient condition that resolves with maturation. Further, this is an age group where SSCD may be present but asymptomatic. Identifying an "active" SSCD in this age group is much more challenging than in adults. So, I would advise extreme caution in the very young.
  - As for the older population, the two factors to consider are (1) the patient's ability to tolerate general anesthesia and (2) the patient's ability to compensate for any vestibular loss or change in the vestibular system. The first factor is common with any other elective surgery in the elderly. The second factor becomes a bigger factor with increasing age. In general, the younger the patient, the more plasticity and capacity for central vestibular compensation. Because of these issues, we sometimes advocate window reinforcement surgery as an alternative for the elderly.
- **Q. What if hearing loss is increasing over time, and tinnitus is getting worse? In those circumstances might a surgery prevent a patient's hearing from deteriorating even further?**
  - **A.** In general, I do not advocate SSCD surgery for hearing loss or tinnitus due to poor reliability of outcome. My main indications for surgical intervention are vestibular symptoms, autophony, and noise intolerance since these symptoms are reliably resolved with surgical intervention.
  - While theoretically surgery to prevent hearing loss/tinnitus progression seems to make sense, currently there does not appear to be any literature to support "prophylactive" surgery in TMWS. Having done my first SSCD surgery in January 1998, I have had the opportunity to follow postoperative patients for more than two decades. Even in successful surgeries with patients who have no TMWS complaints, there are some in whom I have witnessed their hearing to slowly decline. The cause for this may be related to the previously repaired SSCD or it may be a completely unrelated etiology. However, this observation would seem to indicate that hearing may decline despite successful surgery in some patients.
- **Q. Has any research been undertaken to look at whether early intervention might be beneficial, particularly in those diagnosed at a young age? In other words, rather than postponing a surgery until the symptoms become intol-**

erable, proceeding quickly to enable an easier and swifter return to an asymptomatic life.

- **A.** There is no research yet that I have seen regarding this issue. Given that many patients will be asymptomatic or minimally symptomatic throughout their life, intervention in an asymptomatic patient would seem unwise at this point. Every intervention comes with risk, and I would argue that putting an asymptomatic patient at risk of a complication or side effect does not make sense. The old rule of "First, do no harm" applies here.

Post-surgery

- **Q. Are there factors in a patient's past history that will determine the extent and speed of their recovery from surgery? Will a ballet dancer with their excellent poise, for example, generally do better than a rather sedentary office worker?**
  - **A.** Multiple factors play into recovery from surgery—some within our control and some not. It has long been known that recovery from a vestibular deafferentation procedure correlates with the process of central vestibular compensation. The requirement for central compensation is brain plasticity and an active patient—both of which tend to decline with age. Vestibular exercises enhance this process. Vestibular surgery of any kind will change the vestibular function to some degree and require central compensation. The more drastic the change in function, the more prolonged the recovery. The surgical procedure employed and the preoperative residual vestibular function both factor into time for central compensation. A patient with no measurable vestibular function will not see a dramatic change with a labyrinthectomy, and hence will not have near as prolonged recovery as a patient with normal preoperative vestibular function. So, in this example the patient with normal preoperative vestibular function will generally have the longer and more difficult recovery. One wild card with SSCD surgery is the possibility of an inflammatory reaction that can alter vestibular function much more than the intent of the surgeon. These patients will take much longer to recover in general than those who do not have an inflammatory response. However, if everything else were equal, a ballet dancer will recover much more quickly than a sedentary office worker.
- **Q. Does the timeline for recovery after surgery vary considerably? Would you expect most patients to be able to return to their normal activities after six weeks, with no straining or heavy lifting during that period?**
  - **A.** As noted in the prior question and answer, there are several variables at play, but in general, most patients will be able to return to normal activities within six weeks. Many will have postoperative BPPV. This usually is noted the first week after surgery and most resolve spontaneously within the first

couple of weeks. If not, they respond well to canalith repositioning. Further improvement with vestibular compensation throughout the first postoperative year is the general rule, although the bulk of symptomatic improvement is noted within the first three months.

- **Q. Could you explain what postoperative symptoms, such as autophony and ear fullness, are caused by fluid, blood, and swelling in the ear, and how long they may be expected to last.**
  - **A.** The most common reason for autophony is a conductive hearing loss—much more common than TMWS. Postoperatively, virtually all patients will have a conductive hearing loss due to hemotympanum and associated swelling. Patients who have window reinforcement surgery will also have some additional temporary conductive hearing loss due to the repair material utilized. How quickly the middle ear aerates and the conductive gap resolves will vary to a great degree for individual patients, often depending on whether there is any eustachian tube dysfunction. The resolution of the above middle ear problems correlates with reduction of the autophony and fullness sensation postoperatively.
- **Q. Post-surgery vertigo and disequilibrium can cause patients anxiety about whether or not their operation has been successful. Is BPPV often at the root of this, and needs to be addressed with Epley maneuvers? Can any damage be caused by doing these maneuvers when the problem is actually not BPPV?**
  - **A.** Postoperative BPPV is so common after surgery for TMWS that I tell patients to expect it, especially the first week. It usually resolves without treatment but will respond to canalith repositioning. Performing canalith repositioning in the immediate postoperative period is not deleterious but I am reticent to use mastoid oscillation in the early weeks after surgery. I am unaware of any potential damage that can occur in performing an Epley maneuver when BPPV is not the cause of the patient's vertigo. I have performed Epley maneuvers on patients where I was not sure if they had BPPV simply because it has such a favorable risk/benefit ratio. Another cause for postoperative vertigo is edema and inflammation, both of which will resolve with time.
- **Q. In the case of a bilateral patient, after their first surgery on one side are symptoms from the other side often unmasked? Could you estimate the percentage of bilateral patients to whom this may happen?**
  - **A.** Certainly there are patients with bilateral disease who have their better side "unmasked" after the first procedure. The typical symptoms that are unmasked are the auditory symptoms—fullness, tinnitus, autophony—rather than the vestibular symptoms. While the phenomenon of unmasking certainly occurs, most bilateral patients seem to identify bilateral symptoms. I would estimate that I have seen this unmasking in perhaps 10% bilateral patients.

- **Q. How important is post-surgery vestibular therapy? Would a patient have an equally successful long-term outcome without it, and it just speeds up that recovery process?**
  - **A.** Vestibular exercises are routinely employed after surgery and many studies support their benefits in hastening a more complete recovery. The exact form of vestibular therapy is not yet defined and is being actively investigated. Are there some patients who would have successful long-term outcome without vestibular therapy? Almost certainly, but there are many who would struggle without it. It could also be argued that those who "do well" without vestibular therapy may have had a better outcome with it.
- **Q. The fear of having an unsuccessful surgery for TMWS is a very real one for many patients. Is it appropriate to wait at least six months from the surgery before any investigations are undertaken to determine whether the operation really has failed?**
  - **A.** My general rule is that three months is a reasonable time to assess surgical success even though they have not attained maximal improvement. At three months, the wounds are well healed, a fair degree of swelling has resolved, and even though patients will note improvement in central compensation for a year, the bulk of that improvement is seen in the first three months.
- **Q. When it comes to a revision surgery, are there increased risks, such as hearing loss being more likely? Could you please summarize what is known about a revision surgery's success rate being lower?**
  - **A.** As with most revision surgeries, complications tend to be higher, and success tends to be lower. Specific to SSCD surgery, the literature suggests a higher rate of hearing loss and a higher risk of CSF leak. Scarring and distorted landmarks are inevitably encountered in revision surgery and may be the cause for some of this. Success in revision SSCD surgery has been reported to be lower than primary surgery. I suspect the reason for this may have more to do with diagnosis than surgical technique. The current diagnostic criteria for SSCD includes (1) history compatible with SSCD, (2) testing compatible with SSCD, and (3) CT findings of SSCD. However, just arriving at the diagnosis of SSCD is not enough. Some of these patients undergoing revision surgery will have other problems not addressed with the surgery. Some of the more common concomitant problems are second dehiscent sites, elevated intracranial pressure, perilymphatic fistula, endolymphatic hydrops, and migraine. A thorough evaluation of the patient from the start will help obviate the need for revision surgery and the very unfortunate event of failed revision surgery.

The Future

- **Q. An important question for future treatment relates to whether stem cells could be used clinically to help replace damaged or missing bone. An important discovery in 2018 was the identification of the human skeletal stem cell. Professor Charles Chan at Stanford University School of Medicine explained, "The skeletal stem cell we've identified possesses all of the hallmark qualities of true, multi-potential, self-renewing, tissue-specific stem cells. They are restricted in terms of their fate potential to just skeletal tissues, which is likely to make them much more clinically useful." Do you foresee any potential uses within the scope of TMWS?**
  - **A.** I do not. Currently, surgeons use autologous bone and bone dust that result in bone formation in this area. Use of differentiated material such as this would seem much safer since we know the end result of its use. Skeletal stem cell use in this area may provide a similar benefit but has a few drawbacks. The first is the unpredictability of the outcome compared to the autologous grafts that have been used for decades, of which the outcomes are very predictable. The second would be the cost. Undoubtably, skeletal stem cells would add significant cost to a surgical procedure where the cost of an autologous graft is mostly just a few minutes of time in the OR.

References

1. Chien WW, Janky K, Minor LB, Carey JP. Superior canal dehiscence size: multivariate assessment of clinical impact. Otol Neurotol. 2012;33(5):810–5. https://doi.org/10.1097/MAO.0b013e318248eac4. PMID: 22664896; PMCID: PMC3620043.
2. Yuen HW, Boeddinghaus R, Eikelboom RH, Atlas MD. The relationship between the air-bone gap and the size of superior semicircular canal dehiscence. Otolaryngol Head Neck Surg. 2009;141(6):689–94. https://doi.org/10.1016/j.otohns.2009.08.029. Epub 2009 Oct 31. PMID: 19932839.
3. Yuen HW, Boeddinghaus R, Eikelboom RH, Atlas MD. 15th Yahya Cohen Memorial Lecture - the relationship between the air-bone gap and the size of superior semicircular canal dehiscence. Ann Acad Med Singap. 2011;40(1):59–64. PMID: 21369635.
4. Maheu M, Elblidi A, Saliba I. Investigating performance of cVEMP and oVEMP in the identification of superior canal dehiscence in relation to dehiscence location and size. Audiol Res. 2021;11(3):452–62. https://doi.org/10.3390/audiolres11030042. PMID: 34562880; PMCID: PMC8482095.
5. Formeister EJ, Zhang L, Dent J, Aygun N, Carey JP. Predictive factors for concurrent tegmen dehiscence in superior canal dehiscence syndrome. Otol Neurotol. 2022;43(4):494–9. https://doi.org/10.1097/MAO.0000000000003481. PMID: 35213476.

6. Ward BK, van de Berg R, van Rompaey V, Bisdorff A, Hullar TE, Welgampola MS, Carey JP. Superior semicircular canal dehiscence syndrome: diagnostic criteria consensus document of the committee for the classification of vestibular disorders of the Bárány Society. J Vestib Res. 2021;31(3):131–41. https://doi.org/10.3233/VES-200004. PMID: 33522990.
7. Bhatt AA, Vibhute P, Gupta V, Zapala DA, Pooley RA, Lundy LB. New bone formation over dehiscent semicircular canal with cartilage cap. Neuroradiol J. 2022;19714009221096820 https://doi.org/10.1177/19714009221096820. Epub ahead of print. PMID: 35506568.
8. Santosh UP, Rao MS. Incidence of hypothyroidism in Ménière's disease. J Clin Diagn Res. 2016;10(5):MC01–3. 10.7860/JCDR/2016/17587.7759. Epub 2016 May 1. PMID: 27437251; PMCID: PMC4948427.
9. Tikka T, Slim MAM, Gaggini M, Kontorinis G. Video Head Impulse Test (vHIT) findings in patients with superior semicircular canal dehiscence: a case-control study. J Int Adv Otol. 2021;17(2):103–8. https://doi.org/10.5152/JIAO.2021.8572. PMID: 33893778.
10. Mantokoudis G, Saber Tehrani AS, Wong AL, Agrawal Y, Wenzel A, Carey JP. Adaptation and compensation of vestibular responses following superior canal dehiscence surgery. Otol Neurotol. 2016;37(9):1399–405. https://doi.org/10.1097/MAO.0000000000001196. PMID: 27556420; PMCID: PMC5025376.

Part VI
The Future

Introduction

One of the things that attracts aspiring clinicians to the field of medicine is its dynamism. Medicine is constantly evolving and trying to improve itself. Our field is no different than the rest of medicine. I know that there is a large swath of hardworking, motivated, and innovative professionals pushing the boundaries of what we know now and what we will know in the future. This last chapter will focus on what research is being done and what should be done to further the body of knowledge on Third Mobile Window Syndrome disorders. The authors do an impressive job reviewing multiple aspects of TMWD with recommendations for future research. Young clinicians and researchers would do well to let this chapter guide them to future endeavours.

Chapter 30
Future Research

Bradley W. Kesser and Daniel R. Morrison

Introduction

The concept of the mobile third window was first described by Tullio in the early twentieth century when he found that fenestration of the lateral semicircular canal in pigeons would produce a characteristic sound-induced vertigo [1]. It was not until the late 1990s, however, that superior semicircular canal dehiscence (SSCD), the most common pathologic third mobile window syndrome (TMWS), was described [2, 3]. Over the last quarter century, SSCD has attracted an increasing amount, if not explosion, of interest within the neurotology and neurology communities. The number of publications regarding SSCD has risen exponentially, and it is a topic now discussed annually at national meetings. For example, for the last two years, the annual American Neurotology Society meeting has had a dedicated panel geared towards SSCD and other TMWS. Searching the PubMed database for "superior semicircular canal dehiscence" reveals a steadily increasing number of annual publications (Fig. 30.1). The disease entity "Semicircular canal dehiscence" is now a term in the Medical Subject Headings (MeSH) database, added in 2021.

Past research has significantly advanced our understanding of third mobile window syndromes (TMWS) such as SSCD. For example, vestibular evoked myogenic potentials (VEMP) have been extensively studied and VEMP testing is now considered essential for the diagnosis of SSCD. Research is conducted both from a clinical and basic science standpoint, and there are now multiple animal models of third window syndromes used by investigators around the world. Conducting clinical research on TMWS is challenging for several reasons. First, the diagnosis of TMWS is often elusive, and TMWS has only recently become more widely recognized by

B. W. Kesser (✉) · D. R. Morrison
UVA Health, Charlottesville, VA, USA
e-mail: BWK2N@uvahealth.org; BEK7PS@uvahealth.org

G. J. Gianoli, P. Thomson (eds.), *Third Mobile Window Syndrome of the Inner Ear*, https://doi.org/10.1007/978-3-031-16586-3_30

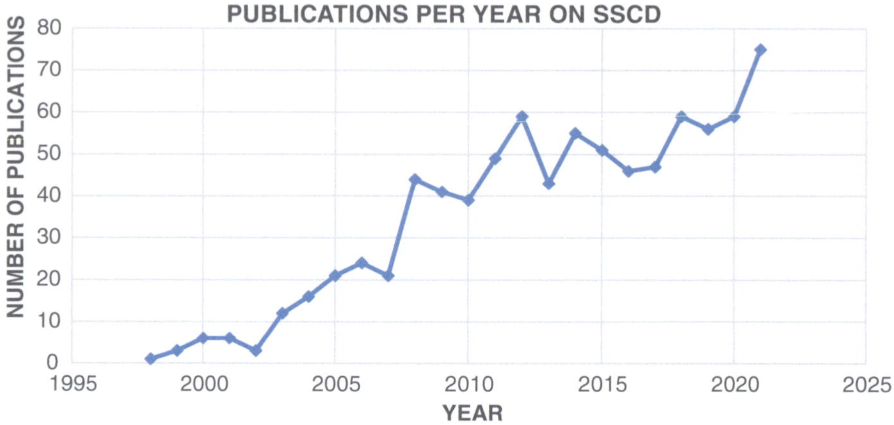

Fig. 30.1 Number of publications in PubMed database on the topic of SSCD per year. PubMed search was performed using the term "superior semicircular canal dehiscence"

clinicians. Additional factors include the heterogeneity of patient presentations, the lack of standardized diagnostic and treatment protocols across institutions, and the lack of standardized outcome measures regarding patient satisfaction and quality of life. There remain several TMWS management controversies including proper diagnostic workup, indications for surgery, and techniques for repair, as evidenced by a recent survey of members of the American Otologic Society and the American Neurotologic Society [4].

This final chapter will recapitulate some of the recent research on TMWS. We will touch on etiology, pathophysiology, diagnosis, treatment modalities, and outcomes. Current experimental models of TMWS will be briefly reviewed. We hope to provide a framework for conducting future investigation on third window disorders.

Prevalence, Etiology, Pathophysiology, Natural History

Prevalence

The true population prevalence of TMWS is difficult to determine. However, there have been excellent cadaveric studies, notably from the Johns Hopkins temporal bone library showing a 0.5% incidence of SSCD and a 0.6% cochlear-facial dehiscence [5, 6]. The introduction of this textbook, in fact, asserts that TMWS is not truly a rare disorder as defined by the Rare Disease Act of 2002 (affecting 0.06% of the population or less). Several studies focus on radiographic evidence of SSCD or near-dehiscence in patients undergoing temporal bone imaging for a variety of reasons, with prevalence rates ranging from 1.7% to 9% [7–10]. The prevalence of radiographic cochlear-facial dehiscence has been reported to be 1.4–9% [11, 12]. Due to the inherent flaws of imaging, these rates are very likely overestimations of the real prevalence rate. Additionally, these rates represent primarily incidental findings in patients who underwent high-resolution computed tomography imaging (HRCT) for unrelated reasons. The true prevalence of TMWS in the general population remains uncertain.

Etiology

There are multiple theories regarding the underlying etiology of SSCD. Certainly, there is no one single underlying, unifying etiology which explains every patient's SSCD. A primary tenet in clinical medicine is to treat the disorder underlying the patient's illness. Therefore, it stands to reason that an attempt to understand why a patient developed TMWS is warranted. At present time, unless the history is highly suggestive, this is not a straightforward task.

SSCD is thought to potentially arise from a congenital thinning of the bone of the middle cranial fossa and that overlying the superior semicircular canal [5, 13]. In some patients, there may be either a traumatic event or chronic dural pulsations causing a "second hit" leading to symptomatic SSCD. Multiple studies have found a relatively high prevalence of radiographic SSCD in infants that then decreases with age, suggesting that some patients likely are left with thin bone of the middle cranial fossa (MCF) [14–16].

Idiopathic Intracranial Hypertension

The relationship between idiopathic intracranial hypertension (IIH) and SSCD has been investigated by multiple groups with mixed results [17–21]. Most of these studies are retrospective in nature and assess patients undergoing procedures related to their IIH (CSF leak repair) evaluating concomitant radiographic presence of SSCD. Other studies assess skull base thickness along the floor of the MCF in patients undergoing SSCD repair, with the assumption that those patients with IIH will have tegmen thinning as well.

Obesity is the greatest risk factor for IIH, so, if there is indeed a relationship between SSCD and IIH, one would suspect most SSCD patients to be obese. Yet, there is conflicting evidence regarding the relationship between obesity and SSCD [22–24]. Rizk et al. retrospectively found that MCF bone thickness in SSCD patients was lower than control groups with both increased and normal BMIs, indicating that SSCD is not more common in obese patients [25]. Schutt et al. found a higher incidence of spontaneous tegmen defects, obesity, and OSA in SSCD patients versus controls [24]. Kuo et al. retrospectively reviewed a cohort of patients undergoing lumber puncture for a variety of reasons and examined HRCT from this cohort, finding that the rate of radiographic SSCD was not higher in patients with elevated opening pressure [19]. It is worth noting that none of the patients in their cohort with radiographic SSCD had symptoms.

Clearly, larger population-based, likely multi-institutional studies are needed to clarify this relationship. Currently there are no published data regarding treatment of TMWS with medications like acetazolamide. Our review of the literature also shows a paucity of collaborative work between specialties who deal with IIH (i.e., neurology, ophthalmology). We believe it is in our collective interest to create a common vocabulary and promote interdisciplinary management of patients in whom IIH is suspected.

Metabolic Disorders

Osteoporosis has also been investigated as a potential underlying factor in the development of SSCD. Yu et al. reported a case series of female patients of East Asian descent with SSCD who all had osteoporosis or osteopenia based on bone mineral density scans [26]. Nguyen et al. reported similar findings in a group of female patients, also noting that serum calcium levels postoperatively after repair correlated negatively with the need for revision surgery. Serum levels of 25-hydroxyvitamin D negatively correlated with preoperative hyperacusis in SSCD patients and positively correlated with postoperative autophony [27]. These data support further investigation into the role of chronic metabolic issues and especially bone loss as an underlying etiology in SSCD in female patients.

Genetics

To date, there is no strong evidence supporting routine genetic testing in patients with SSCD. There are small published series showing familial SSCD, raising the suspicion for a genetic component. For example, Heidenreich et al. reported on three families, each with multiple first-degree relatives who had symptomatic SSCD. One of these families included a set of monozygotic twins [28]. Niesten et al. reported a similar case series with three affected families [29]. DFNA9, an autosomal dominant disorder resulting in progressive cochleovestibular dysfunction, has been associated with SSCD [30, 31]. Patients with COCH mutations have been found to have sclerotic lesions on HRCT affecting the semicircular canals with corresponding T2 signal loss on MRI [32]. Noonan et al. reviewed HRCT in patients with CDH23 pathogenic variants (Usher syndrome type 1D) and found a significantly higher risk of radiographic SSCD compared with age-matched controls [33]. Overall, much more work is needed to clarify whether there are clear genetic correlates with TMWS.

Symptoms and Natural History

Classic symptoms of TMWS include autophony, amplification of body sounds, sound- or pressure-induced vertigo, aural fullness, conductive hearing loss, and pulsatile tinnitus. However, not all patients present in the same way, even if their radiographic and audiometric testing are identical. There is evidence that size and location of the dehiscence in SSCD influence patient presentation, with larger dehiscences producing more cochleovestibular symptoms as well as reduced VEMP thresholds. Patients with bilateral SSCD tend to have more symptoms corresponding with the side of the larger dehiscence [34].

There is some evidence indicating cognitive and neurobehavioral dysfunction in patients with TMWS with improvement after repair [35]. There is a body of literature describing the interaction between the vestibular system and cognitive function in general, reviewed by Gurvich et al. [36]. These interesting findings should prompt inclusion of cognitive measures in studies examining TMWS to obtain a more "global" picture of these patients. Such cognitive studies could also serve as outcome measures following SSCD repair.

There is very little in the literature addressing the natural history of TMWS. Thus, it is difficult to counsel patients accurately on the likelihood of spontaneous improvement or progression of symptoms. Longitudinal studies of patients, both pediatric and adult, electing to forego surgical treatment for TMWS are needed, with particular focus on patient-described symptoms and quality of life measures.

Pathophysiology

The mechanisms of both the depression in air conduction threshold and the elevation in bone conduction thresholds in TMWS, primarily SSCD, have been the topic of several studies. Guan et al. [37] used a human cadaveric model to calculate the difference in sound pressure level during bone conduction stimulation between the scala vestibuli and scala tympani both before and after creation of a SSCD. They found that the pressure inside the scala vestibuli was increased in the SSCD condition, whereas the pressure was unchanged in the scala tympani, thus increasing the pressure differential between the spaces. A lumped element impedance model of the inner ear was used by Stenfelt to show that fluid inertia is the most important factor in both air and bone conduction, both in healthy ears and in ears with simulated pathologic third windows. Essentially, the low impedance created by a third window such as SSCD is in parallel to the normal cochlear impedance. This improves the conduction of sound energy between the vestibular and cochlear fluids, thus improving the bone conduction efficiency [38].

The low frequency effect of third window phenomena on air conduction values has been thoroughly investigated and is well understood. To summarize, shunting of the intralabyrinthine pressure wave through the pathologic third window on the vestibular side of the inner ear reduces the impedance at the oval window, causing a decrease in the intracochlear pressure which in turn decreases the vibration of the basilar membrane [38–42]. Iversen et al. have published a comprehensive review of the biomechanics of TMWS [43].

While much is known about the audiologic findings in TMWS, it remains unclear why there is such considerable variation among patients. While there is recent evidence supporting the contribution of dehiscence size in the air-bone gap, two patients with SSCD may have quite different audiograms [44]. Location of dehiscence may also have implications for clinical symptoms and signs (see below). Furthermore, patients' experience of SSCD symptoms is likely to be very distinct. More work is needed to shed light on these issues.

Classification

The topic of TMWS classification schemes is covered in detail in Chap. 4. In recent years, several research groups have shown that the site of the otic capsule dehiscence in TMWS may indeed be more variable than previously thought. For example, cochlea-facial nerve dehiscence has been reported in the literature and has been shown to be amenable to round window reinforcement [45, 46].

In addition, there is likely a subset of patients with TMWS who will not have a radiographic dehiscence on HRCT [47]. There is a push by some research groups to use a more general term such as otic capsule dehiscence syndrome to describe patients with symptoms consistent with SSCD or other third window syndromes. Along the same lines, Reynard et al. have recently proposed a classification scheme to categorize patients with TMWS by location and structures involved in the otic capsule dehiscence. Type 1 describes a dehiscence between the otic capsule and the meninges, type II between the otic capsule and a vascular structure, and type III between the otic capsule and the petrous bone (Table 30.1) [48]. While this classification scheme may be useful anatomically, it does not differentiate clinical signs and symptoms, as the incidence of audiological and vestibular symptoms appears to be the same among the anatomical types.

Size and location of the dehiscence in SSCD have also been investigated: increased size of the dehiscence in SSCD has been shown to increase the air-bone gap with a plateau effect at a certain dehiscence size [42]. Lookabaugh et al. proposed a radiographic classification scheme for SSCD which focuses on the location of the dehiscence in relation to the slope of the middle cranial fossa as well as whether the superior petrosal sinus is involved with the dehiscence (Fig. 30.2) [49].

Table 30.1 Proposed classification system for TMWS with accompanying clinical and c-VEMP characteristics [48]

Reynard et al. A Third Window's Abnormalities Classification

TABLE 1 | Third Mobile Window Abnormalities (TMWA): classification and clinical elements.

	Interface	Type	Number of patients	Clinical features	cVEMP thresholds
Extralabyrinthine TMWA (OCD)	OC-Meningeal	I	48	Vertigo (42%) Auditory symptoms (35%)	Decreased (20%)
	OC-Vascular	II	28	Vertigo (64%) Auditory symptoms (64%)	Decreased (14%)
	OC-Petrosal	III	17	Vertigo (47%) Auditory symptoms (52%)	Decreased (21%)
Intralabyrinthine TMWA -like	Vestibular aqueduct - Posterior SC		4	Vertigo (50%) Auditory symptoms (25%)	Decreased (0%)
Multiple OCD	Multiple locations (on the same ear)	/	11	Vertigo (80%) Auditory symptoms (100%)	Decreased (40%)

SC, Semicircular Canal; OCD, Otic capsule dehiscence.

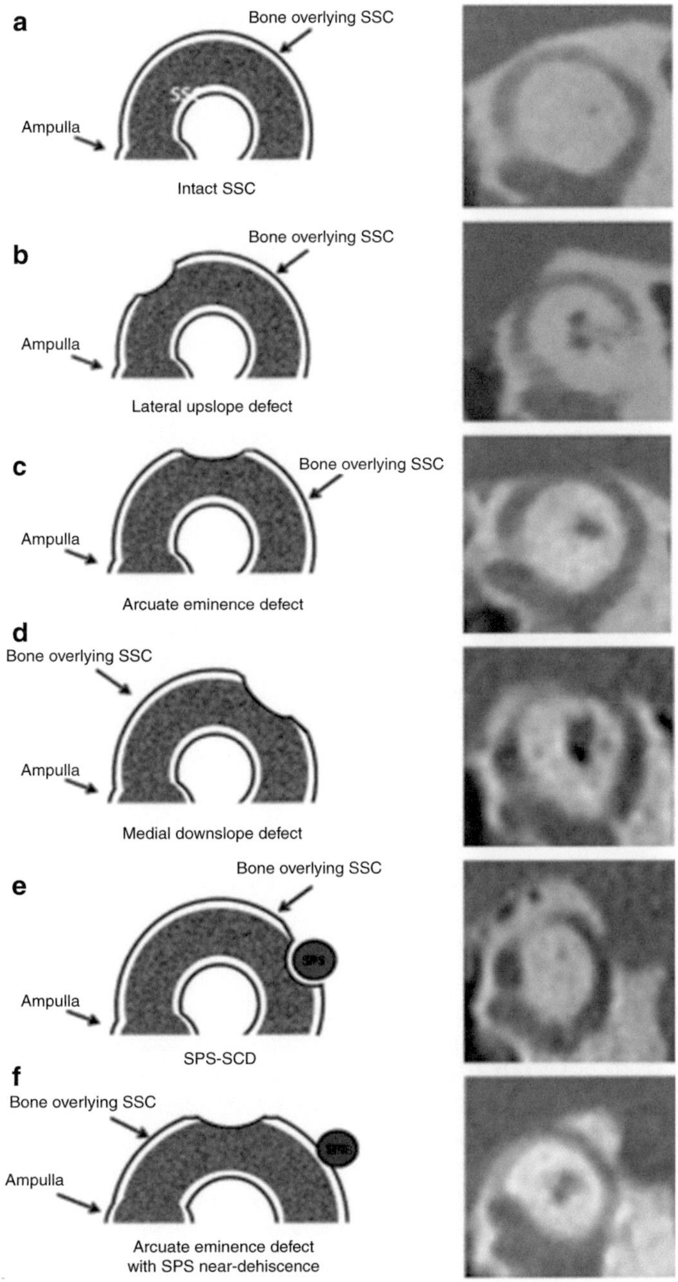

Fig. 30.2 SSCD classification scheme accounting for involvement of superior petrosal sinus. (Reprinted with permission from [49].) (**a**). Intact superior semicircular canal (SSC). (**b**) Dehiscence of the lateral upslope of the SCC, adjacent to the ampullated end. (**c**) Dehiscence of the SCC at the arcuate eminence. (**d**) Dehiscence of the medial downsloping SCC. (**e**) Superior petrosal sinus-associated SSCD. (**f**) Arcuate eminence dehiscence with near-dehiscent superior petrosal sinus

Cochlear-carotid dehiscence is rare and has yet to be fully described. Classification schema such as these create a common vocabulary among clinicians and have the potential to influence surgical decision-making, as well as allow a more unified investigatory effort, especially when tracking natural history. Time will tell if these schemas will be adopted and aid in our communication about this disease.

Diagnosis

History

Diagnosis of TMWS can be challenging, and patients may go undiagnosed for prolonged periods of time, particularly when being evaluated by clinicians less familiar with TMWS. The history is the most important piece of the diagnostic puzzle and will guide the practitioner down a path of further investigation. Classically, the patient is asked to describe the onset, quality, duration, frequency, and associated factors of their dizziness. Recent studies have suggested an overreliance on these factors on our diagnosis, and purport that *timing* of symptoms and *triggering factors* should be more thoroughly investigated and more heavily weighted when taking a history [50, 51]. Evidence-based strategies may avoid misdiagnosis and ultimately result in more expedient diagnosis and improved outcomes for all dizzy patients.

Audiometric Testing

In addition to a thorough history, diagnosis of TMWS is aided by audiometric and radiographic testing. These topics have been discussed thoroughly in previous chapters. We will review some recent noteworthy data and attempt to direct new research avenues.

Vestibular evoked myogenic potentials (VEMP) have been studied extensively and are commonly used in diagnostic algorithms. Data have shown that the combination of VEMP (c-VEMP or o-VEMP) with audiometric data is more reliable for detecting true third window phenomena than VEMP alone [52]. Noij et al. developed a "third window indicator" by subtracting the air-bone gap at 250 Hz from the c-VEMP threshold, yielding a positive predictive value of 100% in diagnosis of SSCD [53]. A multicenter analysis of patients who underwent SSCD repair showed a slight advantage of c-VEMP sensitivity and specificity when compared with o-VEMP, although there may be some institutional variability [54]. VEMPs likely have lower diagnostic utility in a postoperative setting, i.e., if a surgeon is considering a revision. While VEMPs have been well established in the diagnosis of SSCD, there is, however, a lack of standardization among institutions making data comparison difficult. Additionally, there is not much data examining VEMP testing in both the pediatric and elderly populations. Less is known about VEMP testing in other third window syndromes.

Electrocochleography (ECoG) has also been studied in the context of third window syndromes, primarily SSCD. Elevated SP/AP ratio has shown high sensitivity and specificity in detecting ears with symptomatic SSCD [55, 56]. ECoG has also been examined intraoperatively as a predictor of satisfactory occlusion of the dehiscence [55]. Recently, intraoperative reduction in SP/AP ratio <0.4 was shown to correlate with postoperative reduction in symptoms, particularly auditory symptoms [57]. These studies elegantly correlate anatomy with physiology in the plugging of the third window; however, use of ECoG is not currently widespread, and more data are needed to determine its utility.

Wideband acoustic immittance (WAI) has been examined in SSCD and has shown promise, both in initial diagnosis and in the postoperative setting. WAI is akin to tympanometry, as it measures the impedance of the middle and inner ear. However, as the name implies, it uses a range of frequencies (standard tympanometry uses a single frequency). WAI is dependent on normal middle ear physiology, and alterations therein will confound its results. The typical pattern of WAI in TMWS is one of decreased resonance frequency compared with normal ears, and a characteristic peak in middle ear absorbance around 1000 Hz [58]. Currently available data show WAI may be an effective screening tool for SSCD and that the absorbance at low frequencies tends to normalize after effective surgical treatment [58, 59]. This technology is not widely utilized but certainly merits further investigation, particularly as a screening tool that could indicate a need for further workup.

The issue of reducing healthcare cost and maximizing efficiency is one that needs exploration in any clinical situation, and TMWS is no exception. For example, a diagnostic algorithm using high-frequency c-VEMP, patient symptoms (primarily autophony), and HRCT has been proposed for diagnosis of SSCD. This algorithm also accounts for the patient's theoretical desire to undergo surgery if SSCD is found and has the potential to reduce cost (Fig. 30.3) [60]. Interestingly, the percentage of radiographic SSCD on HRCT in symptomatic patients was only 43.1% in this study; migraine was more prevalent in patients with symptoms but without SSCD.

Video head impulse testing (vHIT) is a relatively new diagnostic tool that may aid in the diagnosis of TMWS. Reduced VOR gain in the plane of the affected superior canal has been described in SSCD [61–63]. This phenomenon is potentially thought to be related to "auto-plugging," wherein the superior semicircular canal is occluded by the patient's own tissues (e.g., dura), thus impeding canal function. In small dehiscences, one would not expect this phenomenon to occur. Recent data support this supposition [62]. Despite these findings, the clinical utility of vHIT in evaluation of SSCD and other TMWS remains unclear.

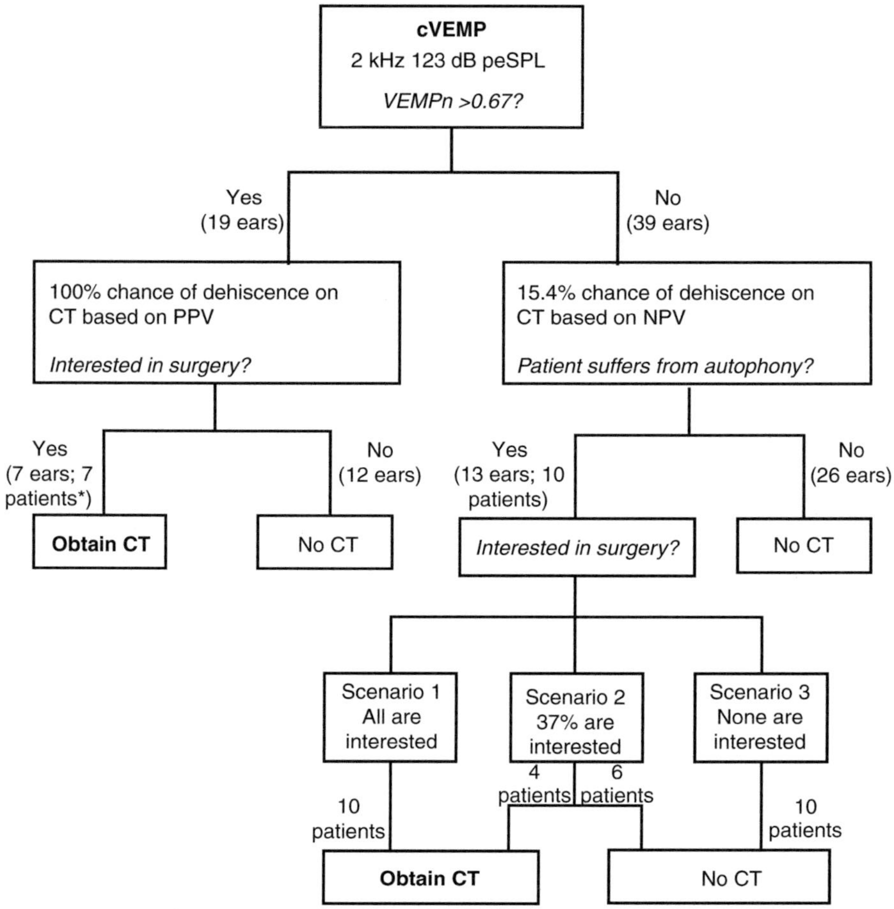

Fig. 30.3 Proposed algorithm for clinical decision-making in workup for SSCD. (Reprinted with permission from [60])

Imaging

High-resolution computed tomography (HRCT) has emerged as the gold standard for the diagnosis of a bony defect, its presence and location, in TMWS and is instrumental in surgical planning. Advances in technology have significantly improved the spatial resolution of CT imaging, and newer innovations will continue to improve this resolution. For example, the gray-scale inversion technique, which the clinician

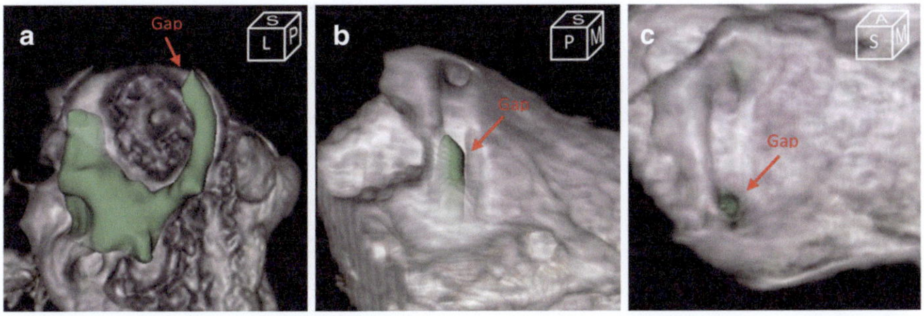

Fig. 30.4 Novel 3D reconstruction technique using fused CT-MRI in the postoperative setting after plugging, showing residual dehiscence. (Reprinted with permission from [66].) 33-year-old man with left ear SCD following SSC plugging via MCF. A residual defect is noted in the posterior limb on combined 3D reconstruction of CT and MRI imaging. T2-weighted MRI signal represents the fluid in the SSC with the surrounding bony CT. (**a**) parallel view of SSC (Poschl view). (**b**) posterior–superior view of SSC. (**c**) Superior view of SSC. *A* indicates anterior; *CT*, computed tomography; *L*, lateral; *M*, medial

can apply to images within the DICOM or PACS systems, may be useful in detecting subtle findings in suspected TMWS [64]. A relatively new imaging technique, flat panel CT (FPCT), is quick to obtain, displays higher resolution images with lower radiation dose, and is promising in TMWS diagnosis. The lower radiation dose is noteworthy, particularly in the pediatric population [65].

Heavily T2-weighted, high-resolution magnetic resonance (MR) sequences are complementary to HRCT in diagnosis and may be used to exclude SSCD. MR is particularly helpful in evaluation of treatment failures as the presence or lack of fluid signal will provide information regarding the extent and location of plugging, particularly when used in combination with HRCT (Fig. 30.4) [66]. Lee et al. used a novel 3D MR reconstruction technique to calculate the volume of the labyrinth after superior SCC plugging. They were able to accurately correlate clinical outcomes with volumetric changes based on this imaging technique. Patients with volumetric analyses indicating incomplete plugging (higher volumes) were significantly more symptomatic postoperatively (Fig. 30.5) [67]. New MR techniques are now able to detect endolymphatic hydrops, using delayed post-gadolinium 3D-FLAIR and T2-weighted sequences. A study by Ray et al. showed that endolymphatic hydrops was present in 27.3% of ears with SSCD, indicating that medical treatment of the endolymphatic hydrops may be indicated [68].

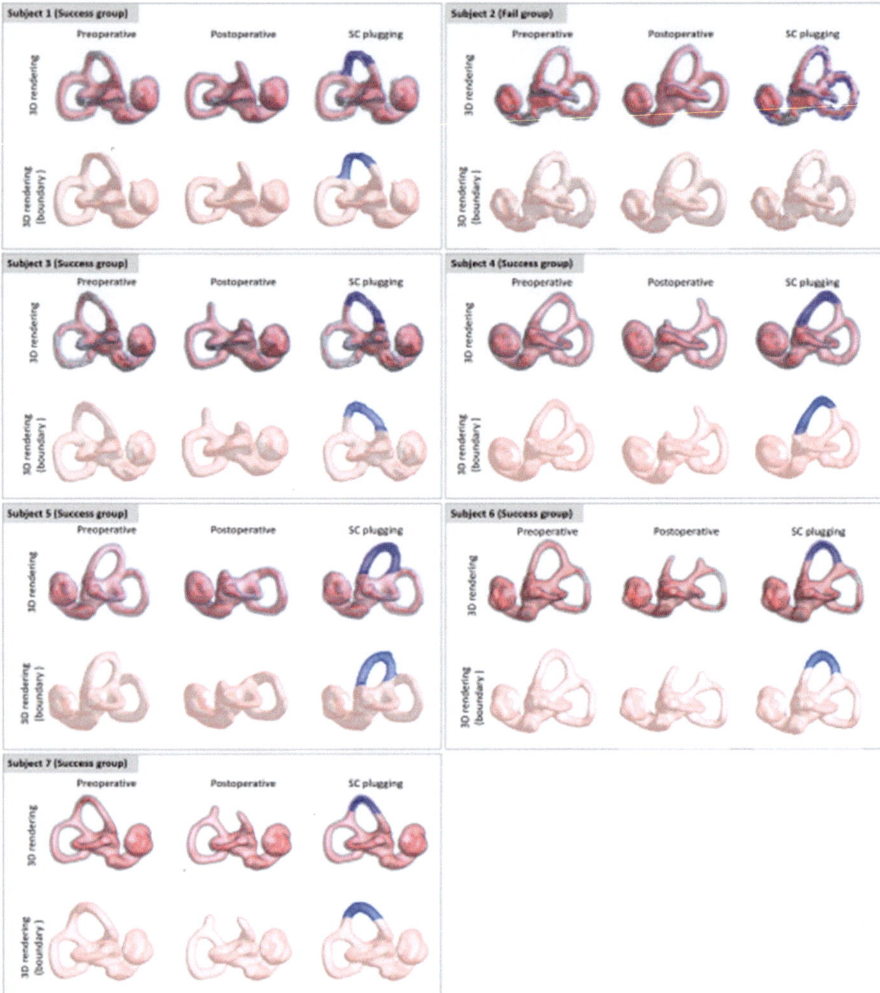

Fig. 30.5 3D reconstruction of the labyrinth using MRI techniques after SSCD plugging, blue shaded areas showing the extent of the plug [67]

Treatment

Clinical research has been instrumental in our understanding of best practices and treatment recommendations for patients with SSCD and more recently TMWS. Whether resurfacing vs. plugging, MCF vs. transmastoid vs. round window reinforcement, and what material to use, careful clinical research has given us important answers in the management of patients with TMWS.

Yet, many questions remain unanswered. It is difficult for single institutions to accumulate large cohorts of TMWS patients. Multi-institutional clinical studies will be better positioned to offer further treatment recommendations. For example, one meta-analysis showed no difference in technique between canal plugging and resurfacing [69]; yet, other studies have clearly shown plugging to have a lower recurrence rate [70–72]. A multi-institutional study comparing transmastoid and MCF approaches for SSCD repair showed no significant difference in outcomes between the two approaches, although there was a higher revision rate for the MCF group as well as longer hospital stay. These authors reported combinations of plugging and resurfacing in both approaches. Notably, there are no patient-reported outcome measures included in the study [73]. A systematic review by Ossen et al. effectively highlights the significant heterogeneity of available studies with regard to outcome measures, making definitive conclusions difficult to ascertain [74].

Models for Study

A variety of animal models have been utilized by research groups around the world to investigate TMWS. Most studies using animal models are focused on elucidating the underlying mechanisms of the audiometric phenomena of TMWS. With these models, treatment modalities can be tested and compared, although the auditory physiology is much easier to assay than the vestibular. A gerbil model of SSCD showed that bone wax had higher adverse tissue reactions and that muscle and fat were less successful in plugging SSCD, therefore favoring autologous bone and teflon [75]. A combination of bone pate and fibrinogen sealant is thought to reduce the risk of postoperative hearing loss due to labyrinthitis [76].

An animal model of SSCD has also been created in the fat sand rat. Bony fenestration has been performed in the superior SCC, demonstrating postoperative air-bone gaps [77]. Fenestration of the posterior SCC in these rats also demonstrates expected decrease in air conduction threshold, consistent with expected TMWS pathophysiology [78]. Similarly, cochlear third windows have also been created in a sand rat model [79].

Dlugaiczyk et al. recorded action potentials from superior canal neurons both before and after creation of superior canal dehiscence in a guinea pig model, observing an increase in firing after creation of the dehiscence [80]. Guinea pig models have been used by multiple other groups, primarily in investigating the underlying pathophysiologic mechanisms of hearing loss in SSCD as well as in treatment outcomes [81, 82].

Finally, chinchillas have easily accessible SCCs and hearing that is in a similar range to humans, making them ideal animal models for TMWS [42, 83–87].

Human temporal bone banks remain a vital resource in the study of various otologic disorders, and TMWS is no exception. Our understanding of the prevalence of SSCD in the general population came about through cadaveric studies [5]. More recently, human temporal bones were used in a feasibility study examining the potential for SSCD repair with exoscopic assistance and image guidance [88]. Our field will undoubtedly continue to lean on this valuable resource for further study of TWMS.

Pang et al. created a computational model of inner ear dynamics in patients with enlarged vestibular aqueduct and a predominantly conductive hearing loss [89]. Stenfelt used a computational model to investigate the pathophysiology of SSCD, confirming prior research as to the reduced cochlear impedance and its subsequent effect on bone and air conduction seen in TMWS [38].

Advanced Technology

Several groups have reported the use of new technology such as exoscopes for otologic surgery, including MCF approaches [88, 90, 91]. Endoscopic repair of SSCD is being performed at several centers around the world, both with transmastoid and MCF approaches. Multiple groups have reported on endoscopic-assisted repair of SSCD, particularly when the dehiscence is present in the more downsloping medial portion of the middle cranial fossa [92].

Surgeons have reported using an "underwater" technique with balanced salt solution in attempts to minimize perilymph loss and improve hearing outcomes compared with traditional microscopic technique (https://cdnlinks.lww.com/permalink/mao/a/mao_00_00_2020_01_30_carey_on-18-589_sdc1.mp4) [93, 94]. Totten et al. reviewed their institution's outcomes and found no difference in outcomes between microscopic and endoscopic repair techniques [95].

Special Situations

Challenging clinical situations, including bilateral SSCD, otosclerosis, elevated intracranial pressure, migraine, and others have been addressed elsewhere in this book (see Part IV); further research will elucidate best options for managing these difficult clinical scenarios.

Patient Outcome Measures

To define best practices in the management of TMWS, clinicians need validated outcome measures, including patient-reported outcome measures (PROM). Currently, there is no validated PROM measure specific to TMWS. Creation of such an instrument would simplify and standardize our assessment of patients' response to treatment. The Dizziness Handicap Inventory (DHI) is a tool used commonly in reporting outcomes from TMWS treatment. This tool is nonspecific and may capture other etiologies underlying a patient's dizziness aside from TMWS. 11-point Likert scales specific to third window symptoms have also been used [96]. Ohman et al. interviewed patients with known SSCD and described their experiences in their own words, shedding light on some of the less tangible TMWS symptoms such as mental fatigue [97].

These PROMs must be applied not only to surgical treatment of this condition, but also to medical management and simple observation. Basic hearing outcomes are easily assessed by comprehensive audiometry, but electrophysiologic parameters also have a role in the diagnosis and assessment of adequacy of treatment in SSCD. In assessing vestibular outcomes, the Dizziness Handicap Inventory has been used along with postop VEMP testing [46, 74, 98, 99]. An Autophony Index has been created but is nonspecific to TMWS [100].

Quality of life metrics should be evaluated in patients with TMWS, both before and after treatment, and especially in those electing not to undergo treatment. Just as the ETD-7 has been developed for Eustachian Tube Dysfunction, a TMWS-specific Quality of Life questionnaire should be developed and validated [101, 102]. Studies are also needed to follow children with SSCD and other third mobile windows—both symptomatic children and children in whom a third mobile window has been identified incidentally—from a young age through adulthood, to determine how symptoms progress (if at all) and which forms of treatment optimally minimize symptoms in this population.

Conservative/Medical Management

To date, there are no published studies reporting outcomes from conservative or medical management of TMWS. However, it certainly seems reasonable to attempt a trial of habituation strategies such as vestibular therapy and avoidance of triggers. Strategies such as migraine diet and prophylactic migraine medications could certainly be beneficial as well, particularly in patients with a history of migraine or multifactorial dizziness with components of vestibular migraine. These strategies have been described in a previous chapter.

Round Window Reinforcement

Round window reinforcement is an alluring option in TMWS, wherein the surgeon eliminates one of the three mobile windows of the inner ear. There is variance in technique reported in the literature and the currently available evidence generally demonstrates less predictable outcomes [103–105]. Gona recently reported a single case of "soft reinforcement" of the round window in a patient with predominantly auditory symptoms of SSCD. They used fat and perichondrium in the round window niche and reported a good postoperative outcome in their patient [106]. Round window reinforcement is a potentially efficacious option in cases of less recognized TMWS such as cochlear-facial dehiscence [46]. More patient data over long-term follow-up are needed to establish the role of round window reinforcement in treatment of TMWS.

Migraine

Migraine and TMWS are addressed in Part IV, and while there is no known causal association between migraine and TMWS, several studies have examined their relationship. Patients with comorbid migraine have less improvement in their vestibular symptoms after SSCD repair [57, 96]. There are data showing that treatment of TMWS improved headache-specific quality of life measures [48]. The mechanism for this improvement is unclear. If vestibular input can act as a trigger for migraine headache, then in theory treatment of a pathologic vestibular input may in turn improve the patient's migraine symptoms. The connection between TMWS and migraine certainly merits further investigation.

Conclusion

In the years since SSCD was described and clinician awareness of TMWS has increased, high quality research using a variety of retrospective, preclinical, and clinical models has shed light on prevalence, pathophysiology, diagnosis, treatment options, and surgical outcomes. However, many aspects of TMWS remain incompletely understood. A definitive link between comorbid conditions such as IIH and migraine with TMWS has not been established. Much more research is needed regarding prevalence, diagnosis, and treatment of non-SSCD TMWS. In addition, there are very likely novel sites of cochlear dehiscence/TMWS that have yet to be described in the literature. There remains controversy surrounding the ideal approach for surgical treatment as well as the utility of novel technologies such as endoscopes, exoscopes, and underwater techniques. The natural history of SSCD and other TMWS has not been reported and merits investigation. Uncommon special situations such as bilateral SSCD, cognitive dysfunction, and comorbid otosclerosis and SSCD are increasingly being recognized and merit investigatory effort as well. Accumulating a large number of subjects is difficult, indicating a need for collaboration among specialties and institutions. Finally, validated patient-reported outcomes and quality of life surveys ensure uniformity, concordance, and validity across institutions, approaches, treatment modalities, and surgical techniques.

References

1. Addams-Williams J, Wu K, Ray J. The experiments behind the Tullio phenomenon. J Laryngol Otol. 2014;128(3):223–7. https://doi.org/10.1017/S0022215114000280.
2. Minor LB, Solomon D, Zinreich JS, Zee DS. Sound- and/or pressure-induced vertigo due to bone dehiscence of the superior semicircular canal. Arch Otolaryngol Head Neck Surg. 1998;124(3):249–58. https://doi.org/10.1001/archotol.124.3.249.
3. Smullen JL, Andrist EC, Gianoli GJ. Superior semicircular canal dehiscence: a new cause of vertigo. J La State Med Soc. 1999;151(8):397–400. https://www.ncbi.nlm.nih.gov/pubmed/10554474.
4. Cozart AC, Kennedy JT III, Seidman MD. A basis for standardizing superior semicircular canal dehiscence management. Ear Nose Throat J. 2021;100(10):444–53. https://doi.org/10.1177/0145561320927941.
5. Carey JP, Minor LB, Nager GT. Dehiscence or thinning of bone overlying the superior semicircular canal in a temporal bone survey. Arch Otolaryngol Head Neck Surg. 2000;126(2):137–47. https://doi.org/10.1001/archotol.126.2.137.
6. Fang CH, Chung SY, Blake DM, Vazquez A, Li C, Carey JP, Francis HW, Jyung RW. Prevalence of cochlear-facial dehiscence in a study of 1,020 temporal bone specimens. Otol Neurotol. 2016;37(7):967–72. https://doi.org/10.1097/MAO.0000000000001057.
7. Berning AW, Arani K, Branstetter BFT. Prevalence of superior semicircular canal dehiscence on high-resolution CT imaging in patients without vestibular or auditory abnormalities. AJNR Am J Neuroradiol. 2019;40(4):709–12. https://doi.org/10.3174/ajnr.A5999.
8. Crovetto M, Whyte J, Rodriguez OM, Lecumberri I, Martinez C, Elexpuru J. Anatomo-radiological study of the Superior Semicircular Canal Dehiscence Radiological considerations of Superior and Posterior Semicircular Canals. Eur J Radiol. 2010;76(2):167–72. https://doi.org/10.1016/j.ejrad.2009.05.038.
9. Klopp-Dutote N, Kolski C, Biet A, Strunski V, Page C. A radiologic and anatomic study of the superior semicircular canal. Eur Ann Otorhinolaryngol Head Neck Dis. 2016;133(2):91–4. https://doi.org/10.1016/j.anorl.2015.11.001.
10. Williamson RA, Vrabec JT, Coker NJ, Sandlin M. Coronal computed tomography prevalence of superior semicircular canal dehiscence. Otolaryngol Head Neck Surg. 2003;129(5):481–9. https://doi.org/10.1016/s0194-5998(03)01391-3.
11. Schart-Moren N, Larsson S, Rask-Andersen H, Li H. Anatomical characteristics of facial nerve and cochlea interaction. Audiol Neurootol. 2017;22(1):41–9. https://doi.org/10.1159/000475876.
12. Song Y, Alyono JC, Bartholomew RA, Vaisbuch Y, Corrales CE, Blevins NH. Prevalence of radiographic cochlear-facial nerve dehiscence. Otol Neurotol. 2018;39(10):1319–25. https://doi.org/10.1097/MAO.0000000000002015.
13. Ward BK, Carey JP, Minor LB. Superior canal dehiscence syndrome: lessons from the first 20 years. Front Neurol. 2017;8:177. https://doi.org/10.3389/fneur.2017.00177.
14. Chen EY, Paladin A, Phillips G, Raske M, Vega L, Peterson D, Sie KC. Semicircular canal dehiscence in the pediatric population. Int J Pediatr Otorhinolaryngol. 2009;73(2):321–7. https://doi.org/10.1016/j.ijporl.2008.10.027.
15. Meiklejohn DA, Corrales CE, Boldt BM, Sharon JD, Yeom KW, Carey JP, Blevins NH. Pediatric semicircular canal dehiscence: radiographic and histologic prevalence, with clinical correlation. Otol Neurotol. 2015;36(8):1383–9. https://doi.org/10.1097/MAO.0000000000000811.
16. Saxby AJ, Gowdy C, Fandino M, Chadha NK, Kozak FK, Sargent MA, Lea J. Radiological prevalence of superior and posterior semicircular canal dehiscence in children. Int J Pediatr Otorhinolaryngol. 2015;79(3):411–8. https://doi.org/10.1016/j.ijporl.2015.01.001.
17. Allen KP, Perez CL, Isaacson B, Roland PS, Duong TT, Kutz JW. Superior semicircular canal dehiscence in patients with spontaneous cerebrospinal fluid otorrhea. Otolaryngol Head Neck Surg. 2012;147(6):1120–4. https://doi.org/10.1177/0194599812457545.

18. Arsenault JJ, Romiyo P, Miao T, Monteiro K, De Jong R, Kaur T, Johanis M, Duong C, Sheppard JP, Sun MZ, Ferraro R, Salamon N, Yang I, Gopen Q. Thinning or dehiscence of bone in structures of the middle cranial fossa floor in superior semicircular canal dehiscence. J Clin Neurosci. 2020;74:104–8. https://doi.org/10.1016/j.jocn.2020.01.082.
19. Kuo P, Bagwell KA, Mongelluzzo G, Schutt CA, Malhotra A, Khokhar B, Kveton JF. Semicircular canal dehiscence among idiopathic intracranial hypertension patients. Laryngoscope. 2018;128(5):1196–9. https://doi.org/10.1002/lary.26795.
20. Oh MS, Vivas EX, Hudgins PA, Mattox DE. The prevalence of superior semicircular canal dehiscence in patients with mastoid encephalocele or cerebrospinal fluid otorrhea. Otol Neurotol. 2019;40(4):485–90. https://doi.org/10.1097/MAO.0000000000002155.
21. Stevens SM, Hock K, Samy RN, Pensak ML. Are patients with spontaneous CSF otorrhea and superior canal dehiscence congenitally predisposed to their disorders? Otolaryngol Head Neck Surg. 2018;159(3):543–52. https://doi.org/10.1177/0194599818769875.
22. Formeister EJ, Zhang L, Dent J, Aygun N, Carey JP. Predictive factors for concurrent tegmen dehiscence in superior canal dehiscence syndrome. Otol Neurotol. 2022;43:494. https://doi.org/10.1097/MAO.0000000000003481.
23. Jan TA, Cheng YS, Landegger LD, Lin BM, Srikanth P, Niesten ME, Lee DJ. Relationship between surgically treated superior canal dehiscence syndrome and body mass index. Otolaryngol Head Neck Surg. 2017;156(4):722–7. https://doi.org/10.1177/0194599816686563.
24. Schutt CA, Neubauer P, Samy RN, Pensak ML, Kuhn JJ, Herschovitch M, Kveton JF. The correlation between obesity, obstructive sleep apnea, and superior semicircular canal dehiscence: a new explanation for an increasingly common problem. Otol Neurotol. 2015;36(3):551–4. https://doi.org/10.1097/MAO.0000000000000555.
25. Rizk HG, Hatch JL, Stevens SM, Lambert PR, Meyer TA. Lateral skull base attenuation in superior semicircular canal dehiscence and spontaneous cerebrospinal fluid otorrhea. Otolaryngol Head Neck Surg. 2016;155(4):641–8. https://doi.org/10.1177/0194599816651261.
26. Yu A, Teich DL, Moonis G, Wong ET. Superior semicircular canal dehiscence in East Asian women with osteoporosis. BMC Ear Nose Throat Disord. 2012;12:8. https://doi.org/10.1186/1472-6815-12-8.
27. Nguyen T, Lagman C, Sheppard JP, Duong C, Ong V, Poon J, Alkhalid Y, Azzam D, Romiyo P, Prashant GN, Gopen Q, Yang I. Bone metabolic markers in the clinical assessment of patients with superior semicircular canal dehiscence. World Neurosurg. 2018;114:e42–50. https://doi.org/10.1016/j.wneu.2018.02.017.
28. Heidenreich KD, Kileny PR, Ahmed S, El-Kashlan HK, Melendez TL, Basura GJ, Lesperance MM. Superior canal dehiscence syndrome affecting 3 families. JAMA Otolaryngol Head Neck Surg. 2017;143(7):656–62. https://doi.org/10.1001/jamaoto.2016.4743.
29. Niesten ME, Lookabaugh S, Curtin H, Merchant SN, McKenna MJ, Grolman W, Lee DJ. Familial superior canal dehiscence syndrome. JAMA Otolaryngol Head Neck Surg. 2014;140(4):363–8. https://doi.org/10.1001/jamaoto.2013.6718.
30. Hildebrand MS, Tack D, Deluca A, Hur IA, Van Rybroek JM, McMordie SJ, Muilenburg A, Hoskinson DP, Van Camp G, Pensak ML, Storper IS, Huygen PL, Casavant TL, Smith RJ. Mutation in the COCH gene is associated with superior semicircular canal dehiscence. Am J Med Genet A. 2009;149A(2):280–5. https://doi.org/10.1002/ajmg.a.32618.
31. Khetarpal U. DFNA9 is a progressive audiovestibular dysfunction with a microfibrillar deposit in the inner ear. Laryngoscope. 2000;110(8):1379–84. https://doi.org/10.1097/00005537-200008000-00030.
32. de Varebeke SP, Termote B, Van Camp G, Govaerts PJ, Schepers S, Cox T, Deben K, Ketelslagers K, Souverijns G. Focal sclerosis of semicircular canals with severe DFNA9 hearing impairment caused by a P51S COCH-mutation: is there a link? Otol Neurotol. 2014;35(6):1077–86. https://doi.org/10.1097/MAO.0000000000000283.
33. Noonan KY, Russo J, Shen J, Rehm H, Halbach S, Hopp E, Noon S, Hoover J, Eskey C, Saunders JE. CDH23 related hearing loss: a new genetic risk factor for semicircular canal dehiscence? Otol Neurotol. 2016;37(10):1583–8. https://doi.org/10.1097/MAO.0000000000001210.

34. Pfammatter A, Darrouzet V, Gartner M, Somers T, Van Dinther J, Trabalzini F, Ayache D, Linder T. A superior semicircular canal dehiscence syndrome multicenter study: is there an association between size and symptoms? Otol Neurotol. 2010;31(3):447–54. https://doi.org/10.1097/MAO.0b013e3181d27740.
35. Wackym PA, Balaban CD, Mackay HT, Wood SJ, Lundell CJ, Carter DM, Siker DA. Longitudinal cognitive and neurobehavioral functional outcomes before and after repairing otic capsule dehiscence. Otol Neurotol. 2016;37(1):70–82. https://doi.org/10.1097/MAO.0000000000000928.
36. Gurvich C, Maller JJ, Lithgow B, Haghgooie S, Kulkarni J. Vestibular insights into cognition and psychiatry. Brain Res. 2013;1537:244–59. https://doi.org/10.1016/j.brainres.2013.08.058.
37. Guan X, Cheng YS, Galaiya DJ, Rosowski JJ, Lee DJ, Nakajima HH. Bone-conduction hyperacusis induced by superior canal dehiscence in human: the underlying mechanism. Sci Rep. 2020;10(1):16564. https://doi.org/10.1038/s41598-020-73565-4.
38. Stenfelt S. Investigation of mechanisms in bone conduction hyperacusis with third window pathologies based on model predictions. Front Neurol. 2020;11:966. https://doi.org/10.3389/fneur.2020.00966.
39. Cheng YS, Raufer S, Guan X, Halpin CF, Lee DJ, Nakajima HH. Superior canal dehiscence similarly affects cochlear pressures in temporal bones and audiograms in patients. Ear Hear. 2020;41(4):804–10. https://doi.org/10.1097/AUD.0000000000000799.
40. Kim N, Steele CR, Puria S. Superior-semicircular-canal dehiscence: effects of location, shape, and size on sound conduction. Hear Res. 2013;301:72–84. https://doi.org/10.1016/j.heares.2013.03.008.
41. Niesten ME, Stieger C, Lee DJ, Merchant JP, Grolman W, Rosowski JJ, Nakajima HH. Assessment of the effects of superior canal dehiscence location and size on intracochlear sound pressures. Audiol Neurootol. 2015;20(1):62–71. https://doi.org/10.1159/000366512.
42. Songer JE, Rosowski JJ. A superior semicircular canal dehiscence-induced air-bone gap in chinchilla. Hear Res. 2010;269(1–2):70–80. https://doi.org/10.1016/j.heares.2010.07.002.
43. Iversen MM, Rabbitt RD. Biomechanics of third window syndrome. Front Neurol. 2020;11:891. https://doi.org/10.3389/fneur.2020.00891.
44. Yuen HW, Boeddinghaus R, Eikelboom RH, Atlas MD. The relationship between the air-bone gap and the size of superior semicircular canal dehiscence. Otolaryngol Head Neck Surg. 2009;141(6):689–94. https://doi.org/10.1016/j.otohns.2009.08.029.
45. Blake DM, Tomovic S, Vazquez A, Lee HJ, Jyung RW. Cochlear-facial dehiscence--a newly described entity. Laryngoscope. 2014;124(1):283–9. https://doi.org/10.1002/lary.24223.
46. Wackym PA, Balaban CD, Zhang P, Siker DA, Hundal JS. Third window syndrome: surgical management of cochlea-facial nerve dehiscence. Front Neurol. 2019;10:1281. https://doi.org/10.3389/fneur.2019.01281.
47. Wackym PA, Wood SJ, Siker DA, Carter DM. Otic capsule dehiscence syndrome: superior semicircular canal dehiscence syndrome with no radiographically visible dehiscence. Ear Nose Throat J. 2015;94(8):E8–E24. https://doi.org/10.1177/014556131509400802.
48. Reynard P, Idriss S, Ltaief-Boudrigua A, Bertholon P, Pirvan A, Truy E, Thai-Van H, Ionescu EC. Proposal for a unitary anatomo-clinical and radiological classification of third mobile window abnormalities. Front Neurol. 2021;12:792545. https://doi.org/10.3389/fneur.2021.792545.
49. Lookabaugh S, Kelly HR, Carter MS, Niesten ME, McKenna MJ, Curtin H, Lee DJ. Radiologic classification of superior canal dehiscence: implications for surgical repair. Otol Neurotol. 2015;36(1):118–25. https://doi.org/10.1097/MAO.0000000000000523.
50. Newman-Toker DE, Edlow JA. TiTrATE: a novel, evidence-based approach to diagnosing acute dizziness and vertigo. Neurol Clin. 2015;33(3):577–99. https://doi.org/10.1016/j.ncl.2015.04.011, viii.
51. Stanton VA, Hsieh YH, Camargo CA Jr, Edlow JA, Lovett PB, Goldstein JN, Abbuhl S, Lin M, Chanmugam A, Rothman RE, Newman-Toker DE. Overreliance on symptom quality in

diagnosing dizziness: results of a multicenter survey of emergency physicians. Mayo Clin Proc. 2007;82(11):1319–28. https://doi.org/10.4065/82.11.1319.
52. Milojcic R, Guinan JJ Jr, Rauch SD, Herrmann BS. Vestibular evoked myogenic potentials in patients with superior semicircular canal dehiscence. Otol Neurotol. 2013;34(2):360–7. https://doi.org/10.1097/mao.0b013e31827b4fb5.
53. Noij KS, Duarte MJ, Wong K, Cheng YS, Masud S, Herrmann BS, Curtin HD, Kanumuri VV, Guinan JJ Jr, Kozin ED, Tarabichi O, Jung DH, Lee DJ, Rauch SD. Toward Optimizing Cervical Vestibular Evoked Myogenic Potentials (cVEMP): combining air-bone gap and cVEMP thresholds to improve diagnosis of superior canal dehiscence. Otol Neurotol. 2018a;39(2):212–20. https://doi.org/10.1097/MAO.0000000000001655.
54. Hunter JB, Patel NS, O'Connell BP, Carlson ML, Shepard NT, McCaslin DL, Wanna GB. Cervical and ocular VEMP testing in diagnosing superior semicircular canal dehiscence. Otolaryngol Head Neck Surg. 2017;156(5):917–23. https://doi.org/10.1177/0194599817690720.
55. Adams ME, Kileny PR, Telian SA, El-Kashlan HK, Heidenreich KD, Mannarelli GR, Arts HA. Electrocochleography as a diagnostic and intraoperative adjunct in superior semicircular canal dehiscence syndrome. Otol Neurotol. 2011;32(9):1506–12. https://doi.org/10.1097/MAO.0b013e3182382a7c.
56. Park JH, Lee SY, Song JJ, Choi BY, Koo JW. Electrocochleographic findings in superior canal dehiscence syndrome. Hear Res. 2015;323:61–7. https://doi.org/10.1016/j.heares.2015.02.001.
57. Ellsperman SE, Telian SA, Kileny PR, Welch CM. Intraoperative electrocochleography correlates to outcomes in transmastoid and middle cranial fossa superior semicircular canal dehiscence repair. Otol Neurotol. 2022;43(1):120–7. https://doi.org/10.1097/MAO.0000000000003350.
58. Merchant GR, Roosli C, Niesten ME, Hamade MA, Lee DJ, McKinnon ML, Ulku CH, Rosowski JJ, Merchant SN, Nakajima HH. Power reflectance as a screening tool for the diagnosis of superior semicircular canal dehiscence. Otol Neurotol. 2015;36(1):172–7. https://doi.org/10.1097/MAO.0000000000000294.
59. Velikoselskii A, Papatziamos G, Smeds H, Verrecchia L. Wideband tympanometry in ears with superior canal dehiscence before and after surgical correction. Int J Audiol. 2021;61:1–6. https://doi.org/10.1080/14992027.2021.1964041.
60. Noij KS, Remenschneider AK, Herrmann BS, Guinan JJ Jr, Rauch SD. Optimized diagnostic approach to patients suspected of superior semicircular canal dehiscence. Ear Hear. 2021;42(5):1295–305. https://doi.org/10.1097/AUD.0000000000001015.
61. Castellucci A, Brandolini C, Del Vecchio V, Giordano D, Pernice C, Bianchin G, Maiolo V, Ferri GG. Temporal bone meningocele associated with superior canal dehiscence. Otol Neurotol. 2018;39(6):e506–8. https://doi.org/10.1097/MAO.0000000000001843.
62. Castellucci A, Piras G, Del Vecchio V, Crocetta FM, Maiolo V, Ferri GG, Ghidini A, Brandolini C. The effect of superior canal dehiscence size and location on audiometric measurements, vestibular-evoked myogenic potentials and video-head impulse testing. Eur Arch Otorhinolaryngol. 2021;278(4):997–1015. https://doi.org/10.1007/s00405-020-06169-3.
63. Mukherjee P, Chiarovano E, Cheng K, Manzari L, McGarvie LA, MacDougall HG. Video-head impulse test in superior canal dehiscence. Acta Otolaryngol. 2021;141(5):471–5. https://doi.org/10.1080/00016489.2021.1884287.
64. Schwartz TR, Lindemann TL, Mongelluzzo G, Wackym PA, Gadre AK. Gray-scale inversion on high resolution computed tomography of the temporal bone: an observational study. Ann Otol Rhinol Laryngol. 2021;130(10):1125–31. https://doi.org/10.1177/0003489421996844.
65. Tunkel AE, Carey JP, Pearl M. Flat panel computed tomography in the diagnosis of superior semicircular canal dehiscence syndrome. Otol Neurotol. 2019;40(2):213–7. https://doi.org/10.1097/MAO.0000000000002076.
66. Chemtob RA, Epprecht L, Reinshagen KL, Huber A, Caye-Thomasen P, Nakajima HH, Lee DJ. Utility of postoperative magnetic resonance imaging in patients who fail supe-

rior canal dehiscence surgery. Otol Neurotol. 2019;40(1):130–8. https://doi.org/10.1097/MAO.0000000000002051.
67. Lee SY, Lee Y, Choi JY, Bae YJ, Kim M, Song JJ, Choi BY, Jeong WK, Koo JW. Quantitative three-dimensional image analysis of the superior canal after surgical plugging to treat superior semicircular canal dehiscence. Sci Rep. 2021;11(1):16112. https://doi.org/10.1038/s41598-021-95063-x.
68. Ray A, Hautefort C, Guichard JP, Horion J, Herman P, Kania R, Houdart E, Verillaud B, Vitaux H, Attye A, Eliezer M. MRI contribution for the detection of endolymphatic hydrops in patients with superior canal dehiscence syndrome. Eur Arch Otorhinolaryngol. 2021;278(7):2229–38. https://doi.org/10.1007/s00405-020-06282-3.
69. Gioacchini FM, Alicandri-Ciufelli M, Kaleci S, Scarpa A, Cassandro E, Re M. Outcomes and complications in superior semicircular canal dehiscence surgery: A systematic review. Laryngoscope. 2016;126(5):1218–24. https://doi.org/10.1002/lary.25662. Epub 2015 Sep 15. PMID: 26371952.
70. Kontorinis G, Gaggini M. Transmastoid superior semicircular canal plugging: a prospective analysis of surgical outcomes. Otol Neurotol. 2021;42(8):1216–22. https://doi.org/10.1097/MAO.0000000000003191.
71. Limb CJ, Carey JP, Srireddy S, Minor LB. Auditory function in patients with surgically treated superior semicircular canal dehiscence. Otol Neurotol. 2006;27(7):969–80. https://doi.org/10.1097/01.mao.0000235376.70492.8e.
72. Friedland DR, Michel MA. Cranial thickness in superior canal dehiscence syndrome: implications for canal resurfacing surgery. Otol Neurotol. 2006;27(3):346–54. https://doi.org/10.1097/00129492-200604000-00010. PMID: 16639273.
73. Schwartz SR, Almosnino G, Noonan KY, Banakis Hartl RM, Zeitler DM, Saunders JE, Cass SP. Comparison of transmastoid and middle fossa approaches for superior canal dehiscence repair: a multi-institutional study. Otolaryngol Head Neck Surg. 2019;161(1):130–6. https://doi.org/10.1177/0194599819835173.
74. Ossen ME, Stokroos R, Kingma H, van Tongeren J, Van Rompaey V, Temel Y, van de Berg R. Heterogeneity in reported outcome measures after surgery in superior canal dehiscence syndrome-a systematic literature review. Front Neurol. 2017;8:347. https://doi.org/10.3389/fneur.2017.00347.
75. Kwok P, Gleich O, Spruss T, Strutz J. Different materials for plugging a dehiscent superior semicircular canal: a comparative histologic study using a gerbil model. Otol Neurotol. 2019;40(5):e532–41. https://doi.org/10.1097/MAO.0000000000002205.
76. Agrawal SK, Parnes LS. Transmastoid superior semicircular canal occlusion. Otol Neurotol. 2008;29(3):363–7. https://doi.org/10.1097/mao.0b013e3181616c9d.
77. Attias J, Nageris BI, Shemesh R, Shvero J, Preis M. Superior canal dehiscence effect on hearing thresholds: animal model. Otolaryngol Head Neck Surg. 2011;145(4):648–53. https://doi.org/10.1177/0194599811410535.
78. Nageris BI, Attias J, Shemesh R, Hadar T, Preis M. A third window of the posterior semicircular canal: an animal model. Laryngoscope. 2010;120(5):1034–7. https://doi.org/10.1002/lary.20831.
79. Attias J, Preis M, Shemesh R, Hadar T, Nageris BI. Animal model of cochlear third window in the scala vestibuli or scala tympani. Otol Neurotol. 2010;31(6):985–90. https://doi.org/10.1097/MAO.0b013e3181e3d49a.
80. Dlugaiczyk J, Burgess AM, Goonetilleke SC, Sokolic L, Curthoys IS. Superior canal dehiscence syndrome: relating clinical findings with vestibular neural responses from a guinea pig model. Otol Neurotol. 2019;40(4):e406–14. https://doi.org/10.1097/MAO.0000000000001940.
81. Brockenbrough JM, Marzo S, Wurster R, Young MR. Bone wax prevents nystagmus after labyrinthine fenestration in guinea pigs. Otolaryngol Head Neck Surg. 2003;128(5):726–31. https://doi.org/10.1016/s0194-5998(02)23289-1.

82. Tong BS, He ZY, Ding CR, Yang JM, Wang J, Han Z, Huang YB, Gao N, Jia XH, Chi FL, Ren DD. Mechanisms of hearing loss in a guinea pig model of superior semicircular canal dehiscence. Neural Plast. 2018;2018:1258341. https://doi.org/10.1155/2018/1258341.
83. Carey JP, Hirvonen TP, Hullar TE, Minor LB. Acoustic responses of vestibular afferents in a model of superior canal dehiscence. Otol Neurotol. 2004;25(3):345–52. https://doi.org/10.1097/00129492-200405000-00024.
84. Rosowski JJ, Songer JE, Nakajima HH, Brinsko KM, Merchant SN. Clinical, experimental, and theoretical investigations of the effect of superior semicircular canal dehiscence on hearing mechanisms. Otol Neurotol. 2004;25(3):323–32. https://doi.org/10.1097/00129492-200405000-00021.
85. Songer JE, Rosowski JJ. The effect of superior canal dehiscence on cochlear potential in response to air-conducted stimuli in chinchilla. Hear Res. 2005;210(1-2):53–62. https://doi.org/10.1016/j.heares.2005.07.003.
86. Songer JE, Rosowski JJ. The effect of superior-canal opening on middle-ear input admittance and air-conducted stapes velocity in chinchilla. J Acoust Soc Am. 2006;120(1):258–69. https://doi.org/10.1121/1.2204356.
87. Songer JE, Rosowski JJ. A mechano-acoustic model of the effect of superior canal dehiscence on hearing in chinchilla. J Acoust Soc Am. 2007;122(2):943–51. https://doi.org/10.1121/1.2747158.
88. Kaul VF, Fan CJ, Perez E, Schwam ZG, Hadjipanayis C, Wanna GB. 3D Exoscope navigation-guided approach to middle cranial fossa. Otol Neurotol. 2021;42(8):1223–7. https://doi.org/10.1097/MAO.0000000000003185.
89. Pang J, Wang Y, Cheng Y, Chi F, Li Y, Ni G, Ren D. Conductive hearing loss in large vestibular aqueduct syndrome -clinical observations and proof-of-concept predictive modeling by a biomechanical approach. Int J Pediatr Otorhinolaryngol. 2021;146:110752. https://doi.org/10.1016/j.ijporl.2021.110752.
90. Colombo G, Di Bari M, Canzano F, De Virgilio A, Cugini G, Mercante G, Spriano G, Ferreli F. 3D-4K exoscope-assisted temporal bone dissection: a new frontier in surgical training. Eur Arch Otorhinolaryngol. 2021a;279:3875. https://doi.org/10.1007/s00405-021-07137-1.
91. Colombo G, Ferreli F, Di Bari M, Cugini G, Miceli S, De Virgilio A, Spriano G, Poletti A. Introducing the High-definition 3D exoscope in ear surgery: preliminary analysis of advantages and limits compared with operative microscope. Eur Arch Otorhinolaryngol. 2021b;278(11):4217–23. https://doi.org/10.1007/s00405-020-06510-w.
92. Cheng YS, Kozin ED, Lee DJ. Endoscopic-assisted repair of superior canal dehiscence. Otolaryngol Clin N Am. 2016;49(5):1189–204. https://doi.org/10.1016/j.otc.2016.05.010.
93. Creighton F Jr, Barber SR, Ward BK, Sharon JD, Carey JP. Underwater endoscopic repair of superior canal dehiscence. Otol Neurotol. 2020;41(4):560. https://doi.org/10.1097/MAO.0000000000002277.
94. Creighton FX Jr, Zhang L, Ward B, Carey JP. Hearing outcomes for an underwater endoscopic technique for transmastoid repair of superior semicircular canal dehiscence. Otol Neurotol. 2021;42(10):e1691–7. https://doi.org/10.1097/MAO.0000000000003238.
95. Totten DJ, Smetak MR, Manzoor NF, Perkins EL, Cass ND, Hatton K, Santapuram P, O'Malley MR, Haynes DS, Bennett ML, Rivas A. Endoscope-assisted superior semicircular canal dehiscence repair: single institution outcomes. Ann Otol Rhinol Laryngol. 2021;131:743. https://doi.org/10.1177/00034894211041223.
96. Alkhafaji MS, Varma S, Pross SE, Sharon JD, Nellis JC, Santina CCD, Minor LB, Carey JP. Long-term patient-reported outcomes after surgery for superior canal dehiscence syndrome. Otol Neurotol. 2017;38(9):1319–26. https://doi.org/10.1097/MAO.0000000000001550.
97. Ohman J, Forssen A, Sorlin A, Tano K. Patients' experiences of living with superior canal dehiscence syndrome. Int J Audiol. 2018;57(11):825–30. https://doi.org/10.1080/14992027.2018.1487086.
98. de Wolf MJF, Dawe N, Jervis S, Kumar R, Dalton CL, Lindley K, Irving R. Transmastoid occlusion surgery for superior semicircular canal dehiscence syndrome improves patient-

reported quality-of-life measures and corrects cVEMP thresholds and amplitudes. Otol Neurotol. 2021;42(10):1534–43. https://doi.org/10.1097/MAO.0000000000003329.

99. Noij KS, Wong K, Duarte MJ, Masud S, Dewyer NA, Herrmann BS, Guinan JJ Jr, Kozin ED, Jung DH, Rauch SD, Lee DJ. Audiometric and cVEMP thresholds show little correlation with symptoms in superior semicircular canal dehiscence syndrome. Otol Neurotol. 2018b;39(9):1153–62. https://doi.org/10.1097/MAO.0000000000001910.
100. Crane BT, Lin FR, Minor LB, Carey JP. Improvement in autophony symptoms after superior canal dehiscence repair. Otol Neurotol. 2010;31(1):140–6. https://doi.org/10.1097/mao.0b013e3181bc39ab. PMID: 20050268.
101. Mehta NK, Ma C, Nguyen SA, McRackan TR, Meyer TA, Lambert PR. Medical management for eustachian tube dysfunction in adults: a systematic review and meta-analysis. Laryngoscope. 2021;132:849. https://doi.org/10.1002/lary.29878.
102. Poe D, Anand V, Dean M, Roberts WH, Stolovitzky JP, Hoffmann K, Nachlas NE, Light JP, Widick MH, Sugrue JP, Elliott CL, Rosenberg SI, Guillory P, Brown N, Syms CA III, Hilton CW, McElveen JT Jr, Singh A, Weiss RL Jr, et al. Balloon dilation of the eustachian tube for dilatory dysfunction: a randomized controlled trial. Laryngoscope. 2018;128(5):1200–6. https://doi.org/10.1002/lary.26827.
103. Ahmed W, Rajagopal R, Lloyd G. Systematic review of round window operations for the treatment of superior semicircular canal dehiscence. J Int Adv Otol. 2019;15(2):209–14. https://doi.org/10.5152/iao.2019.6550.
104. Nieto P, Gallois Y, Molinier CE, Deguine O, Marx M. Surgical treatments of superior semicircular canal dehiscence: a single-centre experience in 63 cases. Laryngosc Investig Otolaryngol. 2021;6(6):1414–20. https://doi.org/10.1002/lio2.684.
105. Succar EF, Manickam PV, Wing S, Walter J, Greene JS, Azeredo WJ. Round window plugging in the treatment of superior semicircular canal dehiscence. Laryngoscope. 2018;128(6):1445–52. https://doi.org/10.1002/lary.26899.
106. Gona A, Phillips JS. 'Soft reinforcement' of the round window for superior semi-circular canal dehiscence syndrome. J Laryngol Otol. 2020;134(4):366–8. https://doi.org/10.1017/S0022215120000353.

Index

G. J. Gianoli, P. Thomson (eds.), *Third Mobile Window Syndrome of the Inner Ear*, https://doi.org/10.1007/978-3-031-16586-3

MIX
Papier aus verantwortungsvollen Quellen
Paper from responsible sources
FSC® C105338

If you have any concerns about our products,
you can contact us on
ProductSafety@springernature.com

In case Publisher is established outside the EU,
the EU authorized representative is:
Springer Nature Customer Service Center GmbH
Europaplatz 3, 69115 Heidelberg, Germany

Printed by Libri Plureos GmbH
in Hamburg, Germany